Pediatric Laboratory Medicine

Pediatric Laboratory Medicine

Patricia M. Jones, PhD

Professor of Pathology
University of Texas Southwestern Medical Center
Clinical Director, Chemistry and Metabolic
  Disease Laboratory
Children's Medical Center
Dallas, Texas

Dennis J. Dietzen, PhD, DABCC

Professor of Pediatrics and Pathology &
  Immunology
Washington University School of Medicine
Core Laboratory Director
St. Louis Children's Hospital
St. Louis, Missouri

Shannon Haymond, PhD, DABCC, FACB

Assistant Professor of Pathology
Northwestern University Feinberg School
  of Medicine
Chicago, Illinois
Department of Pathology
University of Texas Southwestern Medical Center
Dallas, Texas

Michael J. Bennett, PhD

Department of Pathology
University of Texas Southwestern Medical Center
Dallas, Texas

New York   Chicago   San Francisco   Athens   London   Madrid
Mexico City   Milan   New Delhi   Singapore   Sydney   Toronto

Pediatric Laboratory Medicine

1 2 3 4 5 6 7 8 9   DSS   22 21 20 19 18 17

ISBN 978-0-07-184099-6
MHID 0-07-184099-0

This book was set in Minion Pro by Thomson Digital.
The editors were Andrew Moyer and Regina Y. Brown.
The production supervisor was Richard Ruzycka.
Production management was provided by Jyoti Kalra, Thomson Digital.
The cover designer was Randomatrix.
RR Donnelley Shenzhen was printer and binder.

This book was printed on acid-free paper.

Library of Congress Cataloging-in-Publication Data

Names: Jones, Patricia M., 1954- author. | Dietzen, Dennis J., 1964- author.
  | Haymond, Shannon, author. | Bennett, Michael J., 1951- author.
Title: Pediatric laboratory medicine / Patricia Jones, Dennis J. Dietzen,
  Shannon Haymond, Michael J. Bennett.
Description: New York : McGraw-Hill Education, [2017] | Includes
  bibliographical references and index.
Identifiers: LCCN 2016056885| ISBN 9780071840996 (pbk. : alk. paper) | ISBN
  0071840990 (pbk. : alk. paper)
Subjects: | MESH: Pediatrics—methods | Clinical Laboratory
  Techniques—methods
Classification: LCC RJ51.L3 | NLM WS 25 | DDC 618.92/0075—dc23

Contents

Contributors

Sarah Brown, PhD
Assistant Director of Pediatrics and
    Pathology and Immunology
Washington University School of
    Medicine
Assistant Medical Director, Core
    Laboratory
St. Louis Children's Hospital
St. Louis, Missouri
Chapters 1, 11

Irene De Biase, MD, PhD, FACMG
Department of Pathology and ARUP
    Laboratories
University of Utah
Salt Lake City, Utah
Chapter 5

Dennis J. Dietzen, PhD, DABCC
Professor of Pediatrics and Pathology
    & Immunology
Washington University School of
    Medicine
Core Laboratory Director
St. Louis Children's Hospital
St. Louis, Missouri
Chapters 3, 4

**Christopher D. Doern, PhD,
D(ABMM)**
Associate Director of Clinical
    Microbiology
Assistant Professor of Pathology
Virginia Commonwealth University
    Health System
Richmond, Virginia
Chapter 14

Uttam Garg, PhD
Department of Pathology and
    Laboratory Medicine
Division of Clinical Pharmacology
    and Medical Toxicology, Children's
Mercy Hospitals and Clinics
Kansas City, Missouri
Chapter 9

Ann M. Gronowski, PhD
Professor of Pathology &
    Immunology and Obstetrics &
    Gynecology
Washington University School of
    Medicine
St. Louis, Missouri
Chapter 8

**Shannon Haymond, PhD, DABCC,
FACB**
Assistant Professor of Pathology
Northwestern University Feinberg
    School of Medicine
Chicago, Illinois
Department of Pathology
University of Texas Southwestern
    Medical Center
Dallas, Texas
Chapter 10

Patricia M. Jones, PhD
Professor of Pathology
University of Texas Southwestern
    Medical Center
Clinical Director, Chemistry and
    Metabolic Disease Laboratory
Children's Medical Center
Dallas, Texas
Chapter 1

Janna Journeycake, MD
University of Texas Southwestern
    Medical Center
Department of Pediatrics
Division of Hematology
Dallas, Texas
Chapter 16

Nathalie Lepage, PhD
Laboratory Head, Biochemical
    Genetics Laboratory
Children's Hospital of Eastern Ontario
Professor
Department of Pathology and
    Laboratory Medicine
University of Ottawa
Ottawa, Ontario Canada
Chapter 7

Stanley F. Lo, PhD, DABCC, FACB
Associate Director Clinical
    Laboratories
Technical Director Clinical
    Chemistry, Point of Care, and
    Biochemical Genetics
Director Reference Standards
    Laboratory
Children's Hospital of Wisconsin
Associate Professor Pathology
Medical College of Wisconsin
Milwaukee, Wisconsin
Chapter 6

Jennifer Lowry, MD
Division of Clinical Pharmacology
    and Medical Toxicology, Children's
Mercy Hospitals and Clinics
Kansas City, Missouri
Chapter 9

Hung S. Luu, PharmD, MD
University of Texas Southwestern
    Medical Center
Department of Pathology
Division of Pediatric Pathology
Dallas, Texas
Chapters 15, 16

John V. Mitsios, PhD
Assistant Professor of Pathology and
    Laboratory Medicine
Department of Pathology and
    Laboratory Medicine
Weill Cornell Medical College
    Cornell University
New York, New York
Chapter 3

Jon Nakamoto, MD, PhD
Laboratory Medical Director
Quest Diagnostics – Nichols Institute
San Juan Capistrano, California
Chapter 12

Robert D. Nerenz, PhD
Postdoctoral Fellow in Clinical
    Chemistry
Department of Pathology and
    Immunology
Washington University School of
    Medicine
St. Louis, Missouri
Chapter 4

Daniel K. Noland, MD
Assistant Professor of Pathology
University of Texas Southwestern
    Medical Center
Dallas, Texas
Chapter 17

Zaher K. Otrock, MD
Department of Pathology and
  Immunology
Washington University School of
  Medicine
St. Louis, Missouri
Chapter 8

Jason Y. Park, MD, PhD
Assistant Professor
Pathology and the Eugene
  McDermott Center for Human
  Growth and Development
UT Southwestern Medical Center
Director, Advanced Diagnostics
  Laboratory
Children's Medical Center – Dallas
Dallas, Texas
Chapter 13

Marzia Pasquali, PhD, FACMG
Department of Pathology and ARUP
  Laboratories
University of Utah
Salt Lake City, Utah
Chapter 5

Khushbu Patel, PhD
Clinical Chemistry Fellow
Department of Pathology and
  Immunology
Washington University School of
  Medicine
St. Louis, Missouri
Chapter 11

Amy L. Pyle-Eilola, PhD, DABCC
Assistant Director of Core Laboratory
  Services
Department of Pathology and
  Laboratory Medicine
Nationwide Children's Hospital
Columbus, Ohio
Chapter 2

Julie Shaw, PhD, FCACB
Clinical Biochemist
The Ottawa Hospital
Assistant Professor
Department of Pathology and
  Laboratory Medicine
University of Ottawa
Ottawa, Ontario Canada
Chapter 7

**Kaede Sullivan, MD, MSc, FRCPC,
FAAP, FCCM, D(ABMM)**
Associate Director of Clinical
  Microbiology, Immunology, and
  Virology Laboratories
Associate Professor of Pathology &
  Laboratory Medicine
Temple University
Philadelphia, Pennsylvania
Chapter 14

David J. Thornton, PhD, DABCC
Director of Core Laboratory
  Services
Department of Pathology and
  Laboratory Medicine
Nationwide Children's Hospital
Columbus, Ohio
Chapter 2

Charles F. Timmons, MD, PhD
University of Texas Southwestern
  Medical Center
Department of Pathology
Division of Pediatric Pathology
Dallas, Texas
Chapter 15

Jason Wang, MD
Assistant Professor, Pathology
UT Southwestern and Children's
  Medical Center – Dallas
Dallas, Texas
Chapter 13

Ayesha Zia, MD
University of Texas Southwestern
  Medical Center
Department of Pediatrics
Division of Hematology
Dallas, Texas
Chapters 15, 16

Preface

In the field of pediatric laboratory medicine (PLM), one of the truisms that you hear over and over is that "children are not small adults." This saying is a truism for a reason. Metabolically and biochemically children are often as different from adults as it is possible to be. The basic chemical and hematological components of blood, urine, cerebral spinal fluid, and other body fluids are often more diverse and almost always more dynamic than comparable components in adults. A pediatric patient is rarely static in any way. Even when physically well, an infant and child is constantly growing and changing, and analytes that we measure in blood and other body fluids reflect those changes. In contrast to infants and children, a chemical component in an adult may not change much over multiple decades unless the person has a pathophysiological problem occurring; however, in an infant these parameters may change hourly. Total bilirubin measurements are a good example of this type of rapid changes in infancy.

In addition, especially in infancy, the body can change much more rapidly from a critical state to a well state and vice versa. Infants have very little in the way of reserves, such as stored fats and/or glycogen, and a higher percentage of their body is water. Thus, for example, infants can easily become critically hypoglycemic with even short periods of fasting. Critical electrolyte imbalances can occur with a relatively brief intake of improperly made formula, and dehydration is common after fairly short periods without fluid intake, or of vomiting and diarrhea. At the same time, infants possess a great deal of plasticity – an enormous ability to deal with rapid internal as well as environmental changes. For example, infants can survive brief periods of blood pH values in the 6.8 range with no lasting physical harm. All of these scenarios are uncommon in the adult population.

Other aspects of PLM also cause this part of laboratory medicine to be special. Infants and children are subject to some disease processes not found routinely in adults, and conversely some diseases are found only in adults. These differences in disorders require that different tests be offered in pediatric labs and in adult labs. Thus serum protein electrophoresis for diagnosing multiple myeloma is not found in pediatric laboratories, as multiple myeloma is not a disease of childhood. On the other hand catecholamines, such as vanillylmandelic acid and homovanillic acid are rarely analyzed in adult labs, but not uncommon in pediatric ones, as neuroblastoma is a childhood cancer. While most basic testing such as that included in a basic or comprehensive metabolic panel is essentially identical between children and adults, some of the tests found in those panels have different significance in the pediatric population. Thus test menu differences will be found between the two types of labs and test interpretation may differ as well.

Along with the different disorders found between the two populations, some diseases have begun crossing over between the age-groups in recent years. Disorders that used to be considered pediatric are now being found in the adult population as improving medical treatment for pediatric diseases allows these children to survive to adulthood. For example, cystic fibrosis and many other inborn errors of metabolism (IEM) now require clinics to treat adults with these disorders. Pediatric labs commonly are asked to provide IEM testing for some adult patients now, and pregnant women who themselves were born with an inborn error of metabolism are requiring close monitoring of their own disease and prenatal testing for their unborn child.

Conversely, some disorders that were at one time considered adult-only are now being increasingly seen in the pediatric population, like the spectrum associated with obesity and type 2 diabetes. The obesity epidemic in children will cause more and more testing once considered part of the adult realm, such as lipid analyses, to be necessary in children.

Thus laboratory medicine practiced at a pediatric institution has unique characteristics specific to pediatrics. In addition, infants and children have a limited blood supply. This particular issue affects many of the basic day-to-day mechanics of running a pediatric laboratory, as will be seen in the chapters of this book. Many aspects of laboratory medicine are affected by the differences seen in the pediatric population, all the way from basic, day-to-day operational issues through test selection for pediatric-specific disorders, and on up to age-related reference intervals and changes in basic tests during growth and changing metabolism. Specialty areas also abound in PLM, including such areas as testing for inborn errors of metabolism, testing of hormones during puberty, and prenatal and maternal-fetal testing. Training a new practitioner in PLM must incorporate various aspects specific to children. This book is intended as a resource for the combined knowledge needed for basic PLM training.

Acknowledgment

I would like to gratefully acknowledge all the help and support from my coeditors, Shannon Haymond, Dennis Dietzen, and Michael Bennett.

DAILY ISSUES IN THE PRACTICE OF PEDIATRIC LABORATORY MEDICINE

1

Patricia M. Jones and Sarah Brown

LEARNING OBJECTIVES

1. Describe issues related to collection sample volume in pediatric patients.
2. Describe the optimal ages and usages for venipuncture versus capillary sampling.
3. List the proper order of multi-tube blood collection for venipuncture and for capillary collection.
4. Explain how mislabeled specimens might arise and how they might be handled in a pediatric laboratory.
5. Describe "add-on" samples and the factors which affect them.
6. Define issues that may arise in test validation in a pediatric laboratory.

INTRODUCTION

The operation of a clinical laboratory requires a wide knowledge base and a considerable variety of skills. Expertise is necessary in: 1) operating, maintaining, and trouble-shooting a large array of instrumentation types ranging from particle counters and spectrophotometers to mass spectrometers and molecular diagnostics; 2) understanding chemical and immunological reactions and being able to trouble shoot and explain them to physicians; 3) handling of a variety of patient sample types and explaining acceptable versus unacceptable samples to other medical professional; and 4) being aware of the spectrum of tests available to medical professionals and appropriateness of test utilization patterns under different conditions.

A pediatric clinical laboratory adds another layer of complexity to the knowledge base requirements. Many of the regular day-to-day activities of operating a clinical laboratory are quite different between laboratories that provide services for pre-dominately adult populations and those whose patient base is primarily pediatric. Although the majority of the tests performed are the same or similar, many aspects of performing those tests must be tailored differently for the pediatric population and their unique needs. In addition, many pre-analytical aspects are quite different and specialized training and handling skills are required to understand these differences.

This chapter will deal with the pediatric-specific aspects of day-to-day laboratory operations.

BLOOD VOLUME AND VOLUME OF DRAW

The small total blood volume of infants and children limits the amount of blood that can safely be drawn from a pediatric patient. Current guidelines vary considerably between institutions, however most recommend that no more than 3% of total body volume be drawn per day, and 10% over 2 months in healthy children. Smaller amounts are recommended for ill and hospitalized children.[1] Table 1-1 shows the calculated average total blood volumes and permissible collection volumes as a function of body weight and average blood volume.

The volume of blood required for any testing is a sum of a number of volumes, including the volume needed to perform the assay, the volume necessary to measure hemolysis, lipemia, and icterus indices on chemistry analyzers, and the volume below which the instrument cannot accurately pipet that sample, also called the instrument dead volume. These volumes vary from instrument to instrument, as described in the section, Instrument Issues later. In a pediatric facility, it is not uncommon for healthcare professionals to collect the absolute minimum volume required, as opposed to appropriately filling a vacuum tube, in an effort to reduce the volume of draw. Often, this practice results in sub-optimal volumes collected. Another means of reducing the blood volume requirement is to combine test orders as much as possible. Combining tests that require the same tube type and will be performed on the same instrument reduces the total blood requirement because it uses the dead volume and volume for indices only once. Efforts should be made to coordinate lab requests from all health care providers and research protocols. It is important to maintain open communication between the laboratory and the health care team when minimum volume initiatives are undertaken, as these initiatives benefit from education regarding specimen collection, tube additives, and impact of minimum volume draws on the ability to repeat or add-on tests. In contrast to adult labs, it is not uncommon to have insufficient volume for repeat testing, for adding on additional tests, or sometimes even for measuring the indices.

Table 1-1	**MAXIMUM BLOOD COLLECTION VOLUMES (ML) FROM PATIENTS UNDER 100 LBS AS PERCENT OF AVERAGE TOTAL BLOOD VOLUME**					
			Healthy Patients		Hospitalized Patients	
			Collection (mL)		Collection (mL)	
	Weight	Average Total Blood Volume	Single	Over 2 month	Single	Over 2 month
(lbs)	(kg)	(mL)	3%	10%	2.5%	5%
< 4	< 1.8	< 207	< 6	< 20	< 5	< 10
4 – 6	1.8 – 2.7	220	7	22	6	11
6 – 8	2.7 – 3.6	300	9	30	8	15
8 – 10	3.6 – 4.5	380	11	38	10	19
10 – 15	4.5 – 6.8	540	16	54	14	27
15 – 20	6.8 – 9.1	700	21	70	18	35
20 – 25	9.1 – 11.4	900	27	90	22	45
25 – 30	11.4 – 13.6	1100	33	110	28	55
30 – 35	13.6 – 15.9	1300	39	130	32	65
35 – 40	15.9 – 18.2	1500	45	150	38	75
40 – 45	18.2 – 20.4	1700	51	170	42	85
45 – 50	20.4 – 22.7	1850	56	185	46	92
50 – 55	22.7 – 25.0	1920	58	192	48	96
55 – 60	25.0 – 27.2	2100	63	210	52	105
60 – 65	27.2 – 29.5	2280	68	228	57	114
65 – 70	29.5 – 31.8	2460	74	246	62	123
70 – 75	31.8 – 34.0	2500	75	250	63	125
75 – 80	34.0 – 36.3	2560	77	256	64	128
80 – 85	36.3 – 38.6	2720	82	272	68	136
85 – 90	38.6 – 40.9	2900	87	290	72	145
90 – 95	40.9 – 43.1	3050	92	305	76	152
95 – 100	43.1 – 45.4	3220	97	322	80	161

Drawing minimal volumes increases the risk of a quantity not sufficient (QNS) specimen, without enough volume to perform the requested assay, especially for serum chemistries. Some QNS samples occur even when a seemingly adequate volume of whole blood has been drawn. This may occur because the total whole blood drawn does not contain enough plasma/serum for testing. Infants have a high hematocrit at birth and therefore a lower percentage of the total blood volume as serum.[2] Table 15-1 in Chapter 15 shows age-dependent hematocrit reference intervals. Thus, a larger volume of draw is required to obtain sufficient sample for laboratory testing, at a time when the patient has a lower total blood volume.

SAMPLE COLLECTION

The quality of a lab result is only as good as the sample being tested. In this day and age of precise and accurate automated instrumentation, the majority of the errors in lab results are now derived from pre-analytical events.[3-5] Actual analysis of the sample has become relatively error-free, however, everything that happens to a specimen before it gets to the on-instrument analysis step can affect the final result. In a pediatric setting, additional care must be taken to properly collect and label samples the first time to avoid having to re-collect blood.

Blood collection, commonly referred to as phlebotomy, is a skill set that requires even more expertise in a pediatric population.[6] Adults for the most part will hold still when you are performing a venipuncture. Children and infants as a rule will frequently not hold still. Thus proper training for pediatric phlebotomists includes not only the mechanics of the collection, but also tips on dealing with infants and children in various age groups.[7-10] Skilled pediatric phlebotomists can enlist the child's "help" with the process and often manage to accomplish the procedure with a minimum of restraint. It is not possible to over-emphasize the importance of good pediatric phlebotomy on the whole process of laboratory testing.

Basic Phlebotomy

Like all phlebotomy procedures at any age, a few procedural steps are standard when collecting a blood sample. Universal precautions are always used, which means treating each patient and his samples as if they could be infectious. Gloves are always worn during phlebotomy and scrubs or protective clothing such as a lab coat are also a requirement. No matter whether the child being collected is an inpatient in the hospital or an outpatient at a clinic or draw station, each patient is positively identified. Positive identification of patients requires verification of two unique identifiers such as name, date of birth, medical record number, and social security number. Patient identification can be verified by asking the patient or their parent/guardian for their name and date of birth and then matching that information against the orders for the blood collection. Another verification method is to match two pieces of information on an armband which is worn by the patient to the information on the blood collection orders. Blood collection should not proceed until the patient identification has been positively verified using two separate identifiers. Although medical staff frequently refer to patients by their room number, room number is not a unique identifier since rooms can change. An armband attached to a crib, bed or stroller is also not an acceptable identification.[6]

Beyond the standard procedural steps, pediatric phlebotomy is very different from adult phlebotomy. For venipuncture, it is not uncommon to use a topical anesthetic applied to the skin before the needle stick in the pediatric population. In adults, this is an uncommon practice. Immobilization may also be necessary.[10] The parent or guardian accompanying the infant or child will usually be called upon to hold or help restrain a young child during the phlebotomy process. Occasionally a parent will not be asked to help due to the anxiety of the parent causing more anxiety in the child. In these cases another phlebotomist may assist. Although the need for medical restraints beyond merely holding is highly unusual, it can occur. Pediatric hospitals will have policies in place on the use of medical restraints on non-violent patients that will cover these types of eventualities. Well trained and experienced pediatric phlebotomists are adept at reading the needs of each situation and knowing when NOT to collect samples if the child is too combative, and there is a risk of injury to the child or phlebotomist.[7] The skillful pediatric phlebotomist receives training in and is very good at establishing a rapport with children of various ages and successfully collecting samples without emotional or physical trauma to the child or parent.[7,10]

Another difference in basic pediatric phlebotomy is that children have smaller veins. The vacuum in adult collection tubes may be too strong and result in vein collapse and preclude blood collection. Two different ways of dealing with this issue are commonly employed. Pediatric phlebotomy is often recommended to be performed using a winged needle (butterfly) collection device (Figure 1-1) and a syringe. The phlebotomist can easily control the amount of pressure on the syringe and insure that the vein is not collapsed by excessive pressure. Another way to deal with this issue is that many collection tube manufacturers produce "reduced volume" tubes. These tubes are designed for lower collection volumes and have a lower vacuum and also contain less additive in the tube. For this reason a tube with a vacuum should never have the top removed in order to fill the tube. It should always be filled using the vacuum to ensure the appropriate amount of blood in the tube for the amount

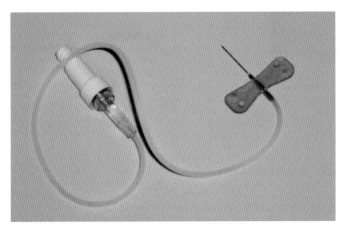

Figure 1-1 ▪ Example of a winged needle (butterfly) venipuncture device

of additive. When a butterfly and syringe are used to collect a sample, vacuum tubes are then filled using a "needleless" transfer device (Figure 1-2) and again the vacuum is not broken but used to fill the tube appropriately.

Heel-stick and Finger-stick Collections—Capillary Blood

If a large volume of blood needs to be collected at any age, a venipuncture will be the default collection type, and at least one study has suggested that it is always the preferred collection.[10] For routine blood collection in children under two years old, finger- and heel-stick samples are often recommended.[11]

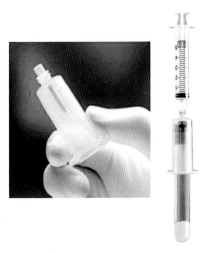

Figure 1-2 ▪ A transfer device that can be used to transfer blood collected in a syringe into tubes with vacuums

Table 1-2	**TYPE OF COLLECTION THAT SHOULD BE USED AT SPECIFIC AGES**
Age	Type of Collection
< 6 months old	Heel-stick
6 months – 1 year old	Heel-stick preferred Finger-stick can be done
1 – 2 years old	Finger-sticks
> 2 years old	Finger-sticks Venipuncture

This is because heel and finger-sticks tend to be easier on both the phlebotomist and the patient than a venipuncture in this age group. Also, small blood volumes are collected from infants and young children whenever possible due to total volume constraints. A general rule for types of collection can be seen in Table 1-2. Once a child is walking, heel-stick sampling should not be routinely performed as calluses may begin to build up, and finger-stick samples are preferred.

There is a proper and recommended way to perform a heel-stick collection, and attention must be paid to doing it correctly. First of all, the heel should always be warmed prior to blood collection, which can be done with a heel warmer made for this purpose. Warming the heel ensures that the capillary blood is free-flowing and not only increases the likelihood of obtaining an adequate sample volume, but also makes the component analytes in the sample better reflect venous or even arterial blood. A capillary sample from a properly warmed heel for a blood gas analysis reflects arterial blood in gas content and capillary blood is acceptable for measuring most analytes.[12-16]

Second, the puncture must be performed on the lateral or medial plantar surface of the heel as shown in Figure 1-3. A heel-stick should never be performed at the back of the heel as the bone is closer to the surface there and hitting the bone will not only cause pain, but can cause osteomyelitis.[17] For this same reason, the toes should never be used for a blood collection and finger-sticks are not recommended in children under one year of age.

Lancets designed for performing either heel-sticks or for finger-sticks are commercially available. Heel-stick devices should never be used to perform a finger-stick or vice versa. Devices designed for finger-sticks puncture the finger. Many devices designed for heel-sticks slash the heel with a blade moving in quick pendulum motion. Slashing the finger in this manner may result in a larger wound than necessary resulting in unnecessarily excessive bleeding.

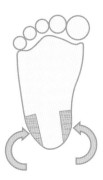

Figure 1-3 ▪ Diagram of the correct positions to perform a heel-stick (shaded areas)

Finger-stick and heel-stick devices are manufactured with puncture "tip lengths" that range from 0.85 mm up to 2.2 mm and thus they deliver a puncture to different depths. In general the deeper the puncture, the more likely a good flow of blood will be achieved, however, the more painful it will be also. In addition in infants and young children a tradeoff must be made for safety and not hitting bone upon puncturing. The distance from the skin surface to the bone in a normal birth weight (roughly 7 pound or 3 kg) infant averages 3.32 mm on the sides of the heel, 2.33 mm at the back of the heel and 2.19 mm on the toes.[9] Recommended tip lengths for use in finger- and heel-stick blood collection are shown in Table 1-3.

Urine Collection

Collecting a urine sample has its own set of difficulties in infants and children, especially in infants. The proper way to collect a urine sample from an infant is to "bag" the infant.[18] Figure 1-4 shows a urine collection bag. This device is

Table 1-3	COLLECTION DEVICE TIP LENGTH RECOMMENDED FOR HEEL-STICK AND FINGER-STICK COLLECTIONS	
Age	Collection Type	Tip Length
Pre-mature newborn	Heel-stick	0.85 mm
Term neonate-6 months	Heel-stick	1.5 mm
6 months – 8 years	Finger-stick	1.5 mm
> 8 years	Finger-stick	2.2 mm

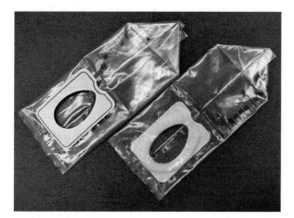

Figure 1-4 ▪ Pediatric urine bag

essentially a plastic bag with a mild adhesive around the outside edge of the central hole. The infant's genital area is cleaned and allowed to dry and the bag is secured over the area, with the diaper then being placed over the bag. The difficulty lies in that the adhesive does not hold well when wet, so the baby must be monitored for when urine has collected in the bag and the bag and sample should be retrieved immediately. The only other approved method for collecting urine in an infant is catheterization. In addition, if the urine sample is being collected for evaluation of a urinary tract infection, catheterization is the recommended sample collection technique.[19]

Nursing personnel and other caregivers are often creative about collecting urine samples on infants, with a commonly used practice being to place cotton balls in the diaper, and then retrieve them and wring the urine sample out of them. Wringing out diapers has also been used. These two methods are not appropriate for collecting urine samples because fiber and chemical contamination can occur in both instances.

Occasionally a 24-hour or other timed urine sample is necessary in the pediatric population, for example to assess prophyrins, catecholamines, or urinary free cortisol. Collecting a 24-hour or other timed urine sample is probably one of the sample collections most frequently done incorrectly, despite being non-invasive. For a 24-hour urine collection on an infant, hospitalization and catheterization will be necessary although a 24-hour urine collection is rarely necessary in infants. The proper way to collect a 24-hour urine sample for children and adults is to get up in the morning and empty the bladder as usual, discarding this first morning void. After this first voiding, collect and keep all the rest of the urine output for the rest of the day until going to bed. When arising the next morning, collect and keep the first morning void as the bladder is emptied. This completes the 24-hour collection. The same principles apply to other timed collections. All the collected urine should be kept mixed together in a single 24-hour urine collection container. These collection containers are obtained from the laboratory and sent home with the patient family. In general, caustic additives are not added to the container before collection as they pose a safety risk. The container should be kept refrigerated or in an ice chest during the collection, and can be acidified or other additives added once the sample is returned to the lab.

Pediatric Blood Micro-Collection Tubes

Because the volume of sample being collected in pediatric patients is often small, tubes that hold smaller volumes are used for the collections. These small tubes (micro-collection tubes) generally hold 500 µL to 1 mL and are often referred to as "bullets". As much as 60 – 70% of the collections arriving in a pediatric laboratory may be in this size of tube. Figure 1-5 shows a variety of manufacturer's small volume tubes. These tubes are intended to be used for finger-stick and heel-stick samples. Reduced volume tubes have already been mentioned.

Samples collected in bullets effect a multitude of operations of the pediatric lab which are discussed in sections, Pediatric Sample Processing; Instrument Issues; Miscellaneous Pediatric-Specific Issues below. In addition, collecting small samples volumes, many of them by capillary blood collection in micro-collection tubes, causes a higher rate of sample rejection than other tube sizes.[20] Several factors may result in this higher sample rejection rate. These factors include: 1) inadequate volume; 2) higher likelihood of hemolysis

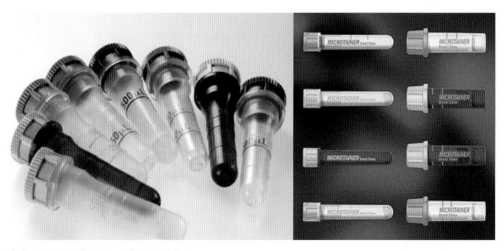

Figure 1-5 ▪ Types of micro-collection tubes

occurring during collection, usually from improper collection technique such as milking or squeezing the heel or finger; and 3) higher likelihood of clotting caused by slow blood flow rates from tiny veins or by delayed mixing of tubes after collection. Thus pediatric labs often find themselves with higher sample rejection rates than adult laboratories, requiring more recollection of samples. A pediatric lab may also report results on hemolyzed specimens that adult labs in general will not report, such as potassium. This will depend on the laboratory, but because of the frequency of hemolyzed samples in a pediatric population and the issues surrounding inability to recollect samples due to limited blood volume, very often results will be reported on hemolyzed samples, with a disclaimer about the presence of hemolysis.

The order in which tubes are collected is important when multiple tube types are being collected. Because all the tubes contact the needle, butterfly or transfer device in a venipuncture, additive in the tube can contaminate the device and subsequently contaminate the next tube. Thus the tubes must be collected in such an order that if the contamination occurs it will not affect the sample in the next tube collected. As a general rule, tubes without additives are collected first, followed by tubes with weak anti-coagulants such as sodium citrate, followed by tubes with stronger anticoagulants such as EDTA. In addition, samples being collected for blood culture are often collected first in order to minimize the risk of bacterial contamination of the sample. For a heel- or finger-stick sample the order of tube collection is different than for a venipuncture sample. Blood from a skin puncture starts clotting immediately, so anticoagulated tubes are collected first with tubes needing clotted samples (serum) collected last.[21-23] Table 1-4 shows the order of collection for capillary blood and venipuncture.

Table 1-4 **ORDER OF BLOOD COLLECTION**			
Venipuncture		**Capillary Blood**	
Usage or additive	Tube top color	Usage or additive	Tube top color
Blood culture bottles or tubes	Yellow	Blood gases (heparin)	Microhematocrit tubes
Coagulation /sodium citrate	Light blue	EDTA	Lavender
Serum/clot activator or gel	Red, Tiger	Heparin	Green
Plasma/Heparin	Green	Other additives	Light blue, gray
CBC/EDTA	Lavender	Non additives	Red, Tiger, yellow
Oxalate/fluoride	Grey		

PEDIATRIC SAMPLE PROCESSING

Usually arriving in the lab in bullets or reduced volume vacutainers, pediatric samples require considerable manual processing compared to specimens from adults. This includes manual accessioning, transfer from the primary sample tube and dividing in to aliquots, and manual entry into the analyzer. The manual processing requirement can add significantly to the turn-around-time as well as impact the number of employees, or full-time equivalents (FTEs) needed.

Pediatric bullets do not fit on most analyzers, let alone automated robotic systems. These small tubes aren't compatible with most bar coding systems and the sample information often must be manually entered in the LIS and the analyzer. While some manufacturers do make false-bottom tubes that fit on some systems, more often the sample must be transferred to a compatible sample cup prior to analysis. On some instruments[24] the pediatric tube can be dropped into a larger tube, and a bar-coded label placed around the larger tube. Measures taken to accommodate small volumes, such as the use of false-bottom tubes, sample cups, or tube-within-a-tube, need to be validated prior to reporting patient results (see section, Test Validation in a Pediatric Lab). Careful attention is required during manual processing, especially pour-offs, to reduce the risk of sample mix-up.

Evaporation is another concern. Smaller sample volumes have greater surface area to total volume, allowing for evaporation to have significant effects. For example, a sample containing 5 mL of serum (typical adult volume) that sits open to the air will show an increase in glucose concentration that is approximately 10% higher than the initial measurement after several hours. A sample containing 0.1 mL under the same conditions will show a 50% increase in glucose measurement over the initial analysis.[25] Another effect of the large surface to volume ratio in small samples is the enhanced rate of gas diffusion between the sample and the room air, which can cause significantly decreased total CO_2 concentrations in these small samples. Thus small samples must be kept tightly capped, and evaporation and gas diffusion must be considered before adding-on tests.

INSTRUMENT ISSUES

When considering the acquisition of any instrumentation, the following should always be assessed: test menu, footprint, utility requirements, connectivity, service agreements (including availability of customer support), and cost. In addition, there are considerations specific to pediatrics to be evaluated, including: instrument dead volume, sample volume required for testing, whether or not bullets will fit on the system and how pediatric samples are handled, for example, whether it is necessary to interrupt an automated system to load pediatric samples.

Small sample volume requirements are a high priority when selecting pediatric laboratory instrumentation. Careful attention needs to be paid when assessing a manufacturer's claims for sample volume requirements - the total sample volume consists of the volume required for the assay plus hidden volume requirements for the dead volume and integrity indices. The instrument dead volume is essential a wasted volume that is required for instrument function, for example, the amount below which the instrument cannot pipette. Dead volumes can significantly increase the sample volume requirement for a test. An assay may require 30 μL but the dead volume of the instrument may be 240 μL, bringing the total sample volume to 270 μL. The dead volume needs to be validated in-laboratory as it may vary from the manufacturer's specifications. When validating the dead volume, the tube size that will be used most often should be tested. The dead volume may vary considerably between a 10 mL primary tube and a 0.5 mL sample cup. Table 1-5 shows some representative dead volume requirements, as dependent on sample cup size. In addition to the dead volume, another "hidden" volume that needs to be considered is the volume required for specimen integrity parameters such as the hemolysis, icterus, or turbidity indices. These parameters are usually measured prior to assays on chemistry and hematology instruments and can add 10 μL to the volume requirement.

Table 1-5 **INSTRUMENT DEAD VOLUMES**			
Instrument	Sample Cup Size (mL)	Dead Volume (μL)	Assay Volume (μL)
Abbott Architect c4000		50	1 – 35
Beckman Coulter® Au480	0.5	40	1 – 25
	2.0	360	
Ortho-Clinical Diagnostics Vitros 5600		35	2 – 17
Roche Cobas® 6000	1.5	50	1 – 35
	2.5	100	
Siemens Healthcare Dimension Vista 500	0.5	10	1 – 25

If pediatric samples are being tested in an automated lab that also performs testing on adult samples, the impact on automation needs to be considered. In general bullets do not fit on the tracks of automated systems; therefore the lab should have a plan for interrupting the automated system to load smaller pediatric samples in a timely manner. As previously mentioned, barcodes can't always be read when the label is on a pediatric tube. Patient and test information needs to be manually entered, or a new label printed and placed around a larger tube and the patient specimen transferred to this larger tube. The manual processing involved in testing pediatric specimens may require additional FTEs to complete the process and meet turnaround times.

MISCELLANEOUS PEDIATRIC-SPECIFIC ISSUES

There are a number of random, frequently occurring day-to-day issues that are very specific for pediatric laboratories and which require some discussion.

Handling of Mislabeled Samples

As a general rule of good laboratory practice, a sample that is mislabeled or unlabeled is considered unsuitable, discarded and the sample is recollected. This is true for a wide range of incidents, from as simple as a misspelled name, through having a name on the label that does not match the orders and all the way up to having no labeling at all. This practice is especially important in areas like transfusion medicine, where the possibility of doing a type and cross match and dispensing blood of the wrong type on a patient has considerable risk of harm to the patient. It is also true of other area of the laboratory however, where treatment decisions may be made on the basis of a sample that does not belong to the child being treated. Therefore good laboratory practice mandates a recollection of the sample for mislabeled samples.

Specimens that cannot be recollected without significant harm to the patient are considered irreplaceable. Upon approval by the lab medical director, mislabeled irreplaceable specimens might be processed. The laboratory must have a procedure that clearly defines mislabeled and irreplaceable specimens. In adult laboratories, irreplaceable specimens may include such samples as cerebrospinal fluid (CSF), wound drainage and biopsy specimens. Blood and urine are generally not considered irreplaceable because these specimens can be recollected without significant harm to the patient. In pediatric labs the list of irreplaceable specimens may extend to blood samples when the patient cannot afford to lose additional blood volume by phlebotomy, for example, low birth weight infants. The Lab Medical Director must be notified of and approve these exceptions.

In order to be considered properly labeled, a sample that arrives in the laboratory should have on its label at least two unique patient identifiers as outlined earlier plus the date and time of collection, and the initials or identification of the person who collected the sample. In addition, any or all of this information can be hand-written on the tube label as long as it is all legible. It is not uncommon to receive tubes in the lab which are totally unlabeled because the label printer on the nursing unit or the computer system was down. In a laboratory that deals predominately with adult patients, these mislabeled tubes are discarded and the samples are re-collected. Section, Blood Volume and Volume of Draw above deals with issues surrounding pediatric blood volume and why mislabeled samples may need to be corrected rather than recollected in babies due to low blood volumes.

There is an extensive list of reasons why mislabeled samples tend to be more common in a pediatric setting than in a predominately adult one. One of the primary reasons is that patient identification may be suboptimal. Keeping an armband on an infant is often problematic. Healthcare providers have been known to place the armband on the crib rather than the infant, and neglect to remove the old armband when a location change occurs. In addition, many times the patient is too young to identify themselves. The patient is identified by a parent or guardian who may be distraught and not paying attention. Another common occurrence in pediatric institutions is that the patient changes names. A child may be adopted, or a newborn may be admitted under the mother's name. Children without names may be generically identified as "Baby Boy", "Baby Girl", or "Twin A" and "Twin B" then receive a new name while in the hospital. Name changes are less common in adult institutions. And finally, siblings may all come to the ED together with a single parent and be seen in the same ED room, providing significant opportunity for mislabeling samples.

Other opportunities for mislabeling occur when a sheet of pre-printed labels is generated upon admittance. These labels accompany the patient and are intended to make things flow more smoothly and decrease the risk of misspelled names or incorrectly numbered medical record numbers. Yet these sheets of labels can find their way into places and be used by mistake on the incorrect patient. Using a system that allows labels to be printed at the time and place of blood collection is designed to print only those labels needed at exactly the time they are needed, with the correct information. Interestingly, healthcare providers have been known to pre-print even these labels to save themselves some time. Unfortunately, the system may be designed to print the collection time as the time the label is printed. If the labels are pre-printed four hours before the sample is collected, the sample will arrive in the lab and appear to be 4-hours old, when in fact it is 10 minutes old. Blood gas samples that are 4-hours old will probably be rejected.

Once the sample arrives in the lab, there are also increased opportunities for mislabeling errors to occur.[20] Since small bullet tubes do not allow primary tube sampling, aliquots must be made and labeled. In an adult lab, the primary tube is spun and place in a robotic system which reads the bar-coded label; in a pediatric lab the sample is spun, transferred over into a small tube that must be labeled, which in turn may be placed into a larger tube (also labeled) to fit the robotic and barcode systems. Not only is more work required, more opportunity for human error is available.

Add-On Samples

Add-on tests are those ordered on to a sample that has already been collected and is already in the lab. Although this practice occurs in an adult setting, it is much more common in a pediatric setting where blood volume is at a premium and healthcare workers prefer not to collect additional samples if it can be avoided. This practice is handled in different ways by different laboratories. A verbal request for an add-on to an existing sample may be called to the lab, followed by a written or computer generated order arriving. The hospital computer system can also be designed to have an "add-on" priority, as an ordering priority on a test. When a test is ordered as an "add-on", it generates an automatic order in the lab.

However the practice is handled, it generates extra work for the laboratory. The laboratory personnel must locate the original sample and determine if it is appropriate for the new tests being added on to it. That determination will include the following aspects of the existing sample: sample type, ie., serum vs plasma vs whole blood; sample volume—enough to perform additional test?; sample quality—hemolyzed sample may be okay for original test but not for requested add-on; sample age—a sample that has been on an instrument and evaporating for a few hours or degrading in other ways may give inaccurate results.

Informatics Issues

There are a few issues related to computers that are specific to the pediatric lab, and should be considered whenever a laboratory information system (LIS) is being evaluated for a pediatric institutions. The flexibility and adaptability of the LIS may become an issue.

The most obvious need for a good pediatric institution LIS is an ability to deal with age-stratified reference intervals. Proper interpretation of laboratory tests is impossible without appropriate reference intervals. This is nowhere more apparent than in the pediatric population where reference intervals can sometimes change hourly, as does bilirubin concentration after birth. The computer system must have the capability of determining the patient's age and applying the appropriate age-related reference interval when available to all tests. It is important to be aware of how the LIS accomplishes this however, as not all LIS handle it the same way. The most ideal way is for the LIS to essentially hard-wire a reference interval to each result, so that the reference interval on that result never changes. Some systems are set up to change the reference intervals as the patient age changes but also change the reference intervals on all previous results, with the unintended consequence of incorrect reference intervals on past results when the past results were pulled up for viewing.

SEND OUT TESTING

Testing that is not performed in-house and is sent out to reference laboratories is commonly referred to as send out testing. There are literally hundreds of reference labs that perform anywhere from a few tests to several hundred tests. With the fast advancement of molecular diagnostics, reference lab test menus have grown overnight. In general, pediatric laboratories have a large send out test volume because many tests needed for diagnosing constitutional genetic disease and monitoring developing children are very specialized. It is important to manage reference lab usage for accreditation, patient quality and safety, and financial reasons.

There are regulatory requirements for reference labs, and it is the responsibility of the referring lab to ensure these requirements are met before sending specimens. The College of American Pathologists requires laboratories to have a procedure for use of reference laboratories. The reference lab must be Clinical Laboratory Improvement Act (CLIA) certified, and molecular diagnostic laboratories must have an American College of Medical Genetics (ACMG) board certified medical director. If the reference lab does not meet the requirements, the result must be clearly noted as research use only.

Other issues with reference laboratory testing include sample volume and cost. Reference laboratory specimens generally require larger sample volumes than in-house testing and care should be taken that too much blood is not drawn when multiple reference laboratory tests are ordered, especially when multiple services are consulting on a complicated patient. Cost must be considered, as high-cost molecular testing generally makes up a significant portion of the send out volume. Laboratory test utilization management is a growing area of interest and requirement in lab medicine. Utilization management practices remain individualized by institution, and include gatekeeping of expensive and/or low utility reference lab tests, formularies of allowed reference lab testing, and preventing specific tests from being sent out.[26] These protocols can be developed in collaboration with the providers, but require the expertise of laboratorians. Genetic counselors have also been shown to be very helpful in reviewing and adjudicating requests for esoteric molecular diagnostics.[27] Whether or not the hospital has a reference lab utilization policy, reference laboratory usage should be closely monitored.

Send out testing presents additional processing issues. Some reference laboratory tests have special requirements. For example, they might need to arrive at the reference laboratory within 24 hours of draw and the reference lab might not be open on the weekend. Therefore the specimen cannot be shipped on a Saturday. Some tests may require a control specimen to be shipped with the patient sample as well. Although some reference labs can be electronically interfaced with hospital computer systems, results from reference labs often have to be manually entered into the LIS. This is an area of potential risk for reporting errors and must be done carefully.[28] Therefore, between processing and resulting, more FTEs and knowledge of send out test requirements and procedures are generally required.

TEST VALIDATION IN A PEDIATRIC LAB

When a new test is introduced into a clinical lab, whether it is an FDA-approved reagent addition to a multi-analyte chemistry platform, or a test developed completely from scratch in the laboratory (laboratory developed test or LDT) itself, the test must be validated. The parameters that must be validated are outlined in the CLIA, specifically in the Federal Register, 42 CFR Part 493, Subpart K – Quality System for Non-waived Testing Section. 493.1253. In a pediatric lab these same regulations hold true, and test validation is much more commonly necessary in a pediatric lab than in an adult lab. The reason for this is that many tests for diagnosing infants and children are performed using LDTs. For example, metabolic disease testing is usually done using LDTs and this testing for diagnosing inborn errors of metabolism is common in pediatric laboratories.

There are often issues involved in pediatric lab test validation that may not be encountered when validating tests in an adult lab. Often test validations are performed using left over samples from patient testing that will be discarded. It can be problematic to find enough excess sample after patient testing in a pediatric lab to allow for adequate validation testing. In some instances it may be easier to find samples which span the reportable range of the assay, for instance with bilirubin. In an adult population samples with high bilirubin concentrations may be difficult to find, but are usually not so in a pediatric population. In other instances, it may be very difficult to find the necessary samples, like samples with elevated troponin or positive drugs of abuse. Occasionally it may be necessary to buy samples from a reference lab to complete a test validation.

For FDA-Approved Assays

FDA-approved tests have fairly straight-forward validations. Essentially the lab must show that the assay performs in their hands in the manner the manufacturer says it does. The lab must validate precision, accuracy, reportable range, which includes the linearity or analytical measurement range (AMR) and the maximum dilution or concentration, and the reference interval.[29] As long as patient samples are available, these parameters can usually be validated with a few easily performed experiments, even in a pediatric lab.

1. Imprecision: The Clinical and Laboratory Standards Institute (CLSI) has guidelines for evaluating these validation parameters, including imprecision.[30] Basically, imprecision, or assay reproducibility, can be validated by assaying 20 low and 20 high quality control (QC) samples in a single run, and then assaying a low and a high QC every day for 20 days. This will provide the within-run and the between-run imprecision, and at the same time will provide data to set QC ranges for when the test goes live. The imprecision is calculated as percent coefficient of variation (%CV), which is the standard deviation obtained from the data divided by the data mean times 100. An acceptable CV depends on the assay. For totally automated assays, a CV of 5% or less is generally expected and considered to be good precision. Manual assays like HPLC or LC-MS/MS generally have wider CVs, with 10 – 20% not being uncommon. In addition, the lower end of nearly all assays will have poorer precision than the higher concentrations, simply because the standard deviation is a higher percentage of the mean. Some assays define their lower limit of assay quantitation, or functional lower limit, as the lowest measurable value where the CV is less than 20%.

2. AMR: The analytical measurement range used to be defined by the assay calibrators, in that the assay was known to be linear within the range between the lowest and highest calibrator. Presently many assays have a single calibrator or a two point calibration, thus the laboratory must verify the AMR. In addition, if the laboratory wishes to extend an AMR on either end of this range, the laboratory must validate the extended range with a high or low sample of known concentration every 6 months. Beyond the established AMR, the laboratory establishes its reportable range, which is how far a sample can be diluted out and still give a linear response. This reportable range can be established with high samples diluted serially and checked for linear results. If the laboratory does not establish a reportable range, then the AMR is the reportable range and anything outside the AMR must be reported as greater than the highest calibrator value or less than the lowest

calibrator value. CLSI has guidelines for linearity and accuracy assessment as well.[31,32]

3. Accuracy: For an FDA-approved assay, accuracy is generally validated by comparing the new assay to an existing assay. This is usually accomplished by assaying at least 20 patient samples, ideally ones that span the reportable range, on the new and the old assay. The more poorly the assays compare, the more samples should be assayed. Once the data has been obtained from both assays, a linear regression, a bias plot and a correlation are performed on the paired data. The linear regression is the calculated mathematical line which describes the relationship between the two sets of data. The line takes the form of $Y = mx + b$, where X is the old assay values, y are the new assay values, m = the slope if the line and b equals the intercept. In a data set with perfectly matching values, the slope will be 1.0 and the intercept will be 0. Thus the closer to 1.0 the slope is, the closer to identical the two sets of values are. A slope greater than 1.0 suggests the new assay overestimates the old assay, and a slope less than one indicates that the new assay gives lower values than the old. The correlation coefficient, although often misused to determine how well two assays match, actually only tells you if they are related, not how well they match.

4. Reference interval: For an FDA-approved assay, in general existing pediatric reference intervals (PRI) can be either validated for use or transferred to the new assay using relatively small (20 – 60 samples) patient correlation studies. Running a 20 sample patient correlation will usually determine whether existing PRI are appropriate for the new assay, and if so this correlation study validates them. If the correlation study shows enough of a bias that the existing PRI cannot be used, assaying additional samples can allow the existing reference intervals to be adjusted to fit the new assay. This adjustment is called transferring a reference interval. For additional information on PRI, see Chapter 7.

For Non-FDA Approved Assays

These assays are also referred to as laboratory developed tests (LDTs). Any FDA-approved assay that is being used in a manner not specified by the manufacturer becomes an LDT. In a pediatric laboratory, this may be considered to encompass the majority of the testing performed since most tests are not validated using pediatric samples. In general LDTs are tests that are completely or partially developed by the laboratory itself. Validating an LDT requires validation of the same parameters as an FDA-approved assay, plus adds on some extra parameters.

1. Precision: The assay should be reproducible, even if it is developed from scratch. Precision studies are a good place to start in assay validation because if it is not possible to get reproducible results with an assay, it's not necessary to put any more work into it. With a completely home brew LDT, it may be necessary to make QC material or calibrators to use for precision studies.

2. AMR: Again, the AMR of the assay will be determined by the calibrators, however with an LDT, it's also necessary to establish a lower limit of quantitation, rather than simply validating a manufacturer's claim. This is often accomplished by diluting a calibrator to the lowest value that can be reproducibly recovered and measured.

3. Accuracy: Accuracy in a LDT may be established in a number of ways. If the assay has been developed and is being assayed elsewhere and samples can be obtained from the other assay, a correlation is done against the other assay to try to determine the accuracy of the new method. If the LDT being developed is not being assayed anywhere else, is essentially a one of a kind assay, accuracy is usually established using recovery studies. Samples are spiked with known concentrations of the analyte of interest and then analyzed by the assay to determine if the assay measures the amount of analyte known to be there. Samples used for recovery studies may not be the calibrators used in the assay, or made from those calibrators. These samples must be made separately.

4. Reference intervals: With LDTs it may be possible to validate or transfer a PRI if correlation samples can be obtained from a lab performing a similar assay. Often with LDTs however it is necessary to establish a PRI from scratch. Ideally, 120 samples from healthy individuals for each sub-population (gender or age sub-group) is used to establish a reference interval, which can be quite problematic in a pediatric laboratory. There are methods available, referred to as "robust" methods, which allow the use of smaller sample sizes. These samples may be collected a priori, meaning they are collected from individuals for the express purpose of establishing a reference interval, or a posteriori, meaning they are samples collected for another purpose and excess sample is used to establish the reference interval if the individual can be shown to be healthy. For a more information on pediatric reference intervals, see Chapter 7.

5. Interferences: In FDA-approved assays it is allowable to accept the manufacturer's claims for interfering substances. When validating a LDT, studies to determine interferences are necessary. Most frequently samples are spiked with hemolyzed, icteric and lipemic samples as these are the three most common interferences encountered in laboratory

testing. In general the sample will be spiked with a high concentration of the interferent to begin. If there is no interference, then the study is done. If there is interference, the sample is spiked again with a lesser concentration of the interferent and this can be repeated until a level of the interferent is found that has no affect. Interference studies for icterus and hemolysis are especially important in the pediatric population as high bilirubin and hemolyzed samples are very common.

SUMMARY

In summary, there are a number of day-to-day issues that are different in operating a pediatric laboratory versus a laboratory whose clientele is essentially adult. These differences include factors which can affect many of the operations of the lab, ranging from types of instruments to number of staff to test menu to computer systems. Being aware of these differences and their affects is an important part of pediatric laboratory medicine.

TRAINING MODULE

1. Which of the following is true about small sample volumes?
   a. They can be routinely collected in regular sized collection tubes
   b. They can affect sample integrity for add-on tests
   c. They do not influence the instrumentation a lab can use
   d. When mislabeled, they are treated the same as in any other lab

2. Heel-stick samples:
   a. Should be collected from the side of the heel
   b. Should be collected before warming the heel
   c. Should not be used for blood analysis
   d. Should be collected with lances designed for finger-stick.

3. When collecting multiple samples involving multiple tubes in a single blood collection opportunity:
   a. The order is the same for micro-collection tubes as for regular sized tubes
   b. For a venipuncture in regular tubes, collect non-anticoagulated tubes last
   c. For a capillary collection in micro-collection tubes, collect non-anticoagulated tubes last
   d. Anticoagulation contamination of the needle will not occur if you are careful

4. Send out testing:
   a. Is unlikely to be extensive in a pediatric lab
   b. Should be managed to prevent over-utilization
   c. Includes tests performed in-house
   d. Does not comprise a large portion of the lab budget

5. A CLIA validation of LDTs includes:
   a. A precision study, a patient correlation and/or recovery study, a study to determine reportable range and an interferences study
   b. A. plus a reference interval study
   c. B. minus the reportable range study
   d. B. plus a study of clinical utility

REFERENCES

1. Howie SR. Blood sample volumes in child health research: review of safe limits. *Bull World Health Organ.* 2011;89(1):46-53.
2. Jopling J, Henry E, Wiedmeier SE, Christensen RD. Reference ranges for hematocrit and blood hemoglobin concentration during the neonatal period: data from a multi-hospital health care system. *Pediatrics.* 2009;123(2):e333-e337.
3. Hawkins R. Managing the pre- and post-analytical phases of the total testing process. *Ann Lab Med.* 2012;32(1):5-16.
4. Laposata M, Dighe A. "Pre-pre" and "post-post" analytical error: high-incidence patient safety hazards involving the clinical laboratory. *Clin Chem Lab Med.* 2007;45(6):712-719.
5. Bonini P, Plebani M, Ceriotti F, Rubboli F. Errors in laboratory medicine. *Clin Chem.* 2002;48(5):691-698.
6. WHO Guidelines on Drawing Blood: Best Practices in Phlebotomy. *Geneva: World Health Organization*;2010.
7. Garza D, Becan-McBride K. Pediatric Procedures. In: Garza D, Becan-McBride K, eds. *Phlebotomy handbook: blood collection essentials.* 7th ed. Upper Saddle River, NJ: Pearson Prentice Hall; 2005:327-359.
8. Meites S. Skin-puncture and blood-collecting technique for infants: update and problems. *Clin Chem.* 1988;34(9):1890-1894.
9. Buckbee KM. Implementing a pediatric phlebotomy protocol. *MLO: Med Lab Obs.* 1994;26(4):32-35.
10. Ogawa S, Ogihara T, Fujiwara E, et al. Venepuncture is preferable to heel lance for blood sampling in term neonates. *Arch Dis Child Fetal Neonatal Ed.* 2005;90(5):F432-F436.
11. Hoeltke LB. Caring for the Pediatric Patient. In: Hoeltke LB, ed. *The Complete textbook of Phlebotomy.* 3rd ed. Clifton Park, NY: Thomas Delmar Learning; 2006:249-264
12. Meites S, Lin SS, Thompson C. Studies on the quality of specimens obtained by skin puncture of children 1. Tendency to hemolysis, and hemoglobin and tissue fluid as contaminants. *Clin Chem.* 1981;27(6):875-878.
13. Meites S, Glassco KM. Studies on the quality of specimens obtained by skin-puncture of children. 2. An analysis of blood-collecting practices in a pediatric hospital. *Clin Chem.* 1985;31(10):1669-1672.
14. Blumenfeld TA, Hertelendy WG, Ford SH. Simultaneously obtained skin-puncture serum, skin-puncture plasma, and venous serum compared, and effects of warming the skin before puncture. *Clin Chem.* 1977;23(9):1705-1710.
15. Dar K, Williams T, Aitken R, Woods KL, Fletcher S. Arterial versus capillary sampling for analysing blood gas pressures. *BMJ.* 1995;310(6971):24-25.

16. Graham G, Kenny MA. Changes in transcutaneous oxygen tension during capillary blood-gas sampling. *Clin Chem.* 1980;26(13):1860-1863.

17. Yuksel S, Yuksel G, Oncel S, Divanli E. Osteomyelitis of the calcaneus in the newborn: an ongoing complication of Guthrie test. *Eur J Pediatr.* 2007;166(5):503-504.

18. Hoeltke LB. Specimen considerations and special procedures. Urine, semen and culture collection. In: Hoeltke LB, ed. *The Complete Textbook of Phlebotomy.* 3rd ed. Clifton Park, NJ: Thomas Delmar Learning; 2006:290-295.

19. Schroeder AR, Newman TB, Wasserman RC, Finch SA, Pantell RH. Choice of urine collection methods for the diagnosis of urinary tract infection in young, febrile infants. *Arch Pediatr Adolesc Med.* 2005;159(10):915-922.

20. Jones BA, Calam RR, Howanitz PJ. Chemistry specimen acceptability: a College of American Pathologists Q-Probes study of 453 laboratories. *Arch Pathol Lab Med.* 1997;121(1):19-26.

21. Hoeltke LB. Phlebotomy technique. In: Hoeltke LB, ed. *The Complete Textbook of Phlebotomy.* 3rd ed. Clifton Park, NJ: Thomas Delmar Learning;2006:165-226.

22. Hoeltke LB. The Challenge of Phlebotomy. In: Hoeltke LB, ed. *The Complete Textbook of Phlebotomy.* 3rd ed. Clifton Park, NJ: Thomas Delmar Learning;2006:227-248.

23. Green A MI, Gray J. *Neonatology & Laboratory Medicine.* London, UK: ACB Venture Publications; 2003.

24. Rautenberg MW, van Solinge WW, Heunks JJ, Stokwielder RH, Lentjes EG, Kemperman H. Pediatric tube direct sampling by the Abbott Architect integrated ci8200 chemistry/immunochemistry analyzer. *Clin Chem.* 2006;52(4):768-770.

25. Hicks JM. Pediatric Clinical Biochemistry: Why is it different? In: Soldin SJ, Rifai N, Hicks JM, eds. *Biochemical basis of pediatric disease.* Washington, DC: AACC Press; 1992:xi, 564

26. Dickerson JA, Cole B, Conta JH, et al. Improving the value of costly genetic reference laboratory testing with active utilization management. *Arch Pathol Lab Med.* 2014;138(1):110-113.

27. Miller CE, Krautscheid P, Baldwin EE, et al. Genetic counselor review of genetic test orders in a reference laboratory reduces unnecessary testing. *Am J Med Genet A.* 2014;164A(5):1094-1101.

28. Cole B, Dickerson JA, Graber ML, et al. A prospective tool for risk assessment of sendout testing. *Clin Chem Acta.* 2014;434:1-5.

29. DB E. Method Evaluation. In: WC, ed. *Professional Practice in Clinical Chemistry.* 2nd ed. Washington DC: AACC Press; 2011:43-53.

30. EP05-A3 Evaluation of Precision of Quantitative Measurement Procedures; Approved Guideline. 3rd ed. *Clinical and Laboratory Standards Institute.* 2014.

31. EP06-A Evaluation of the Linearity of Quantitative Measurement Procedures: A Statistical Approach; Approved Guideline. 1st ed. *Clinical and Laboratory Standards Institute.* 2003:62.

32. EP09-A3 Measurement Procedure Comparison and Bias Estimation Using OPatient Samples; Approved Guideline. 3rd ed. *Clinical and Laboratory Standards Institute.* 2013:98.

COMMON TESTS AND CONSIDERATIONS IMPORTANT IN PEDIATRIC MEDICINE | 2

Amy L. Pyle-Eilola and David J. Thornton

LEARNING OBJECTIVES

1. Distinguish laboratory tests that require specific interpretation or extra attention in children than adults.
2. Recognize pediatric-specific situations which may affect lab results.
3. Identify laboratory assays which have age-dependent reference intervals.
4. Discuss the signs and symptoms of lead poisoning, as well as treatment options.
5. Summarize the causes and associated testing of hyperbilirubinemia in infants.

INTRODUCTION

There are numerous tests routinely ordered in pediatric practice which, while not exclusive to pediatrics, have special significance in young populations. Conversely, other tests, such as prostate specific antigen, which are commonplace in adult practice, are rarely used in pediatrics. This chapter will review the most common tests which are particularly important in pediatric medicine, and special considerations for evaluating laboratory results in this unique population.

| TESTS AND CONDITIONS IMPORTANT IN PEDIATRICS

Bilirubin

Plasma bilirubin circulates primarily in two forms, the water-insoluble unconjugated bilirubin (Bu), which circulates non-covalently bound to albumin, and water-soluble conjugated bilirubin (Bc) in which bilirubin is covalently bound to one or two glucuronide molecules. Bc is sometimes referred to as direct bilirubin because in most common diazo-based methods, the form of bilirubin which reacts directly is mostly Bc. Bu was then referred to as "indirect" bilirubin and was the total bilirubin minus the direct. The term indirect bilirubin is no longer used. A third form of circulating bilirubin, delta bilirubin, is composed of conjugated bilirubin bound covalently to albumin and will not be discussed further here. Total serum bilirubin (TSB) is the sum of all forms of bilirubin in circulation. Bu is a by-product of the catabolism of the heme moiety in hemoglobin and is transported by albumin to the liver where glucuronosyl transferases conjugate glucuronide molecules to Bu, thereby converting it to Bc. Bc is then excreted through the bile duct into the gastrointestinal tract where it is further broken down by intestinal bacteria into urobilinogens and excreted.[1]

Following birth, there is a rise in oxygen tension in the newborn's circulation, resulting in a downregulation of erythropoietin.[2] That, along with the relatively short lifespan of red cells containing fetal hemoglobin results in significant physiological hemolysis and decrease in hematocrit.[3] The resulting release of hemoglobin and its breakdown leads to a physiological increase in Bu. The immature neonatal liver lacks sufficient glucuronosyl transferases to match the demand for bilirubin conjugation, thereby restricting conversion to Bc and excretion. Consequently, the newborn has a relatively high normal range for Bu and TSB. Generally, no additional intervention is required for this mild jaundice, termed "neonatal jaundice" (marked primarily by yellowing of the skin), which usually resolves within 3-4 weeks after birth. However, in some newborns, the bilirubin concentration can rise to dangerous concentrations in the first 24-72 hours of life. In these cases, medical intervention such as phototherapy or, much more rarely, exchange transfusion is required to lower the bilirubin concentration and prevent life-threatening acute bilirubin encephalopathy.[4] The lipid-solubility of Bu enables it to cross the blood brain barrier of the developing neonate, causing significant neurological complications and encephalopathy. Acute bilirubin encephalopathy symptoms may include lethargy, hypotonia followed by hypertonia, poor sucking, fever, and development of a high pitched cry. As the symptoms become more serious, irreparable brain damage may occur, leading to apnea, stupor, seizures, and even death. Those who survive the acute encephalopathy with permanent neurologic sequelae

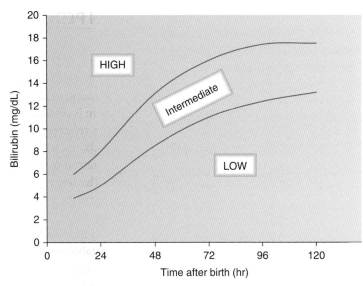

Figure 2-1 ▪ Total serum bilirubin nomogram for risk assessment of newborns based on age in hours. The low risk zone is defined by the 40th percentile and the high risk zone by the 95th percentile tracks, adapted from Bhutani.[5]

have chronic bilirubin encephalopathy or kernicterus. Hallmarks of kernicterus are athetoid cerebral palsy and spasticity, auditory dysfunction, impairment of upward gaze, and dental enamel dysplasia.[6]

Due to the risks associated with jaundice in the newborn, in 2009, the American Academy of Pediatrics published a statement recommending universal screening for hyperbilirubinemia in newborns prior to hospital discharge. Total serum bilirubin (which in most infants is almost exclusively unconjugated) or transcutaneous bilirubin were previously evaluated relative to age in hours using a nomogram from Bhutani, et al. (Figure 2-1).[5] The 2009 recommendations add several risk factors for severe hyperbilirubinemia in addition to the bilirubin concentration. Such risk factors include low gestational age, exclusively breastfeeding, hemolytic disease, previous sibling with jaundice, significant bruising from birth trauma, and East Asian descent.[7] Treatment decisions are made based on the combination of bilirubin concentration and risk factors.

It should be noted that not all bilirubin assays are directly comparable, and there are significant biases reported among different testing platforms. The Bhutani risk nomogram is based on a diazo-based bilirubin assay.[5] Diazo-based assay are the most widely-used assays in laboratories in general and measure direct-reacting bilirubin (mostly Bc) and then after adding an accelerant, measure total bilirubin. However, a very popular testing platform in pediatrics uses a reflectance spectrophotometric quantitation, which measures Bu, Bc, and TSB directly and produces higher results. Transcutaneous bilirubin measurements use a type of reflectance spectrophotometry and measure only TSB. Care should be taken when evaluating bilirubin values in the newborn.[4] Additionally, samples with high concentrations of bilirubin (icteric samples) may not give accurate results for certain other commonly requested laboratory tests, depending on the testing method. Bilirubin can interfere with certain reactions, particularly peroxidase-based methods, such as uric acid, cholesterol, and triglycerides, decreasing the results by up to 10%, as bilirubin serves as a substrate for peroxidase.[8] Bilirubin may also simply interfere with absorbance of light at specific wavelengths. Generally, laboratories will not report results on very icteric for those tests known to be affected by bilirubin.

Lead

Lead poisoning, formerly known as plumbism, of children was first described in Australian children in the towns where dwellings were covered with lead paint. Very few cases of lead poisoning in children were found from children living in the countryside where buildings were not painted.[9] Lead poisoning was described in children being evaluated for peripheral paralysis consisting of bilateral wrist and foot drop who recovered when removed from the lead-containing environment. By the 1940s, it was established that children who had recovered from acute lead poisoning still developed neurological sequelae including intellectual impairment.

Symptoms of Lead Poisoning

In overt acute lead poisoning, generally associated with blood lead levels >70 μg/dL, children present with an encephalopathy with ataxia, developmental regression, poor coordination, apathy, vomiting, seizures, altered mental state, and/or coma. Physical examination may show diminished deep tendon reflexes, increased intracranial pressure, facial nerve palsy, and/or papilledema. Milder presentations include anorexia, constipation, abdominal pain, irritability, and altered behavior. Lower-level, chronic lead exposure (15-70 μg/dL) is associated with slowed reactions and anemia. More subtle symptoms may be mistakenly attributed to "normal childhood behavior" (eg, "Terrible Twos"). These include poor attention span, behavioral problems, and irritability. Other symptoms may include seizures without encephalopathy, developmental delay, colicky abdominal pain, myalgias, and vomiting.[10,11]

The symptoms of lead poisoning in children are nonspecific and are very subtle for lead concentrations less than 25 μg/dL. A report from the Centers for Disease Control (CDC) in 2012 on chronic low-level lead exposure showed decrements in IQ and academic achievement at blood lead levels of less than 10 µg/dL. Studies have shown a decrease of approximately 5 IQ points for every 10 µg/dL increase in blood lead. However, in low-range lead poisoning (1-10 µg/dL), IQ dropped by 7 points, suggesting that the rate of IQ loss is greatest at the lower levels.[12] Based on these findings, the CDC advisory committee recommended that the lowest limit of acceptability for lead be <5 µg/dL.[13]

The wide range of symptoms, particularly in children with low-to-mid level lead exposure, has prompted the American Academy of Pediatrics to recommend regular lead screening for patients deemed at risk for lead exposure.[14,15] In the 1970s and 1980s, patients were screened for elevated lead levels using free erythrocyte protoporphyrin or zinc protoporphyrin. Lead interferes with the production of heme, which normally consists of iron and protoporphyrin. Lead inhibits the insertion of iron into protoporphyrin leading to a buildup of protoporphyrin, which combines non-enzymatically with zinc, to make the fluorescent compound zinc protoporphyrin. Zinc protoporphyrin can be measured in a drop of blood in specially designed instruments called hematofluorometers. Unfortunately, zinc protoporphyrin does not increase until blood lead levels are around 25 µg/dL. With findings that lead levels less than 10 µg/dL can cause decreases in IQ, this test is no longer a viable method for screening patients for lead poisoning. Preferred methods for the measurement of lead in blood include graphite furnace atomic absorption, anodic stripping voltammetry, and inductively coupled plasma-mass spectrometry, which perform batch analysis. The capital costs for this testing is high, but the cost per test is low as reagent requirements are minimal. The LeadCare point of care instrument, which is based on anodic stripping voltammetry, can perform testing at clinics and its results are reliable. The capital cost for this test is low, but the individual cost is high compared to the other two methods.

Treatment

To treat patients with elevated blood lead, oral or intravenous chelation therapy may be administered. Oral chelation should be used for patients with lead concentrations >45 and <69 µg/dL, and may be accomplished with succimer, an analog of dimercaprol, a compound which chelates heavy metals. Succimer binds lead, and the resulting water-soluble compound is excreted in the urine. The efficacy of this drug is modest for patients with mild to moderately elevated blood lead levels, and some studies have shown little difference compared to placebo.[16] In general, lead chelation only removes about 1-2% of total body lead content as chelators cannot access lead stored in some organs, such as the brain.[10] A side effect of oral succimer is that a patient can smell of rotten eggs due to the sulfur content of the drug, which can hinder compliance with taking the drug. With higher lead levels, the use of intravenous chelation with $CaNa_2EDTA$ may be used.[17] While $CaNa_2EDTA$ can very rapidly decrease lead levels, extreme caution must be used, as EDTA can chelate other essential metals, such as zinc, calcium, and magnesium. Therefore, this type of therapy should only be administered in a hospital.

Since the late 1990s, there has been a national effort to decrease childhood lead poisoning in the United States. This program has consisted of identification of housing which may have lead paint and education of the public and physicians to the dangers of lead poisoning. The removal of lead from gasoline and paint beginning in the mid-1970s has decreased the amount of lead in the environment.

The CDC tracks cases of lead poisoning, and in 1998 reported that approximately 7% of children tested in the United States had a confirmed blood lead level of $>10\,\mu g/dL$. That statistic dropped to $<1\%$ by 2011, suggesting that cleanup efforts, public education, and awareness have worked to decrease lead exposure in children. Additional information on lead can also be found in Chapter 9.

Renal Function Tests

Glomerular filtration rate (GFR) is the most widely used indicator of kidney function. GFR defines the volume of plasma that is completely filtered by the kidneys in a unit of time for a given body surface area, and is determined by following the plasma concentration of a physiologically inert compound that is freely-filtered by the glomerulus and not secreted, reabsorbed, or metabolized by other parts of the nephron. The healthy adult reference range for GFR is >90 mg/min/1.73 m^2, and reflects the filtration rate relative to the normal surface area of an adult. A low GFR indicates that kidney function is sub-optimal.[18]

The gold standard for determining GFR is inulin clearance, but this test is only performed in specialized centers. GFR can also be measured by assessing the clearance of other compounds, such as iohexol and radioactive tracers, including Chromium-51 and Technetium-99m.[19,20] Though more common than inulin clearance, special equipment and personnel are required for these tests, making them not appropriate for routine monitoring.[18] Thus, surrogate markers for GFR have been developed. One of the more common alternatives to GFR is a 24-hour creatinine clearance, which requires a 24-hour urine collection for creatinine measurement in addition to measuring a plasma level of creatinine. However, proper collection of a timed urine sample, especially over a 24-hour period is challenging, particularly in children. Therefore, it would be appropriate to have a surrogate marker which is an endogenous substance that can be measured from a single blood sample.

Creatinine

Creatinine, a waste product from the breakdown of the muscle protein creatine, is freely-filtered by the glomerulus, and is the most commonly used marker of kidney function. Numerous formulas have been developed to estimate GFR (eGFR) based a serum creatinine measurement, but many have failed to account for all the parameters which affect GFR, including age, gender, body mass, and ethnicity. In 1999, the Modification of Diet in Renal Disease (MDRD) study proposed the MDRD equation for eGFR.[21]

eGFR by MDRD:

$$\text{eGFR} = 186 \times \text{Serum Creatinine}^{-1.154} \times \text{Age}^{-0.203} \times [1.210 \; \textit{if Black}] \times [0.742 \; \textit{if Female}].$$

Serum creatinine is in mg/dL in this formula. Creatinine results in μmol/L can be converted to mg.dL by dividing by 88.4. This equation is based on serum creatinine measured by assays which are *not* calibrated to isotope dilution mass spectrometry. If the assay is calibrated to isotope dilution mass spectrometry, the eGFR results should be multiplied by 0.95.[22]

This calculated value has been shown to be a fairly good estimate of GFR in most adults. However, because the MDRD equation was developed using patients with chronic kidney disease, it consistently underestimates GFR in patients with high GFRs. Subsequently the CKD-EPI equation was developed and has been shown to perform more accurately than the MDRD equation.[23,24]

eGFR by CKD-EPI:

$$\text{eGFR} = 141 \times \min(\text{Scr}/\kappa)^{\alpha} \times \max(\text{Scr}/\kappa)^{-1.209} \times 0.993^{\text{Age}} \times 1.018 [\textit{if female}] \times 1.159 [\textit{if black}]$$

where, κ = 0.7 if female, 0.9 if male,
α = −0.329 if female, −0.411 if male,
min = The minimum of Scr/κ or 1,
max = The maximum of Scr/κ or 1, and
Scr = serum creatinine (mg/dL).

Despite the widespread use of creatinine to determine eGFR, there are limitations to eGFR, particularly in pediatrics. The amount of creatinine in plasma is dependent upon the muscle mass of the individual and thus varies with age and body habitus; children usually have the lowest serum creatinine concentrations. Individuals with low muscle mass, such as neonates, patients with spina bifida, anorexia nervosa, liver cirrhosis, and muscular dystrophy will have abnormally low plasma creatinine concentrations. Additionally, creatinine is secreted in small amounts in the proximal tubules. As plasma creatinine concentrations increase, so does the secretion, leading to falsely decreased serum creatinine values. The lower creatinine value may mask kidney disease in patients with falsely low creatinine concentrations.[18,25] Another circulating marker with a concentration independent of age and muscle mass would be better for estimating GFR in pediatrics.

Cystatin C

Cystatin C is a low molecular weight protease inhibitor that is made consistently and ubiquitously secreted by all nucleated cells in the body. It is freely-filtered by the glomerulus and entirely reabsorbed and mostly catabolized by the proximal tubules. No pathophysiological states have been shown to consistently affect cystatin C blood levels. Some studies, but not all have shown an increase in cystatin C in some patients with hyperthyroidism, and a decrease in some patients with hypothyroidism.[26,27] Additionally, high-dose glucocorticoid use has an been shown to elevate cystatin C.[27] It is not affected by muscle mass, age, gender, or race. Therefore, cystatin C holds much promise as a marker of kidney function in children and other populations with low muscle mass.[23,27]

Several equations have been developed to calculate the eGFR using measured serum cystatin C levels, including several equations for use in children. Accuracy of eGFR estimation is improved by incorporating more factors, such as serum creatinine, gender, height, and blood urea nitrogen, and incorporating these additional components has demonstrated accuracy >90% compared to gold-standard GFR determinations.[23,28] However, these equations are still not widely used. Until recently, there have been few methods available for measuring cystatin C, and poor agreement across methods. Equations based on cystatin C by one method will not work with cystatin C results by another method. Better standardization of cystatin C assays will be needed for more widespread use of eGFR based on cystatin C.[23,28]

Transient Hyperphosphatasemia

Transient hyperphosphatasemia (TH) is a temporary condition in children under 5 years old, in which serum alkaline phosphatase activity (AP) is elevated 3-20 times the upper reference range with no clinical indications for the elevation. TH is estimated to occur in 2-5% of healthy children.[29,30] Patients are usually asymptomatic, with unremarkable history, physical exam, and laboratory results. Some patients have had a mild viral condition in the recent past. Isoenzyme analysis is non-specific, with both bone and liver isoenzymes usually elevated. The hyperphosphatasemia will usually resolve within 1-20 weeks without treatment.[29,31] Although clinically benign, it is important for this condition to be recognized to prevent undue follow-ups, such as bone scans, liver biopsies, or other workups to try and identify the cause of the elevation. It is recommended that in patients under the age of 5, who have elevations in both bone and liver ALP isoenzymes, and with otherwise normal lab results for liver or bone disease, an isolated elevation in ALP be attributed to TH. In these cases, ALP should be repeated in 4 months to ensure ALP has returned to normal.[32]

Potassium and Hemolysis

The utility of measuring potassium in pediatrics is similar to that of adult populations. Due to the critical nature of potassium for proper cardiac function and normal physiologic homeostasis, especially of the muscle and nervous systems, it is measured in serum/plasma as part of a basic metabolic panel or may be ordered on its own. For patients at high risk of potassium and other electrolyte imbalances, potassium is followed very closely.[33] Such high-risk patients include those with renal disease, diabetic ketoacidosis, and tumor lysis syndrome following chemotherapy for leukemia. Given the critical nature of this analyte, it is very important that results for potassium be accurate. Since red cells have an intracellular potassium concentration about 20 times higher than plasma, even small degrees of hemolysis can increase the potassium content in a blood sample. In newborns and infants, capillary heel-stick is the recommended method of blood collection, and capillary finger-stick is often used with older children (see Chapter 1). Although these methods are less painful and invasive than venipuncture, they can cause more hemolysis. Consequently, potassium results (and other hemolysis-affected tests including aspartate amino transferase (AST), iron, lactate dehydrogenase, haptoglobin, phosphate, and bilirubin) are often inaccurate in pediatrics and must be interpreted carefully.[34] In serum and plasma samples, the degree of hemolysis is easily detected by visually or spectrophotometrically detecting an increase in red-colored hemoglobin. For these sample types, laboratories should have established guidelines to restrict reporting of specific results on hemolyzed samples. Some have proposed the use of correction factors to estimate the true potassium concentration in hemolyzed samples. For example, Mansour et al., derived two correction factors: 0.51 or 0.40 meq/L increased potassium for every 0.1 g/dL increase in plasma hemoglobin. However, most studies have found that such factors are insufficiently accurate for use.[35] Potassium may be tested in whole blood using point of care instruments. In this situation, hemolysis cannot be identified, and results must be interpreted with caution. It is wise to repeat and verify an unexpected high potassium result from a whole blood sample before making any treatment decisions. Likewise, a normal point of care potassium value in a patient who was expected to be hypokalemic, should also alert the clinician that hemolysis may have falsely elevated the result.[36,37]

Hemolysis and Plasma Hemoglobin

In addition to using visual means to assess the degree of hemolysis in a plasma or serum sample, plasma hemoglobin can be measured directly with a spectrophotometer using several hemoglobin-specific wavelengths or using chemical reactions to cause a color change, which can also be measured spectrophotometrically.[38] In this way, the amount of hemoglobin in a plasma sample can be quantified. While this is not routinely used to determine the degree of hemolysis caused by sample collection, it is used to follow hemolysis from a transfusion reaction, or due to mechanical fragmentation of red cells. Extracorporeal membrane oxygenation (ECMO) is a cause of red cell fragmentation and hemolysis seen more commonly in pediatrics than in adult practice. ECMO is an effective means of providing emergency cardiac and pulmonary aid. The process of ECMO requires circulating blood from the patient through a series of pumps which may mechanically lyse red cells, causing an increase in free circulating hemoglobin, which puts children at risk for renal impairment and death. High plasma hemoglobin may indicate the presence of a clot in the pumps, prompting modification of anticoagulation and maintenance of the ECMO circuit.[39]

DIABETES TESTING

Glucose concentrations in the blood of a normal individual are the result of the tightly regulated interplay between dietary intake, cellular uptake, glycogenesis, glycogenolysis, and gluconeogenesis. These pathways and processes are regulated by hormones, including insulin, glucagon, growth hormone, cortisol, and epinephrine. Of these hormones, insulin is the only one which lowers blood glucose and increases cellular uptake of glucose and formation of glycogen. Diabetes is a group of disorders in which glucose regulation has been lost and glucose concentration in the blood remains high.

Diabetes in the pediatric population has seen a shifting paradigm for the type of diabetes commonly encountered. Between 2001 and 2009, both type 1 and type 2 diabetes have increased in the pediatric population, however type 2 has increased 30.5% during that time, as opposed to a 21.1% increase in type 1.[40] Type 2, or adult onset diabetes, was rarely diagnosed in a pediatric setting. Now its diagnosis in pediatrics is not uncommon. The increasing prevalence of obesity in the pediatric population is believed to contribute to this trend.

Diabetes mellitus, most commonly simply referred to as diabetes, is defined by elevated blood glucose concentrations over extended periods of time. It comprises a group of metabolic disorders that are broadly classified into four categories, type 1, type 2, gestational, and other specific types.[41]

Type 1

Type 1 diabetes makes up approximately 10% of diabetes patients. It is characterized by insulin deficiency due to destruction of the insulin-producing beta cells in the islets of Langerhans in the pancreas. The majority of cases are immune-mediated with autoimmune attacks on the beta cells resulting in beta cell loss. Type 1 is also at least partially inherited, but the inheritance mode is complex and not fully understood.[41] Multiple genes have been shown to be involved in conferring a predisposition to diabetes. Genetically susceptible individuals may have diabetes onset triggered by environmental factors. Type 1 diabetes occurs in both adults and children and is also referred to as autoimmune diabetes or immune-mediated diabetes. It was traditionally called "juvenile onset" because the majority of cases presented and were diagnosed in children. It has also been called "insulin-dependent" diabetes, as treatment usually requires insulin administration. The onset of type 1 diabetes tends to be sudden and accompanied by ketoacidosis in an often thin, ill-appearing individual.

Type 2

Type 2 diabetes is by far the more common form, making up approximately 90% of diabetes patients. It is characterized by a progressive defect in insulin production and secretion on the background of insulin resistance. Type 2 diabetes causation is complex and is believed to be related to a combination of genetics and lifestyle, and is strongly associated with obesity, and to a lesser degree, genetic predisposition, lipid distribution, low physical activity, stress, and poor diet.[41,42] This type of diabetes occurs in both adults and children, but was traditionally referred to as "adult onset" and was relatively rare in the pediatric population. With the rising incidence of pediatric obesity and sedentary lifestyle, type 2 diabetes is now more common in the pediatric population than ever before.[40] The onset of type 2 diabetes tends to be gradual and ketoacidosis is rare. Initial treatment often involves changes in diet and lifestyle, including weight-loss programs. There are also several drugs available to treat hyperglycemia in type 2 diabetes.

The American Diabetes Association recommends that diagnostic testing for type 2 diabetes should be performed in children that are overweight (BMI >85th percentile for age and sex, or weight >120th percentile for height) and in addition have any two of the following risk factors: 1) family history of type 2 diabetes in 1st or 2nd degree relative, 2) ethnicity is Native American, African American, Latino, Asian American, or Pacific islander, 3) signs or conditions associated with insulin resistance (acanthosis nigricans, hypertension, dyslipidemia, polycystic ovary disease, small for gestational age birth weight), or 4) maternal history of diabetes or gestational diabetes during the patient's gestation. This testing should begin at age of 10 and be repeated every 3 years.

Gestational

As its name suggest, gestational diabetes (GDM) occurs during pregnancy. Normal pregnancy is associated with increased insulin resistance, especially in the latter half of the pregnancy. In pregnancy, glucose levels are maintained by increased production of insulin, and women who cannot meet the increased demand for insulin production develop gestational diabetes mellitus. This topic is covered in detail in Chapter 8.

Other Specific Types

Other types of hyperglycemia not clearly type 1 or 2 or GDM used to be referred to as "secondary diabetes." Included among this group are genetic defects in β-cell function and insulin action causing disorders like neonatal diabetes and maturity-onset diabetes of the young (MODY), diseases of the exocrine pancreas like cystic fibrosis, endocrinopathies like Cushing's and acromegaly, infections, and drug or hormone induced beta-cell or insulin dysfunction. Cystic fibrosis-related diabetes occurs in 20% of adolescents and up to 50% of adults with cystic fibrosis, and is associated with worse nutritional status, more severe inflammatory lung disease and increased mortality in this population.

Diagnosis

Regardless of the type of diabetes, diagnosis is made by demonstrating hyper-glycemia. This can be accomplished by measuring glucose and/or hemoglobin A1C (HbA1C) concentrations. Glucose measurement provides a snapshot of current glucose levels at the time of blood collection. HbA1C is a measure of the percentage of hemoglobin molecules which have had glucose attached covalently due to elevated glucose concentrations over time. The extent of hemoglobin glycosylation thus reflects glucose concentration over the lifespan of hemoglobin-containing red cells—approximately 3 months.

In adults, the following criteria are used for the diagnosis of diabetes:

- HbA1C ≥6.5%;
- Fasting plasma glucose ≥126 mg/dL (7.0 mmol/L) with fasting for at least 8 hours before blood collection;
- Oral glucose tolerance test with the 2 hour timed glucose ≥200 mg/dL (11.1 mmol/L); and
- Patient with classic symptoms of hyperglycemic or hypoglycemic crisis with a random plasma glucose ≥200 mg/dL (11.1 mmol/L).

Unless there is a clear clinical presentation consistent with the onset of diabetes, diagnosis should not be made on the basis of a single result; a second test is required to confirm a diagnosis. If any of these tests yield equivocal results, the result should be confirmed by repeat testing.[42]

There are several considerations regarding the methods used for testing. Despite the convenience of point-of-care glucometers, most are not sufficiently accurate to be used in establishing a diagnosis of diabetes. Therefore, until glucometer manufacturers improve the assay performance, diagnostic glucose testing should be performed on plasma samples in a clinical laboratory.[43] Likewise, HbA1C used for diagnosis of diabetes should not be performed with a point-of-care method, but a laboratory assay that is standardized against or traceable to the Diabetes Control and Complications Trial reference assay. There are other issues regarding the use of HbA1C for the diagnosis of diabetes, particularly in children. For example, the threshold for using HbA1C to diagnose diabetes is not as clear in the pediatric population, as the studies recommending its use in diagnosis were only performed in adults.[44] In addition, HbA1C should not be used to diagnose cystic fibrosis related diabetes nor acute onset type 1diabetes. Hemoglobinopathies may cause falsely low or high HbA1C values depending on the variant hemoglobin and the method used for determination. If the presence of an abnormal hemoglobin is not known, false HbA1C results may be interpreted incorrectly, resulting in inaccurate diagnoses. Hemoglobin variants are not detected by immunoassay methods for HbA1C. Therefore, HbA1C methods without interference by these other hemoglobins, such as chromatography methods, are recommended for use when establishing a diagnosis of diabetes.

Autoantibodies

Not all cases of diabetes follow the classic presentation or allow clear-cut classification into type. Determining type 1 or 2 or other is important however, as treatments differ and persons with type 1 diabetes are also prone to other autoimmune conditions. Measuring autoantibodies can provide useful information, especially in the less than straightforward cases, or when a person with type 2 diabetes is suspected of actually having type 1. In more than 85% of type 1 diabetics, one or more autoantibodies are present, and measuring these can aid in making a diagnosis. The presence of multiple autoantibodies however is associated with a >90% risk of type 1 diabetes, and studies in children with more than two autoantibodies showed that roughly 70% developed type 1 diabetes within 10 years and 84% developed it within 15 years.[45,46] The primary autoantibodies involved in diabetes are described here.

Islet cell cytoplasmic autoantibodies (ICA) are present in 75-85% of new-onset type 1 diabetics, a percentage which declines to 5-10% by 10 years post-diagnosis. ICA can be present before the onset of type 1 diabetes, and ICA presence in a non-diabetic indicates a markedly increased risk of type 1 diabetes. ICA that are detected in a type 2 diabetic suggest that the person actually has a form of diabetes known as latent autoimmune diabetes of adulthood (LADA), and that beta cell destruction is on-going.

Glutamic acid decarboxylase autoantibodies (GAD65/GAD67/GADA), including the 65 KD and 67 KD forms, may also be found in type 1 diabetics. GADA are present in roughly 70-80% of newly diagnosed type 1 diabetics. Their presence in normal individuals are predictive of development of type 1 diabetes, and in type 2 diabetics, indicate that the patients may in fact have type 1. However, they are not as specific indicators for type 1 diabetes as ICA: GADA are also found in up to 3% of the general population, whereas ICA are rare in the general population.

Insulin autoantibodies (IA2 or IAA) are the autoantibodies which are least commonly present at onset of type 1 diabetes, occurring in 50-60% of children and uncommonly in adults with new onset type 1 diabetes. They are also the least disease-specific of the autoantibodies. Measuring IA2 is problematic because assays do not distinguish between antibodies produced against endogenous versus exogenous insulin.

Insulinoma-associated-2 autoantibodies (IA-2A) can be found in approximately 60% of new-onset type 1 diabetes. They are more prevalent than IA2 in the general population.

Zinc transporter 8 autoantibodies (ZnT8A) have recently been identified in association with type 1 diabetes. It appears to be raised against the transporter that moves zinc from the cytoplasm to the insulin-containing secretory granules in the beta cells. ZnT8A autoantibodies are present in 60-70% of new onset type 1 diabetics under the age of 20, and about 40% of new onset type 1 diabetics diagnosed after 20 years old. They are also present in 14% of cases which are negative for GADA, IA2, and IA-2A and are common in LADA patients. In addition, patients who are positive for ZnT8A have a more aggressive disease process, with more frequent ketoacidosis and requiring higher insulin doses.[47]

LAB TESTS WITH PEDIATRIC-SPECIFIC CONSIDERATIONS

Normal concentrations of many analytes change with age; some reference intervals vary widely between childhood and adulthood. Those assays with significantly different reference intervals in pediatric versus adulthood are generally related to body systems that change throughout development: skeletal, endocrine, and hematologic. Often, the reference intervals change in parallel with major shifts in physiology: early postnatal life, in which the infant's body is transitioning from the in utero environment to ex utero, bone development in early childhood, and changes at adolescence with growth velocity changes and sexual maturation, at which time there are significant fluctuations in the measured concentrations of various hormones described later. Reference intervals which reflect these changes are necessary for proper interpretation of lab values. Pediatric reference intervals are covered in detail in Chapter 7.

Newborn Specific Considerations

In the newborn, there are several circumstances which can significantly alter the concentration of certain analytes. For example, birth trauma contributes to red cell turnover and elevated unconjugated bilirubin. Additionally, due to the postnatal change in oxygen tension, red cells and hemoglobin turnover and degrade within days of birth, also contributing to a rise in unconjugated bilirubin and mild physiological jaundice. Nutritional indicators are often different in the newborn due to lack of body stores of lipids and glycogen. Consequently, glucose and lipid concentrations are usually lower than adult levels within the first 2 weeks after birth. Frequently, a metabolic acidosis may be observed in newborns due to the accumulation of lactic acid and other organic acids within the first 24-hours after birth.

Hemoglobin F (HbF) and alpha-fetoprotein (AFP) are vital for normal fetal physiology. HbF, with a higher oxygen affinity than adult hemoglobin A, helps pull oxygen from the maternal to fetal circulation. The expression of the gamma globin chain which is characteristic of HbF, is highly expressed starting around 3 month gestation, falls off rapidly after birth, and within 6-12 months stabilizes to adult concentrations.[48] The presence of high concentrations of HbF can interfere with certain assays, such as screens for sickled red cells and hemoglobin A1C, which may be affected by numerous hemoglobin variants as noted in the earlier section. Due to altered affinity for carbon monoxide of HbF, infants and others with high HbF that have been exposed to carbon monoxide, may have different concentrations of carboxyhemoglobin than a normal adult with a similar exposure.[49]

AFP is the fetal equivalent to albumin, and decreases after birth as an infant's liver matures and produces albumin in lieu of AFP. Postnatally, AFP is highest immediately after birth, and may be 10,000 times higher than a normal adult. Concentrations drop off rapidly and reach near-adult concentrations by 18-24 months of life.[1,50] Persistent elevation in AFP may indicate liver or bone disease.[32] Similar to AFP, B-type Natriuretic Peptide (BNP) and NT-Pro BNP, biomarkers of cardiac failure, are very elevated in the first few days of life, but fall off rapidly thereafter. Due to the difficulty in obtaining blood samples from healthy neonates, many laboratories have not established a newborn reference range for BNP or NT-Pro BNP. Again, without proper knowledge of the high concentration in the healthy neonate, results can be easily misinterpreted, leading to an unnecessary cardiac workup.[51,52]

Endocrine Considerations

The hypothalamic-pituitary-thyroid axis undergoes significant maturation starting as a mid-gestation fetus continuing through infancy, as the hypothalamus, pituitary, and thyroid develop. At birth, there is a surge of hypothalamic thyrotropin releasing hormone and pituitary thyroid stimulating hormone (TSH). TSH, which is most commonly used to screen for thyroid disorders, including for congenital hypothyroidism on most state newborn screens, is quite high in the first week of life, with ranges 2-3 times higher than that of an adult. TSH equilibrates within 2-20 weeks post-birth, and continues to decline through puberty. Thyroxine and free thyroxine follow a similar though more subtle pattern: highest following birth (1.5-2 times adult upper limit of normal) and declining through adolescence.[53,54]

Reproductive hormones, such as testosterone, estrogen, luteinizing hormone, and follicle stimulating hormone, all change with sexual maturation, as mediated by gonadotropin releasing hormone (GnRH) secretion at the initiation of puberty. In both males and females, pubertal changes begin with pituitary secretion of GnRH that promotes the release of luteinizing and follicle stimulating hormones, which stimulate the synthesis of gonadal hormones, such as estrogen and testosterone. These gonadal hormones mediate many of the physical changes and development of secondary sexual characteristics associated with puberty.[55] Clinical testing for hormones is generally done by immunoassay, and there is currently poor standardization between most routine assays and manufacturer's. However, there is effort underway to create better standards and methods to provide consistency in reporting.[56] Laboratories should supply lab- and method-specific reference intervals to account for the differences in analytical methods and provide consistency in interpretation across methods.

Since the development of secondary sexual characteristics and onset of puberty can occur at a range of ages, biochemical markers are best interpreted in light of developmental stage, rather than age. Originally developed by James Tanner, the Tanner stages describe physical development based on sexual characteristics, such as breast and genital size, testicular volume, and pubic hair development.[57] Establishing reference intervals requires samples from hundreds of normal individuals, which can be challenging for small and medium sized labs to establish any reference interval. Because Tanner stage determination is fairly invasive, it is incredibly difficult for most labs to determine Tanner-specific ranges. Recent large-scale studies have established

Tanner stage-specific reference intervals for many hormones, and will provide means to adapt these intervals to labs using various methodologies.

Growth-Related Considerations

Alkaline phosphatase (AP) is expressed in nearly all organs, and exists in circulation as multiple isoforms. The predominant isoforms are liver and bone, though kidney, intestinal, and placental isoforms are sometimes observed as well. In the young children and infants, there is a benign, transient elevation in AP, primarily liver and bone, which can be up to 10 times higher than in adults. This is believed to be due to decreased clearance of the enzyme from circulation.[1,32] Failure to recognize this elevation as part of normal physiology (which should be reflected by age-specific reference intervals), could result in unnecessary testing and interventions for bone or liver disease. AP concentrations decline through childhood, but rise again at the start of puberty and are closely associated with bone growth. As discussed earlier, transient elevations in AP occur in 2-5% of healthy children under 5 years old, and do not warrant an extensive clinical work-up.[30]

Likewise, other bone markers, such as osteocalcin and the amino-terminal propeptide of type I procollagen may change significantly throughout childhood in parallel with bone growth, though not as robustly as AP.[58,59] Similarly, growth hormone, insulin-like growth factor-1 (IGF-1), and IGF binding proteins (IGF-BP) 1-3, all change throughout childhood, especially during periods of significant growth. These analytes are covered in detail in Chapter 12.

With growth and muscle development, there is an increase in serum creatinine, since creatinine is derived from creatine phosphate in muscle. The normal concentration of serum creatinine in children is generally about two-thirds to half that of adult serum creatinine.[60] In newborns, expected concentrations of creatinine may be higher due to remaining maternal creatinine in newborn circulation.[61] All of these markers should be interpreted during infancy and childhood using age-appropriate pediatric reference intervals.

SUMMARY

Care should be used when ordering and interpreting laboratory tests on children, as many tests reference intervals are quite different in children than adults. Specific ordering differences occur because some tests are more useful in pediatrics than adults. Differences in interpretation may be due to the altered physiology following birth, during periods of significant growth, and in puberty.

TRAINING MODULE

1. As part of a work up for abdominal pain in a 4 years old female, a complete metabolic panel is ordered. Physical exam was unremarkable. All the results are normal, except for alkaline phosphatase, which was 1,238 U/L (normal range: 85-370 U/L). What should the physician do with these results?

    a. Nothing. The alkaline phosphatase result is probably a lab error. Ignore it and move on.

    b. Refer the patient to a pediatric gastroenterologist to work up a liver problem.

    c. Order alkaline phosphatase isoenzymes. If bone and liver isoenzymes are equally elevated, then retest the patient in 4 months.

    d. Prescribe antibiotics.

2. A 3 month old male presents with suspected new-onset diabetes type 1. To confirm the diagnosis, an A1C is ordered for this patient. However, the lab rejects the sample. Why?

    a. The laboratory's A1C instrument wasn't working.

    b. The value of HbF is too high in a 3 month old to report an accurate A1C.

    c. A1C is not an acceptable test for children.

3. Which of the following is a common problem specifically encountered in pediatric laboratory testing?

    a. Need for age-specific reference intervals.

    b. Low rate of hemolyzed specimens.

    c. Adequate sample volume.

    d. Hemoglobin A may affect certain test results.

4. A 3-day old newborn is screened for kernicterus risk prior to discharge. His total serum bilirubin at the hospital places him in the intermediate risk zone, and he is discharged with orders to have total serum bilirubin measured 24 hours later as an outpatient. The result from the outpatient laboratory is 3.5 mg/dL higher than at the hospital, moving him to the high risk zone. What could explain this increase?

    a. The patient has a hemolytic disease and his red cells are continuing to release hemoglobin, so bilirubin continues to rise.

    b. The outpatient laboratory uses a spectrophotometric method which produces higher results than the hospital lab's diazo-based method.

    c. The patient has developed liver disease.

    d. All of the above.

5. Which of the following is true about lead exposure?

    a. Lead poisoning has no treatment.

    b. Blood lead levels as low as 10 µg/dL have no impact on a child's IQ.

    c. Historically, many children were exposed to lead from leaded gasoline.

    d. Mild lead poisoning has dramatic symptoms which are easily recognizable as lead poisoning.

REFERENCES

1. Higgins T, Beutler E, Doumas BT. Hemoglobin, iron and Bilirubin, In: Burtis CA, Ashwood ER, Bruns DE, eds. *Tietz Textbook of Clinical Chemistry and Molecular Diagnostics*. 4th ed. St. Louis MO, Elsevier Saunders; 2006:1165-1208.

2. Kett JC. Anemia in infancy. *Pediatr Rev*. 2012;33:186-187.

3. National Collaborating Centre for Women's and Children's Health, *Neonatal Jaundice*, London: Royal College of Obstetricians and Gynaecologists, 2010.

4. Greene DN, Liang J, Holmes DT, Resch A, Lorey TS. Neonatal total bilirubin measurements: still room for harmonization. *Clin Biochem*. 2014;47:1112-1115.

5. Bhutani VK, Johnson L, Sivieri EM. Predictive ability of a predischarge hour-specific serum bilirubin for subsequent significant hyperbilirubinemia in healthy term and near-term newborns. *Pediatrics*. 1999;103:6-14.

6. Kaplan M, Hammerman C. Understanding severe hyperbilirubinemia and preventing kernicterus: adjuncts in the interpretation of neonatal serum bilirubin. *Clin Chim Acta*. 2005;356:9-21.

7. Maisels MJ, Bhutani VK, Bogen D, Newman TB, Stark AR, Watchko JF. Hyperbilirubinemia in the newborn infant ≥35 weeks' gestation: an update with clarifications. *Pediatrics*. 2009;124:1193-1198.

8. Kroll MH, McCudden CR. *Endogenous Interferences in Clinical Laboratory Tests: Icteric, Lipemic and Turbid Samples*. Berlin: De Gruyter, 2013.

9. Turner AJ. On lead poisoning in childhood. *Br Med J*. 1909;1:895-897.

10. Henretig FM. Lead. In: Nelson LS, Lewis, N.A., Howland M., Hoffman, R.S., Goldfrank, L.R., Flomenbaum, N.E., eds. *Goldfrank's Toxicologic Emergencies*. 9th ed. New York, NY: McGraw-Hill, 2011.

11. Abadin H, Ashizawa A, Stevens YW, Llados F, Diamond G, Sage G, et al. Toxicological profile for lead. Atlanta (GA), 2007.

12. Canfield RL, Henderson CR, Cory-Slechta DA, Cox C, Jusko TA, Lanphear BP. Intellectual impairment in children with blood lead concentrations below 10 μg per deciliter. *N Engl J Med*. 2003;348:1517-1526.

13. Betts KS. Cdc updates guidelines for children's lead exposure. *Environ Health Perspect*. 2012;120:a268.

14. Screening for elevated blood lead levels. American academy of pediatrics committee on environmental health. *Pediatrics*. 1998;101:1072-1078.

15. Committee on Practice and Ambulatory Medicine, BFPSW. 2014 recommendations for pediatric preventive health care. *Pediatrics*. 2014;133:568-570.

16. Mortensen ME, Walson PD. Chelation therapy for childhood lead poisoning. The changing scene in the 1990s. *Clin Pediatr*. 1993;32:284-291.

17. Ellis MR, Kane KY. Lightening the lead load in children. *Am Fam Physician*. 2000;62:545-554, 559-560.

18. Laterza OF, Price CP, Scott MG. Cystatin c: an improved estimator of glomerular filtration rate? *Clin Chem*. 2002;48:699-707.

19. Stevens LA, Levey AS. Measured gfr as a confirmatory test for estimated gfr. *J Am Soc Nephrol*. 2009;20:2305-2313.

20. Payne SR, Eardley I, O'Flynn K. *Imaging and Technology in Urology: Principles and Clinical Applications.* Dordrecht; New York: Springer, 2012:xvi, 385.

21. Levey AS, Bosch JP, Lewis JB, Greene T, Rogers N, Roth D. A more accurate method to estimate glomerular filtration rate from serum creatinine: a new prediction equation. Modification of diet in renal disease study group. *Ann Intern Med.* 1999;130:461-470.

22. Levey AS, Coresh J, Greene T, Marsh J, Stevens LA, Kusek JW, Van Lente F. Expressing the modification of diet in renal disease study equation for estimating glomerular filtration rate with standardized serum creatinine values. *Clin Chem.* 2007;53:766-772.

23. Delanaye P, Mariat C. The applicability of egfr equations to different populations. *Nat Rev Nephrol.* 2013;9:513-522.

24. Levey AS, Stevens LA, Schmid CH, Zhang YL, Castro AF, 3rd, Feldman HI, et al. A new equation to estimate glomerular filtration rate. *Ann Intern Med.* 2009;150:604-612.

25. Shlipak MG, Matsushita K, Arnlov J, Inker LA, Katz R, Polkinghorne KR, et al. Cystatin c versus creatinine in determining risk based on kidney function. *N Engl J Med.* 2013;369:932-943.

26. Manetti L, Pardini E, Genovesi M, Campomori A, Grasso L, Morselli LL, et al. Thyroid function differently affects serum cystatin c and creatinine concentrations. *J Endocrinol Invest.* 2005;28:346-349.

27. Filler G, Huang S-HS, Yasin A. The usefulness of cystatin c and related formulae in pediatrics. *Clin Chem Lab Med.* 2012;50:2081-2091.

28. Schwartz GJ, Schneider MF, Maier PS, Moxey-Mims M, Dharnidharka VR, Warady B, et al. Improved equations estimating gfr in children with chronic kidney disease using an immunonephelometric determination of cystatin c. *Kidney Int.* 2012;82:445-453.

29. Huh SY, Feldman HA, Cox JE, Gordon CM. Prevalence of transient hyperphosphatasemia among healthy infants and toddlers. *Pediatrics.* 2009;124:703-709.

30. Ridefelt P, Gustafsson J, Aldrimer M, Hellberg D. Alkaline phosphatase in healthy children: reference intervals and prevalence of elevated levels. *Horm Res Paediatr.* 2014;82:399-404.

31. Gualco G, Lava SA, Garzoni L, Simonetti GD, Bettinelli A, Milani GP, et al. Transient benign hyperphophatasemia. *J Pediatr Gastroenterol Nutr.* 2013;57:167-171.

32. Otero JL, Gonzalez-Peralta RP, Andres JM, Jolley CD, Novak DA, Haafiz A. Elevated alkaline phosphatase in children: an algorithm to determine when a "wait and see" approach is optimal. *Clinical Med Insights Pediatr.* 2011;5:15-18.

33. Lanham-New SA, Lambert H, Frassetto L. Potassium. *Adv Nutr.* 2012;3:820-821.

34. Oostendorp M, van Solinge WW, Kemperman H. Potassium but not lactate dehydrogenase elevation due to in vitro hemolysis is higher in capillary than in venous blood samples. *Arch Pathol Lab Med.* 2012;136:1262-1265.

35. Mansour MM, Azzazy HM, Kazmierczak SC. Correction factors for estimating potassium concentrations in samples with in vitro hemolysis: a detriment to patient safety. *Arch Pathol Lab Med.* 2009;133:960-966.

36. Kazmierczak SC, Robertson AF, Briley KP. Comparison of hemolysis in blood samples collected using an automatic incision device and a manual lance. *Arch Pediatr Adolesc Med.* 2002;156:1072-1074.

37. Algeciras-Schimnich A, Cook WJ, Milz TC, Saenger AK, Karon BS. Evaluation of hemoglobin interference in capillary heel-stick samples collected for determination of neonatal bilirubin. *Clin Biochem.* 2007;40:1311-1316.

38. Fairbanks VF, Ziesmer SC, O'Brien PC. Methods for measuring plasma hemoglobin in micromolar concentration compared. *Clin Chem*. 1992;38:132-140.

39. Butt W, Heard M, Peek GJ. Clinical management of the extracorporeal membrane oxygenation circuit. *Pediatr Crit Care Med*. 2013;14:S13-S19.

40. Dabelea D, Mayer-Davis EJ, Saydah S, et al. Prevalence of type 1 and type 2 diabetes among children and adolescents from 2001 to 2009. *JAMA*. 2014;311:1778-1786.

41. Sacks DB. Carbohydrates. In: Burtis CA, Ashwood ER, Bruns DE, eds. *Tietz Textbook of Clinical Chemistry and Molecular Diagnostics*, 4th ed. Elsevier Saunders, St. Louis MO. 2006, 837-901.

42. Classification and diagnosis of diabetes. *Diabetes Care*. 2016;39:S13-S22.

43. Vucic Lovrencic M, Radisic Biljak V, Bozicevic S, Pape-Medvidovic E, Ljubic S. Validation of point-of-care glucose testing for diagnosis of type 2 diabetes. *Int J Endocrinol*. 2013;2013:206309.

44. Nowicka P, Santoro N, Liu H, Lartaud D, Shaw MM, Goldberg R, et al. Utility of hemoglobin a(1c) for diagnosing prediabetes and diabetes in obese children and adolescents. *Diabetes Care*. 2011;34:1306-1311.

45. Ziegler AG, Rewers M, Simell O, Simell T, Lempainen J, Steck A, et al. Seroconversion to multiple islet autoantibodies and risk of progression to diabetes in children. *JAMA*. 2013;309:2473-2479.

46. Sosenko JM, Skyler JS, Palmer JP, Krischer JP, Yu L, Mahon J, et al. The prediction of type 1 diabetes by multiple autoantibody levels and their incorporation into an autoantibody risk score in relatives of type 1 diabetic patients. *Diabetes Care*. 2013;36: 2615-2620.

47. Juusola M, Parkkola A, Harkonen T, Siljander H, Ilonen J, Akerblom HK, Knip M. Positivity for zinc transporter 8 autoantibodies at diagnosis is subsequently associated with reduced beta-cell function and higher exogenous insulin requirement in children and adolescents with type 1 diabetes. *Diabetes Care*. 2016;39:118-121.

48. Huehns ER, Dance N, Beaven GH, Hecht F, Motulsky AG. Human embryonic hemoglobins. *Cold Spring Harb Symp Quant Biol*. 1964;29:327-331.

49. Liebelt EL. Hyperbaric oxygen therapy in childhood carbon monoxide poisoning. *Curr Opin Pediatr*. 1999;11:259-264.

50. Ashwood ER, ed. Pediatric Testing. In: *ARUP's guide to pediatric clinical laboratory testing*. Salt Lake City, UT: ARUP Laboratories; 2004.

51. Nir A, Lindinger A, Rauh M, Bar-Oz B, Laer S, Schwachtgen L, et al. Nt-pro-b-type natriuretic peptide in infants and children: reference values based on combined data from four studies. *Pediatr Cardiol*. 2009;30:3-8.

52. Mir TS, Laux R, Hellwege HH, Liedke B, Heinze C, von Buelow H, et al. Plasma concentrations of aminoterminal pro atrial natriuretic peptide and aminoterminal pro brain natriuretic peptide in healthy neonates: marked and rapid increase after birth. *Pediatrics*. 2003;112:896-899.

53. Fisher DA, Nelson JC, Carlton EI, Wilcox RB. Maturation of human hypothalamic-pituitary-thyroid function and control. *Thyroid*. 2000;10:229-234.

54. Fisher DA, Schoen EJ, La Franchi S, Mandel SH, Nelson JC, Carlton EI, Goshi JH. The hypothalamic-pituitary-thyroid negative feedback control axis in children with treated congenital hypothyroidism. *J Clin Endocrinol Metab*. 2000;85:2722-2727.

55. Styne DM, Grumbach MM. Puberty: ontogeny, neuroendocrinology, physiology and disorders. In: Melmed SP, Polonsky KS, Larsen PR, Kronenberg HM, eds. *Williams Textbook of Endocrinology.* 12th ed., Philadelphia: Elsevier Saunders; 2011;1054-1201.

56. Stenman UH. Standardization of hormone determinations. *Best Pract Res Clin Endocrinol Metab.* 2013;27:823-830.

57. Tanner JM. Normal growth and techniques of growth assessment. *Clin Endocrinol Metab.* 1986;15:411-451.

58. Gracia-Marco L, Ortega FB, Jimenez-Pavon D, Rodriguez G, Valtuena J, Diaz-Martinez AE, et al. Contribution of bone turnover markers to bone mass in pubertal boys and girls. *J Pediatr Endocrinol Metab.* 2011;24:971-974.

59. Kanbur NO, Derman O, Sen TA, Kinik E. Osteocalcin. A biochemical marker of bone turnover during puberty. *Int J Adolesc Med Health.* 2002;14:235-244.

60. Boer DP, de Rijke YB, Hop WC, Cransberg K, Dorresteijn EM. Reference values for serum creatinine in children younger than 1 year of age. *Pediatr Nephrol.* 2010;25: 2107-2113.

61. Guignard JP, Drukker A. Why do newborn infants have a high plasma creatinine? *Pediatrics.* 1999;103:e49.

INBORN ERRORS OF METABOLISM | 3

John V. Mitsios and Dennis J. Dietzen

LEARNING OBJECTIVES

1. List laboratory results associated with a variety of inborn errors of metabolism.
2. Explain the molecular basis for a broad array of inborn errors of metabolism.
3. Describe the clinical presentation of an array of inborn errors of metabolism.
4. Describe the various effective treatment modalities for inborn errors of metabolism.

INTRODUCTION

The clinical recognition and eventual laboratory diagnosis of many inborn errors of metabolism (IEMs) is challenging due to an often long presymptomatic phase and nonspecific clinical presentation. Missed or delayed diagnoses can have severe and long-lasting consequences. In 2006, the American College of Medical Genetics (ACMG) reported on its examination of dozens of metabolic conditions and their suitability for newborn screening. The report recommended screening for 29 core conditions and a number of secondary targets.[1] The following chapter will primarily focus on the clinical presentation, molecular genetic basis, and diagnosis of the "core panel" IEMs. These include branched-chain and aromatic aminoacidopathies, some urea cycle disorders, mitochondrial fatty acid oxidation disorders, and cofactor metabolism abnormalities. The final section will summarize the treatment strategies associated with these disease states. The reader should be aware that currently there are over 500 single gene IEMs and that these 29 ACMG recommended conditions for screening represent some of the more significant conditions in terms of diagnosis and treatment. For an extensive review of all IEM's, the reader is recommended to read the online version of Metabolic and Molecular Bases of Inherited Diseases (oMMBID).

Branched-Chain Aminoacidopathies

The branched-chain amino acids (BCAA) are leucine, isoleucine, and valine. These amino acids are "essential" because they cannot be synthesized by mammals and must be obtained through the diet. The branched-chain amino acids comprise approximately 35% of the total essential amino acids in muscle protein and 40% of the dietary amino acids required by mammals.[2] The carbon skeletons of BCAAs can generate ketone bodies or provide succinate for TCA cycle function, thus providing substrates for energy production. Derived carbon skeletons from these amino acids also provide precursors for fatty acid and cholesterol synthesis. Some of the most common signs and symptoms of branched-chain amino acid disorders include encephalopathy, coma, or death if not diagnosed and treated promptly. Common biochemical findings include but are not limited to metabolic acidosis, hyperammonemia, hypoglycemia with appropriate or increased ketosis, liver dysfunction, and the presence of reducing substances in the urine. A high level view of branched-chain amino acid catabolism is shown in Figure 3-1. Some of the most common disorders are described here.

Maple Syrup Urine Disease (MSUD)

Maple syrup urine disease (MSUD; OMIM #248600) also known as branched-chain ketoacidemia/uria, is an autosomal recessive disorder affecting the catabolism of branched-chain amino acids as a result of decreased branched-chain keto-acid dehydrogenase (BCKDH; EC 1.2.4.4) activity. The catabolism of these amino acids occurs via BCKDH, the second enzyme in the metabolic pathway of the three branched-chain amino acids leucine, isoleucine, and valine. BCKDH is located in the inner mitochondrial membrane and consists of three catalytic components (E1, E2, and E3) and two regulatory enzymes (BCKD phosphatase and BCKD kinase).[3] The genes encoding the BCKDH complex components E1-α (19q.13.1-q13.2), E1-β (6p22-p21), E2 (1p31), and E3 (7q31-q32) have been sequenced.[4-7] The incidence of MSUD in the general population is approximately 1 in 185,000 newborns[8-10] and 1 in 200 live births in the older Mennonite population in Pennsylvania.[11] Onset of symptoms typically occurs in the newborn period but clinical presentation can range from childhood to that of adulthood. Symptoms include psychomotor retardation, feeding problems, and maple syrup odor in urine.

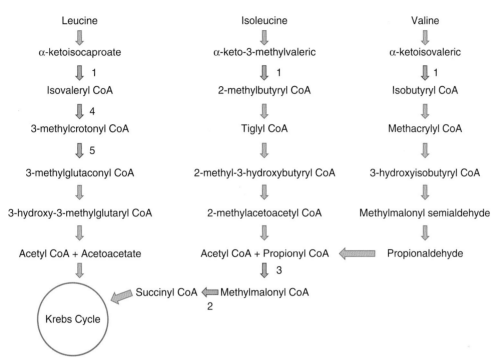

Figure 3-1 ▪ **Normal catabolism of branched-chain amino acids.** All enzymatic steps not necessarily included. Red arrows indicate sites of enzymatic deficiencies discussed in the text: 1) Branched-chain α-ketoacid dehydrogenase (MSUD); 2) methylmalonyl-CoA mutase; 3) propionyl-CoA carboxylase; 4) isovaleryl-CoA dehydrogenase; 5) 3-methylcrotonyl-CoA carboxylase.

Clinical Presentation: Decreased BCKDH results in accumulation of branched α-keto-acids and branched-chain amino acids in plasma and urine. Clinical manifestations of MSUD include body fluid odor that resembles maple syrup (urine and particularly strong in cerumen and sweat), and overwhelming illness in the first days of life, beginning with vomiting and lethargy, and progressing to seizures and eventually to death if left untreated. Neurotoxicity associated with MSUD is predominantly a result of increased concentrations in branch-chained amino acids (predominantly leucine) in both plasma and organs.[11,12] On the basis of clinical and biochemical features, MSUD patients can be categorized into four different phenotypes: classic, intermediate, intermittent, and thiamine responsive. The E3 subunit (lipoamide dehydrogenase) is shared by the pyruvate and α-ketoglutarate dehydrogenase complexes. Deficiency of lipoamide dehydrogenase is a phenotypically distinct defect, which includes additional deficiency of the other two enzymes and appears more like pyruvate dehydrogenase deficiency with lactic acidosis. *Classic MSUD* is the most common and severe phenotype, with BCKDH enzyme activity <2%

of normal activity. Newborns within the first 48 hours of life develop keto-nuria with irritability, poor feeding, vomiting, lethargy, and dystonia.[11] By the day 4 of life, neurological abnormalities include alternating lethargy and irritability, dystonia, apnea, seizures, and signs of cerebral edema. In addition, the development of symptoms may be delayed from 4 to 7 days depending on the feeding regimen; breast feeding may further delay the onset of symptoms for approximately 2 weeks. The clinical manifestations include hypertonia, seizures, and death. Other forms of MSUD may have up to 30% of normal enzyme activity and typically present with failure to thrive or late onset of neurological involvement.

Diagnosis: The most important diagnostic test in the diagnosis of MSUD is the plasma amino acid profile. Patients with MSUD will have markedly elevated concentrations of BCAA (leucine, isoleucine, and valine). An isomer of isoleucine, alloisoleucine, also uniquely accumulates and persists even in treated patients. Urine organic acids also display elevated concentrations of branched-chain keto-acids, α-ketoisovaleric acid, α-ketoisocaproic acid, and α-keto-3-methylvaleric acid. Detection of branched-chain keto-acids in a urinary organic acid profile requires stabilization through oximation. Without oximation the major urinary metabolite is α-hydroxyvaleric acid. BCAA can also be increased in urine, but typically to a lesser degree during fasting or postprandial states. BCKDH enzyme activity may be measured in lymphocytes and cultured fibroblasts, however, these tests are not necessary for diagnosis. Molecular testing is also routinely available.

Methylmalonic Acidemia

Methylmalonic acidemia (MMA) is a disorder characterized by impaired metabolism of methylmalonyl-CoA generated during the metabolism of isoleucine, methionine, threonine, valine, and odd-chain fatty acids. These disorders are caused by genetic errors in a number of genes encoding either the adenosylcobalamin-dependent enzyme methylmalonyl-CoA mutase (EC 5.4.99.2) or enzymes important for the metabolism of cobalamin (vitamin B12). The gene for the mutase enzyme is located on chromosome 6p21. Patients with a mut(0) defect have no enzyme activity, while patients with mut(-) have reduced enzyme activity but with some residual function. Other forms of methylmalonic acidemia affect cofactor metabolism and are commonly classified by complementation group (cbl). Mutations that impact only the metabolism of adenosylcobalamin (eg, cbl A, cbl B) result in isolated accumulation of methylmalonic acid. Upstream mutations that impact the metabolism of both adenosyl-and methyl cobalamin (eg, cbl C, cbl D, cbl F, cbl J) result in accumulation of both methylmalonic acid and homocysteine. The mut(0), mut(-), cblA, and cblB defects collectively account for approximately 90% of isolated methylmalonic acidemia cases.[13,14] In screening of 3-4 week old infants in Massachusetts, the incidence of MMA was found to be 1 in 48,000,[15] and the cumulative incidence is approximately 1 in 100,000 newborns. All genetic forms of MMA are autosomal recessive traits and occur more frequently in populations with increased rates of consanguinity.

Clinical Presentation: MMA typically presents within the first months of life with severe metabolic acidosis, ketosis, and lactic acidemia. Almost all patients with MMA mut(0) or mut(-) present with failure to thrive, poor growth, feeding problems, and some developmental delay. Metabolic decompensation in all forms of MMA is often accompanied by vomiting, lethargy, seizures, and hepatomegaly. Some patients may present with acute neurological deterioration and multisystem disease. Microcephaly, pigmentary retinopathy, nystagmus, secondary reduced visual acuity, hydrocephalus, or megaloblastic anemia may also develop during infancy depending upon the site of the genetic defect but in particular in patients with cblC disease.[13,16]

Diagnosis: The diagnosis of MMA is made by measurement of urine organic acids in which large amounts of methylmalonic acid are present as well as methylcitrate and 3-hydroxyproprionic acid. Concentrations of plasma methylmalonic acid and propionylcarnitine (C3) are also elevated. Hyperammonemia, sometimes severe, is also a common presenting feature of MMA, particularly during a metabolic crisis. In patients presenting with combined MMA and homocystinuria, plasma homocysteine levels are typically increased while methionine is low.

Propionyl-CoA Carboxylase Deficiency (Propionic Acidemia)

Propionic acidemia (PA, OMIM #232000) results from deficient propionyl-CoA carboxylase (EC6.4.1.3), the enzyme that converts propionyl-CoA to D-methylmalonyl-CoA. Propionyl-CoA is an intermediate by-product of the catabolism of branched-chain amino acids isoleucine and valine, as well as threonine, methionine, odd-chain fatty acids, thymidine, uracil, and cholesterol. Significant amounts of propionic acid can also be generated by gut bacteria. Propionyl-CoA accumulates when the carboxylase is deficient, resulting in accumulation of urinary 3-hydroxypropionic acid, methylcitrate, propionylglycine, and plasma propionylcarnitine. The increased concentrations of these metabolites directly lead to toxic effects and inhibit other metabolic pathways leading to hyperglycinemia, hyperammonemia, ketosis, and lactic acidosis. Propionyl CoA carboxylase consists of an A (13q32) and B (3q21-q22) subunit.[17,18] Pathologic mutations have been noted in both. The incidence of PA in the general population is approximately 1 in 200,000 newborns and has an autosomal-recessive mode of inheritance.

Clinical Presentation: Patients typically present in the neonatal period although there have been reports of patients presenting at an older age.[19] Common signs and symptoms include hypotonia, vomiting, lethargy, coma, ketoacidosis, hypoglycemia, hyperammonemia, bone marrow suppression, growth delay, intellectual disability, and physical disability. Hyperammonemia in patients with PA and MMA is thought to be due to compromised synthesis and function of *N*-acetylglutamate, an obligate activator of carbamoyl phosphate synthase, an early step in the synthesis of urea.[20] Cardiomyopathy, both dilated and hypertrophic, has been shown to develop in about one-quarter to one-half of patients independent of a specific metabolic profile.[21-23] As a result of this cardiomyopathy conduction abnormalities may develop and therefore electrocardiograms should be performed on a regular basis.[24,25] Other reported clinical manifestations include pancreatitis[26] and optic nerve atrophy (particularly in male patients).[27] Some infants with PA have similar dysmorphic facial features as seen in patients with MMA, such as a high forehead, broad nasal bridge, epicanthal folds, a long smooth philtrum, and a triangular mouth.

Diagnosis: Measurement of organic acids shows elevated concentrations of 3-hydroxypropionic and methylcitric acids, as well as propionyl- and tiglylglycine. Plasma acylcarnitine analysis shows elevated concentrations of propionyl (C3) carnitine. Plasma and/or urine amino acid analysis reveals elevated concentrations of glycine in some patients, which is a result of inhibition of the glycine cleavage enzyme by propionyl-CoA, leading to reduced glycine oxidation.[19] Hyperglycinemia does not likely contribute to toxicity as elevated glycine often persists in patients who are clinically well.

Isovaleryl-CoA Dehydrogenase Deficiency (Isovaleric Acidemia)

Isovaleric acidemia (IVA; OMIM #243500) results from a deficiency of isovaleryl-CoA dehydrogenase (EC 1.3.99.10; 15q14-q15). This enzyme converts isovaleryl-CoA to 3-methylcrotonyl-CoA, a step in the catabolic pathway of the ketogenic branched-chain amino acid leucine.[28] The incidence of IVA is approximately 1 in 62,500 newborns in Germany and 1 in 250,000 newborns in the United States.

Clinical Presentation: Patients with IVA can be classified into two categories: a) those that present in early neonatal life with a sudden onset of symptoms and b) those that have a chronic intermittent disease and present at a later date in life. The former typically present within the first few days of life with lethargy, difficulty feeding, dehydration, and weight loss. Many affected neonates do not survive the acute phase of illness and die of acidosis, cerebral edema, infections, and/or bleeding. Those patients that do survive the initial acute phase go on to follow a chronic intermittent course. The acute presentation can be brought about when a patient experiences minor stress like an upper respiratory infection or can even be triggered by the increased intake of protein-rich foods. Patients with chronic intermittent IVA typically have had their first acute phase by the age of one.

Diagnosis: IVA is characterized by the accumulation of isovaleric acid resulting in a characteristic odor described as "sweaty feet."[19] Measurement of organic acids in the urine by GC-MS demonstrates increased concentrations of oxidation and conjugated derivatives of isovaleryl-CoA accumulation, including 3-hydroxyisovaleric acid and isovalerylglycine. Acylcarnitine profile in plasma shows increased concentrations of isovaleryl (C5) carnitine. IVA can be diagnosed prior to the onset of symptoms by newborn screening. Newborn screening has also resulted in identifying potentially asymptomatic forms of IVA along with cases of short branched-chain acyl CoA dehydrogenase that may also be benign. These cases dictate genotyping of the isovaleryl CoA dehydrogenase locus and careful follow-up observation in both affected infants and potentially affected siblings.[29]

3-Methylcrotonyl-CoA Carboxylase Deficiency (3-Methylcrotonylglycinuria)

3-Methylcrotonylglycinuria (3MCC, OMIM #212200) results from deficiency of 3-methylcrotonyl-CoA carboxylase (MCC, EC6.4.1.4), the enzyme responsible for the conversion of 3-methylcrotonyl-CoA to 3-methylglutaconyl-CoA in the leucine catabolic pathway.[30] MCC is a biotin-dependent carboxylase and can be affected secondarily by defects in biotin metabolic pathways mediated by holocarboxylase synthetase and biotinidase.

Clinical Presentation: This disorder has a wide range of clinical presentations ranging from clinically benign to acute exacerbation that may lead to death. Asymptomatic women have been diagnosed with 3MCC when metabolites in their infant's blood spots are detected by newborn screening. Symptomatic patients present between the ages of 6 months and 3 years of age with vomiting, feeding difficulties, hypotonia, hyperreflexia, spasms, and seizures. In addition, patients may present with hypoglycemia, hyperammonemia, carnitine deficiency, mild metabolic acidosis, and ketosis.

Diagnosis: The diagnosis of 3MCC is dependent on the detection of 3-hydroxyisovaleric acid and 3-methylcrotonylglycine by urine organic analysis. The urine concentration of 3-methylcrotonylglycine may range between significantly elevated to barely detectable. Total and free plasma carnitine concentrations are decreased and the concentration of plasma 3-hydroxyisovalerylcarnitine (C5-OH) is increased. These biochemical abnormalities along with increased urinary 3-hydroxypropionic acid, propionylglycine, and methylcitric acid may indicate holocarboxylase synthetase deficiency rather than isolated 3MCC deficiency.

Aromatic Aminoacidopathies

The aromatic amino acids include phenylalanine, tryptophan, histidine, and tyrosine. All of these amino acids except tyrosine are also essential amino acids and must be obtained from the diet. Tyrosine is considered as semi-essential amino acids, since it can be synthesized in mammals directly from phenylalanine. In the following section, we will focus on two of the most common aromatic aminoacidopathies: phenylketonuria and tyrosinemia.

Phenylketonuria

Phenylketonuria (PKU, MIM#261600) is caused by deficiency in phenylalanine hydroxylase (PAH) which is responsible for the conversion of phenylalanine to tyrosine. The incidence of PKU is 1 in 13,500 to 19,000 live births.[31] Nearly all cases are caused by mutations in the gene encoding PAH (12q24.1), which are inherited in an autosomal recessive pattern.[32] More than 400 mutations have been identified including deletions, insertions, splicing defects, missense, and nonsense mutations.[31] PAH requires tetrahydrobiopterin (BH4) for its activity. This pathway is responsible for the disposition of 75% of dietary phenylalanine with the remainder used in protein synthesis.[32] Deficiency in BH4 can result from impaired synthesis or decreased regeneration via dihydropteridine reductase or pterin-4-carbinolamine dehydratase. Approximately 2% of patients with elevated phenylalanine can be attributed to defects in BH4 metabolism, which effects tyrosine hydroxylase and tryptophan hydroxylase in addition to phenylalanine hydroxylase and results in impaired neurotransmitter production. PKU results in elevated concentrations of blood and urine phenylalanine and its organic acid metabolites, phenylpyruvic, and phenyllactic acids. Complete enzyme deficiency results in classic PKU, with serum phenylalanine concentrations >1,200 μmol/L. Patient's with residual enzyme activity can be classified into two groups: those that have mild PKU (600-1,200 μmol/L) and those with benign hyperphenylalaninemia (360-600μmol/L). Even "benign" hyperphenylalaninemia, however, may not be so during pregnancy. Maternal hyperphenylalaninemia may result in serious neonatal and developmental sequelae including microcephaly, facial dysmporphism, in utero growth retardation, and intellectual disability.

Clinical Presentation: Newborn infants are typically asymptomatic before the initiation of feeding. If PKU goes undetected by newborn screening, symptoms do not develop until early infancy. Left untreated, patients develop intellectual disability due to severe white matter damage. Progressive neurological impairment manifests as seizures, mental retardation, and motor dysfunction. Many patients also present with light skin pigmentation due to tyrosine deficiency and abnormal melanocyte metabolism or may have an eczematous rash. Maternal PKU syndrome is a severe long-term risk in affected females. Elevated maternal phenylalanine concentrations can result in toxic embryo-/fetopathy with an increased risk of fetal loss. The embryopathic effects include intrauterine growth restriction, permanent intellectual disability, microcephaly, and cardiac malformations. Specific dietary restrictions are needed in women with PKU for the duration of pregnancy.[33]

Diagnosis: The diagnosis of PKU is assessed by measuring plasma or serum concentrations of phenylalanine (>120 μmol/L) and an elevated phenylalanine/tyrosine ratio (>3). Before initiation of treatment, measurement of urinary biopterin or neopterin as well as assessment of blood dihydropteridine reductase (DHPR) activity should be assessed to exclude defects in BH4 metabolism. This testing is important since the treatments for PKU and BH4 deficiency require different approaches. The mainstay of treatment for PKU is dietary restriction of phenylalanine, while BH4 defects require additional dietary BH4 supplementation along with provision of neurotransmitter precursors for dopamine and serotonin synthesis.

Tyrosinemia

Tyrosine is an important molecular precursor for the synthesis of thyroxine, catecholamines, dopamine, and melanin. Tyrosine is derived from dietary intake and hydroxylation of phenylalanine and catabolized by five enzymatic reactions ultimately yielding acetoacetate and fumarate. Hepatocytes and renal proximal tubular cells express the complete pathway. Hypertyrosinemia results from defects in tyrosine metabolism but is also seen as secondary to severe hepatocellular dysfunction. Four autosomal recessive disorders result from deficiencies in specific enzymes in the tyrosine catabolic pathway: hereditary tyrosinemia type I, II, III, and alkaptonuria. Tyrosinemia Type I (HT1, MIM#276700), also referred as hepatorenal tyrosinemia, is due to fumarylacetoacetate hydrolase (FAH) deficiency. FAH is the last step in the pathway of tyrosine catabolism. Fumarylacetoacetate (FAA) accumulates in FAH-deficient hepatocytes and proximal renal tubular cells, leading to liver and kidney injury. HT1 has a prevalence of 1 in 100,000 individuals of Northern European descent[34] and the gene encoding HT1 has been mapped and sequenced to chromosome 15q23-q25.[35,36] Tyrosinemia type II (HT2, MIM#276600), also referred as oculocutaneous tyrosinemia, or is characterized by early development of eye and skin symptoms. HT2 results from defective tyrosine aminotransferase (16q22.1-22.3).[37] Tyrosinemia type III (HT3, MIM#276710) is a rare autosomal recessive disorder resulting from a deficiency in 4-hydroxyphenylpyruvate dioxygenase (HPD), the second step in the tyrosine catabolism pathway. HT3 is an inherited autosomal recessive disorder with an unknown prevalence and the gene encoding HT3 has been mapped and sequenced to chromosome 12q24. Finally, alkaptonuria (MIM#203500) results from a deficiency in homogentisic acid dioxygenase, the third enzyme in the tyrosine degradation pathway.[38] The homogentisic acid dioxygenase gene has been mapped to chromosome 3q21-q23.[39,40]

Clinical Presentation: HT1 typically presents with acute liver failure, cirrhosis, hepatocellular carcinoma, renal Fanconi syndrome, glomerulosclerosis, and peripheral neuropathy. Most patients with HT1 present in early infancy with failure to thrive and hepatomegaly. When discovered early, therapy with nitisinone (Orfadin) effectively spares liver and kidney function. Later clinical presentation of HT1 may manifest as childhood rickets secondary to a chronic Fanconi syndrome. HT2 is characterized by early development of eye (eg, corneal erosions) and skin (eg, palmoplantar keratosis) abnormalities with photophobia and mental retardation in 50% of patients that are apparent in the first year of life. HT3 is a rare disorder that is characterized by skin and ocular changes often associated with neurological dysfunction (ataxia, seizures, mild psychomotor retardation). Patients with alkaptonuria are typically asymptomatic in childhood but during the third decade of live develop deposits of brownish or bluish pigments in the ear cartilage and sclera. Deposition of homogentisic acid in alkaptonuria results in joint pain and arthritis later in life. Transient tyrosinemia of newborn is a common but benign cause of increased tyrosine concentrations[41,42] associated with immaturity of 4-hydroxyphenylpyruvate dioxygenase.

Diagnosis: Hypertyrosinemia is considered when values of tyrosine are >200 μmol/L (normal newborn concentrations are 30-120 μmol/L). Tyrosine accumulation by any mechanism is accompanied by increased urinary excretion of deaminated tyrosine derivatives, p-hydroxyphenyllactate and p-hydroxyphenylpyruvate. HT1 is characterized by elevations of circulating tyrosine but in many cases the increased blood concentration is mild (200-600 μmol/L). Succinylacetone, derived from reduction and decarboxylation of fumarylacetoacetate, is pathognomonic for HT1. Patients presenting with HT2 are distinguished by markedly elevated plasma concentrations (>1000 μmol/L). The diagnostic findings of HT3 include isolated elevations of plasma tyrosine concentrations (300-700 μmol/L). It is important to note that patients with HT2 and HT3 do not have increased urinary excretion of succinylacetone differentiating them from HT1. Alkaptonuria is characterized by the excretion of urine that appears normal when fresh, but turns brown or black if left standing or after alkalinization. This phenomenon is due to the increased concentrations of homogentisic acid, which polymerizes to give rise to dark urine color upon oxidation (alkapton). Diagnosis is confirmed by quantitative measurement of homogentisic acid in urine; alkaptonuria patients typically have normal circulating tyrosine concentrations. The discoloration of urine may be apparent in infancy due to discoloration of diapers but diagnosis is typically made in adulthood during routine urinalysis or during an evaluation for arthritis.[43]

Glutaric Aciduria Type I

Glutaric aciduria type I (GAI) is the result of defects in glutaryl-CoA dehydrogenase (EC1.3.99.7, 19p13.2), a mitochondrial enzyme responsible for the conversion of glutaryl-CoA derived from lysine and tryptophan to glutaconyl-CoA.

Clinical Presentation: Patients with GAI typically present with acute encephalopathic episodes between the ages of 4 and 18 months. These episodes are often triggered by common infections, fasting, routine immunizations, and/or minor trauma. Affected babies develop irreversible dystonic movement disorder (loss of head control, hypotonia, and seizures). During acute crisis, the basal ganglia are damaged resulting in permanent disability but cognitive function is preserved.[44-46] The clinical picture often progresses to a severe dystonic and dyskinetic disorder. MRI imaging of affected patients may reveal subdural and retinal hemorrhage leading to suspicion of non-accidental trauma.

Diagnosis: Excretion of glutaric acid may be quite variable (<100 mmol/mol creatinine in low excreters and >100-4000 mmol/mol creatinine in high excreters). 3-hydroxyglutaric acid excretion is uniquely increased in patients with GAI.[47,48] In addition, plasma total carnitine levels may be low and plasma glutarylcarnitine (C5DC) will be increased.

Urea Cycle Disorders

The urea cycle consists of five catalytic reactions (Figure 3-2), with the main purpose of detoxifying waste nitrogen. The major urea cycle disorders are caused by deficiencies of: carbamoyl phosphate synthetase I (CPSI, MIM#237300), *N*-acetyl glutamate synthetase (NAGS, MIM#237310), ornithine transcarbamoylase (OTC, MIM#311250), argininosuccinate (ASA) synthase (MIM#215700, type I citrullinemia), ASA lyase (MIM#207900, argininosuccinic aciduria), and arginase (MIM#207800). The cumulative incidence of urea cycle disorders in the United States is approximately 1 in 8,200 live births.[49] Specifically, deficiencies of CPS I, NAGS, OTC, ASA synthase, ASA lyase, and arginase affect 1 in 50,000, 100,000, 30,000, 50,000, 50,000, and 100,000 births, respectively. The mode of inheritance for the urea cycle disorders is autosomal recessive with the exception of OTC deficiency which is X-linked. The impact of OTC deficiency, therefore, is much more severe in males and is both biochemically and clinically variable in females depending upon the degree of X-chromosome inactivation.

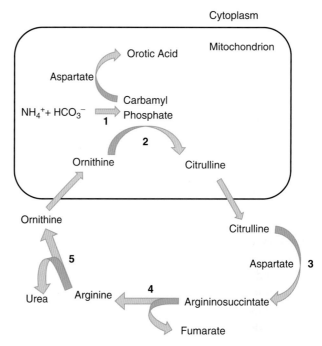

Figure 3-2 ▪ **Enzymatic reactions and transport steps of the urea cycle.**
1) Carbamoyl phosphate synthase; 2) ornithine transcarbamoylase; 3) argininosuccinate synthase; 4) argininosuccinate lyase; 5) arginase.

Clinical Presentation: The onset and severity of the urea cycle disorders is variable depending on the specific mutation and the amount of residual enzyme function. The infant becomes symptomatic after feeding has started since breast milk and infant formula provide a nitrogen load provoking an increase in ammonia and glutamate. Typical signs include somnolence, inability to maintain body temperature, poor feeding, vomiting, lethargy, and coma.[50,51] This presentation is also very similar to an infant in sepsis.[52] Hyperammonemia may lead to cerebral edema, brainstem compression, and eventually death, if not treated promptly. Approximately 50% of all infants with hyperammonemia have seizures.[49] On the other hand, patients with partial enzyme deficiencies have less acute presentations after the newborn period.[53,54] Signs and symptoms in these patients with partial enzyme deficiency include: chronic vomiting, developmental delay, seizure disorder, sleep disorders, or psychiatric disorders.[55-57] These patients may also exhibit chronic hyperammonemia or intermittent hyperammonemia during states of metabolic decompensation associated with stress.[58,59] Some affected patients tend to prefer a vegetarian diet since increased protein intake often leads to symptoms like headache, lethargy, ataxia, or behavioral abnormalities.[53,54,60] Patients with arginase deficiency typically present later in infancy to preschool years with mental retardation and progressive spastic quadriplegia.

Diagnosis: The primary laboratory hallmark of urea acid cycle disorders is elevated plasma ammonia concentrations (>100-150 up to 3000 µmol/L in acute cases). It is important that specimens be drawn in ammonia-free collection tubes containing heparin (green top) or EDTA (purple top) as an anticoagulant and processed promptly. Ammonia concentrations may be falsely elevated due to hemolysis, delayed processing, and exposure to room air where ammoniacal cleaning agents have been used. The preferred specimen for ammonia concentration determination is arterial or venous blood rather than the capillary samples that are commonly utilized for infants. In the initial evaluation of patients with suspected urea cycle disorders laboratory determination of arterial pH, carbon dioxide, lactate, glucose, electrolytes, and plasma amino acids (increased concentrations of lysine, citrulline, and arginine and the presence of argininosuccinic acid) are important. Orotic acid is increased in urine in proximal disorders of the urea cycle (NAGS, CPS, OTC, citrullinemia) but not typically elevated in the downstream defects of the urea cycle. Accumulation of orotic acid results from diversion of carbamoyl phosphate from citrulline formation to the alternate pathway of pyrimidine synthesis. Orotic acid may also accumulate in primary disorders of pyrimidine synthesis, such as deficiencies of dihydropyrimidine dehydrogenase (MIM#274270) or uridine 5′-monophosphate synthase (MIM#258900). Patients presenting with elevated plasma ammonia and normal blood glucose as well as a normal anion gap strongly suggest a urea cycle disorder.

Fatty Acid Oxidation Disorders

Mitochondrial fatty acid oxidation disorders are a group of genetic metabolic diseases in which the body is unable to oxidize fatty acids as an alternate energy source during periods of fasting. Fatty acids constitute the largest energy reserve in the body and play a crucial role in supplying energy-yielding substrates especially in situations where carbohydrate metabolism is insufficient for energy needs. In brief, long-chain fatty acids are broken down by the β-oxidation pathway in the mitochondria to form acetyl-CoA. The number of acetyl-CoA molecules depends on the carbon length of the fatty acid that is being oxidized. There are four enzyme activities involved in the process of generating one molecule of acetyl CoA (Figure 3-3): 1) Acyl-CoA dehydrogenase, 2) enoyl-CoA hydratase, 3) hydroxyacyl-CoA dehydrogenase, and 4) keto-acyl-CoA thiolase. The resulting acetyl-CoA enters the Krebs cycle to facilitate energy production or is utilized for ketone body production in the liver.

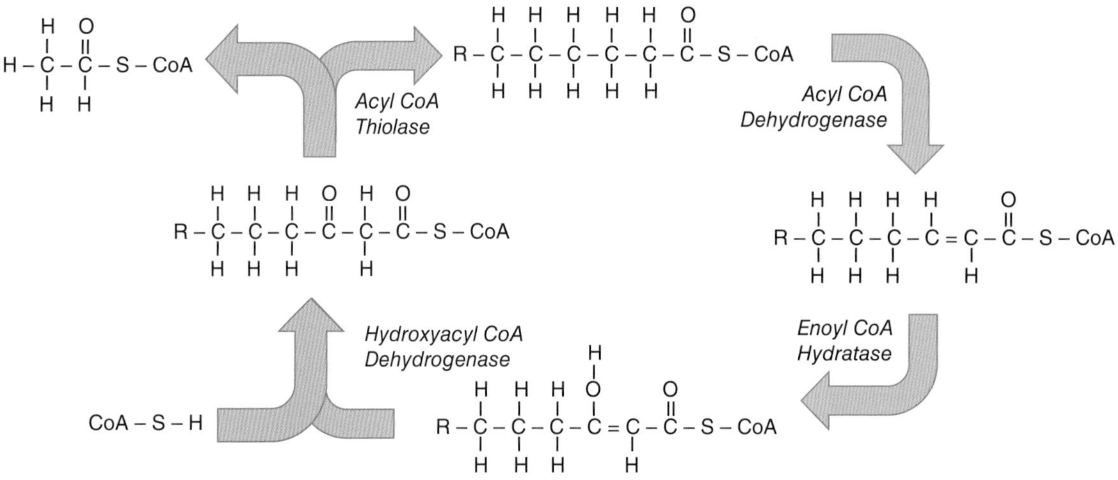

Figure 3-3 ▪ **Reactions of the fatty acid β-oxidation spiral.** The four basic enzymatic reactions involved in the sequential generation of acetyl-CoA are displayed. Each reaction is catalyzed by multiple enzymes with varying chain-length specificity.

Carnitine plays a particularly important role in transporting long-chain fatty acids into the mitochondria. Prior to β-oxidation, long-chain fatty acyl CoA are converted to fatty acyl carnitine esters via carnitine palmitoyltransferase 1 (CPT1), which traverse the inner membrane through the activity of the carnitine:acylcarnitine translocase. Carnitine esters are then converted back to fatty acyl CoA esters via carnitine palmitoyltransferase 2 (CPT2). More than 20 defects in fatty acid transport and mitochondrial β-oxidation have been identified and are inherited as autosomal recessive disorders.[61] The incidence of fatty acid oxidation disorders varies from 1:8000 to 1:100,000. As a group fatty acid oxidation disorders are considered among the most common metabolic disorders associated with potentially severe consequences in affected individuals.

Clinical Presentation: The hallmark clinical presentation of fatty acid oxidation disorders is hypoketotic hypoglycemia but other signs and symptoms may include life-threatening encephalopathy, lactic acidosis, hyperammonemia, cardiomyopathy, rhabdomyolysis, liver failure, and sudden death. Fatty acid oxidation disorders are exacerbated under conditions of increased energy demands, such as prolonged fasting, febrile illness, or any other stressful situation in which the body requires excess energy. The inability to generate energy from fatty acids when carbohydrate supplies are limited ultimately causes metabolic decompensation. Prior to the expansion of newborn screening in the last decade, fatty acid oxidation disorders were implicated as the cause of death in 5-8% of cases of sudden unexpected death during infancy.[62]

Diagnosis: The primary biochemical feature of fatty oxidation disorders is hypoglycemia without evidence of appropriate ketone body formation. Diagnosis of fatty acid oxidation disorders using urine organic acid analysis is limited by the types of metabolites detected and by episodic excretion of diagnostically informative metabolites. Medium-chain dicarboxylic aciduria (adipic, suberic, and sebacic acids) is a common but non-specific feature of these disorders while medium chain glycine conjugates, such as hexanoylglycine, suberylglycine, and 3-phenylpropionylglycine may indicate deficiency of medium chain acyl-CoA dehydrogenase (MCAD). Urine organic acid analysis may be uninformative if the patient is healthy and well-fed. Plasma acylcarnitine analysis detects a broader range of short, medium, and long-chain disorders and is nearly always informative when the patient is healthy and well-fed. Table 3-1 lists many fatty acid oxidation disorders and their distinguishing biochemical features.

Cofactor Metabolism

There are circumstances when enzymes involved in key metabolic transformations are transcribed and translated normally but the supply of cofactors for holoenzyme assembly are compromised. These cofactors are non-protein prosthetic groups that play a key role in mediating catalysis. Enzymes that lack these cofactors are referred to as apoenzymes. Mature, fully functional enzymes with appropriately bound cofactors are termed holoenzymes. Some enzymes, such as phenylalanine hydroxylase contain a single type of cofactor (biopterin) but others like BCKDH require multiple cofactors (thiamine, lipoamide, FAD, NAD). Impaired cofactor supply, metabolism, or binding can impair enzyme activity to the same extent as an alteration in the polypeptide backbone. Cofactors that commonly mediate metabolic disorders are discussed later.

Vitamin B12. Also referred to as cobalamin, this vitamin consists of a central cobalt atom coordinated at four positions by a planar corrin ring, by a dimethylbenzimidazole moiety at a fifth position and by a variable moiety at a sixth position. Depending upon the identity of the sixth ligand, vitamin B12 exists as hydroxy-, methyl-, adenosyl-, or cyano-cobalamin. In mammals, vitamin B12 assists with isomerization (eg, methylmalonyl CoA mutase) and methyltransfer (eg, methionine synthase). Methylmalonyl CoA mutase requires adenosylcobalamin while methionine synthase requires methylcobalamin.

Cobalamin is absorbed from the intestine via intrinsic factor and circulates bound to transcobalamin. Following receptor-mediated endocytosis, cobalamin is released into the cytoplasm without a distinguishing component in the sixth coordination position and then is ultimately converted to

Table 3-1 BIOCHEMICAL FINDINGS IN FATTY ACID OXIDATION DISORDERS		
Enzyme Deficiency	Urine Organic Acid Features	Plasma Acylcarnitine Features
Medium-chain acyl CoA dehydrogenase (MCAD)	Medium-chain dicarboxylic aciduria (adipic, suberic, sebacic acids). Hexanoyl-, suberyl-, and 3-phenylpropionyl - glycine conjugates. Ketones inappropriately low.	Increased C6, C8, C8:1, C10, C10:1 carnitine ester species. Elevations typically not isolated.
Very long-chain acyl CoA dehydrogenase (VLCAD)	Possible medium-chain dicarboxylic aciduria. Ketones absent or minimal.	Elevation of multiple saturated and unsaturated esters with chain length ≥12. C14:1 typically elevated to the greatest extent.
Long-chain hydroxyacyl CoA dehydrogenase (LCHAD)/TFP.	Possible medium-chain dicarboxylic and hydroxy-dicarboxylic aciduria. Ketones minimal or absent.	Elevation of multiple hydroxylated carnitine esters with chain length ≥12.
Short-chain acyl CoA dehydrogenase (SCAD)	Increased ethylmalonic and sometimes methylscuccinic acid.	Isolated elevation of C4 carnitine.
Short-chain hydroxyacyl CoA dehydrogenase (SCHAD)	Increased hydroxy-dicarboxylic and 3-hydroxyglutaric acids.	Isolated elevation of C4-OH carnitine.
Carnitine palmitoyl transferase I (CPT I)	Possible medium-chain dicarboxylic aciduria. Otherwise not informative.	Increased free (C0) carnitine relative to longer chain esters.
Carnitine palmitoyl transferase II (CPT II)	Possible medium-chain dicarboxylic aciduria. Otherwise not informative.	Increased long-chain esters relative to free (C0) carnitine.
Carnitine acylcarnitine translocase	Similar to CPT II.	Similar to CPT II
β-ketothiolase	Increased excretion of ketones with 2-methyl-3-hydroxybutyric and 2-methylacetoacetic acids as well as tiglylglycine.	Increased C5-OH and C5:1 (tiglyl) carnitine.

adenosylcobalamin in the mitochondrion or to methylcobalamin in the cytoplasm. Depending on the nature of the defect in cobalamin metabolism, methylmalonic acid, and homocysteine may accumulate in isolation or in a combined fashion. Biochemical and genetic testing is required to pinpoint the specific defect and dictate treatment.

Folate. Also referred to as vitamin B9, folate facilitates the transfer of single carbon moieties including methyl (CH_3), methylene ($-CH_2-$), and methylidine ($-CH=$) groups. Folate consists of 2-amino-4-hydroxypteridine bound to *p*-aminobenzoic acid. Fully reduce folate is referred to as tetrahydrofolate (THF). Intracellular folate is linked to one or more glutamic acid residues. Methyl groups are covalently bound to folate through the N-5 position of the pteroic acid and the N-10 bridge to the *p*-aminobenzoic acid moiety. Molecular species dependent on folate for synthesis include purines, pyrimidines, creatinine, serine, and methionine.

The most common disorder of folate metabolism is deficiency of methylene-tetrahydrofolate reductase (MTHFR). This enzyme is responsible for conversion of methylene THF to methyl-THF. The latter supplies the methyl group necessary for conversion of homocysteine to methionine via methionine synthase. Folate and cobalamin metabolism intersect in this reaction. Biochemically, MTHFR deficiency is characterized by hyperhomocysteinemia with normal or decreased concentrations of methionine. Decreased blood methionine distinguishes patients with MTHFR deficiency from patients with homocysteinemia due to cystathionine-β-synthase deficiency, which exhibit increased methionine concentrations.

Biotin. Biotin (vitamin B7), tetrahydro-2-oxothieno[3,4-d]-imidazoline-4-valeric acid, facilitates transfer of fully oxidized methyl groups (O=C=O) in the four mammalian carboxylase enzymes: acetyl-CoA, propionyl-CoA, 3-methylcrotonyl-CoA, and pyruvate carboxylase. It is found covalently associated with protein via lysine residues or in an extremely high affinity complex with avidin. Protein bound biotin is recovered via the action of biotinidase and incorporated into mature carboxylase enzymes via the activity of holocarboxylase synthetase. Molecular defects in each of the carboxylase enzymes have a characteristic metabolic signature. Defects in biotinidase or holocarboxylase synthetase result in biochemical signatures associated with all four deficiencies and biotinidase deficiency may be effectively treated with dietary biotin supplementation.

Biopterin. Tetrahydrobiopterin (BH4) 2-amino-4-hydroxy-6(L-erythro-1′,2′-dihydroxypropyl)-tetrahydropteridine, is a cofactor in the phenylalanine hydroxylase, tyrosine-3-hydroxylase, tryptophan-5-hydroxylase reactions leading to synthesis of tyrosine, dopamine, and serotonin, respectively. Hydroxylation is mediated by reversible formation of the carbinolamine form of BH4 (BH4-OH). Defects in GTP cyclohydrolase and 6-pyruvoyl-tetrahydrobiopterin synthase inhibit synthesis of BH4. Defects in pterin-4α-carbinolamine dehydratase and dihydropteridine reductase disable the recycling of BH4. Both synthetic and recycling defects lead to hyperphenylalaninemia and decreased formation of dopamine and serotonin. Inborn errors of BH4 metabolism are important to distinguish from mutations in phenylalanine hydroxylase as the former may respond favorably to pharmacologic BH4 supplementation and therapeutic doses of specific neurotransmitter precursors.

Pyridoxine. Pyridoxine (2-methyl-3-hydroxy-4,5-bis(hydroxymethyl) pyridine) and its related dietary precursors, pyridoxal, and pyridoxamine, are collectively referred to as vitamin B6. The active coenzyme form of the vitamin, pyridoxal phosphate (PLP), functions as a carrier of amino groups in over 140 different transamination, deamination, decarboxylation, and racemization reactions. It does so via reversible formation of a Schiff base involving the 4′ aldehyde moiety and a primary amine. Notable enzymes dependent upon PLP include aminotransferases (eg, ALT, AST), glutaminase, asparaginase, aromatic amino acid decarboxylase, ornithine decarboxylase, the glycine cleavage system, and serine dehydratase. In addition to defects in enzymes that require PLP, other metabolic errors that inhibit the synthesis and recycling of PLP exist. Deficiency of pyridoxine phosphate oxidase (MIM#610090) leads to a seizure disorder that is responsive to PLP supplementation. Deficiencies of Δ^1-pyrroline-5-carboxylate dehydrogenase (Type II hyperprolinemia, MIM#239510) and Δ^1-piperidine-6-carboxylate dehydrogenase (MIM#266100) likewise lead to PLP-responsive seizure phenotypes.

Thiamine. Thiamine (2-{3-[(4-amino-2-methylpyrimidin-5-yl)methyl]-4-methylthiazol-5-yl}ethanol), Vitamin B1, is an essential component of mammalian diets. The active form of the vitamin, thiamine pyrophosphate acts as a carrier of active aldehyde groups in decarboxylation reactions (eg, pyruvate dehydrogenase, α-ketoglutarate dehydrogenase, branched-chain α-ketoacid dehydrogenase) as well as the transketolase reaction of the pentose-phosphate pathway. Dietary thiamine deficiency or malabsorption may lead to a constellation of symptoms including high-output heart failure (beriberi) or neurologic consequences ranging from ophthalmoplegia, ataxia, and confusion (Wernicke Encephalopathy) to amnesia and confabulation (Korsakoff Syndrome).

Inborn errors of metabolism associated with thiamine belong to one of two general clusters. First, mutations in various thiamine transport genes (*SLC19A2, SLC19A3, and SLC25A19*) are reported to cause thiamine-responsive megaloblastic anemia, sensorineural hearing loss, diabetes, as well as an array of neurologic symptoms that are also observed in dietary thiamine insufficiency. Second, a subset of patients with deficiencies of α-ketoacid dehydrogenase complexes benefit from thiamine supplementation. In these cases, thiamine is thought to stabilize the E1 (decarboxylase) component of the enzyme complex resulting in decreased protein turnover and enhanced activity.

Riboflavin. Riboflavin, 7,8-dimethyl-10-[(2S,3S,4R)-2,3,4,5-tetrahydroxypentyl] benzo[g]pteridine-2,4-dione, vitamin B2, forms the core of flavin mononucleotide (FMN) and flavin adenine dinucleotide (FAD). The tricyclic benzopteridine moiety of these nucleotides mediates a single electron transfer to form stable semiquinone radicals or a full 2 electron reduction. Flavoprotein dehydrogenases include components of the mitochondrial electron transport chain (NADH dehydrogenase and succinate dehydrogenase), fatty acyl CoA dehydrogenase, the electron transferring flavoprotein, and glutathione reductase just to name a few. Dietary riboflavin deficiency is rare and usually occurs in concert with other dietary inadequacies. Genetic defects in some riboflavin transport genes (*SLC52A1, SLC52A2, and SLC52A3*) causing a constellation of non-specific biochemical and neurologic signs and symptoms have been documented. These conditions, some electron transport defects, and some cases of ETF deficiency (glutaric aciduria type II) are treated with dietary riboflavin supplementation, which has inconsistent clinical benefit.

Treatment

The treatment of inborn errors of metabolism can be accomplished using a combination of four different approaches: 1) decreasing the "fuel" proximal to the metabolic defect; 2) preventing catabolism; 3) boosting residual enzyme activity; and 4) preventing accumulation of metabolic toxins.

Clinical expression of inborn metabolic disorders results in part from accumulation of substrate upstream of an enzymatic defect and/or scarcity of metabolites distal to the enzymatic defect. Dietary restriction of fuel coupled with supplementation of downstream metabolites is a mainstay in the treatment of multiple disorders. In PKU (phenylalanine hydroxylase deficiency), for example, phenylalanine must be restricted to prevent accumulation in the central nervous system. At the same time, the product of phenylalanine hydroxylase, tyrosine, must be added as a dietary supplement as it provides the building block for a number of important metabolites including dopamine, adrenaline, and thyroxine. Restriction of metabolic fuel may be also be accomplished by gut microbiome manipulation. Specific species of gut bacteria, for example, supply significant quantities of propionic acid. In propionic and methylmalonic acidemia, upstream supply of propionate may be limited by decreasing gut bacterial load with antibiotics. All dietary therapy requires constant vigilance and frequent laboratory follow-up during growth and development of the patient.

A number of the pathways compromised in metabolic disease are invoked during periods of metabolic stress. Stressors may include exercise or prolonged fasting associated with vomiting or anorexia. Such prolonged fasting induces the catabolism of branched-chain amino acids that are both ketogenic and fuel the TCA cycle. Likewise, fatty acid oxidation flux is increased when carbohydrate supply or metabolism is limiting. When compensatory metabolic adaptations are impaired, multi-organ failure may result. Thus, a powerful approach to preventing metabolic decompensation is frequent feeding and aggressive nutritional support (eg, parenteral glucose) during illness.

In many metabolic disorders, enzyme activity is significantly diminished but there is often detectable residual activity. For example, mutations may lead to an enzyme with altered binding of substrate or cofactor leaving a small percentage of normal enzyme activity. In these circumstances an effective strategy is to boost the amount of residual enzyme activity via administration of supplemental enzyme cofactors. In some forms of methylmalonic acidemia, for example, pharmacologic doses of cobalamin ameliorate clinical and biochemical abnormalities. In defects of folate metabolism that impair methionine remethylation, betaine (trimethylglycine) may be employed to serve as an alternative methyl donor. Likewise, the phenylalanine hydroxylase cofactor, tetrahydrobiopterin, is increasingly employed to boost residual phenylalanine hydroxylase activity in PKU. The use of cofactor supplementation may lead to reduced intensity of dietary therapy and more sustainable clinical improvement.

Toxins that accumulate secondary to the primary enzyme defect must also be controlled to diminish the morbidity and mortality of metabolic disorders. Severe hyperammonemia is a common complication of propionic acidemia, methylmalonic acidemia, fatty acid oxidation defects, and urea cycle defects. Ammonia may be removed by dialysis or chemical nitrogen scavengers. Benzoic acid and phenylacetic acid are administered to generate excretable forms of nitrogen, hippurate, and phenacetylglutamate, respectively. Such alternate pathways of nitrogen excretion decrease dependence on the urea cycle. Fumarylacetoacetate is the primary toxin that accumulates in type 1 tyrosinemia (fumarylacetoacetate hydrolase deficiency). In this condition, a novel enzyme inhibitor is employed to prevent pathologic accumulation of fumarylacetoacetate. Nitisinone (Orfadin) is administered to inhibit hydroxyphenylpyruvate dioxygenase, the enzymatic step immediately upstream of the hydrolase. Inhibition at this stage of tyrosine catabolism prevents formation of fumarylacetoacetate and its subsequent conversion to succinylacetone. In general, these agents are well tolerated and effectively reduce disease burden.

TRAINING MODULE
Case Study and Review Questions

A 15-year-old female presents to gastroenterology clinic with a chief complaint of a 6 year history of abdominal pain and episodic vomiting. She was born at term to healthy parents and has no siblings. Her height and weight are at the 50-75th percentile and she has no dysmorphic features. Physical exam was notable for "poor coordination" but was otherwise not remarkable. Cognitive development is characterized as normal but she has had bouts of depression and carries a diagnosis of Asperger Syndrome. Blood chemistry including a comprehensive metabolic profile, ammonia, lipase, and amylase were within normal limits. CBC was notable for mild microcytic anemia (hemoglobin 10.4). A plasma acylcarnitine profile was performed and results are displayed below:

Acylcarnitine	Result (μmol/L)		Reference Range (μmol/L)
C2	11.19		5.00-30.00
C3	0.59		0.00-1.20
C4	1.37	HIGH	0.00-0.60
C5	0.49	HIGH	0.00-0.40
C4-OH	0.07		0.00-0.40
C6	0.84	HIGH	0.00-0.30
C5-OH	0.12		0.00-0.20
C6-OH	0.02		0.00-0.20
C8:1	0.30		0.00-0.80
C8	1.42	HIGH	0.00-0.60
C3-DC	0.06		0.00-0.30
C10:1	0.78	HIGH	0.00-0.50
C10	2.80	HIGH	0.00-0.60
C5-DC	0.14		0.00-0.20
C12:1	0.27		0.00-0.40
C12	0.73	HIGH	0.00-0.40
C12-OH	0.01		0.00-0.10
C14:2	0.39	HIGH	0.00-0.30
C14:1	0.47	HIGH	0.00-0.40
C14	0.23		0.00-0.40
C14:1-OH	0.03		0.00-0.20
C14-OH	0.01		0.00-0.10
C16:1	0.17		0.00-0.20
C16	0.13		0.00-0.50
C16:1-OH	0.01		0.00-0.20
C16-OH	0.01		0.00-0.10
C18:2	0.22	HIGH	0.00-0.20
C18:1	0.22		0.00-0.50
C18	0.13		0.00-0.20
C18:2-OH	0.01		0.00-0.10
C18:1-OH	0.00		0.00-0.10

Questions for Further Study

1. Explain how data acquisition in tandem mass spectrometry using precursor ion scanning is performed.
2. What is the precursor ion common to all carnitine esters?
3. What is an isobaric compound when referring to mass analysis?
4. List the two carnitine esters that primarily contribute to the C4 component.
5. List the carnitine esters that might contribute to the C5 component.
6. List the enzymes implicated by elevations of C4, C5, C6, C8, C10, C14, and C18 carnitine esters.
7. What is the difference between a C14 ester and a C14:1 carnitine ester?
8. How likely is it that all of these enzymes are deficient?
9. Is there a diagnosis that can unify these biochemical findings?
10. What molecules would be found in urine organic acid analysis in a patient with this condition?

REFERENCES

1. Watson MS, Lloyd-Puryear MA, Mann MY, Rinaldo P, Rodney Howell R. Main report. *Genet Med.* 2006;8:12S-252S.
2. Harper AE, Miller RH, Block KP. Branched-chain amino acid metabolism. *Annu Rev Nutr.* 1984;4:409-454.
3. Chuang DT. Maple syrup urine disease: it has come a long way. *J Pediatr.* 1998;132: S17-S23.
4. Zhang B, Zhao Y, Harris RA, Crabb DW. Molecular defects in the e1 alpha subunit of the branched-chain alpha-ketoacid dehydrogenase complex that cause maple syrup urine disease. *Mol Biol Med.* 1991;8:39-47.
5. Patel MS, Harris RA. Mammalian alpha-keto acid dehydrogenase complexes: gene regulation and genetic defects. *FASEB J.* 1995;9:1164-1172.
6. Chuang DT, Shih VE. *Disorders of Branched Chain Amino Acids and Keto Acid Metabolism.* New York, NY: McGraw-Hill; 2001.
7. Fisher CW, Chuang JL, Griffin TA, Lau KS, Cox RP, Chuang DT. Molecular phenotypes in cultured maple syrup urine disease cells. Complete e1 alpha cdna sequence and mrna and subunit contents of the human branched chain alpha-keto acid dehydrogenase complex. *J Biol Chem.* 1989;264:3448-3453.
8. Naylor EW. *Newborn Screening in Maple Syrup Urine Disease (Branched-Chain Ketoaciduria).* Berlin: Springer Verlag; 1980.
9. Chuang DT, Shih VE. *Maple Syrup Urine Disease (Branched-Chain Ketoaciduria).* New York, NY: McGraw-Hill; 2001.
10. Quental S, Vilarinho L, Martins E, Teles EL, Rodrigues E, Diogo L, Garcia P, Eusebio F, Gaspar A, Sequeira S, Amorim A, Prata MJ. Incidence of maple syrup urine disease in portugal. *Mol Genet Metab.* 2010;100:385-387.
11. Morton DH, Strauss KA, Robinson DL, Puffenberger EG, Kelley RI. Diagnosis and treatment of maple syrup disease: a study of 36 patients. *Pediatrics.* 2002;109: 999-1008.

12. Korein J, Sansaricq C, Kalmijn M, Honig J, Lange B. Maple syrup urine disease: clinical, eeg, and plasma amino acid correlations with a theoretical mechanism of acute neurotoxicity. *Int J Neurosci.* 1994;79:21-45.

13. Fenton WA, Gravel RA, Rosenblatt DS. Disorders of propionate and methylmalonate metabolism. In: Scriver CR, Beaudet AL, Sly WS, Valle D, eds. *The Metabolic and Molecular Basis of Inherited Disorders.* New York, NY: McGraw-Hill; 2001:2165.

14. Wappner RS. Disorders of amino acids and organic acid metabolism. In: McMillan JA, Feigin JA, DeAngelis C, Jones MD, eds. *Oski's Pediatrics: Principles and Practice.* Philadelphia, PA: Lippincott, Williams & Wilkins; 2006:2153.

15. Coulombe JT, Shih VE, Levy HL. Massachusetts metabolic disorders screening program. II. Methylmalonic aciduria. *Pediatrics.* 1981;67:26-31.

16. Rosenblatt DS, Aspler AL, Shevell MI, Pletcher BA, Fenton WA, Seashore MR. Clinical heterogeneity and prognosis in combined methylmalonic aciduria and homocystinuria (cblc). *J Inherited Metab Dis.* 1997;20:528-538.

17. Ugarte M, Perez-Cerda C, Rodriguez-Pombo P, Desviat LR, Perez B, Richard E, Muro S, Campeau E, Ohura T, Gravel RA. Overview of mutations in the pcca and pccb genes causing propionic acidemia. *Hum Mutat.* 1999;14:275-282.

18. Kraus JP, Spector E, Venezia S, Estes P, Chiang PW, Creadon-Swindell G, Mullerleile S, de Silva L, Barth M, Walter M, Walter K, Meissner T, Lindner M, Ensenauer R, Santer R, Bodamer OA, Baumgartner MR, Brunner-Krainz M, Karall D, Haase C, Knerr I, Marquardt T, Hennermann JB, Steinfeld R, Beblo S, Koch HG, Konstantopoulou V, Scholl-Burgi S, van Teeffelen-Heithoff A, Suormala T, Ugarte M, Sperl W, Superti-Furga A, Schwab KO, Grunert SC, Sass JO. Mutation analysis in 54 propionic acidemia patients. *J Inherited Metab Dis.* 2012;35:51-63.

19. Nyhan WL, Ozand PT. *Atlas of Metabolic Diseases.* London: Chapman and Hall Medical; 1998.

20. Coude FX, Sweetman L, Nyhan WL. Inhibition by propionyl-coenzyme a of n-acetylglutamate synthetase in rat liver mitochondria. A possible explanation for hyperammonemia in propionic and methylmalonic acidemia. *J Clin Invest.* 1979;64:1544-1551.

21. Mardach R, Verity MA, Cederbaum SD. Clinical, pathological, and biochemical studies in a patient with propionic acidemia and fatal cardiomyopathy. *Mol Genet Metab.* 2005;85:286-290.

22. Romano S, Valayannopoulos V, Touati G, Jais JP, Rabier D, de Keyzer Y, Bonnet D, de Lonlay P. Cardiomyopathies in propionic aciduria are reversible after liver transplantation. *J Pediatr.* 2010;156:128-134.

23. Pena L, Burton BK. Survey of health status and complications among propionic acidemia patients. *Am J Med Genet Part A.* 2012;158A:1641-1646.

24. Baumgartner D, Scholl-Burgi S, Sass JO, Sperl W, Schweigmann U, Stein JI, Karall D. Prolonged qtc intervals and decreased left ventricular contractility in patients with propionic acidemia. *J Pediatr.* 2007;150:192-197, 197 e191.

25. Jameson E, Walter J. Cardiac arrest secondary to long qt(c)in a child with propionic acidemia. *Pediatr Cardiol.* 2008;29:969-970.

26. Bultron G, Seashore MR, Pashankar DS, Husain SZ. Recurrent acute pancreatitis associated with propionic acidemia. *J Pediatr Gastroenterol Nutr.* 2008;47:370-371.

27. Ianchulev T, Kolin T, Moseley K, Sadun A. Optic nerve atrophy in propionic acidemia. *Ophthalmology*. 2003;110:1850-1854.

28. Mohsen AW, Anderson BD, Volchenboum SL, Battaile KP, Tiffany K, Roberts D, Kim JJ, Vockley J. Characterization of molecular defects in isovaleryl-coa dehydrogenase in patients with isovaleric acidemia. *Biochemistry*. 1998;37:10325-10335.

29. Ensenauer R, Vockley J, Willard JM, Huey JC, Sass JO, Edland SD, Burton BK, Berry SA, Santer R, Grunert S, Koch HG, Marquardt I, Rinaldo P, Hahn S, Matern D. A common mutation is associated with a mild, potentially asymptomatic phenotype in patients with isovaleric acidemia diagnosed by newborn screening. *Am J Hum Genet*. 2004;75:1136-1142

30. Baumgartner MR, Almashanu S, Suormala T, Obie C, Cole RN, Packman S, Baumgartner ER, Valle D. The molecular basis of human 3-methylcrotonyl-coa carboxylase deficiency. *J Clin Invest*. 2001;107:495-504.

31. National Institutes of Health Consensus Development Panel. National institutes of health consensus development conference statement: phenylketonuria: screening and management, October 16-18, 2000. *Pediatrics*. 2001;108:972-982.

32. Erlandsen H, Stevens RC. The structural basis of phenylketonuria. *Mol Genet Metab*. 1999;68:103-125.

33. Rohr FJ, Lobbregt D, Levy HL. Tyrosine supplementation in the treatment of maternal phenylketonuria. *Am J Clin Nutr*. 1998;67:473-476.

34. Kaye CI, Committee on G, Accurso F, La Franchi S, Lane PA, Hope N, Sonya P, S GB, Michele AL. Newborn screening fact sheets. *Pediatrics*. 2006;118:e934-e963.

35. Phaneuf D, Labelle Y, Berube D, Arden K, Cavenee W, Gagne R, Tanguay RM. Cloning and expression of the cdna encoding human fumarylacetoacetate hydrolase, the enzyme deficient in hereditary tyrosinemia: assignment of the gene to chromosome 15. *Am J Hum Gen*. 1991;48:525-535.

36. Labelle Y, Phaneuf D, Leclerc B, Tanguay RM. Characterization of the human fumarylacetoacetate hydrolase gene and identification of a missense mutation abolishing enzymatic activity. *Hum Mol Genet*. 1993;2:941-946.

37. Barton DE, Yang-Feng TL, Francke U. The human tyrosine aminotransferase gene mapped to the long arm of chromosome 16 (region 16q22-q24) by somatic cell hybrid analysis and in situ hybridization. Hum Genet. 1986;72:221-224.

38. La Du BN, Zannoni VG, Laster L, Seegmiller JE. The nature of the defect in tyrosine metabolism in alcaptonuria. *J Biol Chem*. 1958;230:251-260.

39. Fernandez-Canon JM, Granadino B, Beltran-Valero de Bernabe D, Renedo M, Fernandez-Ruiz E, Penalva MA, Rodriguez de Cordoba S. The molecular basis of alkaptonuria. *Nat Genet*. 1996;14:19-24.

40. Zatkova A. An update on molecular genetics of alkaptonuria (aku). *J Inherited Metab Dis*. 2011;34:1127-1136.

41. Weiner DL. Metaboilc emergencies. In: Fleisher GR, Ludwig S, Henretig FM, eds. *Textbook of Pediatric Emergency Medicine*. Philadelphia,PA: Lippincott, Williams & Wilkins; 2006:1193.

42. Levine SZ, Marples E, Gordon HH. A defect in the metabolism of aromatic amino acids in premature infants: the role of vitamin c. *Science*. 1939;90:620-621.

43. La Du BN. Alkatonuria. In: Scriver CR, Beaudet AL, Sly WS, Valle D, eds. *The Metabolic and Molecular Basis of Inherited Disease*. New York, NY: McGraw-Hill; 1995:1371.

44. Hartley LM, Khwaja OS, Verity CM. Glutaric aciduria type 1 and nonaccidental head injury. *Pediatrics*. 2001;107:174-175.

45. Hoffmann GF, Trefz FK, Barth PG, Bohles HJ, Biggemann B, Bremer HJ, Christensen E, Frosch M, Hanefeld F, Hunneman DH, et al. Glutaryl-coenzyme a dehydrogenase deficiency: a distinct encephalopathy. *Pediatrics*. 1991;88:1194-1203.

46. Gordon N. Glutaric aciduria types i and ii. *Brain Dev*. 2006;28:136-140.

47. Kolker S, Christensen E, Leonard JV, Greenberg CR, Boneh A, Burlina AB, Burlina AP, Dixon M, Duran M, Garcia Cazorla A, Goodman SI, Koeller DM, Kyllerman M, Muhlhausen C, Muller E, Okun JG, Wilcken B, Hoffmann GF, Burgard P. Diagnosis and management of glutaric aciduria type i-revised recommendations. *J Inherited Metab Dis*. 2011;34:677-694.

48. Gregersen N, Brandt NJ. Ketotic episodes in glutaryl-CoA dehydrogenase deficiency (glutaric aciduria). *Pediatr Res*. 1979;13:977-981.

49. Brusilow SW, Maestri NE. Urea cycle disorders: diagnosis, pathophysiology, and therapy. *Adv. Pediatr*. 1996;43:127-170.

50. Burton BK. Inborn errors of metabolism in infancy: a guide to diagnosis. *Pediatrics*. 1998;102:E69.

51. Summar M. Current strategies for the management of neonatal urea cycle disorders. *J Pediatr*. 2001;138:S30-S39.

52. Maestri NE, Clissold D, Brusilow SW. Neonatal onset ornithine transcarbamylase deficiency: a retrospective analysis. *J Pediatr*. 1999;134:268-272.

53. Brusilow SW, Horwich AL. Urea cycle enzymes. In: Scriver CR, Beaudet AL, Sly WS, eds. *The Metabolic and Molecular Bases of Inherited Disorders*. New York, NY: McGraw-Hill; 2001:1909.

54. Leonard JV, Morris AA. Urea cycle disorders. *Semin Neonatol*. 2002;7:27-35.

55. Maestri NE, Lord C, Glynn M, Bale A, Brusilow SW. The phenotype of ostensibly healthy women who are carriers for ornithine transcarbamylase deficiency. *Medicine*. 1998;77:389-397.

56. Serrano M, Martins C, Perez-Duenas B, Gomez-Lopez L, Murgui E, Fons C, Garcia-Cazorla A, Artuch R, Jara F, Arranz JA, Haberle J, Briones P, Campistol J, Pineda M, Vilaseca MA. Neuropsychiatric manifestations in late-onset urea cycle disorder patients. *J Child Neurol*. 2010;25:352-358.

57. Sedel F, Baumann N, Turpin JC, Lyon-Caen O, Saudubray JM, Cohen D. Psychiatric manifestations revealing inborn errors of metabolism in adolescents and adults. *J Inherited Metab Dis*. 2007;30:631-641.

58. Arn PH, Hauser ER, Thomas GH, Herman G, Hess D, Brusilow SW. Hyperammonemia in women with a mutation at the ornithine carbamoyltransferase locus. A cause of postpartum coma. *N Engl J Med*. 1990;322:1652-1655.

59. Tuchman M, Yudkoff M. Blood levels of ammonia and nitrogen scavenging amino acids in patients with inherited hyperammonemia. *Mol Genet Metab*. 1999;66:10-15.

60. Houston B, Reiss KA, Merlo C. Healthy, but comatose. *Am J Med*. 2011;124:303-305.

61. Rinaldo P, Matern D, Bennett MJ. Fatty acid oxidation disorders. *Annu Rev Physiol.* 2002;64:477-502.

62. Boles RG, Buck EA, Blitzer MG, Platt MS, Cowan TM, Martin SK, Yoon H, Madsen JA, Reyes-Mugica M, Rinaldo P. Retrospective biochemical screening of fatty acid oxidation disorders in postmortem livers of 418 cases of sudden death in the first year of life. *J Pediatr.* 1998;132:924-933.

DIAGNOSTIC APPROACH TO THE PATIENT WITH A SUSPECTED INBORN ERROR OF METABOLISM

4

Robert D. Nerenz and Dennis J. Dietzen

LEARNING OBJECTIVES

1. List clinical symptoms that prompt further workup for an inborn error of metabolism (IEM).
2. Define the utility of common laboratory tests in the diagnosis of children with an IEM.
3. Distinguish the features of laboratory test results in the setting of an IEM from those in other pathologic conditions.
4. Describe the indications and limitations of specialized metabolic techniques used in the diagnosis and monitoring of children with an IEM.

INTRODUCTION

Countless biological processes are required to sustain human life, including the synthesis and catabolism of proteins, carbohydrates, and lipids. The bulk of this activity is performed by a tightly regulated network of enzymes and transport proteins, each of which is responsible for performing a specific step in one of many metabolic pathways. These metabolic pathways are highly dynamic and interrelated, allowing individual cells to turn some pathways on and others off during normal growth and aging, following changes in nutritional status and in response to stress. In states of normal health, enzyme activity is continuously turned up or down to maintain cellular concentrations of pathway intermediates within an acceptable range. Deficiencies in any of these enzymes caused by inborn errors of metabolism (IEMs) result in pathway dysregulation, leading to excesses of certain pathway intermediates and deficiencies in others. Depending on the enzyme deficiency, certain IEMs are asymptomatic, others cause significant impairment in the absence of appropriate treatment, while others are incompatible with life.

Because IEMs often cause clinical symptoms during the first days, months, or years of life, patients with IEMs are most frequently encountered in a pediatric setting. Unfortunately, due to the wide range of enzyme deficiencies and phenotypic clinical presentations, IEMs are often difficult to recognize, diagnose, and treat in a timely manner, thus representing a unique set of challenges for the pediatric physician. Metabolic abnormalities observed in many patients with IEMs can cause irreversible damage to the brain, liver, and other essential organ systems if left untreated. Fortunately, neurological damage and other morbidities caused by some IEMs may be avoided if the correct diagnosis is made and treatment initiated in a timely fashion. The goal of this chapter is to provide an introduction to IEMs, describe the role of metabolic genetics in the diagnostic process, and discuss the laboratory techniques most commonly used in diagnosis and disease management.

Newborn Screening

To date, greater than 500 IEMs have been characterized, each of which is associated with a distinct pattern of metabolic abnormalities. Because of the importance of rapidly diagnosing patients with IEMs, newborn screening (NBS) for selected IEMs is now standard practice in all 50 states and many countries around the world. The American College of Medical Genetics (ACMG) has recommended the measurement of biomarkers that strongly suggest the presence of 29 IEMs (Table 4-1).[1] It is likely that this panel will expand to include biomarkers for additional disorders, as indicated by the recommendation by the Department of Health and Human Services (HHS) in 2010 to add screening for severe combined immunodeficiency (SCID) to the Uniform Screening Panel[2] and the addition of Pompe Disease, mucopolyaccharisosis, type 1 (MPS1) and X-linked adrenoleukodystrophy (X-ALD) in 2014 and 2015. Importantly, the specific NBS core panel does not differ from state to state but screening for additional IEMs beyond the ACMG-recommended panel may be performed. Patients with abnormalities identified on NBS should be referred to a metabolic geneticist for further testing and confirmation of the IEM in a specialized metabolic disease laboratory.[3] Despite routine NBS, patients with some IEMs may be missed during initial screening.[4] The conditions evaluated in the ACMG-approved core panel are reliably detected but there are hundreds of additional metabolic diseases that are undetectable during NBS. Furthermore, false negatives may occur due to improper sample collection

Table 4-1	**ACMG RECOMMENDED NEWBORN SCREENING CORE CONDITION PANEL**	

Organic Acidemias
Isovaleric acidemia
Glutaric acidemia type I
3-Hydroxy-3-methylglutaryl-CoA
   lyase deficiency
Multiple carboxylase deficiency
Methylmalonic acidemia (mutase, cbl)
3-Methylcrotonyl-CoA carboxylase
   deficiency
Propionic acidemia
β-ketothiolase deficiency

Fatty Acid Oxidation Defects
Medium-chain acyl-CoA dehydrogenase
   deficiency
Very long-chain acyl-CoA
   dehydrogenase deficiency
Long-chain L-3-hydroxyacyl-CoA
   dehydrogenase deficiency
Trifunctional protein deficiency
Carnitine transporter deficiency

Amino Acidemias
Phenylketonuria
Maple syrup urine disease
Homocystinuria
Citrullinemia
Argininosuccinic acidemia
Tyrosinemia type I

Hemoglobinopathies
Sickle cell anemia Hb (Hb S/S)
Hb S/β-thalassemia
Hb S/C disease

Other
Congenital hypothyroidism
Biotinidase deficiency
Congenital adrenal hyperplasia

Galactosemia
Hearing loss
Cystic fibrosis

or the absence of the diagnostic biomarker at the time of sample collection.[5] For these reasons, a normal NBS profile does not rule out the presence of an IEM in children with suggestive clinical symptoms. Additionally, patients with acute perinatal onset of metabolic decompensation due to IEMs often require treatment before NBS results are available. This may require urgent in-house diagnostic testing. Therefore, it is crucially important that pediatric physicians recognize the symptoms of children with an IEM and understand the test methods that should be used to establish a rapid and correct diagnosis.[6]

Physical Symptoms

Despite characteristic patterns of metabolic intermediates that can be used to ultimately make a definitive diagnosis, neonates, and infants with IEMs may present with one or more nonspecific clinical features. Symptoms consistent with IEMs include neurologic deterioration and lethargy, seizures, hypotonia, unusual odor, tachypnea, failure to thrive, picky or poor diet, cardiomyopathy, skeletal myopathy, ocular symptoms, dermatologic abnormalities, and abnormal urine output.[7] Other features that should raise the clinical suspicion of an IEM are a progressive functional decline in infancy after a normal period immediately following birth or a family history of previous unexplained neonatal or infant death. Parental consanguinity should increase the level of suspicion as many of the IEMs are inherited in an autosomal recessive manner.[8]

Neurologic Deterioration and Lethargy

One symptom with relatively high specificity for an IEM is progressive neurological decline after a normal period immediately following birth. Initial signs include poor sucking and feeding followed by increasing lethargy, which in some cases progresses to coma despite supportive care. Initial workup should consist of cerebrospinal fluid (CSF) analysis, cerebral ultrasound, and chest X-ray to rule out infectious or other causes. If no other cause can be identified, accumulation of toxic metabolic intermediates due to an IEM should be considered. IEMs frequently associated with neurological decline are maple syrup urine disease (MSUD), methylmalonic aciduria (MMA), propionic aciduria (PA), isovaleric aciduria (IVA), and urea cycle defects.[9]

Seizures

Seizures in the neonatal period are most often due to a non-metabolic disorder, such as cerebral ischemia, intracranial infection, brain malformation, or a benign neonatal seizure syndrome.[10] While they constitute a relatively rare cause, untreated metabolic disorders can also result in seizures with the age of onset of symptoms depending on the specific metabolic defect. Fortunately, many of the metabolic causes of neonatal or infantile seizures are treatable with good metabolic control assisted by appropriate dietary restriction or supplementation. In general, seizures constitute an extremely non-specific finding but may suggest an IEM when observed in conjunction with other characteristic symptoms.

Several mechanisms are responsible for causing seizures in patients with IEMs. The first consists of direct neurotoxicity of metabolic intermediates accumulating in the brain, as illustrated by the accumulation of glycine in all body tissues (including the brain) of patients with non-ketotic hyperglycinemia (NKH).[11] Seizures can also occur in the context of decompensation due to the hypoglycemia or hyperammonemia observed in a wide spectrum of metabolic disorders. Other causes include metabolic defects resulting in cerebral energy deficiency in creatine synthetic defects, dysregulated neurotransmitter metabolism, or enzyme cofactor deficiencies. Importantly, seizures do not indicate a specific metabolic defect but require specialized metabolic testing to establish a definitive diagnosis.

Hypotonia

As in the case of other symptoms observed in neonates with IEMs, "floppy" infants with poor muscle tone are most often affected by pathologic conditions unrelated to deficiencies in metabolic enzymes. Oxygen deprivation immediately before or following birth, brain defects, or non-metabolic neuromuscular disorders, including myasthenia gravis or muscular dystrophy are frequently the cause of persistent hypotonia in neonates.[7] Once common causes have been ruled out when evaluating a symptomatic child with a normal pregnancy and delivery, consideration should be given to an IEM as the underlying cause. Hypotonia is a symptom of many IEMs including mitochondrial defects, glycogen storage diseases, organic acidurias, fatty acid oxidation defects, and urea cycle defects. Therefore, progressive hypotonia should suggest an IEM, especially in conjunction with neurologic symptoms, lethargy and seizure.

Unusual Odor

Normal baby odors in a healthy child are rarely cause for alarm but unusual body or urine odors, especially in conjunction with other symptoms, strongly suggest the presence of certain IEMs. These odors are generally observed first by the nursing staff on neonatal care units or parents or other family members within the home and may be reported to pediatricians during the initial clinical evaluation. In conjunction with acute symptoms, maple syrup urine disease (sweet smelling urine), isovaleric aciduria/glutaric acidemia type 2 (sweaty feet) and trimethylaminuria (fishy urine and body odor) are the metabolic diseases most strongly associated with unusual odor.[12] In the presence of other non-specific symptoms, these characteristic odors may be the most helpful initial diagnostic tool in affected patients.

Tachypnea

Rapid short, shallow breathing is frequently observed in both preterm and term infants due to lung immaturity and deficiencies in lung surfactant (preterm infants) or transient retention of lung fluid immediately following delivery (term infants).[13] When immature lung function has been ruled out and respiratory distress persists beyond the initial 24-48 hours following delivery of a term infant, tachypnea may represent respiratory compensation for an underlying metabolic acidosis caused by an organic acidemia.

Failure to Thrive

Failure to thrive is not a specific diagnosis but rather a general symptom frequently encountered by the pediatric physician. Up to 10% of children evaluated in primary care facilities display some form of delayed growth, which can most often be attributed to dietary insufficiency or a genetic predisposition to small size.[14] In these non-pathogenic cases, children should gain weight following increased dietary intake or other appropriate clinical management. When a patient's symptoms persist despite treatment, an IEM may be present. In patients with an IEM who experience failure to thrive, numerous other physical symptoms including recurrent vomiting, lethargy, neurological symptoms, and hypotonia are often present. Patients presenting with multiple symptoms cannot be diagnosed on the basis of physical symptoms alone and should be referred for the specialized metabolic testing that is described under "Specialized Testing", beginning on page 85.

Picky or Poor Diet

In patients with a mild or moderate IEM, a relatively common cause of failure to thrive is a poor or selective diet. Infants and older children may correctly associate certain foods with the onset of vomiting and other symptoms and refuse to eat when presented with meals containing those foods. For example, patients with mild urea cycle defects often avoid eating meat or other foods with a high protein content due to symptoms associated with accumulation of ammonia and other metabolites of amino acid catabolism.[15] These patients are often asymptomatic when the offending macromolecules are absent from the diet but develop symptoms shortly after consumption of foods that require a missing enzyme for proper metabolism. When presented with a patient with no obvious cause of relatively slow growth and small size, detailed evaluation of the child's dietary preferences may provide the first indication of an underlying metabolic defect.

Cardiomyopathy

Cardiomyopathy is occasionally encountered in patients with an IEM and may even be the dominant clinical feature during the initial clinical evaluation, although most often other characteristic symptoms discussed in this section are also present. In particular, serum lactate is often increased due to decreased perfusion of peripheral tissues, resulting in an increased reliance on anaerobic glycolysis rather than oxidative phosphorylation. IEMs constitute only 5% of pediatric cardiomyopathy cases but their symptoms often respond to specific treatment once the correct diagnosis has been made, making these patients particularly important for the pediatric physician to diagnose. Cardiomyopathy due to an IEM is most often hypertrophic with or without dilation while non-hypertrophic dilated cardiomyopathy makes up the remainder of cases. Restrictive cardiomyopathy has not been documented in a patient with an IEM.[16]

There are three pathophysiological mechanisms responsible for cardiomyopathy arising in patients with an IEM. The first consists of infiltration and storage of macromolecules in cardiomyocytes, thereby disrupting the organization of myofibrils and preventing efficient contraction, which ultimately results in cardiac hypertrophy. The second consists of generalized energy deficiency caused by one of many metabolic defects and also leads to inefficient contraction and cardiac hypertrophy. The third mechanism consists of the accumulation of toxic metabolites in cardiac tissue, which progresses to dilated cardiomyopathy when left untreated. Because patients with an IEM constitute a very small percentage of all pediatric cardiomyopathy cases, the presence of cardiomyopathy alone should not increase the clinical suspicion of an IEM. When other characteristic symptoms are present and the suspicion of an IEM is high, the type of cardiomyopathy may help narrow the differential diagnosis. Ultimately, metabolic testing is required to conclusively diagnose the patient.

Skeletal Myopathies

Structural muscular defects constitute the most common cause of neuromuscular disorders in neonates and infants but numerous IEMs have been documented as the cause of different skeletal myopathies. Due to the relatively high rate of energy consumption in muscle, children with a wide range of metabolic deficiencies may experience exercise intolerance, muscle pain, progressive muscle weakness, or myoglobinuria.[17] Glycogen storage diseases, fatty acid oxidation defects, and mitochondrial defects are the classes of IEM most often associated with muscle pain. Unexplained and persistent skeletal myopathy should prompt further evaluation for an underlying IEM.

Ocular Symptoms

Decreased vision is a symptom associated with several IEMs and in some cases may be the initial symptom that brings the patient to the physician's attention.[18] The age of onset and severity of vision loss are variable with decreased vision or bilateral cataract development shortly after birth in some patients while others do not experience symptoms until later in childhood. In general, IEMs contribute to the development of corneal defects, cataracts, retinal degeneration, lens dislocation, and other ocular symptoms through the toxic effects of metabolic intermediates, accumulation of abnormal metabolites, defects in energy production or deficiencies in metabolic processes specific to the eye. The presence of specific ocular symptoms may offer useful diagnostic information but conclusive diagnosis requires metabolic testing.

Dermatologic Abnormalities

Dermatologic abnormalities in neonates and infants are frequent occurrences and are most likely due to either benign causes or non-metabolic pathogenic conditions. Notable exceptions are certain porphyrias in which precursors of heme biosynthesis accumulate in the skin, resulting in photosensitivity and patients with multiple carboxylase or biotinidase deficiency who often present with a characteristic rash in conjunction with seizure and failure to thrive. In the vast majority of cases, dermatologic symptoms in young children do not have a metabolic cause and can be easily treated. However, in conjunction with other symptoms, dermatologic symptoms can significantly narrow the differential diagnosis.

Urine Output/Stones

Urine abnormalities detectable on routine urinalysis are an extremely non-specific finding in metabolic diseases and only rarely the presence of crystals in urine can be attributed to an IEM. Exceptions include Zellweger spectrum disorders (ZSDs) and cystinuria. [19,20] ZSDs are defined by deficient peroxisomal assembly and affected patients exhibit hyperoxaluria and nephrocalcinosis caused by oxalate accumulation due to enzymatic deficiencies. Importantly, these patients most often also experience progressive neurological dysfunction that facilitates diagnosis. Cystinuria arises due to defects in kidney-specific transporters responsible for the reabsorption of cysteine and other amino acids, resulting in abnormally high urine concentrations and the development of cystine crystals in the kidneys or bladder. Cystinuria is unique among metabolic disorders in that patients may present with chronic pain, hematuria or oliguria as the predominant symptoms without other characteristic signs of metabolic disease discussed earlier.

Dysmorphic Features

Dysmorphic features, while visually apparent and easily detectable, are rarely caused by an IEM. Exceptions include peroxisomal disorders and certain cases of glutaric aciduria type II or β-hydroxybutyric aciduria.[21] Unless other symptoms of metabolic disease are present, workup of children with dysmorphic features should begin with a thorough evaluation of non-metabolic syndromic disorders.

Initial Laboratory Evaluation

While a conclusive diagnosis is often dependent on more specialized testing that will be discussed later, the initial laboratory evaluation of patients with a suspected IEM begins with rapidly available routine tests performed in almost every clinical laboratory.[22] Specifically, abnormalities in arterial blood gases, complete metabolic profile (CMP), complete blood count (CBC), liver function tests, plasma glucose, triglycerides, ammonia, homocysteine, cyanocobalamin (vitamin B12), and urine ketones can all indicate the possibility of an underlying IEM. Depending on the IEM, one or more of these biomarkers may be abnormal. To further complicate the diagnostic pathway, many of these abnormalities in basic laboratory tests may also be observed in the neonatal period in healthy infants with no underlying IEM due to immature organ function, particularly liver and kidney. Often the magnitude of the abnormality as well as the timing can help differentiate patients with IEMs from those without. Abnormal laboratory values that are not reproducible may also lessen suspicion for an IEM.

Electrolytes

The most common metabolic abnormality in neonates is metabolic acidosis. In many cases, acidosis is an artifact associated with small blood volumes collected for testing in very small babies. If samples are not transported to the laboratory and tested in a timely fashion, CO_2 diffusion out of the sample results in decreased total CO_2 measurement and inappropriate determination of pH. In cases of non-artifactual metabolic acidosis, common causes including hypoxia, infection, cardiac, and lung disease should first be considered. When these more common causes have been ruled out, metabolic acidosis could indicate the presence of an organic acidemia, disorder of pyruvate metabolism, glycogen storage disease, or respiratory chain disorder.[23] Metabolic acidosis can be easily identified during routine electrolyte analysis performed immediately following birth or during a follow-up visit to investigate the onset of symptoms during the first months of life. In normal neonates, the anion gap (sodium–(chloride + bicarbonate)) should be less than 15-20 mmol/L. In patients with metabolic acidosis, chloride and bicarbonate concentrations are decreased to compensate for the increased concentrations of negatively charged acids, resulting in an increased anion gap. In certain untreated IEMs, it is not uncommon to observe anion gaps of 30 mmol/L or more with very low bicarbonate levels. Administration of bicarbonate is generally effective in the short-term in these patients but long-term treatment requires identification of the enzymatic deficiency and dietary modification to avoid accumulation of the specific acidic pathway intermediates, such as methylmalonic acid in the methylmalonic acidurias.

Lactate

Following the identification of a metabolic acidosis, subsequent measurement of plasma lactate and pyruvate are most useful in the evaluation of patients with mitochondrial disease.[24] An elevation in blood lactate is most likely due to tissue hypoxia caused by sepsis, seizures, or asphyxia or may be attributed to preanalytical error, such as extended tourniquet use during blood drawing. As a result, a single, modestly elevated lactate measurement will frequently occur in the absence of an IEM. In the presence of consistently elevated lactate, mitochondrial respiratory chain defects, and defects of pyruvate metabolism should be suspected.

Glucose

Hypoglycemia is a relatively frequent finding in sick neonates and reflects an inability to balance glucose utilization with replenishment of glucose, either through feeding, breakdown of glycogen stores, or gluconeogenesis.[25,26] Single, isolated glucose measurements below the reference interval constitute the majority of hypoglycemic events in the neonatal period. These newborns often have no metabolic defects but have exhausted their modest glycogen stores. Fortunately, these instances of hypoglycemia can be easily corrected by administration of exogenous glucose. Maternal diabetes is the most frequent cause of hypoglycemia that persists despite glucose supplementation. Neonates born to diabetic mothers experience hyperinsulinemia, which leads to increased glucose requirements. Importantly, glucose metabolism stabilizes in these infants within the first months of life and does not indicate an IEM. However, recurrent hypoglycemia in association with other clinical symptoms, such as lethargy or encephalopathy, with or without other metabolic abnormalities, should increase the suspicion of an IEM.

Ketones

Given the limited ability to mobilize glycogen stores during the first months of life, fatty acid oxidation represents an important energy source in healthy neonates.[27] Fatty acid oxidation in the liver leads to the formation of ketone bodies, specifically acetoacetate and β-hydroxybutyrate. In healthy neonates, acetoacetate, and β-hydroxybutyrate normally exist in a 1:1 ratio but acetoacetate is much more labile than β-hydroxybutyrate and decreases rapidly, if samples are not processed correctly. Importantly, urine dipsticks designed to detect the presence of ketone bodies do not detect β-hydroxybutyrate and generate negative test results in neonates with normal metabolism. Conversely, a positive urine dipstick test indicates the presence of acetoacetate, which is most often associated with abnormalities in fatty acid or ketogenic amino acid metabolism and should prompt further testing to identify the underlying IEM. Consistent elevations in plasma β-hydroxybutyrate measurements are observed in a wide range of IEMs, including organic acidemias, disorders of amino acid metabolism, pyruvate carboxylase deficiency, and disorders of glycogen metabolism and storage. In addition to elevations in plasma ketones, abnormally low plasma ketones may also indicate the presence of certain IEMs.[28] Given the essential role of fatty acid oxidation as an energy source during fasting, modest concentrations of plasma ketones are associated with normal metabolic processes. When plasma ketones remain low in the presence of hypoglycemia, defects in enzymes involved in fatty acid oxidation should be high on the list of differential diagnoses.

Ammonia

Hyperammonemia also serves as an early indicator of abnormal metabolism due to some inherited enzyme deficiencies. Ammonia is formed in the liver during hepatic deamination of amino acids and is normally converted to urea following the series of enzymatic manipulations in the urea cycle before being excreted in urine. As in the case of plasma ketones, modest plasma ammonia concentrations (50-100 µmol/L) are frequently observed in healthy normal neonates presumably due to immature hepatic function but higher concentrations in the newborn and levels around 100 µmol/L in older individuals including adults may indicate a metabolic abnormality. A common artifactual cause of modestly elevated ammonia is ex vivo glutamine deamidation due to delays in sample processing following collection. Ammonia concentrations >200 µmol/L require prompt, aggressive investigation, and intervention. IEMs most often associated with extreme elevations in plasma ammonia are urea cycle defects, hyperornithinemia-hyperammonemia-homocitrullinuria (HHH) syndrome, as well as propionic and methylmalonic acidemias.[29] Modest elevation of ammonia may be seen in some fatty acid oxidation defects.

Liver Function Tests

Because the liver plays a central role in many metabolic processes, toxic pathway intermediates often accumulate in the liver in patients with certain enzymatic deficiencies. These toxic intermediates may cause liver damage which is reflected by abnormalities in liver function tests, increased serum concentrations of conjugated or unconjugated bilirubin, and/or abnormal coagulation tests. In the case of patients with galactosemia, galactose-1-phosphate, and other hepatotoxic intermediates accumulate, resulting in liver dysfunction and jaundice during the first or second week of life.[30] Disease symptoms are compounded by the accumulation of galactose-1-phosphate within erythrocytes, resulting in increased serum concentrations of unconjugated bilirubin due to erythrocyte lysis. Galactose-1-phosphate levels also rise in the kidney, which results in tubular dysfunction and a Fanconi syndrome with loss of glucose, phosphate, and amino acids. Additional sequestration of phosphate as galactose-1-phosphate results in very low plasma phosphate levels. Pyruvate kinase deficiency also results in hemolytic anemia and causes a similar increase in unconjugated bilirubin. Defects in bile acid synthesis or transport, lysosomal disorders, or glycogen storage diseases can cause neonatal cholestasis, resulting in increased serum concentrations of conjugated bilirubin.[31,32] Additionally, because the liver synthesizes most proteins required for proper coagulation, abnormal coagulation tests are also often encountered during the initial laboratory workup of neonates with a suspected IEM. For the same reason, low plasma albumin may reflect the presence of hepatotoxic metabolic intermediates caused by an IEM. Importantly, the liver has an extensive reserve capacity and decreases in protein synthesis and abnormal coagulation tests are generally not observed unless liver damage is severe.

Complete Blood Count

Abnormal CBC results are relatively common in sick neonates and often constitute a non-specific finding. However, in the context of other unusual laboratory results, such as hyperammonemia or acidosis, hematologic abnormalities can often help narrow the differential diagnosis. For example, a number of organic acidurias are associated with decreases in all three cell lineages (erythrocytes, leukocytes, platelets). Megaloblastic anemia or pancytopenia may also be indicators of defects in enzymes involved in folate and vitamin B12 metabolism which may progress to psychomotor retardation, intractable seizures, and cerebral atrophy when left untreated.[33] Elevated concentrations of plasma homocysteine should alert the physician to the possibility of an enzymatic deficiency in the folic acid or vitamin B12 pathways. Automated immunoassays for the quantitation of homocysteine are available for most laboratory analyzers and can provide clinically useful information within hours of sample collection.

Imaging

Metabolic disorders caused by the vast majority of IEMs are not associated with abnormal imaging studies (X-ray, CT, MRI). One notable exception is the finding of subdural hemorrhage and cerebral atrophy on CT scans of patients with glutaric aciduria type 1 (GA1).[34] Given that intracranial bleeding due to GA1 can often be confused with non-accidental injury caused by domestic abuse, a rapid and accurate diagnosis of a metabolic cause of bleeding in these patients has important legal and custodial implications. Another exception is the detection of cardiomyopathies by X-ray or MRI, which may be the initial indicator of an IEM in patients with other suggestive but non-specific symptoms. Beyond excluding other pathologic conditions, imaging studies have limited diagnostic utility in patients with an IEM.

Initial Laboratory Workup Summary

Because of the interrelated nature of metabolic pathways, patients with IEMs often present with multiple abnormalities. Urea cycle defects resulting in hyperammonemia can cause a secondary lactic acidosis through disruption of mitochondrial function. Defects in fatty acid oxidation can shift the cellular machinery toward increased amino acid consumption as the primary energy source, resulting in hyperammonemia. Patients with glycogen storage diseases often present with hypoglycemia and metabolic acidosis but normal plasma ammonia concentrations. Measurement of plasma electrolytes, lactic acid, ketones, and ammonia can often help the pediatrician narrow the list of IEMs on his or her differential diagnosis based on the pattern of metabolic abnormalities identified during initial testing.

It must be noted that individuals with certain IEMs may present with progressively worsening clinical symptoms but only modest abnormalities during the initial laboratory workup mentioned earlier. Referral for specialized testing is warranted in these cases where the clinical suspicion for an IEM remains high despite a relatively normal initial laboratory workup. In some cases, IEMs are only detectable using routine laboratory testing during periods of stress and samples collected during non-catabolic periods will not reflect any metabolic abnormalities. Furthermore, communication between the primary care physician and the laboratory performing the specialized testing can greatly facilitate the diagnostic process in cases where metabolic abnormalities may be subtle. An understanding of the clinical symptoms can help the metabolic specialist differentiate between a healthy patient with isolated, modestly abnormal test results and a patient with similar laboratory results caused by an IEM.

Specialized Testing

Following the identification of abnormalities suggestive of an IEM during the initial laboratory workup, specialized testing must be performed to establish a definitive diagnosis, guide appropriate treatment, and monitor patients once treatment has been initiated. Profiling of urine organic acids, plasma/serum amino acids, and plasma/serum acylcarnitines by mass spectrometry (MS) or other test methods capable of measuring multiple analytes simultaneously provides a comprehensive snapshot of the metabolic state of children with a suspected IEM at the time of sample collection. While the metabolic profile generated by one of the specialized test methods sometimes provides enough information to establish a diagnosis, the metabolic abnormalities identified using only one profiling technique may be consistent with multiple IEMs. Therefore, measurements of urine organic acids, plasma/serum amino acids, and plasma/serum acylcarnitines are often performed in parallel and patterns of metabolic abnormalities identified using each technique are correlated to establish an accurate diagnosis. Importantly, while biochemical testing is diagnostic in many cases, assessment of enzymatic activity or genetic testing may be required to establish a definitive diagnosis in some instances.

As in the case of all laboratory testing, results of multiple-analyte metabolic testing must be interpreted in the context of each patient's clinical presentation. Metabolic profiling is capable of providing invaluable information in the diagnostic process but can lead to an incorrect diagnosis if abnormal test results are not correlated with clinical symptoms. First, modest abnormalities can often be explained by the application of imperfect reference intervals to a patient in a normal state of health. Second, analytical issues may cause falsely elevated measurements of a particular biomarker, leading to the diagnosis of a metabolic disorder that is inconsistent with a patient's symptoms. Third, analytes suggestive of a metabolic disorder may be elevated due to nonmetabolic pathologic conditions. In these patients, incorrect diagnosis of a metabolic disorder would impede discovery of the true underlying cause and delay the administration of appropriate treatment. For all these reasons, it is vitally important that results of metabolic testing are correlated with clinical symptoms in order to establish the correct diagnosis for each patient.

Urine Organic Acids

Organic acids are pathway intermediates defined by one or more carboxyl groups and a typical molecular weight less than 500 Da that accumulate in patients with IEMs. While amino acids fit this description, they are typically measured using a different technique that will be described in detail later. Organic acids accumulate in a variety of dysregulated metabolic processes, including the synthesis and catabolism of proteins, lipids, and carbohydrates.[35] Most diagnostically important organic acids are not reclaimed from the glomerular filtrate and are found at much higher concentrations in urine than plasma. Therefore, urine is the optimal sample type for organic acid measurement. 24-hour urine specimens eliminate pre-analytical concerns involving variations in organic acid excretion throughout the day but extended collection periods often present logistical challenges, especially in pediatric patients.

In practice, random urine specimens are most often used with preference given to samples collected at first morning void. As described earlier, collection of samples during symptomatic periods maximizes the likelihood of detecting abnormal metabolic intermediates that reflect the presence of an IEM.

As of the 2013 College of American Pathologists (CAP) survey, 82 participating laboratories offered urine organic acid testing and all 82 utilized gas chromatography linked with mass spectrometry (GC/MS). MS detection offers optimal sensitivity and, when coupled with GC, generates results with extremely high specificity. Modest differences in derivatization and extraction conditions exist between laboratories offering urine organic acid measurement but the fundamental analytical principle is consistent across laboratories.[36] Briefly, in GC/MS, organic acids are extracted from aliquots of urine containing a standardized quantity of creatinine using organic solvents, dried and derivatized to increase volatility. Small volumes of derivatized sample are introduced into a GC column and organic acids present in the sample are separated by differences in volatility and affinity for the column stationary phase, resulting in different elution times for each organic acid of interest. Upon elution from the column, compounds are ionized by electron impact ionization and fragmented in consistently reproducible patterns into smaller ions to produce a unique "chemical fingerprint" called a mass spectrum. Signal is generated when these ionized fragments come into contact with the MS detector. By combining the retention time provided by GC analysis with the fragmentation pattern provided by MS, GC/MS is capable of simultaneously identifying and quantitating the many organic acids present in urine specimens with high sensitivity and specificity. Using currently available methods, it is possible to detect the presence of thousands of different compounds using a single urine specimen. Hundreds of these compounds are routinely detected in clinical samples. A metabolic specialist is required to interpret these complex metabolic patterns and communicate any follow-up action to caregivers.

The presence of an unusual metabolite that has no role in normal metabolic processes is often a strong indication of underlying metabolic disease. In patients with a metabolic defect, intermediates may accumulate at high enough concentrations to act as substrates for enzymes that normally display very little activity toward the compound at normal concentrations. For example, in patients with propionic acidemia, deficiencies in propionyl-CoA carboxylase activity result in the accumulation of propionyl-CoA, which substitutes for acetyl-CoA in the citrate synthase reaction, forming methylcitrate.[37] Detection of methylcitrate in urine in conjunction with tiglylglycine and propionylglycine is strongly indicative of propionic acidemia as these compounds are not produced in normal metabolic processes and are usually not found in detectable amounts in urine from healthy individuals.

It must also be remembered that the presence of a single organic acid at abnormally high concentrations is not necessarily diagnostic of an IEM. Certain organic acids can accumulate in the urine of normal individuals following intake of specific food products while other organic acids can accumulate in the urine of patients with disease not caused by metabolic deficiencies. Ultimately, successful interpretation of urine organic acid profiles requires the recognition of patterns of multiple metabolic abnormalities as well as an understanding of how the detected analytes fit into specific metabolic pathways. When a specific enzymatic defect is suspected based on metabolic profiling, correlation of the presumed diagnosis with patient symptoms is always required. If patient symptoms are inconsistent with the presumed diagnosis, further evaluation is necessary.

Amino Acids

Amino acids are small molecular weight compounds with an amino group and a carboxyl group that play a primary role as the building blocks of protein synthesis. As proteins are continuously synthesized and degraded, metabolic abnormalities caused by IEMs may result in the accumulation of any of the 20 amino acids involved in protein synthesis or other amino acids that serve as metabolic intermediates in the urea cycle and other biological pathways.[38] Therefore, amino acid profiling offers important information in the diagnosis of many IEMs. In contrast to many organic acids that are not reclaimed from the glomerular filtrate, amino acids are actively and efficiently reclaimed. As a result, plasma/serum is the preferred specimen for amino acid analysis. However, amino acid measurement in urine may be required to detect certain transport defects including cystinuria and lysinuric protein intolerance. Similarly, CSF is the specimen of choice for the evaluation of NKH.

Clinical measurement of amino acids has been performed for over 60 years and as of 2013, 99 institutions offered amino acid measurement by one of the two techniques. The most common technique (employed by 88 laboratories participating in the 2013 CAP survey) consists of amino acid derivatization and separation by ion exchange chromatography, followed by detection and quantitation by visible (ninhydrin derivatization), ultraviolet (phenylisothiocyanate derivatization), or fluorescence (o-phthalaldehyde derivatization) spectroscopy. Derivatization can be performed either before or after the chromatography step, depending on the specific reagent used. Many variations of this method are routinely employed in clinical practice but the most common consists of post-column derivatization with ninhydrin followed by detection at 570 nm. While ninhydrin-based techniques are routinely used, they are time-intensive and relatively non-specific as other ninhydrin-positive compounds may co-elute with amino acids of clinical interest, resulting in falsely elevated measurements.[39,40] As a result, the remaining 11 laboratories offering amino acid measurement employ MS-based methods. The combination of chromatographic separation and mass identification provides appropriate sensitivity while reducing non-specific interference and facilitating the accurate identification of isobaric amino acids like alanine/β alanine/sarcosine and allo-isoleucine/isoleucine/leucine/hydroxyproline. At the author's institution, amino acids are extracted from the patient sample with methanol, butylated, and separated by liquid chromatography (LC). Eluting compounds are ionized and introduced into a tandem mass spectrometer where data are acquired in multiple reaction monitoring mode (MRM). Ultimately, the measurement of specific precursor-product ion pairs combined with a characteristic retention time facilitates the specific identification and quantitation of 32 amino acids simultaneously from a single specimen.[41]

As in the case of urine organic acid testing, modest, isolated elevations of a single amino acid are regularly observed in normal patients. Reference intervals for plasma amino acids are difficult to establish and vary with age,[42] resulting in amino acid measurements that frequently fall slightly outside of the reference interval in individuals without metabolic disease. Furthermore, gross abnormalities in plasma or urine amino acid concentrations are often observed in patients with liver failure or other non-metabolic disorders. Therefore, correct diagnosis of patients with an IEM requires the identification of characteristic patterns of amino acid abnormalities that reflect a specific metabolic defect and correlate with appropriate clinical signs and symptoms.

Plasma Acylcarnitines

In conjunction with urine organic acid and plasma amino acid measurements, plasma acylcarnitine (carnitine ester) measurement can provide essential information in the diagnosis of children and occasionally adults with an IEM. Carnitine esters are a class of molecules consisting of carnitine [3-hydroxy-4-(trimethylammonio)butanoate] conjugated to a fatty acyl group of variable chain lengths. Carnitine plays an essential role in the transport of long-chain fatty acids across the mitochondrial inner membrane, facilitating fatty acid oxidation as an energy source when intracellular glucose concentrations are low. Additionally, carnitine acts as a reservoir for short-chain and medium-chain acyl residues, facilitating the regeneration of reduced CoA (CoASH), which is required for numerous mitochondrial processes.[43] In patients with deficiencies in acyltransferases or enzymes required for fatty acid oxidation, carnitine esters of various sizes (C0-C18) accumulate upstream of the deficient enzyme and are often present at abnormally high concentrations in the plasma of affected individuals. As a result, patterns of abnormally elevated carnitine esters strongly indicate the presence of a fatty acid oxidation defect as well as certain organic acid disorders.

Clinical measurement of carnitine esters is currently offered by 49 participants in the 2013 CAP survey, all of which utilize tandem mass spectrometry. Carnitine esters are extracted from patient samples using methanol, often derivatized by butylation then reconstituted in mobile phase and introduced to the mass spectrometer. As no chromatographic separation is used to increase specificity, individual carnitine esters are identified using a characteristic neutral loss of precursor mass to yield a specific product ion. Using a product ion of mass/charge (m/z) = 85 common to all carnitine esters, scanning of precursor ions in a range of m/z 200-500 identifies the mix of carnitine esters present in the patient sample. This mode of analysis is known as precursor ion scanning.

An important limitation of carnitine ester analysis using precursor scanning is the interference caused by isobaric esters and other substances that generate fragments that are identical to those associated with clinically significant carnitine esters. As one example, the C4 esters, isobutyryl, and butyrylcarnitine ($[M+H]^+$ = 288) cannot be readily distinguished using this approach.[44] Additionally, xenobiotics with precursor-product transitions similar to those of carnitine esters may result in falsely elevated carnitine ester measurements in the absence of underlying metabolic deficiency. Apparent increases in hydroxyhexadecenoylcarnitine (C16:1-OH), for example, are often observed secondary to therapy with the cephalosporin, cefotaxime. Due to these analytical considerations, results of carnitine ester profiling must be correlated with each patient's clinical symptoms before a conclusive diagnosis is established.

SUMMARY

In order to maintain life, metabolic intermediates are continuously shuttled through countless biological pathways throughout the body. These pathways depend on the proper function of many enzymes and transporter proteins and the accumulation of metabolic intermediates in patients with an enzymatic or transporter deficiency often results in progressively worsening clinical symptoms during the first weeks to months of life. While patients with enzymatic deficiencies present with nonspecific clinical features that often overlap with non-metabolic disease states, otherwise unexplained and persistent symptoms should increase suspicion of an IEM. In the presence of appropriate clinical features, underlying metabolic deficiencies are often reflected by consistently abnormal results on routine tests performed in almost all clinical laboratories with minimal turnaround time. Results of the initial laboratory testing often help to narrow the differential diagnosis and suggest particular classes of metabolic deficiencies. If the clinical suspicion of a metabolic disorder remains high following the initial laboratory evaluation, specialized metabolic testing offers a direct measurement of clinically relevant metabolic intermediates and facilitates the establishment of a conclusive diagnosis following correlation with patient symptoms. Once a diagnosis has been established, specialized testing may be necessary at regular intervals to monitor disease progression or response to treatment. By recognizing the clinical symptoms caused by metabolic disease, understanding the effects of metabolic disease on initial laboratory testing and correctly interpreting the results of specialized testing, clinical personnel can rapidly and accurately diagnose children with IEMs and initiate proper treatment that often enables affected children to live a normal life.

TRAINING MODULE

1. List a common reason other than IEM that may lead to the following laboratory results on day of life 2.
   a. Glucose = 40 mg/dL (Reference 50-99)
   b. Plasma ammonia = 150 µmol/L (Reference 10-90 mmol/L)
   c. Lactate = 3.5 mmol/L (Reference 0.5-3.0 mmol/L)
   d. Plasma total CO_2 content = 10 mmol/L (Reference 20-30 mmol/L)

2. Which of the following metabolic disorders is associated with a characteristic odor?
   a. Isovaleric acidemia
   b. Trimethylaminuria
   c. Methylmalonic acidemia
   d. Maple Syrup Urine Disease

3. Which of the following metabolic disorders are associated with hyperammonemia?
   a. Ornithine transcarbamoylase deficiency
   b. Citrullinemia
   c. Propionic acidemia
   d. Homocystinuria

4. Which of the following metabolic disorders are associated with dysmorphic features?
   a. Methylmalonic acidemia
   b. Non-ketotic hyperglycinemia
   c. MCAD deficiency
   d. MSUD
   e. None of the above

5. Amino acid profiles are most commonly performed by which of the following techniques?
   a. LC-MS/MS of butyl derivatives
   b. MS/MS of butyl derivatives using precursor ion scanning
   c. GC/MS
   d. LC-photometric/fluorescent detection

6. Acylcarnitine profiles are most commonly performed using which of the following techniques?
   a. LC-MS/MS of butyl derivatives
   b. MS/MS of butyl derivatives using precursor ion scanning
   c. GC/MS
   d. LC-photometric/fluorescent detection

7. Organic acid profiles are most commonly performed using which of the following techniques?
   a. LC-MS/MS of butyl derivatives
   b. MS/MS of butyl derivatives using precursor ion scanning
   c. GC/MS
   d. LC-photometric/fluorescent detection

8. Which of the following techniques may be employed to detect MSUD?
   a. Acylcarnitine profile
   b. Plasma amino acid profile
   c. Urine amino acid profile
   d. CSF amino acid profile
   e. Urine organic acid profile

9. Which of the following techniques may be employed to detect MCAD deficiency?
   a. Acylcarnitine profile
   b. Plasma amino acid profile
   c. Urine amino acid profile
   d. CSF amino acid profile
   e. Urine organic acid profile

10. Which of the following techniques may be employed to detect methylmalonic acidemia?
    a. Acylcarnitine profile
    b. Plasma amino acid profile
    c. Urine amino acid profile
    d. CSF amino acid profile
    e. Urine organic acid profile

REFERENCES

1. American Academy of Pediatrics Newborn Screening Authoring Committee. Newborn screening expands: recommendations for pediatricians and medical homes-implications for the system. *Pediatrics*. 2008;121:192-217.

2. Kwan A, Abraham RS, Currier R, Brower A et al. Newborn screening for severe combined immunodeficiency in 11 screening programs in the united states. *JAMA*. 2014 Aug 20;312(7):729-738.

3. Dietzen DJ, Rinaldo P, Whitley RJ, Rhead WJ, Hannon WH, Garg UC, et al. National academy of clinical biochemistry laboratory medicine practice guidelines: follow-up

testing for metabolic disease identified by expanded newborn screening using tandem mass spectrometry; executive summary. *Clin Chem.* 2009;55:1615-1626.

4. Sarafoglou K, Banks K, Kyllo J, Pittock S, Thomas W. Cases of congenital adrenal hyperplasia missed by newborn screening in minnesota. *JAMA.* 2012;307:2371-2374.

5. Chan CL, McFann K, Taylor L, Wright D, Zeitler PS, Barker JM. Congenital adrenal hyperplasia and the second newborn screen. *J Pediatr.* 2013;163:109-113.

6. Seashore MR, Seashore CJ. Newborn screening and the pediatric practitioner. *Semin Perinatol.* 2005;29:182-188.

7. Saudubray JM, Nassogne MC, de Lonlay P, Touati G. Clinical approach to inherited metabolic disorders in neonates: an overview. *Semin Neonatol.* 2002;7:3-15.

8. Clarke J. A Clinical Guide to Metabolic Diseases. 2nd ed. Cambridge: Cambridge University Press, 2002.

9. Dionisi-Vici C, Deodato F, Röschinger W, Rhead W, Wilcken B. 'Classical' organic acid-urias, propionic aciduria, methylmalonic aciduria and isovaleric aciduria: long-term outcome and effects of expanded newborn screening using tandem mass spectrom-etry. *J Inherit Metab Dis.* 2006;29:383-389.

10. Rahman S, Footitt EJ, Varadkar S, Clayton PT. Inborn errors of metabolism causing epilepsy. *Dev Med Child Neurol.* 2013;55:23-36.

11. Gropman AL. Patterns of brain injury in inborn errors of metabolism. *Semin Pediatr Neurol.* 2012;19:203-210.

12. Burke DG, Halpern B, Malegan D, McCairns E, Danks D, Schlesinger P, Wilken B. Profiles of urinary volatiles from metabolic disorders characterized by unusual odors. *Clin Chem.* 1983;29:1834-1838.

13. Hermansen CL, Lorah KN. Respiratory distress in the newborn. *Am Fam Physician.* 2007;76:987-994.

14. Ficicioglu C, An Haack K. Failure to thrive: When to suspect inborn errors of metabo-lism. *Pediatrics.* 2009;124:972-979.

15. Gardeitchik T, Humphrey M, Nation J, Boneh A. Early clinical manifestations and eat-ing patterns in patients with urea cycle disorders. *J Pediatr.* 2012;161:328-332.

16. Cox GF. Diagnostic approaches to pediatric cardiomyopathy of metabolic genetic etiologies and their relation to therapy. *Prog Pediatr Cardiol.* 2007;24:15-25.

17. Das AM, Steuerwald U, Illsinger S. Inborn errors of energy metabolism associated with myopathies. *J Biomed Biotechnol.* 2010;2010:340849.

18. Poll-The BT, Maillette de Buy Wenniger-Prick LJ, Barth PG, Duran M. The eye as a window to inborn errors of metabolism. *J Inherit Metab Dis.* 2003;26:229-244.

19. van Woerden CS, Groothoff JW, Wijburg FA, Duran M, Wanders RJ, Barth PG, Poll-The BT. High incidence of hyperoxaluria in generalized peroxisomal disorders. *Mol Genet Metab.* 2006;88:346-350.

20. Chillarón J, Font-Llitjós M, Fort J, Zorzano A, Goldfarb DS, Nunes V, Palacín M. Patho-physiology and treatment of cystinuria. *Nat Rev Nephrol.* 2010;6:424-434.

21. Enns G, Packman S. Diagnosing inborn errors of metabolism in the newborn: clinical features. *Neoreviews.* 2001;2:9.

22. Garganta CL, Smith WE. Metabolic evaluation of the sick neonate. *Semin Perinatol.* 2005;29:164-172.

23. Burton BK. Inborn errors of metabolism in infancy: a guide to diagnosis. *Pediatrics.* 1998;102:E69.

24. Munnich A, Rustin P. Clinical spectrum and diagnosis of mitochondrial disorders. *Am J Med Genet.* 2001;106:4-17.

25. McGowan J. Neonatal hypoglycemia. *Pediatr Rev.* 1999;20:10.

26. de Lonlay P, Touati G, Robert JJ, Saudubray JM. Persistent hyperinsulinaemic hypoglycaemia. *Semin Neonatol.* 2002;7:95-100.

27. Bennett MJ, Rinaldo P, Strauss AW. Inborn errors of mitochondrial fatty acid oxidation. *Crit Rev Clin Lab Sci.* 2000;37:1-44.

28. Saudubray JM, Martin D, de Lonlay P, Touati G, Poggi-Travert F, Bonnet D, et al. Recognition and management of fatty acid oxidation defects: a series of 107 patients. *J Inherit Metab Dis.* 1999;22:488-502.

29. Brusilow SW. Urea cycle disorders: Clinical paradigm of hyperammonemic encephalopathy. *Prog Liver Dis.* 1995;13:293-309.

30. Cuthbert C, Klapper H, Elsas L. Diagnosis of inherited disorders of galactose metabolism. *Curr Protoc Hum Genet.* 2008;Chapter 17:Unit 17.5.

31. Feldman AG, Sokol RJ. Neonatal cholestasis. *Neoreviews.* 2013;14(2):10.1542/neo. 14-2-e63.

32. Setchell KD, Heubi JE. Defects in bile acid biosynthesis-diagnosis and treatment. *J Pediatr Gastroenterol Nutr.* 2006;43 Suppl 1:S17-S22.

33. Banka S, Blom HJ, Walter J, Aziz M, Urquhart J, Clouthier CM, et al. Identification and characterization of an inborn error of metabolism caused by dihydrofolate reductase deficiency. *Am J Hum Genet.* 2011;88:216-225.

34. Hartley LM, Khwaja OS, Verity CM. Glutaric aciduria type 1 and nonaccidental head injury. *Pediatrics.* 2001;107:174-175.

35. Kumps A, Duez P, Mardens Y. Metabolic, nutritional, iatrogenic, and artifactual sources of urinary organic acids: a comprehensive table. *Clin Chem.* 2002;48:708-717.

36. Jones PM, Bennett MJ. Urine organic acid analysis for inherited metabolic disease using gas chromatography-mass spectrometry. *Methods Mol Biol.* 2010;603:423-431.

37. Sweetman L, Weyler W, Shafai T, Young PE, Nyhan WL. Prenatal diagnosis of propionic acidemia. *JAMA.* 1979;242:1048-1052.

38. Camargo SM, Bockenhauer D, Kleta R. Aminoacidurias: Clinical and molecular aspects. *Kidney Int.* 2008;73:918-925.

39. Narayan SB, Ditewig-Meyers G, Graham KS, Scott R, Bennett MJ. Measurement of plasma amino acids by ultraperformance® liquid chromatography. *Clin Chem Lab Med.* 2011;49:1177-1185.

40. Dietzen DJ, Weindel AL, Carayannopoulos MO, Landt M, Normansell ET, Reimschisel TE, Smith CH. Rapid comprehensive amino acid analysis by liquid chromatography/ tandem mass spectrometry: comparison to cation exchange with post-column ninhydrin detection. *Rapid Commun Mass Spectrom.* 2008;22:3481-3488.

41. Dietzen DJ, Weindel AL. Comprehensive determination of amino acids for diagnosis of inborn errors of metabolism. *Methods Mol Biol.* 2010;603:27-36.

42. Lepage N, McDonald N, Dallaire L, Lambert M. Age-specific distribution of plasma amino acid concentrations in a healthy pediatric population. *Clin Chem.* 1997;43:2397-2402.

43. Bieber LL. Carnitine. *Annu Rev Biochem.* 1988;57:261-283.

44. Rinaldo P, Cowan TM, Matern D. Acylcarnitine profile analysis. *Genet Med.* 2008; 10:151-156.

NEWBORN SCREENING | 5

Marzia Pasquali and Irene De Biase

LEARNING OBJECTIVES

1. Describe the components of a newborn screening program.
2. Discuss the Recommended Uniform Screening Panel (RUSP).
3. Describe the disorders included in the RUSP.
4. Discuss follow-up testing for each disorder included in the RUSP.

INTRODUCTION

Newborn screening (NBS) is a public health activity aimed at the early identification of infants affected with conditions for which timely intervention leads to the elimination or reduction of mortality and morbidity associated with these conditions. Universal NBS started in the early 1960s, thanks to the pioneering work of Dr. Robert Guthrie, who developed the first screening test for phenylketonuria using dried blood spots on filter paper. Thanks to the use of filter paper as a collection device, universal NBS for over 30 inherited conditions is now possible world-wide, saving the lives and intellect of hundreds of children every year.

NEWBORN SCREENING

NBS is not just a clinical test, but rather a program that includes several components: laboratory testing, follow-up activities, clinical care, education, and quality assurance. The smooth integration of all components of the program determines the effectiveness of NBS. There are guidelines to assist NBS programs in establishing protocols and procedures dealing with each of the components. These guidelines have been published by the Clinical and Laboratory Standards Institute and include guidelines on blood collection on filter paper (NBS01-A6), testing methodology (NBS04-A, NBS05-A, NBS06-A), follow-up activities (NBS02-A2), sample collection, and follow-up of premature/sick babies (NBS03-A). These documents are available at www.clsi.org. In addition to these guidelines, follow-up algorithms and basic clinical information on the diseases screened have been developed by the American College of Medical Genetics and Genomics (ACMGG) and they are available at http://www.ncbi.nlm.nih.gov/books/NBK55827/.

With new information on the natural history of inherited disorders and new discoveries leading to novel therapies, the number of conditions that could potentially be screened for in the newborn period is dramatically increasing. However, there are specific criteria to be met before a condition is considered for inclusion in a NBS program. These criteria have been developed and applied by the Uniform Panel Work Group convened by the American College of Medical Genetics and Genomics (ACMG), which, at the beginning of the 2000s, was given the task of identifying conditions to be included in NBS programs in the United States. The final report of the work group can be found at http://mchb.hrsa.gov/programs/newbornscreening/screeningreport-pdf.pdf and it outlines the evaluation process. Conditions were evaluated in three different categories: a) clinical characteristics of the disease (incidence, natural history, burden of the disease); b) analytical characteristics of the test (availability, reliability, sensitivity, specificity, cost); and c) follow-up, diagnosis, treatment, and management of the disease (availability, acceptability, efficacy, cost of treatment).

As a result of the work of the Uniform Panel Work Group, a list of 29 conditions meeting all criteria set forth by the workgroup was published[1]; along with this initial list of disorders, other conditions have been thoroughly examined by the Secretary Advisory Committee for Heritable Diseases in Newborns and Children (SACHDNC) and added to the Recommended Uniform Screening Panel (RUSP) (Table 5-1). The committee reviews proposals for the addition of new conditions to the RUSP and, through an evidence-based and expert review, determines whether the proposed condition fits all the criteria for inclusion. If it does, the condition becomes part of the RUSP. States then decide if and how they want to implement the recommendation of the SACHDNC in their programs. Currently, the RUSP includes 22 metabolic disorders, 2 storage disorders (Pompe disease and Mucopolysaccharidosis type I), 2 endocrine disorders, 3 hemoglobinopathies, cystic fibrosis, the severe combined immunodeficiencies, hearing loss, and critical congenital heart disease (Table 5-1). The rapid evolution and adoption of analytic technology, the development of new therapies, and the availability of outcome studies are the main factors in the expansion of newborn screening. For this reason, the number of conditions included in the RUSP is continuously increasing.

Table 5-1 **LIST OF RECOMMENDED UNIFORM SCREENING PANEL (RUSP) CORE AND SECONDARY CONDITIONS WITH THEIR PRIMARY MARKERS*,†**

ACMG Code	Core Conditions	Methodology					MS/MS	Others (HPLC, IEF, EIA, etc.)		
		OA	FAO	AA	Other	Marker(s)	Endo	HgB	Other
PROP	Propionic acidemia	X				C3			
MUT	Methylmalonic acidemia (methylmalonyl-CoA mutase)	X				C3			
Cbl A, B	Methylmalonic acidemia (cobalamin disorders)	X				C3			
IVA	Isovaleric acidemia	X				C5			
3-MCC	3-Methylcrotonyl-CoA carboxylase deficiency	X				C50H (C6DC)			
HMG	3-Hydroxy-3-methyglutaric aciduria	X				C50H			
MCD	Holocarboxylase synthase deficiency	X				C50H (C3)			
βKT	β-Ketothiolase deficiency	X				C50H (C5:1)			
GA1	Glutaric acidemia type I	X				C5DC			
CUD	Carnitine uptake defect/carnitine transport defect		X			Low C0			
MCAD	Medium-chain acyl-CoA dehydrogenase deficiency		X			C8, C6, C10			
VLCAD	Very long-chain acyl-CoA dehydrogenase deficiency		X			C14:1			
LCHAD	Long-chain L-3 hydroxyacyl-CoA dehydrogenase deficiency		X			C160H, C18:10H			
TFP	Trifunctional protein deficiency		X			C160H, C18:10H			
ASA	Argininosuccinic aciduria			X		Cit (ASA)			

(Continued)

Table 5-1   LIST OF RECOMMENDED UNIFORM SCREENING PANEL (RUSP) CORE AND SECONDARY CONDITIONS WITH THEIR PRIMARY MARKERS*,† (Continued)

		Methodology							
		MS/MS					Others (HPLC, IEF, EIA, etc.)		
ACMG Code	Core Conditions	OA	FAO	AA	Other	Marker(s)	Endo	HgB	Other
CIT	Citrulinemia, Type I			X		Cit			
MSUD	Maple syrup urine disease			X		Leu			
HCY	Homocystinuria			X		Met			
PKU	Classic phenylketonuria			X		Phe, Phe/Tyr			
TYR I	Tyrosinemia, type I			X		SUAC (Tyr)			
CH	Primary congenital hypothyroidism						X		
CAH	Congenital adrenal hyperplasia						X		
Hb SS	S, S disease (Sickle cell anemia)							X	
Hb S/βth	S, β-thalassemia							X	
Hb S/C	S, C disease							X	
BIOT	Biotinidase deficiency								X
CCHD	Critical congenital heart disease								X
CF	Cystic fibrosis								X
GALT	Classic galactosemia								X
GSD II	Glycogen storage disease Type II (Pompe)								X
HEAR	Hearing loss								X
SCID	Severe combined immunodeficiencies								X
MPS I	Mucopolysaccharidosis Type I (alpha-iduronidase deficiency)								X
X-ALD	X-linked adrenoleukodystrophy				X	Hexacosanoyl lysophosphatidylcholine			

ACMG Code	Secondary Conditions	Methodology				Others Other Disorder	
		MS/MS					
		OA	FAO	AA	Marker(s)	Hgb	Other
Cbl C, D	Methylmalonic acidemia with homocystinuria	X			C3		
MAL	Malonic acidemia	X			C3DC		
IBG	Isobutyrylglycinuria	X			C4		
2MBG	2-Methylbutyrylglycinuria	X			C5		
3MGA	3-Methylglutaconic aciduria	X			C50H		
2M3HBA	2-Methyl-3-hydroxybutyric aciduria	X			C50H		
SCAD	Short-chain acyl-CoA dehydrogenase deficiency		X		C4		
M/SCHAD	Medium/short-chain L-3-hydroxyacl-CoA dehydrogenase deficiency		X		C40H		
GA2	Glutaric acidemia Type II		X		C4, C5, Multiple Acylcarnitines		
MCAT	Medium-chain ketoacyl-CoA thiolase deficiency		X		C50H		
DE RED	2, 4 Dienoyl-CoA reductase deficiency		X		C10:2		
CPT IA	Carnitine palmitoyltransferase Type I deficiency		X		High C0		
CPT II	Carnitine palmitoyltransferase Type II deficiency		X		C16, C18:1		
CACT	Carnitine acylcarnitine translocase deficiency		X		C16, C18:1		

(Continued)

Table 5-1   LIST OF RECOMMENDED UNIFORM SCREENING PANEL (RUSP) CORE AND SECONDARY CONDITIONS WITH THEIR PRIMARY MARKERS*,† (Continued)

ACMG Code	Secondary Conditions	Methodology					Others	
		MS/MS					Other Disorder	
		OA	FAO	AA	Marker(s)	Hgb	Hgb	Other
ARG	Argininemia			X	Arg			
CIT II	Citrullinemia, Type II			X	Cit			
MET	Hypermethioninemia			X	Met			
H-PHE	Benign hyperphenylalaninemia			X	Phe, Phe/Tyr			
BIOPT (BS)	Biopterin defect in cofactor biosynthesis			X	Phe, Phe/Tyr			
BIOPT (REG)	Biopterin defect in cofactor regeneration			X	Phe, Phe/Tyr			
TYR II	Tyrosinemia, Type II			X	Tyr			
TYR III	Tyrosinemia, Type III			X	Tyr			
Var Hb	Various other hemoglobinopathies					X		
GALE	Galactoepimerase deficiency							X
GALK	Galactokinase deficiency							X
	T-cell related lymphocyte deficiencies							X

*This list includes all the conditions recommended by the Secretary Advisory Committee for Heritable Diseases in Newborns and Children and approved by the Secretary of Health and Human Services.

†Modified from Recommended Uniform Screening Panel http://www.hrsa.gov/advisorycommittees/mchbadvisory/heritabledisorders/recommendedpanel/

METHODOLOGY

Several screening methods have been developed. They are geared toward the detection of metabolites (eg, phenylalanine), direct measurement of enzyme activity (eg, biotinidase), or more recently, DNA analysis (eg, SCID screening). In addition, there are screening methods for conditions, such as hearing loss and critical congenital heart disease, which do not require a blood spot, but are functional tests performed at the birth facility.

Among the disorders included in the RUSP currently, 20 disorders of metabolism of amino acids (aminoacidopathies, urea cycle disorders, and organic acidemias) and fatty acids (fatty acid oxidation defects) are identified using the same technology, tandem mass spectrometry (MS/MS). The ability of MS/MS to simultaneously identify several metabolites and, therefore, enable multiplex analysis of a sample, has played a major role in the expansion of newborn screening panels.

Tandem Mass Spectrometry (MS/MS)

Tandem mass spectrometry measures the ratio of the mass (m) of a chemical compound to its charge (z). A small punch (usually 3 mm diameter) of the blood collected on filter paper provides the sample needed for MS/MS analysis. Two classes of metabolites are monitored and quantified with MS/MS: amino acids and acylcarnitines.[2] Amino acids are markers for aminoacidopathies, such as Phenylketonuria (PKU) and Maple Syrup Urine Disease (MSUD), and urea cycle disorders, such as Citrullinemia type I and Argininosuccinic aciduria (ASA). Acylcarnitines originate from the esterification of carnitine and organic/fatty acids which are products of the intermediary metabolism. The analysis of acylcarnitines reveals organic acidemias, such as Propionic acidemia (PA), Methylmalonic acidemia (MMA), and Glutaric acidemia type I (GA-I), and fatty acid oxidation (FAO) defects, such as Medium Chain Acyl-CoA Dehydrogenase (MCAD) deficiency and Carnitine Uptake Defect (CUD). Amino acids and acylcarnitines are extracted from the blood spot using a solution of methanol containing isotopically labeled internal standards. After drying the extract, amino acids and acylcarnitines can be either derivatized to form butylester derivatives or re-suspended in appropriate solvent prior to MS/MS analysis. All molecules are ionized to allow MS/MS detection, typically by electrospray. Two mass spectrometers are used in tandem to separate and identify amino acids and acylcarnitines according to their mass to charge (*m/z*) ratios. Since most of the ions have one positive charge, their mass to charge ratio corresponds to the mass (molecular weight) of the molecules analyzed. The molecular ions are separated by the first mass spectrometer, and then they enter the "collision cell" where they are fragmented by collision with a neutral gas (eg, nitrogen, argon). The fragments pass through a second mass spectrometer that separates them according to their mass to charge (*m/z*) ratio. Each molecule has a characteristic fragmentation pattern and classes of compounds will fragment in a similar way. MS/MS allows performing class-specific analysis as well as targeted analysis of the compounds of interest. The MS/MS analysis is very fast (approximately 2 minutes/sample) and suitable for high throughput applications, such as NBS.

In addition to amino acids and acylcarnitines, succinylacetone, the diagnostic marker for Tyrosinemia type I, is also detected from the same sample and analysis run.[3,4]

Tandem mass spectrometry is also used for the detection of hexacosanoyl lysophosphatidylcholine (C26:0-LPC), the marker for X-linked adrenoleukodystrophy (X-ALD). The measurement of C26:0-LPC can occur simultaneously with the measurement of amino acids, acylcarnitines, and succinylacetone.[5]

Interpretation of MS/MS Results

Currently, MS/MS is used to screen for metabolic disorders. The cause of a metabolic disorder is a block in a metabolic pathway leading to accumulation of disease-specific substrates upstream from the metabolic block, decreased concentration of products downstream of the metabolic block, and increased production of by-products not normally present (Figure 5-1). The metabolites

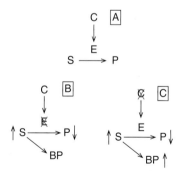

Figure 5-1 ▪ In a metabolic pathway a substrate, S, is converted to a product, P, by the action of an enzyme, E, which, often, is activated by a cofactor, C (1A). Impairment in a metabolic pathway can be due to impaired activity of the enzyme, E (1B), or to a deficiency or impaired metabolism of its cofactor, C (1C). In both cases, there will be a block in the pathway resulting in accumulation of the substrate, S, diminished formation of the product, P, and accumulation of by-products, BP, not normally present, generated by alternative pathways of substrate disposal.

accumulated as a consequence of a metabolic block are the primary markers for identifying metabolic disorders. MS/MS allows the simultaneous detection of many analytes; therefore the interpretation of the results is based also on metabolites' pattern recognition, while their concentration supports the interpretation.[6,7] The advantage of this type of analysis is the ability to use the multiple metabolites simultaneously detected as secondary markers to distinguish true metabolic derangements from iatrogenic causes, such as medications or dietary supplements. For example, in phenylketonuria (PKU) due to phenylalanine hydroxylase deficiency, the concentration of phenylalanine (PHE) increases while tyrosine (TYR) concentration decreases as a result of the metabolic block. The primary marker for PKU is phenylalanine, the ratio PHE/TYR is a secondary marker, important in differentiating between a true PKU case, in which the ratio PHE/TYR will be elevated in addition to elevated PHE, from a case in which PHE is elevated because of total parenteral nutrition, resulting in normal or increased tyrosine concentration and, consequently, normal PHE/TYR.

A limitation of MS/MS is that chemical compounds with the same mass/charge ratio cannot be separated, therefore compounds isomeric/isobaric to a metabolite marker of a specific disease can contribute to a false positive result. It is important to recognize the possible interfering compounds, which may be specific to the method used (derivatized vs non-derivatized), and to develop appropriate second-tier tests, when possible, to reduce the number of false positives.

Second-Tier Tests

One of the major pitfalls in NBS is the number of false-positive results associated with it. The relatively high false positive rate is due to several factors, such as cut-off values too low; presence of isobaric and isomeric compounds that falsely elevate the value of a marker detected through MS/MS; and/or incorrect interpretation of the results. To reduce the number of false positives and, therefore, the number of infants requiring unnecessary confirmatory testing, second-tier tests have been developed. Second-tier tests involve further analysis of the same blood spot that produced an abnormal result on the routine screening. Second-tier tests often target more specific analytes and use a methodology different from the one used in the primary screening test. They include LC-MS/MS analysis for metabolic disorders,[2] DNA analysis for CF,[8] LC-MS/MS steroid profile for congenital adrenal hyperplasia,[9] and other biochemical tests, such as TSH for congenital hypothyroidism.[10] Second-tier testing is a critical component of NBS programs since it increases the specificity of the screening test.

Secondary Conditions

Depending on the algorithm and the method used for screening, it is possible to identify metabolic disorders not included in the RUSP because they can be detected using the same primary markers of those already included in the RUSP. These conditions are included in the Uniform Panel Work Group report as **secondary targets or conditions**, with the recommendation to report them if identified in the course of screening for the RUSP conditions. An example is screening for classic galactosemia. Classic galactosemia is due to deficiency of the enzyme galactose-1-phosphate uridyltransferase and results in the accumulation of the metabolites galactose-1-phosphate and galactose. If the primary screening method relies on the measurement of total metabolites (galactose + galactose-1-phosphate), it will identify infants with classic galactosemia due to galactose-1-phosphate uridyltransferase deficiency (RUSP) as well as infants with galactose kinase and galactose epimerase deficiencies (two other inherited disorders of galactose metabolism, included in the secondary conditions/targets list) because all three enzyme deficiencies will cause increased metabolites.

Time of Screening

The time of collection of the screening sample is crucial. The collection should occur long enough after birth to allow accumulation of abnormal metabolites characteristic of amino acidopathies, urea cycle defects, and organic acidemias, but close enough to birth so that the infant is not anabolic to identify fatty acid oxidation defects.[11] Ideally, the NBS sample should be collected between 24 and 48 hours from birth. In several US states, it is mandatory to routinely perform two screens per newborn, where the first screen is collected at 24-48 hours of life and the second screen is usually collected at 7-28 days of life. While most of the amino acid concentrations do not change significantly with age, acylcarnitines change dramatically; they are usually higher in the first week of life, decreasing rapidly with age.[12] Therefore, age-specific cutoff ranges are essential for the interpretation of screen results.

DISORDERS INCLUDED IN NEWBORN SCREENING PROGRAMS

The disorders included in the RUSP can be classified in four groups:
   a) Metabolic disorders due to impaired activity of an enzyme or a transporter involved in a metabolic pathway. Aminoacidopathies, organic acidemias, defects of fatty acid oxidation, disorders of carbohydrate metabolism, lysosomal storage disorders, peroxisomal disorders, and cystic fibrosis are included in this group.

b) Endocrine disorders, such as congenital hypothyroidism and congenital adrenal hyperplasia.
c) Hemoglobinopathies due to defects in the synthesis of the globin chains of hemoglobin. An example in this group is sickle cell disease (sickle cell anemia or homozygous S disease).
d) Immunodeficiencies due to lack of one or more components of the immune system. Severe Combined Immunodeficiency (SCID) is the most severe example in this group.

Because of advances in therapeutic interventions for IEMs NBS panels are continuously expanding. However, we need to remember that NBS does not identify all infants with conditions included in the panel, and some patients can be missed. Therefore, a symptomatic patient, at any age, should be investigated despite normal NBS results.

The next section will briefly describe the characteristics of each of the disorders currently included in the RUSP and screened by dry blood spot (DBS), their primary markers, and the secondary markers (ratios) when applicable. The acylcarnitine species are indicated with the letter C followed by a number that indicates the number of carbon atoms of the acyl group esterified with carnitine. The presence of additional functional groups and/or double bonds is indicated as well (eg, C3-carnitine means carnitine esterified with an organic acid of 3 carbon atoms chain length; C5OH-carnitine indicates a 5-carbon atoms organic acid hydroxylated, esterified with carnitine). The US incidence of the conditions listed in the next section is derived from a comprehensive study summarizing 10 years of newborn screen data (2001-2010) and over twenty million infants screened, by the National Newborn Screening Information System (NNSIS).[13]

Disorders Screened for Using Tandem Mass Spectrometry

Propionic Acidemia

Propionyl-CoA is an intermediate in the catabolism of isoleucine, valine, threonine, methionine, pyrimidines (uracil and thymine), and cholesterol, and is the final product of the β-oxidation of odd-chain fatty acids. Propionic acidemia (PA) is a defect of propionate catabolism, caused by a deficient propionyl-CoA carboxylase, which converts propionyl-CoA to methylmalonyl-CoA.[14,15] Lacking enzyme activity, propionyl-CoA and its metabolites accumulate, interfering with several cellular processes, including the mitochondrial energy metabolism and the urea cycle.

The incidence of propionic acidemia in the United States of America is 1:238,000[13] live births, with higher frequencies in other populations, such as 1 in 2,000 to 5,000 in Saudi Arabia.[14-16] Patients with PA typically present in the neonatal period with severe metabolic decompensation, characterized by vomiting, irritability, temperature instability, muscular hypo or hypertonia, seizures, lethargy progressing rapidly to coma, and routine investigations consistent with severe metabolic acidosis, ketonuria, lactic acidemia, and severe hyperammonemia. Late-onset forms with variable clinical presentation have been described. Complications, including cardiomyopathy, renal failure, and pancreatitis, occur frequently with disease progression. Long-term neurodevelopmental outcome is generally poor, and appears influenced by the severity and frequency of the metabolic crises. Emergency treatment during decompensation consists in restricted protein intake, intravenous glucose and lipids to provide calories, insulin (as needed), high dose of carnitine, and extracorporeal detoxification in unresponsive patients. Long-term treatment is based on low-protein diet supplemented with a mixture free of propiogenic amino acids, and carnitine.[15]

Newborn screening: The NBS primary marker for propionic acidemia is C3-carnitine and the ratios C3/C2 and C3/C16 serve as secondary markers. The same markers are elevated in methylmalonic acidemia but higher values are associated with propionic acidemia. Second-tier tests performed on the same blood spot used for the initial screen discriminate between the two conditions by measuring methylmalonic and methylcitric acids,[17,18] where the presence of methylcitric acid without concurrent elevation of methylmalonic acid is suggestive of propionic acidemia.

Diagnosis: Confirmatory tests to follow-up an elevated C3-carnitine in NBS include urine organic acids, plasma acylcarnitines, plasma amino acids, and total plasma homocysteine.[19] Diagnosis is confirmed by analysis of urine organic acids showing elevated concentrations of methylcitric acid with or without other propionate metabolites (3-hydroxypropionic acid, tiglylglycine, propionylglycine). Acylcarnitine analysis shows markedly elevated concentrations of propionylcarnitine and often carnitine deficiency especially if untreated. Similar to the finding in the newborn screen sample, elevated plasma propionylcarnitine can reflect not only propionic acidemia but also methylmalonic acidemia. Therefore, plasma acylcarnitine analysis is supportive of the diagnosis, but not a diagnostic test. Plasma amino acids analysis yields non-specific results, usually hyperglycinemia (even though this is not usually present in newborns), which is also observed in other organic acidurias. Enzymatic studies in white blood cells and/or molecular genetic tests should be performed to confirm the diagnosis.[15]

Methylmalonic Acidemias

There are several enzymatic/transporter defects causing methylmalonic acidemia, they include a primary deficiency of the enzyme methylmalonyl-CoA mutase, converting methylmalonyl-CoA to succinyl-CoA, as well as deficiency of any of the factors involved in the synthesis of adenosylcobal-amin, the cofactor of methylmalonyl-CoA mutase. All of these conditions are characterized by elevated methylmalonic acid in all fluids. The RUSP includes, currently, only methylmalonyl-CoA mutase deficiency and cbl A and cbl B deficiencies (involved in the synthesis of adenosylcobalamin), although deficiencies of other factors involved in the metabolism of vitamin B12, and in the synthesis of adenosylcobalamin and methylcobalamin, can cause methylmalonic acidemia, isolated or combined with homocystinuria. These three conditions (methylmalonyl-CoA mutase, cblA, cbl B deficien-cies) are characterized by isolated elevation of methylmalonic acid in all flu-ids. The incidence of methylmalonyl-CoA mutase deficiency is 1:160,000, the combined incidence of cblA and cblB deficiency is 1:410,000 in the United States of America.[13,20]

Methylmalonic acidemia (Methylmalonyl-CoA mutase deficiency)

Methylmalonyl-CoA mutase deficiency (total, *mut*[0], or partial, *mut*[-], defi-ciency) causes accumulation of methylmalonyl-CoA, the upstream compound propionyl-CoA, and their metabolites, such as methylmalonic acid, 3-hydroxy-propionic acid, methylcitric acid. Most *mut*[0] patients present with neonatal metabolic decompensation, clinically indistinguishable from propionic aci-demia, and similarly require emergency treatment. Rarely, infants with *mut*[-] MMA also present with acute neonatal decompensation; but usually onset of symptoms is later in infancy or childhood, with failure to thrive, hypotonia, and developmental delay.[14,20] These patients are at risk of acute crisis. Out-side of acute episodes, treatment consists in a low-protein, high-calorie diet, restricted in propiogenic amino acids, and supplemented with carnitine and hydroxocobalamin (in vitamin B12 responsive patients). Despite treatment, complications are frequent and include intellectual disability, neurological sequelae, progressive renal failure, pancreatitis, and growth failure.[21,22]

Newborn screening: Similarly to PA, the primary NBS marker for meth-ylmalonyl-CoA mutase deficiency is elevated C3-carnitine with elevated C3/C2 and C3/C16 ratios as secondary markers. Elevated concentrations of methylmalonic acid detected by second-tier tests will discriminate between MMA and PA.[18]

Diagnosis: Markedly elevated concentrations of methylmalonic acid by urine organic acids are diagnostic of methylmalonic acidemia, however, this test cannot discriminate among various types of MMA because of consid-erable overlap. Plasma amino acids and total plasma homocysteine should also be performed to identify cases of combined methylmalonic acidemia/homocystinuria. Establishing the specific defect requires complementation studies in cultured fibroblasts and/or molecular testing using a panel that includes all genes capable of causing elevated methylmalonic acid.

Methylmalonic acidemia (Cbl A, Cbl B)

Cobalamin derivatives are required for the activity of the enzymes methyl-malonyl-CoA mutase (adenosylcobalamin; AdoCbl) and methionine synthase (methylcobalamin; MeCbl). Defects that affect only AdoCbl synthesis cause isolated methylmalonic aciduria (cbl A, cbl B), while defects that affect synthesis of both, AdoCbl and MeCbl, result in combined methylmalonic aciduria and homocystinuria (cbl C, cbl D, cbl F, cbl J, cbl X).[23] Clinical presentation is variable, overlapping to what is seen in methylmalonyl-CoA mutase deficiency patients. Most patients present early with metabolic decompensation, often triggered by catabolic state; however, chronic, progressive forms are observed. Treatment consists of hydroxocobalamin supplementation[24] and a special diet, low in precursor amino acids.

Newborn screening: Elevated C3-carnitine is the primary marker for clblA and cblB deficiencies, in addition to the ratios C3/C2 and C3/C16 as secondary markers. The same markers will identify also other disorders of vitamin B12 metabolism resulting in elevated methylmalonic acid (cbl C, cbl D, cbl F, cbl J, cbl X) although not included in the RUSP.

Diagnosis: Urine organic acids show elevated excretion of methylmalonic acid. Normal total plasma homocysteine will exclude a combined, methyl-malonic acidemia/homocystinuria, defect. Measurement of vitamin B12 level excludes vitamin B12 deficiency. Complementation studies and/or molecular studies are necessary to identify the specific defect.

Isovaleric Acidemia

Isovaleric acidemia (IVA) is caused by a deficiency of isovaleryl-CoA dehy-drogenase, in the leucine catabolic pathway. IVA incidence is estimated at 1:159,150 births.[13] Patients can present with severe, neonatal metabolic acidosis and hyperammonemia, fatal if left untreated; milder forms of the disease present with vomiting and failure to thrive, that can evolve into acute presentation when triggered by stressors like illnesses. Treatment with a low-protein diet, glycine and carnitine supplements greatly improves outcome. Metabolic decompensation may occur at any age, and it remains life threatening.[25]

Newborn screening: The primary NBS marker for IVA is elevated C5-carnitine. Several ratios, such as C5/C0, C5/C2, and C5/C3, are also elevated and can be used as secondary markers. C5-carnitine is also elevated in 2-methylbutyrylglycinuria, a disorder of isoleucine catabolism, which is part of the secondary conditions panel. The two conditions cannot be distinguished at the newborn screening level unless an appropriate second tier test is performed. Certain medications (antibiotics) can also result in elevated C5-carnitine, usually to a lower degree than what is observed in IVA. Recently, the use of topical creams/ointments used by nursing mothers and containing pivalic acid (neopentanoic acid) has been responsible for cases of elevated C5-carnitine.[26]

Diagnosis: Follow-up tests for an elevated C5-carnitine on NBS include urine organic acids, urine acylglycines, and plasma acylcarnitines.[19] The diagnosis of IVA is confirmed by urine organic acid analysis showing elevated excretion of isovalerylglycine and 3-hydroxyisovaleric acid. In several patients identified by newborn screening, excretion of isovalerylglycine is only moderately elevated, possibly because of a milder form of the disease.[25] If urine organic acids are normal, 2-methylbutyrylglycinuria is not excluded, as 2-methylbutyrylglycine is not efficiently extracted with the most conventional organic acids extraction methods. Analysis of acylglycines is a more sensitive and specific tests to exclude 2-methylbutyrylglycinuria and also to evaluate milder forms of isovaleric acidemia.

3-Methylcrotonyl-CoA Carboxylase Deficiency

3-Methylcrotonyl-CoA carboxylase (MCC) deficiency is caused by the deficiency of a biotin-dependent carboxylase involved in leucine catabolism. It is one of the most frequent conditions identified by NBS, with an incidence of 1:38,636.[13] The phenotype is highly variable ranging from severe neonatal onset with severe neurological involvement to asymptomatic adults. However, its clinical significance is still unclear, since only about 10% of patients develop symptoms.[27] Therapy consists of carnitine supplementation and fasting avoidance.

Newborn screening: The primary NBS marker for 3MCC deficiency is elevated C5OH-carnitine, with elevated C5OH/C8 and C5OH/C0 ratios used as secondary markers. However, C5OH is not a marker specific for 3MCC, in fact it is a marker for multiple conditions, several of them included in the RUSP. Asymptomatic 3MCC-deficient mothers can be identified because of elevated C5OH-carnitine in their infants' newborn screen sample.

Diagnosis: Follow-up tests for elevated C5OH-carnitine on NBS include urine organic acids and plasma acylcarnitines.[19] Diagnosis of 3MCC is made by urine organic acid analysis, detecting elevated excretion of 3-hydroxyisovaleric acid and 3-methylcrotonylglycine. Infants of mothers with 3MCC will have elevated C5OH-carnitine on NBS and may have abnormal confirmatory tests (urine organic acids and plasma acylcarnitines) as well, especially, if breast-fed. Therefore, maternal 3-MCC deficiency should always be excluded.

3-Hydroxy-3-Methylglutaric Aciduria

3-Hydroxy-3-methylglutaric aciduria is caused by the deficiency of an enzyme involved in leucine catabolism and ketone synthesis, 3-hydroxy-3-methylglutaryl-coenzyme A (HMG-CoA) lyase. In this condition, the conversion of

3-hydroxy-3-methylglutaryl-CoA, derived from the catabolism of leucine, in acetoacetic acid and acetyl-CoA by the enzyme HMG-CoA lyase is impaired. Its incidence is low in the general population (1:1,528,519)[13]; however, its frequency is very high in the Portuguese population.[28] Patients usually present in the neonatal period with episodes of life-threatening metabolic acidosis with hyperammonemia and hypoketotic hypoglycemia. Treatment consists in avoidance of fasting, carnitine supplementation,[29] and leucine restricted diet in some cases.

Newborn screening: The primary NBS marker for 3-hydroxy-3-methylglutaric aciduria is elevated C5OH-carnitine. C6DC-carnitine may be elevated, even though not all programs monitor this acylcarnitine species.

Diagnosis: Several analytes are detected by urine organic acid analysis in these patients: 3-hydroxy-3-methylglutaric, 3-hydroxyisovaleric, 3-methylglutaric, and 3-methylglutaconic acids. Moderate elevations of C5OH-carnitine and C6DC-carnitine can be detected in plasma by acylcarnitine analysis. Molecular testing should be used to confirm diagnosis.

Multiple Carboxylase Deficiency

Multiple carboxylase deficiency (MCD) is caused by defects in enzymes involved in the biotin cycle: holocarboxylase synthetase and biotinidase. Both of these enzyme deficiencies are included in the RUSP. Holocarboxylase synthetase covalently binds biotin to the biotin-dependent enzymes, acetyl-coA carboxylase, pyruvate carboxylase, propionyl-CoA carboxylase, and 3-methylcrotonyl-CoA carboxylase. Holocarboxylase synthase deficiency is very rare, with an incidence of 1:1,927,913.[13] Patients present with the early-onset variant of multiple carboxylase deficiency, characterized by severe metabolic acidosis, hyperammonemia, tachypnea, feeding problems, hypotonia, seizures, developmental delay, skin rash, alopecia. Treatment consists in high-dose biotin supplementation.[30]

Newborn screening: C5OH-carnitine is the primary NBS marker for holocarboxylase synthase deficiency. C3-carnitine may also be mildly elevated.

Diagnosis: Urinary organic acids analysis shows several diagnostic analytes related to the impaired function of the affected carboxylases, such as 3-hydroxyisovalerate, 3-hydroxypropionate, methylcitrate, tiglylglycine, and 3-methylcrotonylglycine. However, urine organic acids findings vary among patients. Normal serum biotinidase, and decreased activity of all carboxylases (propionyl-CoA carboxylase, pyruvate carboxylase, 3-methylcrotonyl-CoA carboxylase) in leukocytes or fibroblasts should be assessed to confirm the diagnosis. Molecular testing is also available.

β-Ketothiolase Deficiency

β-Ketothiolase deficiency is caused by the deficiency of a mitochondrial enzyme involved in isoleucine catabolism and ketolysis. Its incidence is estimated at 1:2,010,308.[13] Clinically, it is characterized by intermittent keto-acidotic episodes triggered by infections or fasting. The treatment for the disorder includes avoidance of fasting, cornstarch supplements, and carnitine supplementation.[31]

Newborn screening: The primary NBS marker for β-ketothiolase deficiency is C5OH-carnitine usually accompanied by elevated C5:1-carnitine (not monitored in all programs). Milder cases of this condition can be missed by NBS.

Diagnosis: Detection of tiglylglycine, 2-methyl-3-hydroxybutyrate (2M3HB), and 2-methylacetoacetate by urine organic acid analysis is diagnostic of this condition. Molecular testing is necessary to confirm the diagnosis as metabolic abnormalities might disappear in well controlled patients.

Glutaric Acidemia Type I

Glutaric acidemia type 1 (GA-1) is caused by a deficiency of glutaryl-CoA dehydrogenase, an enzyme involved in the degradation of lysine, hydroxylysine, and tryptophan. Patients may present at birth with mild hypotonia and macrocephaly.[32] Metabolic decompensation, usually triggered by fever or other illnesses, can result in acute dystonia, spasticity, hypotonia, and seizures. After a crisis, brain imaging demonstrates degeneration of the basal ganglia superimposed to frontotemporal atrophy.[32,33] Subdural hematomas and retinal hemorrhages can also be part of the symptomatic presentation of glutaric acidemia type I, sometimes leading to suspicion of child abuse. Treatment consists of a diet restricted in lysine and tryptophan and carnitine supplementation. The outcome in patients identified by NBS who did not suffer any metabolic decompensation is excellent.[33]

Newborn screening: The primary NBS marker for GA-1 is elevated C5DC-carnitine with elevated C5DC/C5OH, C5DC/C8, and C5D/C16 ratios used as secondary markers.

Diagnosis: Follow-up confirmatory tests for elevated C5DC-carnitine in NBS include urine organic acids, plasma acylcarnitines, and urine glutaryl-carnitine.[19] GA-1 diagnosis is confirmed by urine organic acids detecting 3-hydroxyglutaric acid, usually accompanied by elevated excretion of glutaric acid, and plasma acylcarnitines confirming elevated C5DC-carnitine. However, there are patients with only minimally elevated or normal urine glutaric acid (low excretors) and 3-hydroxyglutaric acid, in which plasma acylcarnitines may also be normal.[32] In these patients, measurement of urinary glutarylcarnitine is more sensitive and specific and will result in significantly elevated glutarylcarnitine.[34] Enzyme assay in cultured fibroblasts and/or molecular testing should be pursued, especially in low excretors to confirm the diagnosis.

Carnitine Uptake Defect/Carnitine Transport Defect

Carnitine uptake defect (CUD), or primary carnitine deficiency, is caused by the deficiency of the carnitine transporter OCTN2 (organic cation transporter novel 2) that mediates the carnitine re-uptake in the kidneys. Patients with primary carnitine deficiency lose 50-95% of filtered carnitine in urine, and consequently present very low levels in serum (0 to 9 μmol/L, markedly reduced compared to the lower limit of the reference intervals ranging from 15 to 25 μmol/L depending on age).[16] Primary carnitine deficiency has an incidence of 1:142,236 in the general population.[13] Patients typically present with hepatic encephalopathy or cardiomyopathy, often triggered by fasting or infection. Asymptomatic patients have been described. These patients are, however, at risk of sudden death. Therapy consists of high-dose carnitine supplementation.[35]

Newborn screening: The primary NBS marker for primary carnitine deficiency is low free carnitine (C0), with low concentrations of long-chain acylcarnitine species as secondary markers. Low carnitine concentrations can also be seen in infants of mothers with primary or secondary carnitine deficiency. Therefore, appropriate follow-up of an abnormally low free carnitine in a newborn screen sample includes testing of the mother in addition to the infant.

Diagnosis: Follow-up confirmatory tests for low free carnitine in NBS include evaluation of plasma and urine free and total carnitine.[19] Total and free carnitine levels in plasma are remarkably low, with urinary levels of carnitine that are normal or elevated. Diagnosis is confirmed by demonstrating reduced carnitine transport (<15% of normal) in skin fibroblasts and/or by molecular testing. Routine laboratory studies show hypoketotic hypoglycemia and hyperammonemia in symptomatic patients. In the mother, measurement of free and total carnitine in plasma and urine (to estimate reabsorption), plasma acylcarnitines profile and urine organic acids can exclude primary or secondary carnitine deficiency.

Medium-chain Acyl-CoA Dehydrogenase Deficiency

Medium-chain acyl-CoA dehydrogenase (MCAD) deficiency is the most common disorder of fatty acid oxidation in Caucasians, with an incidence of 1:17,759.[13] The enzymatic defect results in impaired β-oxidation of medium-chain fatty acids. Symptoms of the disease are variable, from completely asymptomatic patients to those with hypoglycemic crises under fasting or illness, leading to lethargy, seizures, brain damage, or sudden death. Treatment consists in avoidance of fasting, low-fat diet, carnitine supplementation, and institution of an emergency plan in case of illness or other metabolic stress.[36]

Newborn screening: The primary marker for MCAD deficiency is elevated C8-carnitine with elevations of C6-carnitine, C10-carnitine, and C10:1-carnitine to a lower degree.

Diagnosis: Follow-up confirmatory tests for elevated C8-carnitine in NBS include plasma acylcarnitines, urine organic acids, and urine acylglycines.[19] Diagnosis is confirmed by plasma acylcarnitine analysis, which will show elevated medium chain acylcarnitine species (C6, C8, C10) with C8-carnitine being the highest, and by urine organic acids and acylglycine analyses showing increased excretion of dicarboxylic acids (adipic, suberic, sebacic), hexanoylglycine and suberylglycine, without excess ketones. When patients are metabolically stable, the urinary concentration of these analytes is greatly reduced and urine organic acids and urine acylglycines may be normal; however, plasma acylcarnitine profile is almost always abnormal. About 98% of symptomatic patients carry at least one copy of the common p.K304E mutation in the *ACADM* gene. Molecular testing is routinely used to confirm the diagnosis.

Very Long-chain Acyl-CoA Dehydrogenase Deficiency

Very long-chain acyl-CoA dehydrogenase (VLCAD) deficiency is due to a defect in the first step of fatty acid β-oxidation. The severity of the phenotype is variable. VLCAD deficiency may present as (a) an early-onset severe form with hypoglycemia, hepatic insufficiency, hypertrophic cardiomyopathy, and arrhythmias; (b) a childhood-onset form with a milder phenotype mainly characterized by hypoketotic hypoglycemia; or (c) a late-onset form with muscle weakness and recurrent episodes of rhabdomyolysis after exercise or illness. VLCAD deficiency incidence is estimated at 1:63,481.[13] Untreated VLCAD deficiency may lead to sudden death due to cardiac and/or hepatic involvement. Avoidance of fasting and a low-fat diet containing most of the fats as medium chain triglycerides, if started early, improve the clinical course.[37]

Newborn screening: C14:1-carnitine is the primary NBS marker for VLCAD deficiency, accompanied usually by elevation of C14-carnitine, C14:2-carnitine, and other long-chain acylcarnitine species. Carriers for VLCAD deficiency may show mild elevations of the same markers. Infants with VLCAD deficiency may show an abnormal concentration of the primary and secondary markers only in the first few days of life, when they are still under the metabolic stress of birth. The acylcarnitine profile often normalizes as they become metabolically stable.

Diagnosis: Plasma acylcarnitine analysis is the biochemical confirmatory test used for the diagnosis of VLCAD deficiency. However, because metabolically stable patients can have a normal result, a normal result does not exclude the diagnosis and enzyme assay or fatty acid oxidation studies in vitro, and/or molecular analysis of the VLCAD (*ACADVL*) gene[38] should always be pursued in presence of elevated C14:1-carnitine in NBS.

Long-chain L-3 Hydroxyacyl-CoA Dehydrogenase Deficiency and Trifunctional Protein Deficiency

The trifunctional protein is a multi-enzyme complex that harbors the activities of the second and third steps of fatty acid β-oxidation, long-chain enoyl-CoA hydratase (LCEH) and long-chain 3-hydroxy-acyl-CoA dehydrogenase (LCHAD), and the activity of long-chain 3-oxoacyl-CoA dehydrogenase (LCKAT), which catalyzes the last step in β-oxidation of long-chain fatty acids. The trifunctional protein complex is encoded by 2 separate genes. Mutations in either gene may cause complete TFP deficiency. A genotype-phenotype correlation has emerged for TFP deficiency, with residual enzyme activity being associated with a milder, later-onset phenotype.

Mutations in the catalytic domain of the long-chain 3-hydroxy-acyl-CoA dehydrogenase, which is part of the trifunctional protein, cause isolated LCHAD deficiency. LCHAD deficiency and trifunctional protein deficiency are biochemically very similar. Three clinical phenotypes are known: (1) a severe neonatal presentation with cardiomyopathy, hypoglycemia, hepatic insufficiency, and early death; (2) a hepatic form with recurrent hypoketotic hypoglycemia; and (3) a milder, later-onset neuromyopathic phenotype with episodic myoglobinuria. Patients with LCHAD/TFP deficiencies may also develop pigmentary retinopathy and peripheral neuropathy, whose pathophysiology remains obscure. In addition, mothers of these patients can have significant complications with acute fatty liver of pregnancy or hemolysis, elevated liver enzymes, and low platelet (HELLP) syndrome, possibly due to the transplacental passage of 3-OH-fatty acids and related acylcarnitines.[39] This complication occurs in mothers independently of the fetal phenotype.[40]

Therapy for these conditions consists in avoidance of fasting, prompt treatment of infection, and a low-fat diet with most calories provided by medium-chain triglycerides. Low-dose carnitine supplements (25 mg/kg/d) may be given. The incidence of LCHAD deficiency is 1:363,738 births[13] and the incidence of TFP deficiency is 1:1,822,568 births.[13]

Newborn screening: The primary NBS marker for LCHAD and TFP deficiencies is C16:OH-carnitine with or without elevated C18:1-OH-carnitine.

Diagnosis: Follow-up confirmatory tests for an elevated C16:OH-carnitine in NBS include plasma acylcarnitines and urine organic acids. Plasma acylcarnitine profile confirms the diagnosis of LCHAD/TFP deficiency by showing elevations of long-chain hydroxylated species. Urine organic acids collected at the time of an acute episode show hypoketotic C6-C10-dicarboxylic aciduria and C6-C14-3-hydroxydicarboxylic aciduria with prominent unsaturated species. Concentrations of urine organic acids rapidly normalize with therapy and fall within the reference interval in asymptomatic patients. Diagnostic confirmation requires sequencing of the two genes encoding for the two subunits of the trifunctional protein (*HADHA* and *HADHB*).

Argininosuccinic Aciduria

Argininosuccinic aciduria is caused by the deficiency of the urea cycle enzyme argininosuccinate lyase (ASL) that catalyzes the conversion of argininosuccinic acid (ASA) to arginine and fumarate. Similar to other urea cycle defects, ASL deficiency compromises hepatic ureagenesis, causing hyperammonemia. Additionally, the metabolic block has a complex effect on other cellular processes, because of the argininosuccinate accumulation, which may cause direct hepatic injury, and the deficiency of arginine and its downstream metabolites, such as nitric oxide.[41] The incidence of this condition is estimated to be 1:305,032 live births.[13] Clinically, it can present (1) early as severe, neonatal hyperammonemia that can progress, if untreated, to coma and death or (2) late (with or without hyperammonemia) with neurocognitive deficiencies (intellectual disability, behavioral abnormalities, seizures), liver disease (hepatitis, cirrhosis), and systemic hypertension.[42] Treatment of the acute hyperammonemia consists of promptly discontinuing protein intake, providing calories as intravenous glucose and lipids, supplementing with high-dose arginine and using ammonia scavengers (benzoate, phenylacetate, phenylbutyrate). The long-term therapy comprises a protein restricted diet, phenylbutyrate therapy, and oral arginine supplementation.[42,43]

Newborn screening: The primary NBS marker for argininosuccinic aciduria is elevated citrulline, with elevated argininosuccinic acid, ASA, (although this marker is not widely used) and elevated citrulline/arginine ratio as secondary marker. Elevated citrulline is a primary marker for other conditions, such as citrullinemia type 1 (ASS deficiency), lysinuric protein intolerance,[44-46] and citrullinemia type 2 (citrin deficiency), the latter two conditions not included in the RUSP, however ASA is specific for argininosuccinic aciduria.

Diagnosis: Follow-up confirmatory tests for elevated citrulline (with or without elevated ASA) in NBS include plasma and urine amino acids and urine orotic acid. Argininosuccinic aciduria is confirmed by the detection of ASA in patients' plasma and urine by amino acid analysis. Plasma citrulline is also usually high, while arginine is low; additionally, elevated concentrations of plasma glutamine and alanine may be present and indicate hyperammonemia, a common finding in all urea cycle defects. Orotic aciduria can be observed in this condition.[46] The ASL enzyme assay requires a liver biopsy, and is usually not performed. DNA sequencing of the gene (*ASL*) confirms the diagnosis.

Citrullinemia Type 1

Citrullinemia type 1 is caused by the deficiency of the enzyme argininosuccinate synthetase (ASS) that catalyzes the conversion of citrulline and aspartate to argininosuccinate. Deficiency of this enzyme results in a block of the third, rate-limiting step of the urea cycle with consequent hyperammonemia, accumulation of the substrate citrulline, and deficiency of the downstream product, arginine. Citrullinemia type I incidence is estimated at 1:155,679 births.[13] Most patients present during the early neonatal period with severe hyperammonemia. The direct toxic effects of ammonia on the brain together with the brain edema caused by accumulation of glutamine/glutamate lead to (1) poor feeding, (2) vomiting, (3) lethargy, or (4) irritability progressing to coma and death.[47,48] In milder cases when there is residual enzyme activity, patients can present in infancy with failure to thrive, behavioral problems, protein aversion, and non-specific gastrointestinal symptoms. Some late-onset patients can remain asymptomatic until an episode of metabolic decompensation with severe encephalopathy triggered by excess protein intake or catabolic state. Treatment consists in dietary protein restriction, nitrogen scavengers (phenylbutyrate), and arginine supplementation.[48]

Newborn screening: The primary NBS marker for citrullinemia type I is elevated citrulline with elevated citrulline/arginine ratio as secondary marker. Elevated citrulline is also observed in citrullinemia type 2, lysinuric protein intolerance, and in ASA deficiency; however, citrulline levels tend to be the highest in citrullinemia type 1.

Diagnosis: Markedly elevated plasma citrulline by amino acid analysis is diagnostic for this condition. Milder forms of citrullinemia type 1, characterized by mild increases in plasma citrulline, are also identified by NBS; therefore, DNA testing should be used to confirm or exclude the diagnosis. Urine amino acids are used to exclude argininosuccinic aciduria and lysinuric protein intolerance, which may result in mildly elevated citrulline.

Maple Syrup Urine Disease

A defect in any of the components of the branched-chain alpha-keto acid dehydrogenase complex (BCKDC), which catalyzes the catabolism of the branched-chain amino acids, leucine, isoleucine, and valine, causes maple syrup urine disease (MSUD). MSUD has an incidence of 1:197,714 live births.[13] This complex is composed of four subunits: E1α, E1β, E2, and E3. The E3 subunit is shared by two other dehydrogenases: pyruvate dehydrogenase and 2-oxoglutarate dehydrogenase. Several forms of this disease may occur, depending on the severity of the mutations: (1) the classic form, which is the most severe, is characterized by very high plasma concentrations of branched-chain amino acids; (2) thiamine-responsive MSUD,[49] with a milder phenotype responsive to pharmacological doses of thiamine, a cofactor of the BCKD complex; (3) intermediate or intermittent forms triggered by high consumption of proteins or catabolic state (in which endogenous proteins released mostly by the muscle are degraded to produce energy); and (4) E3 deficiency seen with combined deficiency of pyruvate and 2-oxoglutarate dehydrogenase.[50] Classic MSUD presents with poor feeding and vomiting in the first 2 weeks of life followed by lethargy and coma within a few days. Leucine accumulates within the brain, causing cerebral edema, which is responsible for the progressive worsening of neurologic symptoms. Some patients with significant residual enzyme activity have recurrent episodes of vomiting or a neurologic presentation (developmental delays, seizures) even after 1 year of age with no acute event. Other patients have intermittent episodes of acute decompensation with vomiting, ataxia, and lethargy progressing to coma.[50] Treatment includes dietary restriction of branched-chain amino acids, high-dose thiamine (in responsive cases), valine, and isoleucine supplements. Acute episodes are life threatening and require aggressive treatment of brain edema.

Newborn screening: The primary NBS marker for MSUD is elevated leucine with normal concentrations of other amino acids (such as phenylalanine) whose metabolism is not affected and elevated ratio leucine/alanine as secondary marker. Leucine is isomeric with isoleucine and allo-isoleucine and isobaric with hydroxyproline. These amino acids cannot be resolved by routine NBS, a second tier test can distinguish all amino acids. Presence of elevated allo-isoleucine is diagnostic for MSUD in addition to elevated leucine.

Diagnosis: Follow-up confirmatory tests for elevated leucine/isoleucine in NBS include plasma amino acids and urine organic acids.[19] Diagnosis is confirmed by the detection of elevated leucine (usually the prominent amino acid), isoleucine, and valine, in addition to the pathognomonic presence of L-alloisoleucine. Urine organic acids show the presence of characteristic branched-chain ketoacids, 2-ketomethylvaleric acid, 2-keto-isovaleric acid, 2-ketoisocaproic acid, and increased excretion of 2-hydroxyisovaleric acid. The characteristic organic acid pattern is more evident during episodes of metabolic decompensation, when patients are stable excess excretion of 2-hydroxyisovalerate may be the only abnormal finding.

Homocystinuria

Homocystinuria, characterized by increased concentrations of the sulfur-containing amino acid homocystine in blood and urine, is caused by at least seven genetically different disorders that affect the methylation cycle and the transsulfuration pathway. The most common form, classic homocystinuria, is caused by reduced activity of cystathionine-β-synthase, an enzyme in the transsulfuration pathway. This is the condition included in the RUSP. The other causes of homocystinuria are part of the secondary conditions panel. The incidence classic homocystinuria in the United States is 1:456,726 births.[13] Clinical manifestations are non-specific at first, including failure to thrive and developmental delay. Later, patients present with (1) ophthalmologic problems (lens dislocation), (2) bone abnormalities, (3) osteoporosis, (4) mental retardation, and (5) psychiatric disturbances. Therapy for classic homocystinuria requires high doses of pyridoxine (cystathionine-β-synthase cofactor), a special diet low in methionine, and betaine supplementation.

Newborn screening: The primary NBS marker for classic homocystinuria is elevated methionine. Methionine is also increased in liver disease, in diets rich in proteins, and in other rarer disorders of sulfur amino acid metabolism. Defects in re-methylation of homocysteine could potentially be identified during NBS by very low concentrations of methionine, but most screening programs do not screen for them.

Diagnosis: Follow-up confirmatory tests for elevated methionine in NBS include plasma amino acids and total plasma homocysteine.[19] The biochemical diagnosis is obtained by showing increased plasma methionine (especially in children) and the presence of the disulfide homocystine in plasma amino acids. Total plasma homocysteine (measured after release of the protein-bound homocysteine) is also markedly increased in this condition. Definitive confirmation of the diagnosis requires molecular testing. For disorders of homocysteine remethylation, characterized by low plasma methionine, elevated homocystine, and elevated total plasma homocysteine, evaluation of urine, and plasma methylmalonic acid is also recommended to exclude a combined methylmalonic aciduria/homocystinuria. Complementation studies in fibroblasts may be required to identify the specific defect. Molecular testing using a panel of genes is also available and rapidly becoming the first approach to confirmation of diagnosis.

Classic Phenylketonuria (PKU)

Classic phenylketonuria is caused by the profound deficiency of the enzyme phenylalanine hydroxylase (PAH) that converts phenylalanine to tyrosine. Approximately 2% of the cases of PKU identified by NBS in the United States are due to defect in the biosynthesis or recycling of tetrahydrobiopterin (BH_4), the cofactor of PAH.[51] Overall the incidence of these conditions is 1:16,500.[13] The accumulation of phenylalanine and the deficiency of tyrosine, a precursor of neurotransmitters, lead to the clinical symptoms of PKU: intellectual disability, developmental delay, chronic eczema, acquired microcephaly.[51] In patients with PKU due to phenylalanine hydroxylase deficiency, dietary treatment with a special formula without phenylalanine and low-protein foods should be started as soon as possible, ideally before 3 weeks of age. Treatment needs to be continued for life. Phenylalanine concentrations are monitored periodically and should remain between 60 and 360 µmol/L (reference interval: 30 to 80 µmol/L). Patients with hyperphenylalaninemia due to a deficiency of biosynthesis or recycling of BH_4 require treatment with BH_4 and neurotransmitter precursors, since BH_4 is also a cofactor for tyrosine and tryptophan hydroxylases. Many infants with BH_4 deficiencies can have neurologic involvement despite adequate dietary control of phenylalanine concentrations.[52]

Newborn screening: The primary NBS marker for phenylketonuria, benign hyperphenylalaninemia and biopterin defects is elevated phenylalanine with elevated phenylalanine/tyrosine ratio as secondary marker.

Diagnosis: Follow-up confirmatory tests for elevated phenylalanine in NBS include plasma amino acids. The diagnosis of phenylketonuria/hyperphenylalaninemia is made by the elevated plasma concentration of phenylalanine with low or normal tyrosine. Benign hyperphenylalaninemia (phenylalanine <360 µmol/L) due to partial deficiency of phenylalanine hydroxylase can also be identified by NBS. These patients remain healthy without dietary treatment but need to be monitored periodically. The possibility of an underlying cofactor deficiency (disorders of biopterin metabolism) should always be ruled out in all infants with an elevated phenylalanine by measuring urine pterins and red blood cells DHPR (dihydropteridine reductase) activity. DNA testing is used to confirm the presence of mutations in the *PAH* gene.

Tyrosinemia Type 1

Tyrosinemia type 1 is due to impaired activity of the enzyme fumarylacetoacetate hydrolase. The incidence of this condition in the United States is 1:781,144[13] with a higher frequency of 1:16,000 in the region of Quebec (Canada).[53] The enzymatic block results in accumulation of succinylacetone, the by-product of fumarylacetoacetic acid, which is the intermediate immediately upstream of the enzyme defect. The clinical presentation is characterized by severe liver involvement, failure to thrive, renal Fanconi syndrome and rickets. Patients also have peripheral neuropathy mimicking acute intermittent porphyria, caused by the inhibition of the enzyme δ-aminolevulinic acid (ALA) dehydratase. Untreated patients develop liver cirrhosis and liver cancer.[53]

Therapy consists of a diet low in tyrosine and phenylalanine (the precursor of tyrosine) and NTBC [2-(2-nitro-4-trifluoro-methylbenzoyl)-1, 3-cyclohexanedione], an inhibitor of 4-hydroxyphenylpyruvate dioxygenase, that prevents the synthesis of succinylacetone. The adequacy of the diet is monitored by plasma amino acids. Measurement of alpha fetoprotein is also used to monitor these patients, because liver cancer is a complication of this condition. Liver transplantation is indicated in patients who progress to liver failure and in those with liver cancer.[54]

Newborn screening: The primary NBS marker for tyrosinemia type I is succinylacetone,[55-57] because tyrosine may or may not be elevated at the time of the NBS sample collection.[58] Elevated tyrosine is a primary marker for tyrosinemia type II and III, which are part of the secondary conditions panel (Table 5-1). Transient tyrosinemia of the newborn due to immaturity of a specific enzyme in the tyrosine catabolic pathway, is the most common cause of elevated tyrosine in NBS, however succinylacetone in tyrosinemia type II,

III, and in transient tyrosinemia of the newborn is normal. The incidence of tyrosinemia type I in the United States was obtained using tyrosine and several cases have been missed using this marker. Detection is now improving since most screening labs are changing to succinylacetone.

Diagnosis: Follow-up confirmatory tests for elevated succinylacetone (with or without elevated tyrosine) in NBS include plasma amino acids, plasma alpha-fetoprotein, and urine organic acids. Tyrosinemia type I is confirmed by the detection in urine organic acids of succinylacetone (4,6-dioxanehepta-noic acid). Succinylacetone disappears almost immediately after initiation of treatment with NTBC. Elevated plasma tyrosine can also be present, but this elevation usually is not as marked as in patients with other forms of tyrosinemia. Elevated tyrosine is seen in (1) other forms of tyrosinemia (tyrosinemia types II and III), (2) transient tyrosinemia of the newborn, (3) prematurity, (4) hepatocellular dysfunction of almost any cause (including that caused by gluconeogenesis disorders, galactosemia, fructosemia, peroxisomal disorders, or mitochondrial DNA depletion syndrome), and (5) diets very rich in proteins. Molecular testing is available to confirm the diagnosis of tyrosinemia type I. Molecular testing is also the test of choice to confirm or exclude tyrosinemia type II and type III.

Disorders not Screened by MS/MS or Recently Added to the RUSP

Classic Galactosemia

Classic galactosemia is the only disorder of carbohydrate metabolism included in the RUSP. The enzymatic defect impairs the metabolism of galactose and it is due to deficiency of galactose-1-phosphate uridyltransferase. Galactose is derived from the disaccharide lactose found predominantly in milk and dairy products and it is, therefore, one of the major nutrients in newborns and infants. The metabolism of galactose starts with a phosphorylation step to galactose-1-phosphate by the enzyme galactokinase. Galactose-1-phosphate is then converted by the enzyme galactose-1-phosphate uridyltransferase to UDP-galactose, which is in turn converted back to UDP-glucose by the enzyme galactose-epimerase. In classic galactosemia, galactose is phosphorylated to galactose-1-phosphate, but it is not further metabolized. Elevated concentration of galactose-1-phosphate in cells is toxic. Infants have (1) failure to thrive, (2) jaundice, (3) liver failure, and (4) predisposition to infections with *E. coli* and other Gram-negative bacteria that can cause death.

The treatment of galactosemia involves removal of lactose (contained in human or animal-derived milk, but not in soy milk) and avoidance of all foods containing galactose. In classic galactosemia, intervention early in life provides the best prognosis although some long-lasting effects may continue to be observed, particularly in girls who for unknown reasons develop ovarian failure. Learning disorders are occasionally observed in treated individuals as well. The United States incidence of classic galactosemia is 1:53,554.[13]

Newborn screening: NBS for galactosemia primarily targets the most severe form of the disease, classic galactosemia due to galactose-1-phosphate uridyltransferase deficiency. However, because of the instability of the enzyme, individuals with benign Duarte variant galactosemia are often identified in NBS. The most widely used method of screening uses a fluorescent procedure to measure galactose-1-phosphate uridyltransferase activity in dried blood spots. Low enzyme activity results are followed up with confirmatory tests to distinguish between classic galactosemia and Duarte variant galactosemia. Some programs use screening protocols that include other techniques (microbiological) to test for total galactose (galactose+galactose-1-phosphate), followed by GALT enzyme activity, if abnormal (elevated). Elevated total galactose with normal GALT activity can be seen in galactokinase deficiency and UDP-galactose-4-epimerase deficiency. Additional biochemical and molecular tests are available to confirm the presence of these conditions which are included in the RUSP secondary conditions panel.

Diagnosis: The diagnosis of classic galactosemia is confirmed by measurement of the enzyme, galactose-1-phosphate uridyltransferase, in red blood cells and mutational analysis of the *GALT* gene.

Galactokinase and galactose epimerase deficiencies are confirmed by measurement of enzyme activity in red blood cells and/or by molecular testing.

Biotinidase Deficiency

Biotinidase is the enzyme involved in the recycling of biotin, making it available for activation of the 4 mammalian carboxylases: acetyl-CoA, pyruvate, propionyl-CoA, and 3-methylcrotonyl-CoA. Biotinidase deficiency is an autosomal recessive condition due to impaired activity of this enzyme. There are two forms of biotinidase deficiency, profound, in which the enzyme activity is less than 10% of normal controls, and partial deficiency, in which the activity of the enzyme is 10-30% of normal controls. Clinical symptoms of profound biotinidase deficiency include neurological features, such as hypotonia, lethargy, seizures, ataxia, optic atrophy, hearing loss, and intellectual disability, as well as cutaneous manifestations, such as eczema, alopecia, and conjunctivitis.[59] Patients with partial biotinidase deficiency may develop milder symptoms. Treatment with biotin can prevent all of these manifestations if started before irreversible damage has occurred. The US incidence of profound biotinidase deficiency is 1:67,766, while the incidence of partial biotinidase deficiency is 1:24,957.[13]

Newborn screening: The screening method is based on direct measurement of biotinidase activity using a colorimetric assay. The test can be qualitative, reporting results as negative or positive, or semi-quantitative reporting values for enzyme activity. Prematurity and/or mishandling of the samples (exposure to heat) can lead to false positive results (low enzyme activity).[60]

Diagnosis: Profound or partial biotinidase deficiencies are diagnosed by measurement of enzyme activity in serum. Because of the instability of the enzyme, it is recommended to collect blood from an unrelated control at the same time blood is collected for confirmation of the diagnosis. The two samples should be handled at the same time and in the same way. This can help in identifying mishandling of the specimen. Alternatively, parental testing concurrently with patient's testing can be performed. Molecular testing by targeted sequencing or full gene sequencing of the *BTD* gene is also helpful in distinguishing individuals with partial or profound biotinidase deficiency as well as carriers.[61]

Hemoglobinopathies (Sickle Cell Disease)

Hemoglobinopathies represent a major health problem in the United States and worldwide. Sickle cell disease (SCD) is the most frequent among them. Its incidence is 1:500 in African-Americans and 1:36,000 in Hispanic-Americans. In certain populations (Mediterranean, Middle Eastern, Indian, Caribbean, Central and South American ancestry) the incidence is also increased. The term SCD includes a group of disorders, inherited in an autosomal recessive pattern, associated with pathogenic mutations in the beta-hemoglobin gene (HBB) resulting in abnormal hemoglobin (hemoglobin S), which causes distortion of the red blood cells to a "sickle" shape. Normal hemoglobin is a heterotetramer composed of two α-hemoglobin and two β-hemoglobin chains. Hemoglobin S (sickle) derives from a point mutation in the β-hemoglobin gene leading to a glutamine to valine substitution. Sickle cell anemia (homozygous hemoglobin SS) represents 60-70% of SCD, other SCDs are due to coexistence of hemoglobin S and other variants of the β-hemoglobin chain. The most common are sickle-hemoglobin C disease (Hb SC) and sickle- β-thalassemia (Hb Sβ°- and Hb Sβ⁺-thalassemia).

The severity of the disease depends on the genotype. Clinically, SCDs are characterized by anemia, vaso-occlusive pain crisis, chest pain, stroke, multiorgan damage, and, in infants, increased susceptibility to pneumococcal infections. The management of these patients consists in prevention and supportive therapy (hydration, anti-inflammatory drugs, pain medications, transfusions).[62] Hematopoietic cell transplantation for SCD is a therapeutic option, although not often used because of availability of donors, risk associated with the procedure, and cost.[63]

Newborn screening: NBS for SCDs is performed using two methodologies, isoelectrofocusing (IEF) and high-performance liquid chromatography (HPLC). Both methods have high sensitivity and specificity for detecting abnormal hemoglobin. Hemoglobin is usually expressed as a percentage and in the order of abundance, for example, if a NBS result is "FAS", it means that in that particular sample, HbF is greater than HbA, which is greater than HbS. HbF at birth is the predominant form, therefore most newborns will have a "FA" pattern. Several factors may affect the results of the NBS and they have to be taken into account when interpreting NBS results.[64] Premature infants, for example, may have only HbF at the time of their NBS, therefore hemoglobinopathies affecting HbA can be missed. A repeat screen is recommended for these infants. Transfusion makes the NBS results uninterpretable, therefore a repeat screen should be performed in transfused infants at least 3 months after the last transfusion. NBS can identify also carrier state for one of the hemoglobinopathies and appropriate counseling should be provided.

Diagnosis: Diagnosis is confirmed by molecular testing in addition to hematologic studies, such as complete blood count, serum iron, and total iron binding capacity.

Congenital Hypothyroidism (CH)

Congenital hypothyroidism is a condition resulting from the partial or complete loss of thyroid function. The thyroid gland regulates growth, metabolism, and brain development. In 80-85% of cases of congenital hypothyroidism, the thyroid gland is absent, reduced in size, or misplaced. In the remaining of the cases, the thyroid gland is present, may be normal in size, however its hormone production is impaired. Untreated, congenital hypothyroidism leads to intellectual disability. Clinical symptoms include constipation, poor weight gain, hypotonia, jaundice, lethargy. The majority of the cases are sporadic, with only 15% inherited in an autosomal recessive fashion. Treatment, consisting in administration of levo-thyroxine (hormone replacement therapy), is very effective if initiated early and results in normal development.

Newborn screening: Different strategies are used to screen for CH. Measurement of TSH (Thyroid Stimulating Hormone) is widely used. TSH is produced by the pituitary gland and constitutes a feed-back mechanism to maintain constant levels of thyroxine (T4) and triiodothyronine (T3), two thyroid hormones. In CH the concentration of TSH will be high. Screening for CH can also be done by measurement of T4 by itself or in combination with TSH. The advantage of this strategy is that infants with congenital secondary CH (central CH), and at risk for the same degree of intellectual disability as infants with primary CH, can be detected.[65] Several factors affect the results of the NBS, such as prematurity and unrelated illnesses.

Diagnosis: The diagnosis is confirmed by measuring serum free or total T4 and TSH, typically by chemiluminescent immunoassays, in addition to other specialized tests to determine the etiology. Molecular testing is available as well. NBS can detect about 90% of CH cases, therefore when symptoms are suggestive, CH testing should be performed to exclude this condition even if NBS results were normal.

Congenital Adrenal Hyperplasia (CAH)

Congenital adrenal hyperplasia (CAH) is a group of disorders caused by defects in adrenal steroid biosynthesis. They are inherited as autosomal recessive traits. The most common of this condition is caused by impaired activity of 21-hydroxylase, encoded by the *CYP21* gene and accounts for 90% of CAH cases. 21-Hydroxylase converts 17-hydroxyprogesterone (17-OHP) to 11-deoxycortisol and progesterone to deoxycorticosterone. Impaired activity of this enzyme results in increased 17-OHP, reduced synthesis of cortisol and mineralocorticoids, increased synthesis of androstenedione, and decreased central feedback (increased production of adrenocorticotropic hormone) accompanied by adrenal hyperplasia, virilization, and salt-wasting crisis, which can be lethal. Treatment consists in administration of glucocorticoids and mineralocorticoids, with normalization of ACTH secretion. Optimal treatment requires growth monitoring, bone age assessment, and hormonal levels measurements.[66]

Newborn screening: All states in the United States, screen for CAH using, as a primary screen, commercially available immunoassay kits for the measurement of 17-OHP. However, because of the lack of antibody specificity and the high cross-reactivity with other compounds, the number of false positives using this test can be very high. In addition, 17-OHP can be elevated due to prematurity, stress, illness, causing additional false positive results. To overcome this problem, second tier tests, targeting additional steroid and using a different methodology (LC-MS/MS) have been implemented and have been proven very effective.[9]

Diagnosis: Diagnosis is confirmed by measuring 17-OHP in serum. The preferred method for serum testing for 17-OHP is by LC-MS/MS, as testing using an immunoassay kit might have the same limitations as the NBS test. Additional functional tests and molecular analysis are then performed to clarify the specific defect.

Cystic Fibrosis

Cystic fibrosis (CF) is an autosomal recessive disorder affecting predominantly the lungs and, to a lesser extent, other organs such as the pancreas, liver, kidney, and intestine. Clinical symptoms include failure to thrive, bronchopulmonary infections, biliary cirrhosis, pancreatic insufficiency, and infertility. 10-15% of infants with meconium ileus have CF. The disease is due to mutations in the gene encoding for the cystic fibrosis transmembrane conductance regulator (CFTR) protein, which functions mainly as a chloride channel. CF is the most common lethal disorders among Caucasian of northern European descent, with a birth prevalence of 1:3,000. The prevalence of CF varies with ethnicity, and it is 1:4,000-10,000 in Latin Americans and 1:15,000-20,000 in African Americans. Over 1500 mutations have been identified; the most common is F508del, which accounts for two-thirds of the abnormal alleles in northern American and northern European populations.

Newborn screening: In all NBS programs the initial screening for CF is done by measuring immunoreactive trypsinogen (IRT) in dried blood spots.[67] Different algorithms are followed by the different programs if initial the IRT result is elevated indicating an increased risk of CF. Several programs perform DNA analysis as a second tier test. Others repeat the IRT testing on a second sample and, in case of a second elevated IRT, either perform DNA analysis as a third tier test or refer the baby for confirmatory tests. Because many mutations are not included in NBS DNA panels, infants are referred for confirmatory tests even when only one mutation is detected. Because 10-15% of infants with CF have meconium ileus and may have normal IRT, all infants with meconium ileus are either re-screened or subjected to DNA analysis independently from the IRT results.

Diagnosis: To confirm a CF diagnosis a sweat test is still the gold standard, followed by molecular testing if not already performed. Because of the availability of very promising treatments targeting the underlying defect in CF that are mutation specific, DNA testing is becoming essential not only to the diagnosis but also for treatment options.

Severe Combined Immunodeficiencies (SCID)

SCID comprises a heterogeneous group of conditions with a common phenotype caused by mutations in genes responsible for the development of adaptive immunity through T-lymphocytes and B-lymphocytes.[68,69] These conditions are inherited as X-linked or autosomal recessive traits. All forms of SCID are characterized by defective production of T-cells with (T-B- SCID) or without (T-B+ SCID) defective production of B-cells, and defective production of antibodies. Infants with SCID are asymptomatic at birth, but are susceptible to life-threatening infections. The treatment for SCID is hematopoietic stem cell transplant (HSCT), however the success of the transplant is affected by the age and by the presence of infections. Early diagnosis of SCID prevents complications and increases the success of HSCT which can be curative. SCID was introduced in the RUSP in 2008 and almost all states have implemented NBS for these conditions. From a recent survey of the first few years of screening and including 11 states and over 3,000,000 infants, the incidence of SCID is 1:58,000.[68]

Newborn screening: In all types of SCID, T-cells are absent and there is an abnormal T-cell development in the thymus. During normal development, T-cells undergo T-cell receptor gene splicing and rearrangement resulting in the accumulation of T-cell receptor excision circles (TREC), circular DNA by-products, which are used as markers of normal production of naive T-cells. The NBS test is performed by extracting DNA from the blood spots and quantification of TREC by quantitative or end-point polymerase chain reaction (PCR).[69] Infants with SCID have very low copies of TREC. One of the issues associated with the use of TREC for screening is the fact that other conditions characterized by T-cell lymphopenia can also be identified, resulting in increased burden to NBS programs. The incidence of non-SCID T-cell lymphopenia identified by TREC NBS is 1:6,600.[68]

Diagnosis: Confirmatory tests to follow-up an abnormal NBS for SCID include absolute lymphocyte counts, determination of the presence or absence of T-lymphocytes and B-lymphocytes, and molecular genetic testing.[19]

Pompe Disease

Pompe disease is an autosomal recessive lysosomal storage disorder caused by deficiency of the enzyme acid alpha-glucosidase (GAA),[70] only recently (2015) officially added to the RUSP. In this condition, glycogen accumulates within the lysosomes especially in skeletal muscle and heart. There are two forms of Pompe disease, infantile and late-onset. In infantile Pompe disease, symptoms, hypertrophic cardiomyopathy, muscle weakness, hypotonia, are evident by 2 months of age and patients die within the first year of life. Late-onset Pompe disease is characterized by variable age of onset and presentation, with symptoms including progressive muscle weakness and respiratory insufficiency. Cardiomyopathy is not a feature of late-onset Pompe disease. Enzyme replacement therapy using a recombinant form of GAA is available and seems to ameliorate the manifestations of the disease. The incidence of Pompe disease is approximately 1:40,000 births.[71]

Newborn screening: The screening for Pompe disease is based on the measurement of the enzyme activity.[72] There are prevalently two methods used for NBS for Pompe disease: one LC-MS/MS-based method and a fluorometric method. The screening is not fully implemented in all states and definite data about the performance are not yet available.

Diagnosis: The diagnosis of Pompe disease is confirmed by the measurement of enzyme activity in lymphocytes or in fibroblasts and by DNA testing.

Mucopolysaccharidosis Type I (MPS I, Alpha-iduronidase Deficiency)

Mucopolysaccharidosis type I is an autosomal recessive lysosomal storage disorder cause by deficiency of the lysosomal hydrolase alpha-iduronidase. The incidence is estimated at 0.7-4:100,000.[73] Alpha-iduronidase is involved in the degradation of heparan sulfate and dermatan sulfate, two glycosaminoglycans that accumulate throughout the body as a result of the enzyme deficiency, causing organ dysfunction. There is a wide spectrum of phenotypes, from the most severe, MPS-IH or Hurler, to the attenuated Hurler-Scheie (MPS-IHS) and Scheie (MPS-IS). Patients with MPS-IH disease present early in life, with a rapid disease progression involving the central nervous system (CNS) leading, if untreated, to death in the first two decades of life. At the other end of the spectrum are patients with MPS-IS, in which the disease progression is slower, does not involve the CNS, and life expectancy is normal. Other typical features of MPS I are coarse facial features, hepatosplenomegaly, cardiac involvement, joint stiffness, skeletal deformities, corneal clouding. Enzyme replacement therapy (ERT) is available for MPS I, however it is most effective when initiated early, possibly, before CNS involvement. Intrathecal ERT delivery is being investigated to reach the CNS more effectively. Hematopoietic stem cell transplantation (HSCT) is still, however, the preferred therapy, perhaps in conjunction with ERT.[73]

Newborn screening: NBS methods for MPS I are based on measurement of enzyme activity. As for Pompe disease, there are two methods available for high throughput screening, one is LC-MS/MS based and the other is a fluorometric method. This condition has been only recently added to the RUSP, and only a few states have implemented screening for this condition. Therefore no data are yet available on the performance of this screening.

Diagnosis: The diagnosis is confirmed by measuring enzyme activity in freshly isolated leukocytes and by sequencing of the *IDUA* gene.

X-linked Adrenoleukodystrophy (X-ALD)

X-ALD is caused by mutations in the *ABCD1* gene located on Xq28.[74] The gene encodes for the adrenoleukodystrophy protein (ALDP), located in the peroxisomal membrane, whose function is to carry very long-chain fatty acids inside the peroxisomes where they are degraded.

The phenotypic spectrum of X-ALD is wide, however there are two predominant presentations: adrenomyeloneuropathy (AMN) and cerebral adrenoleukodystrophy (CALD). AMN presents usually in the second-third decade of life with progressive spastic paraplegia. Adrenal dysfunction occurs in about 2/3 of males with AMN. 50-65% of female carriers, develop symptoms similar to AMN, however the onset is much later, in the fourth-fifth decade of life. In the cerebral form of X-ALD, symptoms usually appear before 4-5 years of age, and include emotional lability, hyperactivity, cognitive and neurological deterioration, progressing to a vegetative state, and death in 2-5 years following onset of symptoms. The only effective treatment for X-ALD is hematopoietic stem cell transplantation. X-ALD is the most common of the peroxisomal disorders, with an incidence of 1:17,000 births and 1:20,000 males.[75]

Newborn screening: The biochemical marker for X-ALD used in NBS is C26:0 lysophosphatidylcholine (C26:0 LPC) and it is measured by LC-MS/MS. C26:0 LPC is elevated in DBS of patients with X-ALD, Zellweger spectrum disorders, and in approximately 80% of female carriers for X-ALD.[76]

Diagnosis: Measurement of very long-chain fatty acids (VLCFA) in plasma is diagnostic in all males, however it is elevated only in 80-85% of heterozygous females. Therefore, confirmation by DNA sequencing of the *ABCD1* gene is recommended.

SUMMARY

NBS is, without any doubts, the most successful population screening. Its implementation has reduced mortality, morbidity, and improved the quality of life of thousands of individuals affected with the diseases screened by the program. The development of novel and more sensitive technologies will only increase the power of NBS. Tandem mass spectrometry has allowed the ability to identify several markers of multiple diseases simultaneously. Multiple confirmatory tests are necessary to confirm the condition and to initiate promptly the appropriate treatment. Pilot studies are already under way to expand the NBS panel, without adding additional costs by taking advantage of multiplex analysis.[77,78] Even with the more sophisticated assays, though, it is important to remember that, as it is for all screening assays, the possibility of false negative results cannot be ruled out. Therefore, in the presence of clinical symptoms, a disorder included in NBS panels cannot be dismissed because of a negative newborn screen results and appropriate testing needs to be considered.

TRAINING MODULE

1. The best marker for newborn screening for Tyrosinemia type I is:
   a. Bilirubin
   b. Methionine
   c. Phenylalanine
   d. Succinylacetone
   e. Tyrosine

2. Second-tier tests are helpful to:
   a. Decrease the number of false positive results
   b. Decrease the number of false negative results
   c. Increase the number of false negative results
   d. Increase the number of conditions screened
   e. Monitor the performance of newborn screening

3. The newborn screen results of a 5-days old baby boy, born full term after an uncomplicated pregnancy, are abnormal for an elevated C5-carnitine. What are the possible causes of elevated C5-carnitine? (Select all that apply)
   a. Antibiotic artifacts
   b. Galactosemia
   c. Isovaleric acidemia
   d. 2-Methylbutyrylglycinuria
   e. Phenylketonuria

4. Which metabolic disorder identified by newborn screening may have a clinical presentation that can be seen in non-accidental trauma?
   a. Biotinidase deficiency
   b. Citrullinemia type I
   c. Glutaric acidemia type I
   d. MCAD (Medium Chain Acyl-CoA Dehydrogenase) deficiency
   e. Methylmalonic acidemia

5. Newborn screening for SCID (Severe Combined Immunodeficiencies) is performed by measuring T-cell receptor excision circles (TREC); they are:
   a. Acylcarnitines
   b. Amino acids
   c. Circular DNA byproducts
   d. Enzymes
   e. Sugars

REFERENCES

1. American College of Medical Genetics Newborn Screening Expert G. Newborn screening: toward a uniform screening panel and system-executive summary. *Pediatrics*. 2006;117(5 Pt. 2):S296-S307.
2. Chace DH, Kalas TA. A biochemical perspective on the use of tandem mass spectrometry for newborn screening and clinical testing. *Clin Biochem*. 2005;38(4):296-309.
3. Turgeon C, Magera MJ, Allard P, et al. Combined newborn screening for succinylacetone, amino acids, and acylcarnitines in dried blood spots. *Clin Chem*. 2008;54(4):657-664.
4. la Marca G, Malvagia S, Pasquini E, et al. The inclusion of succinylacetone as marker for tyrosinemia type I in expanded newborn screening programs. *Rapid Commun Mass Spectrom*. 2008;22(6):812-818.

5. Haynes CA, De Jesus VR. Simultaneous quantitation of hexacosanoyl lysophosphatidylcholine, amino acids, acylcarnitines, and succinylacetone during FIA-ESI-MS/MS analysis of dried blood spot extracts for newborn screening. *Clin Biochem*. 2016;49(1-2):161-165.

6. McHugh D, Cameron CA, Abdenur JE, et al. Clinical validation of cutoff target ranges in newborn screening of metabolic disorders by tandem mass spectrometry: a worldwide collaborative project. *Genet Med*. 2011;13(3):230-254.

7. Marquardt G, Currier R, McHugh DM, et al. Enhanced interpretation of newborn screening results without analyte cutoff values. *Gen Med*. 2012;14(7):648-655.

8. Rock MJ, Hoffman G, Laessig RH, Kopish GJ, Litsheim TJ, Farrell PM. Newborn screening for cystic fibrosis in Wisconsin: nine-year experience with routine trypsinogen/DNA testing. *J Pediatr*. 2005;147(3 suppl):S73-S77.

9. Schwarz E, Liu A, Randall H, et al. Use of steroid profiling by UPLC-MS/MS as a second tier test in newborn screening for congenital adrenal hyperplasia: the Utah experience. *Pediatr Res*. 2009;66(2):230-235.

10. Maniatis AK, Taylor L, Letson GW, Bloch CA, Kappy MS, Zeitler P. Congenital hypothyroidism and the second newborn metabolic screening in Colorado, USA. *J Pediatr Endocrinol Metab*. 2006;19(1):31-38.

11. Schymik I, Liebig M, Mueller M, et al. Pitfalls of neonatal screening for very-long-chain acyl-CoA dehydrogenase deficiency using tandem mass spectrometry. *J Pediatr*. 2006;149(1):128-130.

12. Cavedon CT, Bourdoux P, Mertens K, et al. Age-related variations in acylcarnitine and free carnitine concentrations measured by tandem mass spectrometry. *Clin Chem*. 2005;51(4):745-752.

13. Therrell BL, Jr., Lloyd-Puryear MA, Camp KM, Mann MY. Inborn errors of metabolism identified via newborn screening: Ten-year incidence data and costs of nutritional interventions for research agenda planning. *Mol Genet Metab*. 2014;113(1-2):14-26.

14. Deodato F, Boenzi S, Santorelli FM, Dionisi-Vici C. Methylmalonic and propionic aciduria. *Am J Med Genet C Semin Med Genet*. 2006;142C(2):104-112.

15. Carrillo-Carrasco N, Venditti C. Propionic Acidemia. In: Pagon RA, Adam MP, Ardinger HH, et al., eds. *GeneReviews(R)*. University of Washington, Seattle (WA) 1993.

16. Ozand PT, Rashed M, Gascon GG, et al. Unusual presentations of propionic acidemia. *Brain Dev*. 1994;16 suppl:46-57.

17. la Marca G, Malvagia S, Pasquini E, Innocenti M, Donati MA, Zammarchi E. Rapid 2nd-tier test for measurement of 3-OH-propionic and methylmalonic acids on dried blood spots: reducing the false-positive rate for propionylcarnitine during expanded newborn screening by liquid chromatography-tandem mass spectrometry. *Clin Chem*. 2007;53(7):1364-1369.

18. Matern D, Tortorelli S, Oglesbee D, Gavrilov D, Rinaldo P. Reduction of the false-positive rate in newborn screening by implementation of MS/MS-based second-tier tests: the Mayo Clinic experience (2004-2007). *J Inherited Metab Dis*. 2007;30(4):585-592.

19. *ACMG ACT Sheets and Confirmatory Algorithms*. Bethesda (MD) 2001.

20. Manoli I, Venditti CP. Methylmalonic Acidemia. In: Pagon RA, Adam MP, Ardinger HH, et al., eds. *GeneReviews(R)*. University of Washington, Seattle (WA) 1993.

21. Horster F, Garbade SF, Zwickler T, et al. Prediction of outcome in isolated methylmalonic acidurias: combined use of clinical and biochemical parameters. *J Inherited Metab Dis*. 2009;32(5):630-639.

22. O'Shea CJ, Sloan JL, Wiggs EA, et al. Neurocognitive phenotype of isolated methylmalonic acidemia. *Pediatrics*. 2012;129(6):e1541-e1551.

23. Watkins D, Rosenblatt DS. Inborn errors of cobalamin absorption and metabolism. *Am J Med Genet C Semin Med Genet*. 2011;157C(1):33-44.

24. Matsui SM, Mahoney MJ, Rosenberg LE. The natural history of the inherited methylmalonic acidemias. *N Engl J Med*. 1983;308(15):857-861.

25. Vockley J, Ensenauer R. Isovaleric acidemia: new aspects of genetic and phenotypic heterogeneity. *Am J Med Genet C Semin Med Genet*. 2006;142C(2):95-103.

26. Boemer F, Schoos R, de Halleux V, Kalenga M, Debray FG. Surprising causes of C5-carnitine false positive results in newborn screening. *Mol Genet Metab*. 2014;111(1):52-54.

27. Stadler SC, Polanetz R, Maier EM, et al. Newborn screening for 3-methylcrotonyl-CoA carboxylase deficiency: population heterogeneity of MCCA and MCCB mutations and impact on risk assessment. *Hum Mutat*. 2006;27(8):748-759.

28. Cardoso ML, Rodrigues MR, Leao E, et al. The E37X is a common HMGCL mutation in Portuguese patients with 3-hydroxy-3-methylglutaric CoA lyase deficiency. *Mol Genet Metab*. 2004;82(4):334-338.

29. Seashore MR. The Organic Acidemias: An Overview. In: Pagon RA, Adam MP, Ardinger HH, et al., eds. *GeneReviews(R)*. University of Washington, Seattle (WA) 1993.

30. Tammachote R, Janklat S, Tongkobpetch S, Suphapeetiporn K, Shotelersuk V. Holocarboxylase synthetase deficiency: novel clinical and molecular findings. *Clin Genet*. 2010;78(1):88-93.

31. Fukao T, Mitchell G, Sass JO, Hori T, Orii K, Aoyama Y. Ketone body metabolism and its defects. *J Inherited Metab Dis*. 2014;37(4):541-551.

32. Hedlund GL, Longo N, Pasquali M. Glutaric acidemia type 1. *Am J Med Genet C Semin Med Genet*. 2006;142C(2):86-94.

33. Viau K, Ernst SL, Vanzo RJ, Botto LD, Pasquali M, Longo N. Glutaric acidemia type 1: outcomes before and after expanded newborn screening. *Mol Genet Metab*. 2012;106(4):430-438.

34. Tortorelli S, Hahn SH, Cowan TM, Brewster TG, Rinaldo P, Matern D. The urinary excretion of glutarylcarnitine is an informative tool in the biochemical diagnosis of glutaric acidemia type I. *Mol Genet Metab*. 2005;84(2):137-143.

35. Longo N, Amat di San Filippo C, Pasquali M. Disorders of carnitine transport and the carnitine cycle. *Am J Med Genet C Semin Med Genet*. 2006;142C(2):77-85.

36. Lindner M, Hoffmann GF, Matern D. Newborn screening for disorders of fatty-acid oxidation: experience and recommendations from an expert meeting. *J Inherited Metab Dis*. 2010;33(5):521-526.

37. Arnold GL, Van Hove J, Freedenberg D, et al. A Delphi clinical practice protocol for the management of very long chain acyl-CoA dehydrogenase deficiency. *Mol Genet Metab*. 2009;96(3):85-90.

38. Boneh A, Andresen BS, Gregersen N, et al. VLCAD deficiency: pitfalls in newborn screening and confirmation of diagnosis by mutation analysis. *Mol Genet Metab*. 2006;88(2):166-170.

39. Eskelin PM, Laitinen KA, Tyni TA. Elevated hydroxyacylcarnitines in a carrier of LCHAD deficiency during acute liver disease of pregnancy - a common feature of the pregnancy complication? *Mol Genet Metab.* 2010;100(2):204-206.

40. Spiekerkoetter U, Sun B, Khuchua Z, Bennett MJ, Strauss AW. Molecular and phenotypic heterogeneity in mitochondrial trifunctional protein deficiency due to beta-subunit mutations. *Hum Mutat.* 2003;21(6):598-607.

41. Erez A. Argininosuccinic aciduria: from a monogenic to a complex disorder. *Genet Med.* 2013;15(4):251-257.

42. Erez A, Nagamani SC, Lee B. Argininosuccinate lyase deficiency-argininosuccinic aciduria and beyond. *Am J Med Genet C Semin Med Genet.* 2011;157C(1):45-53.

43. Nagamani SC, Shchelochkov OA, Mullins MA, et al. A randomized controlled trial to evaluate the effects of high-dose versus low-dose of arginine therapy on hepatic function tests in argininosuccinic aciduria. *Mol Genet Metab.* 2012;107(3):315-321.

44. Ogier de Baulny H, Schiff M, Dionisi-Vici C. Lysinuric protein intolerance (LPI): a multi organ disease by far more complex than a classic urea cycle disorder. *Mol Genet Metab.* May 2012;106(1):12-17.

45. Sebastio G, Nunes V. Lysinuric Protein Intolerance. In: Pagon RA, Adam MP, Ardinger HH, et al., eds. *GeneReviews(R).* University of Washington, Seattle (WA) 1993.

46. Sebastio G, Sperandeo MP, Andria G. Lysinuric protein intolerance: reviewing concepts on a multisystem disease. *Am J Med Genet C Semin Med Genet.* 2011;157C(1):54-62.

47. Smith W, Kishnani PS, Lee B, et al. Urea cycle disorders: clinical presentation outside the newborn period. *Crit Care Clin.* 2005;21(4 suppl):S9-S17.

48. Nassogne MC, Heron B, Touati G, Rabier D, Saudubray JM. Urea cycle defects: management and outcome. *J Inherited Metab Dis.* 2005;28(3):407-414.

49. Fernhoff PM, Lubitz D, Danner DJ, et al. Thiamine response in maple syrup urine disease. *Pediatr Res.* 1985;19(10):1011-1016.

50. Chuang DT, Chuang JL, Wynn RM. Lessons from genetic disorders of branched-chain amino acid metabolism. *J Nutr.* 2006;136(1 Suppl):243S-249S.

51. Longo N. Disorders of biopterin metabolism. *J Inherited Metab Dis.* 2009;32(3):333-342.

52. Mitchell JJ. Phenylalanine Hydroxylase Deficiency. In: Pagon RA, Adam MP, Ardinger HH, et al., eds. *GeneReviews(R).* University of Washington, Seattle (WA) 1993.

53. Sniderman King L, Trahms C, Scott CR. Tyrosinemia Type I. In: Pagon RA, Adam MP, Ardinger HH, et al., eds. *GeneReviews(R).* University of Washington, Seattle (WA) 1993.

54. Scott CR. The genetic tyrosinemias. *Am J Med Genet C Semin Med Genet.* 2006;142C(2):121-126.

55. la Marca G, Malvagia S, Funghini S, et al. The successful inclusion of succinylacetone as a marker of tyrosinemia type I in Tuscany newborn screening program. *Rapid Commun Mass Spectrom.* 2009;23(23):3891-3893.

56. la Marca G, Malvagia S, Pasquini E, et al. Newborn Screening for Tyrosinemia Type I: Further Evidence that Succinylacetone Determination on Blood Spot Is Essential. *JIMD Rep.* 2011;1:107-109.

57. De Jesus VR, Adam BW, Mandel D, Cuthbert CD, Matern D. Succinylacetone as primary marker to detect tyrosinemia type I in newborns and its measurement by newborn screening programs. *Mol Genet Metab.* 2014;113(1-2):67-75.

58. Schlump JU, Mayatepek E, Spiekerkoetter U. Significant increase of succinylacetone within the first 12 h of life in hereditary tyrosinemia type 1. *Eur J Pediatr.* 2010;169(5):569-572.

59. Jay AM, Conway RL, Feldman GL, Nahhas F, Spencer L, Wolf B. Outcomes of individuals with profound and partial biotinidase deficiency ascertained by newborn screening in Michigan over 25 years. *Genet Med.* 2015;17(3):205-209.

60. Suormala T, Wick H, Baumgartner ER. Low biotinidase activity in plasma of some preterm infants: possible source of false-positive screening results. *Eur J Pediatr.* 1988;147(5):478-480.

61. Cowan TM, Blitzer MG, Wolf B, Working Group of the American College of Medical Genetics Laboratory Quality Assurance C. Technical standards and guidelines for the diagnosis of biotinidase deficiency. *Genet Med.* 2010;12(7):464-470.

62. Bender MA, Douthitt Seibel G. Sickle Cell Disease. In: Pagon RA, Adam MP, Ardinger HH, et al., eds. *GeneReviews(R).* University of Washington, Seattle (WA) 1993.

63. Bhatia M, Sheth S. Hematopoietic stem cell transplantation in sickle cell disease: patient selection and special considerations. *J Blood Med.* 2015;6:229-238.

64. Chandrakasan S, Kamat D. An overview of hemoglobinopathies and the interpretation of newborn screening results. *Pediatr Ann.* 2013;42(12):502-508.

65. LaFranchi SH. Approach to the diagnosis and treatment of neonatal hypothyroidism. *J Clin Endocrinol Metab.* 2011;96(10):2959-2967.

66. Ajish TP, Praveen VP, Nisha B, Kumar H. Comparison of different glucocorticoid regimens in the management of classical congenital adrenal hyperplasia due to 21-hydroxylase deficiency. *Indian J Endocrinol Metab.* 2014;18(6):815-820.

67. Ross LF. Newborn screening for cystic fibrosis: a lesson in public health disparities. *J Pediatr.* 2008;153(3):308-313.

68. Kwan A, Abraham RS, Currier R, et al. Newborn screening for severe combined immunodeficiency in 11 screening programs in the United States. *JAMA.* 2014;312(7):729-738.

69. Gaspar HB, Hammarstrom L, Mahlaoui N, Borte M, Borte S. The case for mandatory newborn screening for severe combined immunodeficiency (SCID). *J Clin Immunol.* 2014;34(4):393-397.

70. Burton BK. Newborn screening for Pompe disease: an update, 2011. *Am J Med Genet C Semin Med Genet.* 2012;160C(1):8-12.

71. Chien YH, Hwu WL, Lee NC. Pompe disease: early diagnosis and early treatment make a difference. *Pediatr Neonatol.* 2013;54(4):219-227.

72. Matern D, Gavrilov D, Oglesbee D, Raymond K, Rinaldo P, Tortorelli S. Newborn screening for lysosomal storage disorders. *Semin Perinatol.* 2015;39(3):206-216.

73. de Ru MH, Boelens JJ, Das AM, et al. Enzyme replacement therapy and/or hematopoietic stem cell transplantation at diagnosis in patients with mucopolysaccharidosis type I: results of a European consensus procedure. *Orphanet J Rare Dis.* 2011;6:55.

74. Mosser J, Douar AM, Sarde CO, et al. Putative X-linked adrenoleukodystrophy gene shares unexpected homology with ABC transporters. *Nature.* 1993;361(6414):726-730.

75. Vogel BH, Bradley SE, Adams DJ, et al. Newborn screening for X-linked adrenoleukodystrophy in New York State: diagnostic protocol, surveillance protocol and treatment guidelines. *Mol Genet Metab.* 2015;114(4):599-603.

76. Matern D, Oglesbee D, Tortorelli S. Newborn screening for lysosomal storage disorders and other neuronopathic conditions. *Dev Dis Res Rev*. 2013;17(3):247-253.

77. Pasquali M, Schwarz E, Jensen M, et al. Feasibility of newborn screening for guanidinoacetate methyltransferase (GAMT) deficiency. *J Inherited Metab Dis*. 2014; 37(2):231-236.

78. Orsini JJ, Martin MM, Showers AL, et al. Lysosomal storage disorder 4+1 multiplex assay for newborn screening using tandem mass spectrometry: application to a small-scale population study for five lysosomal storage disorders. *Clin Chim Acta*. 2012;413(15-16):1270-1273.

CYSTIC FIBROSIS AND SWEAT TESTING 6

Stanley F. Lo

LEARNING OBJECTIVES

1. Describe signs and symptoms associated with Cystic Fibrosis (CF).
2. Explain the genetic basis for CF.
3. Describe an algorithm for diagnosing CF.
4. Delineate the sweat testing process.

INTRODUCTION

Cystic fibrosis (CF) is an autosomal recessive disease that primarily affects young children. CF is considered one of the most common life-shortening genetic diseases in Caucasians. In the classical description of the disease, it usually presents itself with a classic clinical pattern of exocrine pancreatic insufficiency, chronic pulmonary disease, and congenital bilateral absence of the vas deferens in males. Other systems are affected as well including the gastrointestinal and endocrine systems. Upon sweat testing, these patients exhibit chloride concentrations ≥60 mmol/L. Patients with mutations in the CF gene detected by newborn screening programs typically represent the classical form of CF. Many other mutations exhibit a milder, non-classic form of CF in which only one organ system is affected. In these cases, symptoms may or may not develop until beyond the newborn period.

Cystic Fibrosis Transmembrane Conductance Regulator

Cystic fibrosis is caused by mutations found in the cystic fibrosis transmembrane conductance regulator (CFTR) gene, a 250 kb gene composed of 27 exons encoding 1,480 amino acids found on the long arm of chromosome 7. CFTR belongs to a family of ATP-binding cassette subfamily C.[1] The protein is found in all exocrine tissue and commonly in the apical portion of mucosal epithelial cells and functions as a chloride channel regulated by cyclic AMP-dependent phosphorylation. The protein contains three primary domains. One domain interacts with ATP and is identified as nucleotide-binding domain 1 (NBD-1) and NBD-2. The second domain is responsible for anchoring the protein in the membrane and is termed membrane-spanning domain 1 (MSD-1) and MSD-2. The final domain is a regulatory domain, termed the R domain, and contains multiple sites for phosphorylation. Mutations affecting the chloride channel result in changes to the transport of ions such as chloride, sodium, and bicarbonate. The functional outcome is the presence of thick, viscous secretions and an overt inflammatory response in the lungs resulting in the inability to clear microorganisms and severe lung disease.

The incidence of clinical CF in the US population is approximately 1:2,500 for Caucasians, 1:13,500 in Hispanics, 1:15,000 in African Americans, and 1:31,000 in Asian Americans, though the incidence in the Asian American population may be influenced by mixing with other ethnic populations.[2] It is expected that the incidence will continue to increase due to increased detection of CF as inclusion of CF into newborn screening programs increases. Over 2000 mutations are listed in the Cystic Fibrosis Mutation Database with the most common occurring approximately 70% of the time. This mutation results in the deletion of phenylalanine at position 508 (F508del). Due to the founder effect, a high frequency gene mutation found in a specific population due to its presence in a single ancestor or small number of ancestors, specific ethnic groups may have different mutations that are more commonly found.

The mutations identified in the CFTR gene are many. Their phenotypic expression covers a wide spectrum. In general, the degree to which ions are transported is related to the specific mutation's functional effect on the quantity or the stability of CFTR. To assist with the understanding of mutations and their phenotype, six classifications based on the mutations primary functional defect have been created.[3] These classes of mutations are defined in Table 6-1. Class I mutations result in defective CFTR protein production and are caused by frameshift, splicing or nonsense mutations resulting in premature stop codons. Defective protein processing, such as protein misfolding or premature degradation, describes Class II mutations where cell surface has little or no CFTR protein. Class III mutations affect the regulation of opening or gating of the chloride channel. Class III mutations are usually located in NBD-1 and NBD-2. Class IV and V are less severe due to the presence of some CFTR function, though still diminished in activity, and generally results in a less severe CF phenotype. Class IV mutations present with defective chloride conductance, and Class V mutations are categorized as mutations that result in decreased mRNA stability which leads to reduced amounts of functional

Class	Function	Mutation
	Table 6-1 CFTR PROTEIN MUTATION CLASSIFICATION	
I	No functional CFTR protein	G542X, R1162X, R553X, W1282X
II	Little or no functional CFTR protein	F508del, N1303K
III	Defective transport of chloride via regulation or gating	G551D, G551S, G1349D
IV	Defective chloride conductance. Some functional CFTR protein	R117H, R347P, R334W
V	Decreased synthesis of functional CFTR protein	A455E, 3120+1G→A, 2789+5G→A
VI	Decreased stability of CFTR protein	Q1412X

protein, possibly due to alternative splicing or promoter abnormalities. Class VI, has been proposed for mutations that alter the stability of the CFTR protein. These classifications have been identified to provide a better understanding of the primary defect. Unfortunately, the functional defects of some mutations have not been identified and many mutations may affect multiple processes and could be classified into more than one group. A new classification scheme may be in order to address these issues better.

With the acceptance of universal newborn screening of CF in newborns, the patient presentation has significantly changed. Prior to CF screening, most patients presented with one or more of the following symptoms: failure to thrive (28%), respiratory symptoms (45%), or meconium ileus (20%).[4] Patients presenting with meconium ileus are usually diagnosed earlier. Since the implementation of CF newborn screening, more than 61% of newborns are diagnosed prior to the development of symptoms, directly due to screening.[5] With earlier diagnosis of CF, treatment can be initiated more quickly and hopefully lead to a better quality of life.

Signs and Symptoms of CF

Pulmonary complications are many, ranging from persistent cough and wheezing to inflammatory states of bronchiectasis and respiratory failure. The inability of the lungs to remove the viscous respiratory secretions due to the altered CFTR protein, leads to persistent pulmonary infections with *Pseudomonas aeruginosa, Haemophilus influenza,* and *Stapholococcus aureus,* including methicillin-resistant *S aureus.* There is a typical progression of bacterial infection. *H influenza* and *S aureus* are most commonly identified in childhood and persists through adulthood. *P aeruginosa* is isolated in children, but becomes much more prevalent in adulthood. *Burkholderia cepacia* is typically only encountered in advanced CF disease. Because of the high incidence of bacterial infection within this patient population, isolation of those infected or suspected to be infected from other CF patients has been strongly recommended. Bacterial colonization signals neutrophils into the lung. The neutrophil response is ineffective in clearing the infection. It has been suggested that the CFTR protein is necessary for the full effect of these cells.[6] What remains unclear is how the inflammatory lung originates, some studies suggest that the infection causes the inflammation, while others suggest that the inflammatory state existed prior to infection.[7]

P. aeruginosa is unique to CF patients, though other Gram negative bacteria can be acquired. The environment created by the viscous mucosal layer is low in oxygen content which allows *P. aeruginosa* to form a biofilm. Once this stage is encountered, it is nearly impossible to eradicate the infection.[8]

Pancreas involvement will typically manifest itself as either pancreatic insufficiency or pancreatitis. Roughly 66% of CF patients have pancreatic insufficiency at birth and nearly 90% will have evidence of dietary fat malabsorption by 1 year of age.[9] There are several ways to identify pancreatic insufficiency including the observation or measurement of steatorrhea, decreased fecal elastase, and reduction of these entities in response to pancreatic enzyme replacement therapy. Pancreatitis occurs due to the inability of the pancreas to release its enzymes due to the build-up of ductular and acinar enzyme secretions caused by dysfunctional CFTR. This damage results in pancreatitis. The damage to the pancreas may also lead to glucose intolerance and CF-related diabetes (CFRD). Considered a common complication of CF, CFRD has been found in 2%, 19%, and 40-50% of all children, adolescents and adults, respectively, with CF.[10] Because CFTR has been identified to play a role in the regulation of insulin secretion by islet β-cells, CFTR modulators have targeted this process in hopes of improving insulin secretion and eventually treating CFRD.[11] It is speculated that earlier detection through screening and more aggressive treatment improves survival of CFRD patients.[12]

Meconium ileus is the most common cause of bowel obstruction in a newborn. A common assumption is that 80-90% of newborns with meconium ileus have CF, but a recent study in 2010 demonstrates the prevalence of CF at 53.5% in newborns presenting with meconium ileus.[13] The true prevalence of newborns presenting with meconium ileus with a subsequent diagnosis of CF, remains unclear.

Other diseases that may be found in CF patients include chronic rhinosinusitis, rectal prolapse, biliary cirrhosis, infertility, nephrolithiasis, nephrocalcinosis, venous thrombosis, and musculoskeletal disorders.

Treatment of Pulmonary Symptoms

Treatment of CF patients for their impending progression to obstructive lung disease begins with prevention of microbial colonization. Antimicrobial medications are selected based on sensitivity data with the goal of suppressing bacterial infection versus complete eradication. There are exceptions such as the colonization of *P aeruginosa* in young children and atypical organisms.[14] Aminoglycosides, such as tobramycin are commonly used, however the rate of clearance of this antibiotic class is more rapid in CF patients requiring higher doses than usually administered. The mechanism of increased renal clearance is not known. Given the ototoxicity and renal toxicity of these drugs, therapeutic drug monitoring is recommended.[15]

Airway clearance techniques, such as chest percussion, remain common. This form of therapy may or may not be used in combination with medication designed to improve mucous clearance. Airway clearance therapies require the assistance of a caregiver, so devices have been designed to replace the caregiver and provide more independence for older patients. Advanced CF disease observes the progression to obstructive lung disease to respiratory failure. A lung transplant is the only remaining treatment option.

Advancements in the understanding of the molecular mechanisms of CFTR have led to the development of specific small molecules to overcome functional deficiencies due to a specific mutation or mutations. Patients with the class III G551D mutation contain CFTR protein with abnormal channel regulation. The molecule VX-770 (ivacaftor) is the first potentiator to be approved by the US Food and Drug Administration. It is able to overcome the functional mutation and increase the chloride conductance of the channel regardless of mutation presence on one or two alleles.[16] Eight additional class III mutations have been approved for the use of VX-770, as well as one class IV mutation (R117H).[17] Patients with the class II F508del mutation have abnormal protein folding and trafficking.[17] The corrector molecule VX-809 (lumacaftor) is able to return up to 15% of normal CFTR channel activity. Unfortunately, the clinical benefit from VX-809 was not promising, but the combination of VX-809 and VX-770 has shown significant clinical improvement.[18] The combined treatment has been approved for nine class II mutations.[17] PTC-124 (ataluren) is an oral drug intended for CF patients with a nonsense mutation or premature stop codon (Class I) contained in their CFTR gene. This type of mutation is found in roughly 10% of all CF patients. A phase 3 clinical trial has indicated that the drug does not improve lung function but may be useful to treat patients not chronically using inhaled tobramycin.[12]

Classic and Non-Classic CF

Classic CF patients present with one or more of these clinical symptoms and have a sweat chloride ≥60 mmol/L. Typically one CF-causing mutation is identified in each CFTR gene. The involvement of multiple organ disease is common to this class.[19] A small percentage of these patients have positive newborn screen results and are asymptomatic. Non-classic CF patients confirmatory testing by measuring sweat chloride concentrations, a very laborious and difficult task on neonates, often results in intermediate results. Up to two CFTR mutations, at least one of which is not identified as a CF-causing mutation, is commonly found.[20,21] The identification of a CF-causing mutation may occur in expanded newborn screening panels or by prenatal DNA sequencing. The term CFTR-related metabolic syndrome (CRMS) has been applied to this population. Clinical disease is usually milder and limited to one organ. The frequency of F508del mutation is less common compared to the classic form.[22] CRMS patients have milder course of disease in infancy and can develop signs of CF disease, such as pancreatic insufficiency and infertility, and yet others may never develop the CF phenotype. The term CF screen positive, inconclusive diagnosis, or CFSPID, has been introduced to rename CRMS population in order to remove the confusion implied by metabolic syndrome.[23] For CFSPID patients, annual visits with a CF provider are recommended. As the knowledge of this patient group increases, guidelines for diagnosis, monitoring, and management will improve.[21]

Newborn Screening

Currently, all states in United States, screen newborns for CF using dried blood spots ideally collected within 2 days after birth. There are two commonly used serial, or tiered, protocols used. Both begin with a serum immunoreactive trypsinogen (IRT) measurement. After IRT testing, one protocol is followed by DNA analysis for mutations in the CFTR gene (IRT/DNA protocol). The second is an IRT-only protocol where newborn samples above a determine IRT cutoff are followed up with a second IRT measurement from a second sample collected within 2 weeks of the initial sample. This is referred to as the IRT/IRT protocol. Newborns with screen positive results are referred to a CF center for further evaluation and likely sweat testing.

Immunoreactive trypsinogen is a pancreatic enzyme. The two major forms secreted by the pancreas are IRT1 (cationic trypsinogen) and IRT2 (anionic trypsinogen).[11] Secreted in an inactive form, the enzyme is activated by cleavage of a hexapeptide at the N-terminus. In normal physiological conditions IRT1 has a higher concentration, but in pathological conditions, this changes and IRT2 is increased relative to IRT1. Increased concentrations of IRT are found in newborns with CF, however the increase is nonspecific as increases are found in other types of pancreatic injury, prenatal asphyxia, and other stresses. Newborn concentrations will decrease rapidly and are negative at roughly 8 weeks of age. For IRT, a negative result is not informative and a positive result supports a diagnosis of CF.

The measurement of IRT is typically performed using a direct sandwich immunoassay using either monoclonal or polyclonal antibodies. A multiplex immunoassay has been developed.[24] The different forms of IRT along with the specificity issues, IRT-2 is not reliably detected, in immunoassays have made standardization of IRT challenging. There are many other variables that can alter the total IRT concentration including the baby's weight and age at time of specimen collection, environment, seasonal variation, immunoassay reagent variability, prematurity, and ethnicity.[25] Soon after birth, IRT concentrations begin to decrease, however the kinetics of this decrease with age remains unclear. Newborns weighing less than 1500 g, as well as prematrity, are reported to have higher IRT levels.[25] Seasonal variations are reported in the United States, however other states do not detect seasonal variations in their population. Screening programs in WI, MI, and NY indicate that African-Americans have higher IRT levels when compared to Caucasians. [26,27] Another inconsistency in newborn screening is the use of either a fixed or floating IRT cutoff. Further studies are warranted to clarify these issues with IRT testing.

In the IRT/IRT protocol, the initial screen typically uses a high concentration cutoff set in the 99th-99.5th percentile range. Newborns in this range have an additional sample collected within 2 weeks of the first sample and another IRT analysis is performed. The second IRT cutoff is typically in the 95th-97th percentile range. Newborns above the second IRT cutoff are referred to a CF center for diagnosis. In spite of the low specificity and lack of standardization, the overall sensitivity for detecting CF using the IRT/IRT protocol is 80%.[28] Overall, the IRT/IRT protocol is less expensive that an IRT/DNA protocol, but is subject to more system failures, particularly as it relates to collecting a second patient sample.[29] Tracking second IRT sample collections and accurately linking them to the first sample can create logistical problems. In addition, the IRT/IRT protocol poorly detects heterozygous carriers of CFTR mutations due to their decreased IRT concentrations.

The IRT/DNA protocol used in most states uses an initial screening by IRT followed by a secondary screen for specific CFTR gene mutations. The initial IRT screen uses a cutoff around the 96th-99th percentile. Some programs will adjust, or float, the cutoff based on a daily or monthly set of IRT values in their population. With over 2000 identified mutations, the determination of which mutations to screen can be daunting. In 2001, the American College of Medical Genetics Cystic Fibrosis Carrier Screening Working Group recommended a panel of CFTR mutations that could be used in newborn screening programs.[30] A 23 mutation pan-ethnic panel was developed for population screening and remains in widespread use. Because of the differences observed between ethnic groups and the prevalence of CFTR mutations, some screening panels have additional mutations to reflect the ethnic make-up of the population being screened. The state of California is screening high IRT newborns using a 40 mutation panel that reflects the ethnic make-up of their population.[31] The basic 23 mutation panel accounts for roughly 90% of all CF causing mutations and the sensitivity of the IRT/DNA protocol is reported to be 96%.[29,32]

DIAGNOSIS

Regardless of protocol and symptoms, newborns with a positive screen result should have sweat chloride testing to confirm the diagnosis of CF. Newborns that exhibit one or more symptoms of CF or newborns from a family with a CF history should also have their sweat chloride concentration determined. Sweat test guidelines recommend that screen positive, asymptomatic newborns be >2 weeks of age and >2 kg, prior to testing. For symptomatic newborns, such as those with meconium ileus, sweat testing may be performed as young as 48 hours of age. Keep in mind, the younger the infant, the more difficult to collect sweat. It is important to collect an adequate amount of sweat (0.075 g or 15 μL depending on method). Diagnostic criteria require an elevated sweat chloride concentration on at least two occasions or identified mutation in each CFTR gene or characteristic abnormalities determined by nasal potential difference measurements. The sweat test remains the gold standard in diagnosing CF. Molecular testing is often used for confirmation and if there is ambiguity in diagnosing CF. Testing for nasal potential difference is uncommon as it is used when sweat testing and molecular testing is inconclusive. As with sweat testing, the nasal potential difference test is quite laborious to perform. In addition, fewer facilities can perform this test, so its availability is limited.

The interpretation of sweat chloride test results is based on age.[33]

If less than 6 months of age:

≤29 mmol/L: Normal, CF very unlikely
30-59 mmol/L: Intermediate, possible CF
≥60 mmol/L: Abnormal, diagnosis of CF

If ≥6 month of age:

≤39 mmol/L: Normal, CF very unlikely
40-59 mmol/L: Intermediate, possible CF
≥60 mmol/L: Abnormal, diagnosis of CF

The lower normal and increased intermediate range reflects the decreasing sweat chloride concentrations in the first few weeks of life, followed by a gradual rise through childhood.[34]

Rarely does a normal sweat chloride result need to be repeated. However, the test is not perfect as 1% of all CF patients have normal sweat test results.[35] If symptoms are strongly suggestive of CF, then the sweat test may be repeated and/or expanded DNA testing may be performed. Intermediate sweat chloride results should be repeated. If the patient is asymptomatic, this would occur at 1-2 months of age. Intermediate results are followed up with DNA testing for CFTR mutations and repeat sweat testing. Abnormal sweat chloride results are considered diagnostic for CF and a second positive test is needed for confirmation of CF. DNA analysis is useful for confirmatory testing as well as to assist in determining appropriate therapeutic treatment for patients.

DNA analysis of the CFTR gene is usually done by direct mutation analysis. There are a number of methods available that provide expanded multi-mutation panel testing and detect deletions or duplications. Direct DNA sequencing is also an option. As technology continues to develop, the cost of these types of analysis will continue to decrease and possibly influence how screening and diagnosis is determined.

Sweat Test

Patients with a family history of CF, exhibiting clinical symptoms of this disease, or a positive newborn screen, need diagnostic testing to determine whether or not CF is present. Mutations in the CFTR protein lead to dysfunction of ion transport across all exocrine tissue. This results in thick, viscous secretions in many different organs and the increase of salt secretion from eccrine sweat glands. Throughout the United States, CF centers accredited by the Cystic Fibrosis Foundation (CFF) provide the quantification of chloride in sweat, more commonly referred to as the sweat test, for the confirmation or diagnosis of CF. The process of sweat testing involves the stimulation of sweat glands by pilocarpine, collection of sweat, and analysis for chloride concentration.

Guidelines to assist with the standardization of the collection and analysis process are available. The most prominent is provided by the Clinical and Laboratory Standards Institute (CLSI document C34-A3.) Sweat testing: Sample collection and quantitative chloride analysis.[36] Similar guidelines are available for the United Kingdom[37] and Australia.[38] The CFF has created their own guidelines[39] based on the CLSI guidelines and the College of American Pathologists Laboratory Accreditation Program Inspection Checklist.[40]

The basic principles and standardization of the method were developed by Gibson and Cooke in 1959.[41] In this method the collection of sweat requires stimulation of sweat glands by pilocarpine using iontophoresis. Pilocarpine is a cholinergic agonist, which stimulates the production of sweat and saliva. Besides its use in sweat testing, pilocarpine is clinically used to treat dry mouth in patients with Sjögren's syndrome and to treat others with glaucoma. Iontophoresis is a process that uses an electric field to move ions. The pilocarpine iontophoresis, stimulation of sweat, commonly occurs on the flexor surface of the patient's forearm. Once the pilocarpine stimulation is completed, either gauze or filter paper, or microbore tubing is used to collect the sweat. The minimum acceptable amount of sweat collected is 15 μL using microbore tubing and 75 mg if collected on gauze or filter paper over a 30-minute time period. These minimums account for a desired rate of sweat of 1 g/m^2/min. The collected sweat contained in the gauze or filter paper is weighed to determine the amount of sweat collected. The sweat is then eluted from the gauze and the chloride content in the sweat is measured. Sweat collected in microbore tubing is expelled from the tubing for sweat chloride determination. Whether the sweat testing process uses filter paper or gauze, or microbore tubing, it requires a significant amount of time to obtain a complete collection sufficient for analysis.

Sweat Stimulation

In the Gibson-Cooke iontophoresis process, the positively charged pilocarpine ions in the saturated gauze (2″ × 2″) are moved into the skin directly under the positive electrode (1.5″ × 1.5″). The negative electrode uses a dilute electrolyte solution in the gauze to complete the circuit. Both electrodes are placed on the same limb. The options for electrode placement include the lower arm or thigh. If there is enough area on the forearm, both electrodes can be placed there. When an inadequate amount of space is available on the forearm, as occurs with newborns, the positive electrode is placed on the forearm and the negative electrode on the upper arm. Alternatively, the thigh can be used for sweat testing; however, the density of sweat glands in the thigh is decreased and may not be an optimal site for stimulation.[42] For newborns, the positive electrode is placed on the inner thigh and the negative electrode onto the lower leg. The electrodes need to be secured firmly to the limb, if not, less pilocarpine may enter into the skin resulting in a decreased sweat rate and the amount of sweat collected. To transport the pilocarpine, a current of 2.5 to 4.0 mA is used to drive the iontophoresis. After 5 minutes, the iontophoresis is complete and collection process can begin.

There are a few vulnerable steps in the stimulation process. The electrode surfaces must be kept clean, daily inspection is highly recommended. If not properly maintained, the amount of current used in the iontophoresis may be decreased. The power source should also be checked periodically to ensure that the amount of current it delivers is accurate. The electrodes must not touch the skin otherwise the potential for a burn significantly increases. A wet interface between the electrode, gauze, and skin must also be maintained. Saturation of gauze with either pilocarpine or electrolyte solution must be complete to maintain the circuit. Of course, chloride contamination must be avoided, so gloves, forceps, hard surfaces, cleaning agents, gauze, and skin need to be kept clean to avoid any potential for falsely increase chloride results.

Sweat Collection

Once pilocarpine has been delivered to the sweat glands in the skin, the electrodes are removed and the pilocarpine site is thoroughly cleaned and dried. The site should be observed for any severe inflammation. If a burn or urticaria is identified, both rare events, medical attention should be made available and the sweat not collected. With the site dry, a pre-weighed piece of gauze is carefully placed over the site. A piece of paraffin wax is used to cover the gauze and wrapped with disposable stretch bandage. Great care must be taken to prevent evaporation. After 30 minutes, check the bandage for any tampering and promptly remove the bandage and paraffin. Carefully collect the gauze and return it into its pre-weighed container. The gauze should be reweighed promptly to determine if 0.075 g of sweat was collected. Quantities less than 75 mg are considered insufficient and not used any further. Sweat testing using microbore method use pilocarpine-containing gel disc in place of gauze soaked in pilocarpine. The collection of sweat uses a proprietary microbore tubing collector and requires a minimum of 15 µL for the collection to be sufficient in sweat.

There are a number of concerns with this process. Extending the 30 minute collection time may lead to erroneous test results and should be avoided. The skin must be completely cleaned and dry prior to placing gauze over the site. The time required to remove the gauze should be minimized in order to minimize the effect of evaporation. Evaporation may also occur from a poorly wrapped bandage around the collection gauze. Any evaporation during the collection process will result in falsely increased chloride concentrations. When removing gauze, it is important to collect any residual drops of sweat that may be located on the paraffin. Likewise, contamination by chloride must be strictly avoided.

Chloride Analysis

Several methods have been used for chloride analysis. Originally a polarographic method developed by Zimmerman and Layton was used.[43] This method used the reaction between mercury and chloride, which was monitored by measuring the current at a fixed applied voltage. The amount of current measured was directly proportional to the amount of chloride in solution. A second method was developed by Schales and Schales in which deproteinized biological fluids were titrated using mercuric nitrate and using diphenylcarbazone as an indicator. [44] The current methods of measurement use the Cotlove method.[45] This is a coulometric titration in which silver ions are generated from the anode and combine with chloride from the sample to precipitate silver chloride. The length of time the current is applied, resulting from this reaction, is directly proportional to the amount of chloride in the sample. A digital chloridometer is required for this measurement. It is possible to use an ion-selective electrode for measuring sweat chloride. A systematic evaluation for sweat chloride determination would need to be conducted to validate this method, as done for all clinical testing devices. This method is rarely used as its sensitivity at lower chloride concentrations may not provide acceptable accuracy and precision.

Quality Control

There are many details involved in pilocarpine stimulation, sweat collection, and chloride analysis. As with other clinical tests, quality control of at least two different levels is performed as well as participation is proficiency testing. The overall process is partly monitored by tracking whether an adequate amount of sweat is collected for chloride analysis. When an inadequate amount of sweat is collected, the sample is described as "quantity not sufficient" or QNS. QNS rates and their determination are established by the CFF. They are set at <5% for patients older than 3 months of age and <10% for patients ≤3 months of age. The QNS rate does not provide quality monitoring of the analytical measurement process, but proficiency testing and quality controls can fulfill this role.

Other Considerations

Other considerations for a successful sweat test include having a clinically stable patient. Some institutions only test on an outpatient basis. The patient's hydration status should be good and no acute illnesses present. The skin should be clean and free of inflammation, such as eczema or other rashes. If clinically acceptable, testing should be delayed until patient is at least 2 weeks of age or older and weighs more than 2 kg. For immature newborns, the decrease in extracellular fluid is more pronounced. If it is clinically reasonable to delay testing to 4 weeks of age, it may be helpful in reducing the chance of a QNS result and the need for repeat testing.

Maintaining the competency of technologists performing the sweat test is critical to the success of the process. Competency is best maintained by frequently performing the sweat collection process. Limiting the number of technologists involved with the sweat collection process may be necessary.

The relationship between sweat chloride concentration and sweat rate has come into question. The positive correlation between sweat electrolyte concentrations and sweat rate were derived from a study done in 1963 of 29 subjects, including 10 CF patients.[46] Consequently, this study concludes that the concentration of electrolytes determined by conductivity is higher at increased sweat rates. The data in this study is used to support the minimum allowable collection for a sweat test as defined by the use of 2″ × 2″ gauze or filter paper, and collecting sweat for 30 minutes. In 2014, data from over 1300 specimens demonstrate a negligible negative correlation between sweat chloride concentrations and the amount of sweat collected.[47] In addition, the 2014 study puts into question the 75 mg sweat collection requirement. Their data from 101 paired specimens containing 24-74 mg and >75 mg of sweat produced no false positive or false negative results. How this information may affect sweat testing for chloride remains unclear.

Other Conditions

The presence of elevated sweat chloride concentrations can be found associated with other diseases and conditions including concurrent administration of steroids or topiramate,[48] celiac disease, familial cholestasis, systemic lupus erythematosus, pseudohypoaldosteronism, hypogammaglobulinemia, and Munchausen syndrome (including by proxy).[36]

| SUMMARY

Cystic fibrosis is the most common life-shortening disease. Identification of the CFTR gene has advanced the understanding of the pathophysiology of this autosomal recessive disease. With more than 2000 identified mutations in the CFTR gene, our understanding of classic and non-classic CF is becoming clearer. Classification of protein function combined with molecular knowledge has led to the development of small molecules to help CF patients manage their disease. CF is commonly found in newborn screening disease panels. The protocol for screening involves IRT and DNA mutation testing. A number of variables affect the measurement of IRT and until these are better understood, standardization of IRT measurement remains elusive. Diagnosis of CF requires the determination of chloride concentration in sweat. The collection and analysis is both labor intensive and time consuming. Difficulties with sweat collection increase with young and premature newborns. Unfortunately, there is no cure for CF, however the increasing knowledge of CF disease has extended the mean survival to 37 years.

TRAINING MODULE

1. Cystic fibrosis is an autosomal recessive disease, and has a frequency in the Caucasian population of:
   a. 1 in 100,000 live births
   b. 1 in 50,000 live births
   c. 1 in 10,000 live births
   d. 1 in 2,500 live births
   e. 1 in 200,000 live births

2. A 1-month old girl with a sweat chloride result of 35 mmol/L is interpreted as:
   a. Normal, CF not likely
   b. Intermediate, possible CF
   c. Abnormal, CF likely

3. The CFTR mutation F508del results in abnormal protein folding and trafficking. This primary function places this mutation into what Class?
   a. Class I
   b. Class II
   c. Class III
   d. Class IV
   e. Class V

4. Non-classic CF patients
   a. typically have pancreatic insufficiency and upper respiratory tract infections
   b. have elevated (>60 mmol/L) sweat chloride concentrations
   c. have clinical disease limited to one organ system
   d. are newborn screen negative
   e. on average, will have more disease complications

REFERENCES

1. Kerr ID. Structure and association of ATP-binding cassette transporter nucleotide-binding domains. *Biochim Biophys Acta*. 2002;1561:47.
2. Centers for Disease Control and Prevention. National Office of Public Health Genomics, Cystic Fibrosis Clinical Validity. September 10, 2007. Available at http://www.cdc.gov/genomics/gtesting/file/print/FBR/CFCliVal.pdf. Accessed December 5, 2014.
3. Rowe SM, Miller S, Sorscher EJ. Cystic Fibrosis. *N Engl J Med*. 2005;352:1992.
4. Accurso FJ, Sonta MK, Wagener JS. Complications associated with symptomatic diagnosis in infants with cystic fibrosis. *J Pediatr*. 2005;147:S37.
5. Cystic Fibrosis Foundation Patient Registry: annual data report 2012. http://www.cff.org/uploadedfiles/research/clinicalresearch/patientregistryreport/2012-cff-patient-registry.pdf. Accessed December 15, 2014.
6. Zhou Y, Son K, Painter RG, et al: Cystic fibrosis transmembrane conductance regulator recruitment to phagosomes in neutrophils. *J Innate Immun*. 2013;5:219.
7. Khan TZ, Wagener JS, Bost T, et al: Early pulmonary inflammation in infants with cystic fibrosis. *Am J Respir Crit Care Med*. 1995;151:1075.

8. Worlitzsch D, Tarran R, Ulrich M, et al. Effects of reduced mucus oxygen concentration in airway Pseudomonas infections of cystic fibrosis patients. *J Clin Invest.* 2002;109:317.

9. Nousia-Arvanitakis S. Cystic fibrosis and the pancreas: recent scientific advances. *J Clin Gastroenterol.* 1999;29:138.

10. Moran A, Dunitz J, Nathan B, et al. Cystic fibrosis-related diabetes: current trends in prevalence, incidence, and mortality. *Diabetes Care.* 2009;32:1626.

11. Barrio R. Cystic fibrosis-related diabetes: novel pathogenic insights opening new therapeutic avenues. *Eur J of Endocrinol.* 2015;172:R131.

12. Kerem E, Konstan MW, De Boeck K, et al. Ataluren for the treatment of nonsense-mutation cystic fibrosis: a randomized, double-blind, placebo-controlled phase 3 trial. *Lancet.* 2014;2(77):539.

13. Gorter RR, Karimi A, Sleeboom C, Kneepkens CM, Heij HA. Clinical and genetic characteristics of meconium ileus in newborns with and without cystic fibrosis. *J Pediatr Gastroenterol Nutr.* 2010;50(5):569.

14. Montgomery GS and Howenstine M. Cystic Fibrosis. *Pediatr Rev.* 2009;30:302.

15. Tan KH, Mulheran M, Knox AJ, Smyth AR. Aminoglycoside prescribing and surveillance in cystic fibrosis. *Am J Respir Crit Care Med.* 2003;167:819.

16. Van Goor F, Hadida S, Grootenhuis PD, et al. Rescue of CF airway epithelial cell function in vitro by a CFTR potentiator, VX-770. *Proc Natl Acad Sci USA.* 2009;106(44):1882.

17. Veit G, Avramescu RG, Chiang AN, et al. From CFTR biology toward combinatorial pharmacotherapy: expanded classification of cystic fibrosis mutations. *Mol Biol Cell.* 2016;27:424.

18. Wainwright CE, Elborn JS, Ramsey BW, et al. Lumacaftor-Ivacaftor in patients with cystic fibrosis homozygous for Phe508del CFTR. *NEJM.* 2015;373(18):1783-1784.

19. De Boeck K, Wilschanski M, Castellani C, et al. Cystic fibrosis: terminology and diagnostic algorithms. *Thorax.* 2006;61(7):627.

20. Ren CL, Desai H, Platt M, Dixon M. Clinical outcomes in infants with cystic fibrosis transmembrane conductance regulator (CFTR) related metabolic syndrome. *Pediatr Pulmonol.* 2011;46(11):1079.

21. Cystic Fibrosis Foundation, Borowitz D, Parad RB, et al. Cystic Fibrosis Foundation practice guidelines for the management of infants with cystic fibrosis transmembrane conductance regulator-related metabolic syndrome during the first two years of life and beyond. *J Pediatr.* 2009;155(6 suppl):S106.

22. Keating CL, Liu X, Dimango EA. Classic respiratory disease but atypical diagnostic testing distinguishes adult presentation of cystic fibrosis. *Chest.* 2010;137(5):1157.

23. Munch A, Mayell SJ, Winters V, et al. Cystic fibrosis screen positive, inconclusive diagnosis (CFSPID): a new designation and management recommendations for infants with an inconclusive diagnosis following newborn screening. *J Cyst Fibros.* 2015;14:706.

24. Lindau-Shepard BA and Pass KA. Newborn screening for cystic fibrosis by use of a multiplex immunoassay. *Clin Chem.* 2010;56(3):445.

25. Therrell BL, Hannon WH, Hoffman G, et al. Immunoreactive trypsinogen (IRT) as a biomarker for cystic fibrosis: challenges in newborn dried blood spot screening. *Molec Gen Metab.* 2012;106:1.

26. Kloosterboer M, Hoffman G, Rock M, et al. Clarification of laboratory and clinical variables that influence cystic fibrosis newborn screening with initial analysis of immunoreactive trypsinogen. *Pediatrics.* 2009;123:338.

27. Korzeniewski SJ, Young WI, Hawkins HC, et al. Variation in immunoreactive trypsinogen concentrations among Michigan newborns and implications for cystic fibrosis newborn screening. *Pediatr Pulmonol.* 2011;46:125.

28. Fritz A and Farrell P. Estimating the annual number of false negative cystic fibrosis newborn screening tests. *Pediatr Pulmonol.* 2012;47(2):207.

29. Wells J, Rosenberg M, Hoffman G, Anstead M, Farrell PM. A decision-tree approach to cost comparison of newborn screening strategies for cystic fibrosis. *Pediatrics.* 2012;129(2):e339.

30. Watson MS, Cutting GR, Desnick RJ, et al. Cystic fibrosis population carrier screening: 2004 revision of American College of Medical Genetics mutation panel. Policy Statement. *Genet in Medicine.* 2004;6(5):387.

31. Alper OM, Wong LJ, Young S, et al. Identification of novel and rare mutations in California Hispanic and African American cystic fibrosis patients. *Hum Mutat.* 2004;24(4):353.

32. Stern RC. The diagnosis of cystic fibrosis. *N Engl J Med.* 1997:336(7):487.

33. Farrell PM, Rosenstein BJ, White TB, et al. Guidelines for diagnosis of cystic fibrosis in newborns through older adults: Cystic Fibrosis Foundation consensus report. *J Pediatr.* 2008;153(2):S4.

34. Parad RB, Comeau AM, Dorkin HL, et al. Sweat testing infants detected by cystic fibrosis newborn screening. *J Pediatr.* 2005;147(3 suppl):S69.

35. Dreyfus DH, Bethel R, Gelfand EW. Cystic fibrosis 3849+10kb C>T mutation associated with severe pulmonary disease and male fertility. *Am J Respir Crit Care Med.* 1996;153(2):858.

36. LeGrys VA, Applequist R, Briscoe DR, et al. Sweat testing: sample collection and quantitative chloride analysis; Approved guideline – Third Edition. CLSI document C34-A3. Wayne, PA: Clinical and Laboratory Standards Institute; 2009.

37. Green A and Kirk J. Guidelines for the performance of the sweat test for the diagnosis of cystic fibrosis. *Ann Clin Biochem.* 2007;44:25.

38. Coakly J, Scott S, Doery J, et al. Australian guidelines for the performance of the sweat test for the diagnosis of cystic fibrosis. *Clin Biochem Rev.* 2006;27(suppl i):S1.

39. LeGrys VA, Yankaskas JR, Quittell LM, et al. Diagnostic sweat testing: the Cystic Fibrosis Foundation guidelines. *J Pediatr.* 2007;151:85.

40. College of American Pathologists Laboratory Accreditation Program. Chemistry and toxicology checklist. Chicago, IL: College of American Pathologists; 2014.

41. Gibson LE and Cooke RE. A test for concentration of electrolytes in sweat in cystic fibrosis of the pancreas utilizing pilocarpine by iontophoresis. *Pediatrics.* 1959;23:545.

42. Wilke K, Martin A, Terstegen L, et al. A short history of sweat gland biology. *Int J Cosmet Sci.* 2007;29:169.

43. Zimmerman WJ and Layton WM. A polarographic micromethod for the determination of blood chloride. *J Biol Chem.* 1949;181:141.

44. Schales O and Schales SS. A simple and accurate method for the determination of chloride in biological fluids. *J Biol Chem.* 1941;140:879.

45. Cotlove E, Tranthan HV, and Bowman RL. An instrument and method for automatic, rapid, accurate, and sensitive titration of chloride in biologic samples. *J Lab Clin Med.* 1958;51:461.

46. Gibson LE and di Sant'Agnese PA. Studies of salt excretion in sweat. Relationships between rate, conductivity, and electrolyte composition of sweat from patients with cystic fibrosis and from control subjects. *J Pediatr*. 1963;62:855.
47. DeMarco ML, Dietzen DJ, and Brown SM. Sweating the small stuff: adequacy and accuracy in sweat chloride determination. *Clin Biochem*. 2015;48(6):443-447.
48. Guglani L, Sitwat B, Lower D, et al. Elevated sweat chloride concentration in children without cystic fibrosis who are receiving topiramate therapy. *Peadiatr Pulmonol*. 2012;47:429.

PEDIATRIC REFERENCE INTERVALS

7

Nathalie Lepage and Julie Shaw

LEARNING OBJECTIVES

1. Describe the difference between reference intervals and decision limits.
2. Discuss the challenges in the establishment and verification of pediatric reference intervals.
3. Compare traditional and alternative strategies for determining or verifying reference intervals.
4. Summarize current initiatives with successful recruitment strategies of healthy children for reference interval studies.

INTRODUCTION

Reference intervals are primordial to correctly interpret the laboratory data produced from biological samples. Comparison of laboratory test results to decision limits or reference intervals is an important part of medical decision making. Therefore, lack of accurate reference intervals can adversely impact patient care, by delaying diagnosis, treatment procedures, and/or modifying prognosis. Reference intervals need to be established for all age groups, as emphasized by quality standard requirements from various laboratory accreditation organizations, such as the College of American Pathologists (www.cap.org) and the Ontario Laboratory Accreditation, a division of the Institute for Quality Management in Healthcare (iqmh.org). For many laboratory tests, the pediatric reference intervals differ from the adult reference intervals. There is a serious risk to patient safety when reference intervals are not adequately evaluated for children. When attempting to conduct "classic" reference interval studies, laboratories face major challenges in accessing adequate numbers of specimens with sufficient volumes collected from healthy children ranging from the newborn period until past the adolescent years.

Furthermore, reference intervals developed using one analytical platform cannot simply be transferred to another platform. The purpose of this chapter will be to review the most commonly encountered challenges and the statistical tools available to establish pediatric reference intervals. It will also highlight alternative approaches to establish or verify reference intervals with discussion of current initiatives that have been successful in conducting large-scale collection of specimens in healthy children for this purpose.

REFERENCE INTERVALS VERSUS DECISION LIMITS

A reference interval is generally defined as the central 95% (between the 2.5th and 97.5th percentiles) of measured analyte concentrations from a reference or "healthy" population.[1] A reference population refers to a population of healthy individuals. Reference intervals should be calculated specifically for each laboratory method and should be calculated for specific populations.[2] Clinicians use reference intervals to aid in interpreting patient quantitative test results to distinguish patients with results outside of the reference interval (ie, "abnormal") from those with results within the reference interval that are typically considered "normal." However, the reference interval should only be used as a guide, as patient analyte values must be interpreted in the context of the clinical situation.[2,3] This is a very important point that is often misunderstood. Given the way in which reference intervals are calculated using statistical approaches, by design, 5% of analyte results from healthy individuals will fall outside of the reference interval. Figure 7-1 outlines a theoretical distribution of analyte values from a reference (healthy) population. The 2.5th and 97.5th percentile results are taken as the lower and upper reference interval limits, which means that 2.5% of values on either side of these cut-points are outside the reference interval although they represent results from healthy individuals.

Alternatively decision limits are analyte values that indicate the need for clinical action and are based on national or international guidelines from expert groups. Decision limits remain the same regardless of the method used to measure the analyte and regardless of the population of individuals.[4] Examples of decision limits include: glucose concentrations greater than 7.0 mmol/L (126 mg/dL) and HbA1C greater than 6.5% as diagnostic for diabetes[5]; guidelines for acceptable, borderline, and high lipid/lipoprotein concentrations in children and adolescents (published by the National Cholesterol Education Program through the NIH in the United States).

Standardization or harmonization across laboratory methods is essential if clinical decision limits are to be used. Without standardization or harmonization, measured values for analytes cannot be compared between laboratory methods.[6] The use of reference intervals does not require standardization,

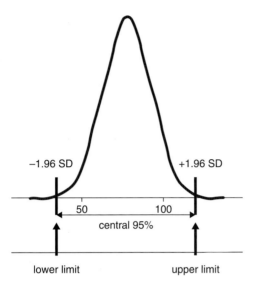

Figure 7-1 ◼ A theoretical normal distribution of analyte values measured in a population of healthy individuals. The central 95% of values are assumed to encompass the reference population and the lower and upper reference interval limits are chosen based on the central 95% of values.

since reference intervals are calculated for each method and if properly validated, will take into account any measurement bias associated with that particular laboratory method.[4]

Common Reference Intervals

Common reference intervals are those that can be applied to a given analyte regardless of the methodology employed. The concept of common reference intervals has been proposed but is difficult to implement given the heterogeneous nature of populations and the lack of analytical method standardization or harmonization. It is important for clinicians to understand that analyte results are not necessarily comparable between laboratories using different methodologies.[7,8] This is especially true of analytes that are measured by immunoassay methods, such as proteins, hormones, and tumor markers. Different immunoassay methods employ different antibodies, which will not recognize the same epitopes on target antigens resulting in differences in measurements of the same analyte. Some proteins, such as β-hCG and growth hormone, can also be heterogeneous molecules, adding further complication. Standardization or harmonization is difficult without standard reference materials which are often not available for proteins, hormones and tumor markers. The difference in laboratory results may directly impact patient safety. Access to results for the same analyte from different platforms and/or reagents may lead to misclassification or inappropriate treatment if the clinician uses common reference intervals when there is a clinically significant method bias. If a clinician wishes to evaluate trends in an analyte concentration measured by immunoassay over time, it is important that the patient be advised to have all testing performed for that analyte in the same laboratory and by the same method. An example of this would be monitoring of tumor marker concentrations in patients treated for cancer.[9]

Challenges in Establishing Pediatric Reference Intervals

Establishing reference intervals is challenging due to the large number of reference samples from healthy individuals that need to be collected for this purpose. The Clinical and Laboratory Standards Institute (CLSI) guideline on reference intervals states that a minimum of 120 reference samples are required to establish a reference interval. This is the minimum number needed to calculate the 90% confidence limit of the upper and lower reference intervals when using non-parametric statistics. If age and gender differences exist for an analyte, this requires the collection of 120 reference samples for each of these groups, adding further challenge (CLSI guidelines EP28-A3). The guidelines do not provide a simple approach to establish pediatric reference intervals in fluids, such as cerebrospinal fluid (CSF) for which specimen collection is invasive, leading to a potential decline in participation from healthy participants and their parents.

Given the dynamic changes occurring during child growth and development, it is not surprising that analyte concentrations change as children grow and develop.[10] This results in the need for many hundreds of samples from healthy children, in order to establish reference intervals for each age and gender partition required. For example, alkaline phosphatase (ALP) concentrations rise rapidly at puberty and concentrations differ between males and females, resulting in multiple reference interval partitions. Pubertal changes impact a variety of analytes, including many hormones. Since the age of puberty onset can vary by up to 5 years in healthy children, further classification is typically required based on pubertal staging. This is most commonly achieved by providing reference ranges that are specific to gender and Tanner staging. The Tanner stage refers to a standardized system that is based on clinical exam findings and describes the extent of pubertal changes in an individual.[11,12] Obtaining sufficient numbers of accurately-staged and truly representative subjects to establish gender-specific, Tanner-staged reference intervals is very difficult.

Other partitions may also be found to be necessary. Recently, a study by the Canadian group, CALIPER, also demonstrated that there are differences in certain analyte values based on ethnicity. This study compared analyte values between Caucasians, East Asians, and South Asians, the three main ethnic groups in Toronto, a large urban center in the heart of Canada, where the study was performed. Ethnic differences were noted for ALT, amylase, IgG, IgM, magnesium, total protein, and transferrin,[13] adding further complexity to the calculation of appropriate reference intervals. Additionally, the epidemic of obesity in most developed countries brings another layer of complexity when designing protocols to establish pediatric reference intervals. There is currently a lack of knowledge on the impact of body mass index (BMI) or waist circumference on the stability of laboratory markers. It is likely that marker levels are impacted by body habitus, hence further increasing the number of partition groups that may need to be taken into account.

Recruitment of healthy children for these studies requires large-scale public campaigns that are time consuming and costly. Consent (parental or patient) is required, depending on the age and jurisdiction. Collecting blood from children may be difficult, requiring phlebotomists with pediatric expertise. Obtaining a sufficient volume of sample can also be an issue and pre-analytical factors, such as diurnal variation and fasting must be taken into account for certain analytes.[14]

Another aspect that should be considered when establishing pediatric reference intervals is the reporting strategy. Currently, most laboratory information systems (LIS) have been designed to allow for partition only by age and gender. However as noted earlier, many hormones depict marked fluctuations during various stages of puberty. These hormones should be interpreted in light of the Tanner stage. One limitation is that most LIS do not have the ability to report reference intervals based on any criteria other than age and gender. However, although a less than ideal solution, interpretive comments referencing clinical guidelines can usually be included with results.

TRADITIONAL APPROACHES FOR CALCULATING REFERENCE INTERVALS

The sections later outline the steps in calculating reference intervals using traditional approaches. The CLSI guideline recommends[1] the collection of a minimum of 120 samples from healthy individuals for each partition (eg, age and gender). When publishing calculated reference intervals or documenting the source of reference intervals for the laboratory method employed, the following should be considered and included: the number of subjects; nature of subjects (how identified as healthy); important exclusions; relevant pre-analytical factors; statistical measures (mean, median, 2.5th and 97.5th percentiles and 90% confidence limits); number of outliers excluded; analytical method; and traceability of method.[15]

Removal of Outlier Results

The first step in establishing reference intervals is to remove any outlier results from the data set of reference samples.[1] Outlier results are extreme values which differ from the majority of values within a population and can skew the data in a population if not removed. There are two statistical approaches that are recommended by CLSI for the detection of outlier results: 1) The approach referred to as the Dixon test; and 2) the Tukey approach. Both approaches require that the data be normally distributed or transformed (logarithmically if not Gaussian) to convert the data distribution as Gaussian, prior to analysis for outliers.[16]

Partitioning of Data

Age-based and gender-based differences in analyte values may require that the data set be partitioned. Partitioning is generally performed initially by visual inspection of the data distribution. Once potential partitions are identified, statistical techniques can be employed to determine whether significant differences exist between subgroups of the distribution. If statistically significant differences exist, the data set should be partitioned.

Two statistical approaches that have been employed are: 1) The method proposed by Lahti; and 2) the method proposed by Harris and Boyd. The Lahti method recommends partitioning when >4.1% of the subgroup data falls outside the central 95% (2.5th-97.5th centiles) of the common distribution.[17] Using the method by Harris and Boyd, partitioning should be performed if the ratio of the subgroup standard deviation to the standard deviation of the common distribution is >1.5.[18]

Statistical Approaches for Calculating the Central 95% of Reference Population Values

Non-parametric statistical approaches are generally preferable to parametric approaches because non-parametric approaches require fewer assumptions about the distribution of data. Using a non-parametric approach, the reference sample data are rank-ordered and from this the 2.5th and 97.5th percentiles calculated as the reference interval limits representing the central 95% of data. These approaches require a large number of samples with CLSI guidelines EP28-A3 recommending at least 120 reference samples in each partition. When large numbers of samples are not available, studies have demonstrated that mathematical models can be employed, such as bootstrapping[19] or robust[20] models in order to calculate reliable reference intervals. Bootstrapping involves repeated re-sampling from the data set for calculation of the 2.5th and 97.5th percentiles. The International Federation of Clinical

Chemistry (IFCC) recommends a minimum of 500 samplings from the data set for these calculations.[21]

Parametric approaches require the assumption that the distribution of data forms a normal or Gaussian distribution. If this is not the case, the data must first be transformed to a normal distribution (eg, by logarithmic transformation) prior to estimation of the 2.5th and 97.5th percentiles.[16]

Occasionally a pediatric reference interval will need to be established that does not use the central 95% as its basis. These types of reference values are generally also set statistically. Examples would include determining a cutoff value for troponin of the 99th percentile of the normal population, or determining a therapeutic range for monitoring certain drugs.

ALTERNATIVE APPROACHES FOR DEFINING PEDIATRIC REFERENCE INTERVALS

Given the challenges associated with establishing reference intervals using classical methods, particularly for pediatrics, alternative approaches have been considered and adopted. These approaches include use of "leftover samples" from selected clinics, statistical approaches applied to hospital databases, and transference of published reference intervals.

Use of "Leftover" Samples from Selected Clinics

Some groups have used "leftover" samples from selected clinics within the hospital to establish reference intervals. These selected clinics are those which would be expected to serve largely "healthy" children, examples being: allergy, elective surgery, dentistry, and orthopedics. Early publications from the CALIPER study in Canada employed this approach.[22-24] A retrospective analysis of the reference intervals calculated from leftover samples indicated that, in general, they were wider than those established from samples from healthy children accumulated prospectively.[13] This makes sense given that these samples are not necessarily from healthy children and the stress of treatment may contribute to differences in analyte values compared to healthy children in the population.

Statistical Approaches Applied to Hospital-Based Data

First proposed by Hoffmann in 1963,[25] these approaches use large amounts of patient data from hospital databases and employ statistical techniques to tease out the data most likely to come from "healthy" individuals. The cumulative frequency of each measured result is plotted against the analyte value and the linear portion around the 50th centile is chosen. The 2.5th and 97.5th centiles are extrapolated from this linear portion as the normal interval. The assumptions made are that 1) the majority of laboratory test values in hospital-based databases are normal; and 2) the data form a Gaussian distribution. A recent study from the CALIPER group[26] employed a modified version of the Hoffmann approach to calculate pediatric reference intervals for several chemistry analytes. These reference intervals were compared to the reference intervals calculated from true reference samples as part of the CALIPER study. The study found that the reference intervals calculated from hospital-based data were wider than those calculated from true reference subjects. The results suggested that hospital-based data may be appropriate for establishing reference intervals for some analytes but not others and should only be used as a guide.

Verification and Transference of Reference Intervals

Given the challenges associated with reference interval establishment studies, many laboratories choose to verify existing reference intervals for their local population. These may be reference intervals published in the literature or provided by the manufacturer of the method in-use in the laboratory. CLSI guidelines EP28-A3 outline a recommended approach to reference interval verification that requires the collection of a minimum of 20 reference samples per partition. A reference interval is said to be verified if no more than 10% of the reference specimen values fall outside the reference interval being verified. This process is less burdensome as it requires fewer samples than a full-scale reference interval establishment study. However, this approach can be problematic when the reference intervals being verified were calculated with measurements made using a different methodology than the laboratory performing the verification, or when the original reference intervals did omit some partition groups.

Another approach that requires fewer samples is to perform a reference interval transference study. This is often the approach used when reference intervals were established using a different methodology. A transference study requires performing a method comparison study to assess the agreement between the method used to establish the reference interval and the local method. CLSI guidelines EP28-A3 recommendations are that a minimum of 40 patient samples be analyzed by each method for a comparison study. These samples should be chosen such that they cover the entire analytical measuring range of the assays. If the methods show acceptable agreement within minimal bias, the reference intervals can be transferred. As an example, if the correlation between the two assays has an $r^2 \geq 0.95$, a slope in the 0.95-1.05 range and a Y intercept that is acceptable for that analyte, the reference interval would be transferred. If bias does exist between the two methods, linear regression can be used to transform the established reference intervals into those applicable to the local method. CLSI EP28-A3 recommends performing a verification study as a follow-up to confirm the validity of the transformation. A multi-instrument transference study was recently performed by the CALIPER study group to provide reference intervals for 40 routine chemistry analytes on five major automated method platforms.[27]

Multi-Centered Trials

To decrease the burden of establishing pediatric reference intervals on all markers reported in the laboratory, it is desirable for laboratories to form a collaborative and pool their data. This requires the following of strict protocols using common quality assurance guidelines. As an example, six laboratories could participate, each center collecting 20 samples per partition group, to achieve the recommended 120 samples per partition as in compliance with CLSI guidelines EP28-A3. The challenge to this approach would be the samples from a mix of different populations potentially resulting in wider reference intervals. It would also require stringent sample collection and processing protocols to ensure a consistent approach.

Sources of Pediatric Reference Intervals

A widely used source of pediatric reference intervals is a book titled "*Pediatric Reference Intervals*," which has been most recently printed in its 7th edition.[28]

Several recent global efforts have been initiated to address the limited resources for reference intervals for pediatrics. The major initiatives in this area will be described briefly below. Similar approaches to participant recruitment have been used in the various initiatives. The most successful approach has been the nationwide advertising campaign like those used by CALIPER in Canada and the KiGGs study in Germany; however, this requires strong commitment from the national organizations and sufficient budget linked to media campaigns. Successful smaller-scale recruitment strategies have involved the direct advertisement and engagement of places and activities that are highly populated with children. Some examples include schools, day care centers, sports teams, religious groups, vaccination clinics, summer camps, etc. There are also hospital-based approaches that may be more feasible for laboratorians. This includes recruitment in outpatient settings serving relatively "healthy" children, (eg, dental, plastic surgery, and orthopedics). Children undergoing elective surgeries may also meet recruitment criteria for reference interval studies. Lastly siblings of children seeking care in hospital settings may be eligible and interested in participating in reference interval studies.

Children's Health Improvement Through Laboratory Diagnostics (CHILDx)

The CHILDx initiative developed through ARUP laboratories in the United States is aimed at prospectively collecting serum and urine specimens from healthy children in two different cohorts, ages 6 months to 6 years and ages 7 years to 17 years. Tanner stage information is also collected for children in the age 7-17 category. The study has calculated reference intervals for many analytes including general chemistries, hormones, and trace metals (www. childx.org). Their findings confirmed the fact that Tanner stage is important when reporting hormones. As an example, androstenedione, dehydroepian-drostenedione and testosterone levels showed a Tanner stage-dependent, an age-dependent and a gender-dependent impact. These three partition groups were mutually exclusive.[29]

Canadian Laboratory Initiative on Pediatric Reference Intervals (CALIPER)

The CALIPER initiative is a nationwide initiative in Canada led by the Hospital for Sick Children. The goal of CALIPER is to establish reference intervals for a variety of analytes through prospective sample collection from healthy children aged 0 to 18 years. Their study protocol includes the collection of several participant characteristics, such as diet for 1 week prior to specimen collection, BMI, height, weight, waist circumference, gender, age, ethnic background. This group has calculated pediatric reference intervals for forty general chemistry analytes on several major platforms. Recently, CALIPER published reference intervals for several hormones and proteins (www.caliperdatabase.org). Their findings provided new information on impact of ethnic background on pediatric reference intervals. Several markers displayed markedly different reference intervals when using ethnicity as the partition group. Total T4 and ferritin are higher in East Asians and lower in South Asians compared to Caucasian. Cobalamin is substantially higher in East Asians, PTH is substantially higher in South Asians, and 25(OH) vitamin D is substantially lower in East Asians.[30]

The German Health Interview and Examination Survey for Children and Adolescents (KiGGs)

This nation-wide study based in German interviewed over 14,000 children and adolescents between the ages of 0 and 17 years. Data collected was a mixture of objective and subjective health parameters, to better assess health risks and expected health requirements in the German pediatric population. As part of the objective aspect of the survey, they collected serum samples from these children to look at the population-based distribution of several laboratory parameters (http://www.kiggs-studie.de/english/home.html).

Publications on their findings have been available in German for few years already; unfortunately complete reference interval data are still not fully available in English. The markers they have evaluated are from the general clinical biochemistry test menu, nutrition status, iron metabolism, thyroid function testing and others.[31]

Pathology Harmony

This group based in the United Kingdom (www.pathologyharmony.co.uk) aims to harmonize adult and pediatric reference intervals through consensus.[32] This initiative restricted their focus to those biomarkers that have been shown to be harmonized, and decided to exclude immunoassays for which several vendors are using non-identical sources of calibrators or antibodies.

Their approach clearly departs from CLSI EP28-A3 recommended approach in that they develop reference intervals by consensus rather than through analyte measurement and calculations. However there are clear benefits to health care providers and decreased impact on patient safety when unified reference intervals are provided from most/all laboratories in delineated geographical environments.

National Children's Study

One of the initiatives that involved the largest number of participants was the National Children's Study (NCS) in the United States. The NCS study design was aimed at evaluating the role of various environmental factors (ie, air, water, etc.) and genetics background on participant phenotype (ie, growth, development, general health status) in the United States. The original plan was for the NCS to be generating data on a prospective basis, following participants from before their birth until 21 years. An expected number of 100,000 participants would have provided biological samples (blood and urine) at regular intervals until 21 years (http://www.nationalchildrensstudy.gov). Unfortunately the NCS was canceled at the end of 2014 and only one reference interval study was accomplished while the NCS was on-going.[33]

Dissemination of Pediatric Reference Intervals

The major initiatives listed earlier and the numerous studies performed locally on a limited number of biomarkers (typically one marker per study design) have produced and will continue to provide invaluable information. Publications are made available on a regular basis as studies are completed. Laboratory professionals can find the compilation of data and results by searching the marker of interest. A useful reference book which summarizes many reference interval studies is that published by Soldin et al.[28] However, the disadvantage of books is their "static" nature. They cannot incorporate newly published results. The use of digital media, such as intelligent applications, could become a wonderful tool, allowing the laboratory professional to stay current with all publications. The CALIPER team is currently working on a commercial app that would address the need to make regular updates.

SUMMARY

Laboratory results must be interpreted in the context of a decision limit or reference interval. Decision limits are analyte values typically measured using methods that have been standardized or harmonized. Decision limits are determined by national or international guidelines from expert groups to indicate the need for clinical action. The use of decision limits based on national or international guidelines depends upon the availability of standardized or harmonized methods for analyte measurement.

Reference intervals are generally defined as the central 95% (between the 2.5th and 97.5th percentiles) of measured analyte concentrations from a reference or "healthy" population and should be calculated for each laboratory method. The classic method for establishing a reference interval is that described in the CLSI guideline, EP28-A3. Many analytes demonstrate age-related, gender-related, and/or growth-related changes with normal development during childhood. Therefore, accurate determination of pediatric-specific reference intervals is important for efficient and effective care in those 0-18 years. Laboratories must also meet regulatory standards related to the definition and verification of reference intervals appropriate for their particular patient population.

Establishing pediatric reference intervals requires consideration of all aspects of the measurement process, including the pre-analytical, analytical, and post-analytical phases. Access to adequate numbers of specimens with sufficient volumes and that meet the defined criteria for inclusion in a "classic" reference interval study is a major challenge for laboratories. This is due to the number of specimens needed per sub-group and the variety of sub-groups required for various analytes. Therefore, alternate approaches and recruitment strategies are commonly employed in pediatrics to establish and validate reference intervals. Published sources of pediatric reference intervals are available and large, prospective trials to establish pediatric-specific reference intervals are underway and may also be used for guidance. However, reference intervals developed using one analytical platform cannot simply be transferred to another testing platform and require transference and further internal verification to apply such ranges to one's own laboratory.

TRAINING MODULE

Your laboratory has proceeded to the purchasing of a new biochemistry analyzer. Addition of this analyzer will require the establishment of a complete set of reference intervals for both genders, from 0 to 99 years.

1. Which statement describes an appropriate approach to determining reference intervals when changing to a new vendor's chemistry analyzer?

   a. The laboratory will be able to apply the manufacturer's stated reference ranges for the new vendor methods without the need to perform a local verification study.

   b. The laboratory will be able to perform transference studies by using a small number of samples in each age/gender sub-group, confirming the validity of this approach using statistical analyses.

   c. The laboratory will be able to analyze 20 specimens from normal male volunteers aged 18-65 years and extrapolate reference intervals for all age/gender sub-groups.

   d. The laboratory will be able to use the current reference intervals since all tests are currently performed in the laboratory and chemistry analytes have less variance across vendors than immunoassay methods.

2. Which of the following statements regarding establishing reference intervals is true?

   a. Decision limits are not available by reviewing national guidelines.

   b. Reference intervals could be established by using left-over samples from the emergency department.

   c. Parametric approach can be used in non-Gaussian distributed parameters.

   d. Common reference intervals across platforms cannot be derived when primary reference material is not available.

3. Which statement regarding reference intervals is true?

   a. The laboratory can exchange specimens with another laboratory for the purpose of establishing reference intervals if the samples have been anonymized.

   b. Reference intervals are not necessary in plasma samples.

   c. Results from national initiatives cannot be transferred to a laboratory located outside the country.

   d. A reference interval taken from a literature source does not need to be verified.

REFERENCES

1. CLSI guidelines EP28-A3. Defining, Establishing, and Verifying Reference Intervals in the Clinical Laboratory; Approved Guideline—3rd ed., 2010.

2. Solberg HE. International federation of clinical chemistry (IFCC), scientific committee, clinical section, expert panel on theory of reference values, and international committee for standardization in haematology (ICSH), standing committee on reference values. Approved recommendation (1986) on the theory of reference values. Part 1. The concept of reference values. *J Clin Chem Clin Biochem.* 1987;25(5): 337-342.

3. Petitclerc C. Normality: the unreachable star? *Clin Chem Lab Med.* 2004;42(7): 698-701.

4. Petersen PH, Jensen EA, Brandslund I. Analytical performance, reference values and decision limits. A need to differentiate between reference intervals and decision limits and to define analytical quality specifications. *Clin Chem Lab Med.* 2011;50(5): 819-831.

5. Goldenberg R, Punthakee Z. Definition, classification and diagnosis of diabetes, prediabetes and metabolic syndrome. *Can J Diabetes.* 2013;37(suppl 1):S8-S11.

6. Gantzer ML, Miller WG. Harmonization of measurement procedures: how do we get it done? *Clin Biochem Rev.* 2012;33(3):95-100.

7. Gowans EM, Hyltoft Petersen P, Blaabjerg O, Horder M. Analytical goals for the acceptance of common reference intervals for laboratories throughout a geographical area. *Scand J Clin Lab Invest.* 1988;48(8):757-764.

8. Fraser CG, Hyltoft Petersen P, Libeer JC, Ricos C. Proposals for setting generally applicable quality goals solely based on biology. *Ann Clin Biochem.* 1997;34 (Pt 1):8-12.

9. Foj L, Filella X, Alcover J, Augé JM, Escudero JM, Molina R. Variability of assay methods for total and free PSA after WHO standardization. *Tumour Biol.* 2014;35(3): 1867-1873.

10. Adeli K. Closing the gaps in pediatric reference intervals: the CALIPER initiative. *Clin Biochem.* 2011;44(7):480-482.

11. Marshall WA, Tanner JM. Variations in pattern of pubertal changes in girls. *Arch Dis Child.* 1969;44(235):291-303.

12. Marshall WA, Tanner JM. Variations in the pattern of pubertal changes in boys. *Arch Dis Child.* 1970;45(239):13-23.

13. Colantonio DA, Kyriakopoulou L, Chan MK, Daly CH, Brinc D, Venner AA, et al. Closing the gaps in pediatric laboratory reference intervals: a CALIPER database of 40 biochemical markers in a healthy and multiethnic population of children. *Clin Chem.* 2012;58(5):854-868.

14. Shaw JL, Binesh Marvasti T, Colantonio D, Adeli K. Pediatric reference intervals: Challenges and recent initiatives. *Crit Rev Clin Lab Sci.* 2013;50(2):37-50.

15. Jones G, Barker A. Reference Intervals. *Clin Biochem Rev.* 2008; 29(Suppl 1):S93-S97.

16. Harris EK, DeMets DL. Estimation of normal ranges and cumulative proportions by transforming observed distributions to gaussian form. *Clin Chem.* 1972;18(7): 605-612.

17. Lahti A, Hyltoft Petersen P, Boyd JC. Impact of subgroup prevalences on partitioning of gaussian-distributed reference values. *Clin Chem.* 2002;48(11):1987-1999.

18. Harris EK, Boyd JC. On dividing reference data into subgroups to produce separate reference ranges. *Clin Chem.* 1990;36(2):265-270.

19. Efron B, Tibshirani R. Boostrap models for standard errors, confidence intervals and other measures of statistical accuracy. *Stat Sci.* 1986;1(1):1-154.

20. Horn PS, Pesce AJ, Copeland BE. A robust approach to reference interval estimation and evaluation. *Clin Chem.* 1998;44(3):622-631.

21. Solberg HE. The IFCC recommendation on estimation of reference intervals. the RefVal program. *Clin Chem Lab Med.* 2004;42(7):710-714.

22. Kulasingam V, Jung BP, Blasutig IM, Baradaran S, Chan MK, Aytekin M, et al. Pediatric reference intervals for 28 chemistries and immunoassays on the roche cobas 6000 analyzer—a CALIPER pilot study. *Clin Biochem*. 2010;43(13-14):1045-1050.

23. Blasutig IM, Jung B, Kulasingam V, Baradaran S, Chen Y, Chan MK, et al. Analytical evaluation of the VITROS 5600 integrated system in a pediatric setting and determination of pediatric reference intervals. *Clin Biochem*. 2010;43(13-14):1039-1044.

24. Chan MK, Seiden-Long I, Aytekin M, Quinn F, Ravalico T, Ambruster D, et al. Canadian laboratory initiative on pediatric reference interval database (CALIPER): pediatric reference intervals for an integrated clinical chemistry and immunoassay analyzer, abbott ARCHITECT ci8200. *Clin Biochem*. 2009;42(9):885-891.

25. Hoffmann RG. Statistics in the practice of medicine. *JAMA*. 1963;185:864-873.

26. Shaw JL, Cohen A, Konforte D, Binesh-Marvasti T, Colantonio DA, Adeli K. Validity of establishing pediatric reference intervals based on hospital patient data: a comparison of the modified hoffmann approach to CALIPER reference intervals obtained in healthy children. *Clin Biochem*. 2014;47(3):166-172.

27. Estey MP, Cohen AH, Colantonio DA, Chan MK, Marvasti TB, Randell E, et al. CLSI-based transference of the CALIPER database of pediatric reference intervals from abbott to beckman, ortho, roche and siemens clinical chemistry assays: direct validation using reference samples from the CALIPER cohort. *Clin Biochem*. 2013;46 (13-14):1197-1219.

28. Soldin S, Wong E, Brugnara C, Soldin O, eds. Pediatric reference intervals, 7th ed. AACC Press, Washington DC, 2011.

29. Kushnir AM, Blamires T, Rockwood AL, Roberts WL, Yue B, Erdogan E, et al. Liquid chromatography-tandem mass spectrometry assay for androstenedione, dehydroepiandrosterone, and testosterone with pediatric and adult reference intervals. *Clin Chem*. 2010;56:1138-1147.

30. Bailey D, Colantonio D, Kyriakopoulou L, Cohen AH, Chan MK, Armbruster D, Adeli K. Marked biological variance in endocrine and biochemical markers in childhood: establishment of pediatric reference intervals using healthy community children from the CALIPER cohort. *Clin Chem*. 2013;59:1393-1405.

31. Kohse K. KiGGs- the German survey on children's health as database for reference intervals and beyond. *Clin Biochem*. 2014;47(9):742-743.

32. Berg J. The Approach to Pathology Harmony in the UK. *Clin Biochem Rev*. 2012;33(3) 89-93.

33. Dietzen DJ, Bennett MJ, Lo SF, Grey V, Jones PM. Dried blood spot reference intervals for steroids and amino acids in a neonatal cohort of the National Children's Study. *Clin Chem*. 2016. DOI:10.1373/clinchem.2016.263434

MATERNAL-FETAL TESTING | 8

Zaher K. Otrock and Ann M. Gronowski

LEARNING OBJECTIVES

1. Define hemolytic disease of the newborn (HDN) and explain how it is diagnosed.
2. Define gestational diabetes mellitus (GDM) and its consequences for the mother and fetus.
3. Explain how ACOG recommends that GDM be diagnosed and discuss the different criteria for screening and diagnosing GDM.
4. Describe the screening methods for fetal aneuploidies during the first and second trimesters.
5. Define the role of cell-free fetal DNA testing in screening for fetal aneuploidies.
6. List the changes in thyroid function tests during pregnancy.
7. Summarize the utility of acid-base and blood gas measurements in umbilical cord blood.
8. Discuss fetal lung maturity testing and the available methods.

INTRODUCTION

Normal physiological changes during pregnancy are reflected in both fetal and maternal hematologic and biochemical parameters. These normal changes can make the diagnosis of disease during pregnancy difficult. This chapter is intended to review the recent clinical and laboratory updates in maternal-fetal screening and diagnosis of hemolytic disease of the newborn (HDN), gestational diabetes mellitus (GDM), fetal aneuploidies, thyroid disease, and other related topics.

HEMOLYTIC DISEASE OF THE NEWBORN

Hemolytic disease of the newborn (HDN) is a hemolytic disorder character-ized by the destruction of fetal red blood cells by maternal antibodies. These antibodies appear in the maternal circulation due to blood group incompat-ibility between the mother and fetus, such as when an Rh(D) negative mother is pregnant with an Rh(D) positive fetus.[1] Other terms used to describe this condition include *isoimmunization disease, Rh isoimmune disease, Rh disease,* or *D isoimmunization.* As this process involves the production of antibodies in one individual (mother) and cell destruction in another (fetus), in vivo HDN is considered the most complex of the three common forms of IgG-mediated red blood cell destruction, that is, HDN, autoimmune hemolytic anemia, and hemolytic transfusion reactions.

The production of maternal antibodies against fetal red blood cell antigens is called sensitization, and it often occurs in a pregnancy in which the fetus' blood cell antigens are foreign to the mother.[2,3] It is widely assumed that fetal and maternal blood compartments are separate during pregnancy; neverthe-less, a few fetal red blood cells manage to enter the maternal circulation con-tinuously. This seemingly harmless antigenic challenge is adequate to provoke an antibody response in some women. Significantly larger antigenic loads may occur with any fetomaternal hemorrhage, such as that seen in (1) spontaneous or induced abortions, (2) ectopic pregnancies, or (3) delivery of an infant.[4] Naturally, the larger the fetomaternal hemorrhage, the higher the possibility that the mother will respond by producing more antibodies. Alloimmuniza-tion usually affects the fetus of the second pregnancy because the exposure to these antibodies typically occurs late during pregnancy or at delivery; thus, the fetus of the first pregnancy is rarely affected.

Maternal IgG antibodies can be actively transported across the placental to the fetus and cause destruction of the fetal erythrocytes.[3] The consequent fetal anemia inflicts an extra load on the fetal heart in an attempt to provide sufficient oxygenation to the fetal tissues. Fetal bone marrow and extramedul-lary erythropoietic tissues in the liver and spleen are also stimulated in order to replace the absent blood cells. With time, extramedullary erythropoiesis destroys the hepatocytes, and accordingly decreases the production of albu-min, with subsequent decrease in oncotic pressure in the intravascular space. When severe, this course ultimately leads to fetal congestive heart failure, with ensuing widespread fetal edema, ascites, severe jaundice, pleural, and peri-cardial effusions. This stage is often referred to as erythroblastosis fetalis or hydrops fetalis, and is life-threatening.[1,5] Clinical manifestations can range from mild hemolysis to severe anemia and fetal demise.

The ABO blood system has four common blood groups: O individuals who have no A or B antigens on their RBC membrane and have both anti-A and anti-B antibodies in their plasma; A individuals have A antigens and anti-B antibodies; B individuals have B antigens and anti-A antibodies; and AB individuals have both A and B antigens but no anti-A or anti-B antibodies.

Numerous alloantibodies have been identified as causative agents in HDN. The most common cause is incompatibility of ABO (major) and minor blood group antigens.[6] It is estimated that 20% of infants have ABO maternal blood group incompatibility, yet the incidence of ABO hemolytic disease in neonates is less than 0.5%. This discrepancy is attributed to the weak expression of major blood group antigens A and B on fetal blood cells and the ability of fetal blood antigens to effectively bind maternal antibodies. Others include antibodies against antigens of the rhesus (Rh) blood group system (c, C, D, e, and E), and those of the Kell (K and k); Duffy (Fya); Kidd (JKa and JKb); and MNSs (M, N, S, and s) systems.[7] The D antigen is the most immunogenic, 50 times more immunogenic than other Rh antigens. The incidence of primary Rh(D) immunization depends on the severity of exposure to Rh(D) positive red blood cells: 15% incidence after 1 mL Rh(D) positive red blood cells and 70-90% after 250 mL.[8,9]

Prophylaxis

One of the greatest successes of modern obstetrics has been the dramatic reduction in the prevalence of Rh(D) alloimmunization and deaths from HDN with the administration of anti-D immunoglobulin. Anti-D immunoglobulin is usually administered to Rh(D) negative (previously non-RhD-sensitized) women within 72 hours of each delivery of an Rh(D) positive fetus; this prevents Rh immunization in the vast majority of cases.[10-12] Rhesus immune globulin has decreased the prevalence of Rh(D) alloimmunization in pregnancy so that approximately six cases occur in every 1,000 live births.[13] Although ante-partum immunoprophylaxis is highly successful, it is not perfect and around 2% of women at risk go on to develop anti-D.[14,15]

In the United States, Rh(D) negative women receive 1500 IU (300 μg) of anti-D between 28 and 32 weeks gestation in all pregnancies.[10,12] If the newborn is Rh(D) positive a similar dose is given after delivery. The same dose of anti-D immunoglobulin is given after any of the following procedures: (1) abortion, (2) fetomaternal hemorrhage, (3) amniocentiesis, or (4) chorionic villi sampling. Anti-D is very safe, and it crosses the placenta and binds to fetal red blood cells, without causing hemolysis, anemia or jaundice. Anti-D reduces the incidence of sensitization during the subsequent pregnancy from 12-16% to 1.6-1.9%.[12] However, ante-partum prophylaxis is not universally administered due to the low incidence of Rh(D) negative women, and the availability and cost of anti-D.[16]

Serologic Screening and Monitoring

Prenatal testing should include a history of pregnancies, surgeries, previous blood transfusions, ABO and Rh(D) grouping, and antibody screening. The ABO group is determined by testing the red blood cells with anti-A and anti-B reagents (forward typing) and by testing the serum or plasma for expected antibodies with A and B red cells (backward typing).[17]

Antigen D is expressed on the surface of red cells of Rh(D) positive subjects, and it is absent from the RBCs of Rh(D) negative subjects. Anti-D does not naturally occur in the plasma of Rh(D) negative individuals and is only detected in some individuals after exposure to Rh(D) positive RBCs. The D antigen is the most immunogenic and thus, most clinically significant antigen in the Rh blood system. It is also the only antigen in which there is a therapeutic intervention to prevent alloimmunization prior to exposure. The Rh blood system consists of numerous other antigens, most commonly C, c, E, and e which have all been implicated in cases of HDN. In addition, antibodies to other blood group antigens may cause mild to severe HDN. Most commonly, these include antibodies to Rh, Kell, Kidd, and Duffy red cell antigens.

The antibody screen is performed to look for unexpected alloantibodies in maternal plasma that may cross the placenta and potentially cause HDN. The antibody screen is performed using the indirect antiglobulin test (IAT) (also known as the Indirect Coombs Test). In general, two drops of maternal plasma are mixed with a 3% solution of reagent red cells with or without the addition of an agglutinating enhancer, incubated for a specific time (per reagent manufactures instruction) centrifuged and then the red cells are washed to remove all maternal plasma and any unbound IgG. The next step is to add an IgM anti-human IgG (Combs reagent) to the red cell to make visible to the naked eye any cross-linked maternal IgG antibody coating the reagent RBC. If the test shows agglutination, it is considered positive. Further work up to identify the specific antibody is required.[17] This is done by repeating the IAT with a panel of 10 or more reagent RBCs which have a combination of all common clinically significant antigens on their surface. The identification is made interpreting as a whole the pattern of reactions.

In addition, the direct antiglobulin test (DAT) may be helpful in the setting of a positive IAT. The DAT is used to detect IgG antibodies bound to the surface of maternal red cells. In brief, after washing to remove any maternal plasma, a 3% suspension of maternal RBCs are directly incubated with Combs Reagent. If agglutination of RBCs occurs, the DAT is positive. Identification of the specific antibodies is done by eluting any IgG antibodies bound to the red cell surface and repeating the IAT with the eluate rather than plasma.

A repeat ABO, Rh(D) typing, and antibody screen is recommended at least once between 28 and 32 weeks of gestation and at the time of delivery.[18]

Identification of maternal antibodies is essential in establishing the risk for HDN and whether further monitoring is required. For example, IgM antibodies, such as anti-P, anti-Le[a], and anti-Le[b], are incapable of crossing the placenta and thus are incapable of causing HDN.[19,20] When clinically significant alloantibodies are detected, IAT titer is performed, and followed up by measuring the titers of antibody and monitoring of any change during the course of pregnancy. The male partner should also have his RBC antigens phenotyped for the relevant antigen(s). The absolute titer of the antibody is not as important as the trend, with a rising titer requiring more frequent monitoring especially with a homozygous partner, and if there is a history of previous alloimmunization.[21]

If there is suspicion of fetomaternal hemorrhage in an RH(D) negative mother, then quantitative assessment of hemorrhage is required by the AABB (formerly known as American Association of Blood Banks) for transfusion services to accurately calculate Rh-Ig dose for Rh-incompatible pregnancies.[17] The Kleihauer-Betke test (also called acid-elution assay) is used to quantify the hemorrhage. The principle utilizes differential resistance to acid elution between fetal hemoglobin F (resistant) and maternal hemoglobin (sensitive). Maternal blood is treated with citric acid-phosphate buffer for 30 minutes, and then examined microscopically for fetal cells which will appear bright pink on staining due to the resistance of fetal hemoglobin F to acid. Maternal red cells will appear as "ghost cells" due to the elution of hemoglobin A from the RBCs leaving only the cell membranes.[22,23] The second step is quantifying the percentage of fetal red blood cells in the mother's blood sample. This is performed by microscopic examination.[6] The standard procedure consists of manually counting the number of darkly stained fetal red blood cells among 2,000 pale-staining adult red blood cells. The third step in determining the volume of a fetomaternal hemorrhage is based on the following formula: Fetomaternal hemorrhage (mL whole blood) = 5,000 mL (represents the mother's arbitrary assigned total blood volume) x acid-elution assay result (%). The fourth step in determining the number of vials of Rh immune globulin required for postpartum Rh immunoprophylaxis. The number of 300 µg vials of Rh immunoglobulin is equal to the volume of fetomaternal hemorrhage divided by 30 (30 mL is the volume of fetal blood that is neutralized by 300 µg of Rh immunoglobulin).[6]

Different flow cytometric methods have also been developed for detecting fetomaternal hemorrhage using fluorescein isothiocyanate-labeled anti D which targets the Rh(D) blood group antigen on fetal red blood cells,[24,25] or using fluorescein isothiocyanate-labeled anti-hemoglobin F which targets fetal hemoglobin.[26,27] Flow cytometric techniques are more expensive and not widespread; they can however be more accurate and objective than the Kleihauer-Betke test in offering guidance for management.[28]

Fetal Assessment in Rh-Immunized Pregnancies

In severely affected alloimmunized pregnancies, the fetus might be at risk of severe anemia and hydrops as early as 17 weeks of gestation. Fetal assessment can start at 16-18 weeks of gestation, depending on the procedure used in the assessment and on the risks and severity of hemolytic disease.[29]

Fetal Blood Sampling

The most accurate method of assessing fetal anemia is to measure the hematocrit of fetal blood directly by cordocentesis. Fetal blood sampling (FBS) is the only procedure that provides direct access to fetal circulation. The procedure is performed when the fetus is suspected of having severe anemia, and it has a high success rate of >98%.[30] In addition to the hematocrit, fetal Rh group can be determined with accuracy. FBS is an invasive procedure and it has risks especially when performed before 18 weeks of gestation. Potential risks of FBS include: bleeding from puncture site; fetal bradycardia; premature labor; pregnancy loss (depending on gestational age and placental penetration); and vertical transmission of hepatitis or human immunodeficiency virus.[30,31] There is no agreement yet on a cutoff hematocrit which indicates the need for fetal transfusion. Ideally, a transfusion is given when the fetal hemoglobin is 4-6 SD below the mean for the gestational age. O-negative unrelated donor blood that is cross-matched with maternal blood should be used for transfusion.[32]

Doppler Ultrasound

Today, Doppler ultrasound offers a non-invasive way to assess fetal anemia.[33] Peak systolic velocity of the fetal middle cerebral artery is measured: If the fetus is anemic, lower blood viscosity and increased cardiac output lead to greater peak blood velocity, and a threshold value of 1.5 multiples of the median predicts moderate-to-severe anemia with 100% sensitivity and 10% false-positive results.[34]

Amniocentesis/Liley and Queenan Charts

Historically, spectrophotometric analysis of amniotic fluid (AF) bilirubin was used to assess fetal red blood cell hemolysis as hemolysis results in accumulation of bilirubin.[35] Concentrations of bilirubin are too low in AF to be assessed by traditional automated enzymatic bilirubin methods. For this reason, bilirubin was measured spectrophotometrically by assessing the OD at 450 nm as a difference from baseline (ΔOD_{450}). Because concentrations of AF bilirubin vary with gestational age,[36,37] ΔOD_{450} measurements had to be interpreted using different methods. The Liley system plotted ΔOD_{450} measurements on a chart that defined three levels of risk: high zone, low zone, and a mid-zone.[38] This system was clinically limited to pregnancies of 27 weeks of gestations and after. This led to development of the Queenan system which could be applied to earlier gestation pregnancies.[39] In Queenan's system, amniotic fluid ΔOD_{450} were charted into four zones of risk: unaffected, indeterminate, affected, and intrauterine death risk zones. Amniocentesis is not without risk, and there was up to 1% fetal mortality directly associated with this procedure. In addition, the ΔOD_{450} method has limited sensitivity and specificity and today is rarely used.[40]

GESTATIONAL DIABETES

During pregnancy, a woman undergoes many anatomic and physiologic changes to accommodate the increasing demands of fetal growth.[41] The maternal physiologic changes are primarily influenced by placental hormones, which affect both glucose and lipid metabolism to ensure an adequate supply of nutrients to the fetus.[42] Although lipids contribute to fetal energy supply, glucose remains the main source of energy. Over 95% of fetal plasma glucose is derived from maternal plasma as shown in studies using isotope-labeled glucose.[43]

Gestational diabetes mellitus (GDM) is defined as any degree of maternal glucose intolerance with the onset or first recognition during pregnancy.[44] The prevalence of GDM is estimated to be 6-7% in the United States with approximately 200,000 new cases annually.[45,46] This prevalence differs between racial and ethnic groups, and it is generally greater in African Americans, Hispanic Americans, Native Americans, Pacific Islanders, and South and East Asian woman.[47] The difference between ethnicities has been attributed to genetic differences. The prevalence has been increasing over the past few decades, probably due to increasing maternal age and weight.[48-50]

The risk factors associated with developing gestational diabetes include: previous gestational diabetes or impaired glucose tolerance, high risk ethnic groups, first degree relatives with diabetes,[51] pre-pregnancy weight and obesity,[52] or excessive gestational weight gain.[53] Other factors include the previous delivery of a baby weighing greater than 9 pounds, or any medical condition associated with diabetes, such as metabolic syndrome, polycystic ovarian syndrome (PCOS), current use of glucocorticoids, and hypertension.[54,55]

GDM-Associated Complications

GDM increases the risk of adverse pregnancy outcomes and has considerable long-term adverse health impacts on both mothers and their offspring. Maternal complications consist of pre-eclampsia, maternal birth trauma, and operative delivery. GDM is also a well-established risk factor for type 2 diabetes mellitus (DM).[56,57] Up to 63% of women with GDM will develop type 2 DM within 5-16 years following pregnancy.[58] These women are also at increased risk for GDM in subsequent pregnancies as most of the risk factors for GDM persist or even become worse in subsequent pregnancies. The recurrence rate is reported to be 35-70%.[59-62]

The fetal complications from GDM are numerous and include hydramnios, macrosomia, and large for gestational age infants, fetal organomegaly, infant birth trauma, perinatal mortality, and other neonatal metabolic problems (hypoglycemia, hyperbilirubinemia, hypocalcemia). The Hyperglycemia and Adverse Pregnancy Outcomes (HAPO) study found a linear relationship between complications, such as fetal macrosomia and the need for primary cesarean delivery and glucose intolerance. This relationship was also seen in patients that were below the threshold for diagnosis of GDM.[63]

Screening and Diagnosis

It is important to identify pregnant women with GDM as treatment can diminish fetal and maternal morbidity, principally macrosomia, shoulder dystocia, and preeclampsia.[64] Although GDM is a well-recognized disorder, there is currently controversy about the proper screening approach.

At present, GDM is most commonly diagnosed in the United States using a two-step process. The two-step approach was originally proposed and recommended by the National Diabetes Data Group (NDDG) and Carpenter and Coustan.[65,66] This approach identifies 5-6% of pregnant women as having GDM. A 1-hour non-fasting screening test is performed with a 50-g glucose load at 24-28 weeks of gestation. The most commonly used cutoff point for serum glucose is 140 mg/dL (7.8 mmol/L) which is 80% sensitive – other used cutoff points are 130 and 135 mg/dL.[67] The diagnostic test consists of a fasting 3-hour 100-g oral glucose tolerance test (OGTT) given to those with elevated glucose concentrations on the screen. The 1-hour, 2-hour, and 3-hour post-load glucose concentrations are measured and evaluated based on Carpenter and Coustan criteria (Table 8-1).[66] The American College of Obstetricians and Gynecologists (ACOG) advises that all pregnant women be screened for GDM, whether by the patient's medical history, clinical risk factors, or laboratory testing using the 2-step approach. ACOG recommends this two-step approach to testing.

It is worth noting that the Canadian Diabetes Association (CDA) proposed a modified two-step approach that relies on the administration of a 50-g glucose challenge test with a diagnostic cutoff at 140 mg/dL (7.8 mmol/L), followed by a 75-g 2-hour OGTT for the second step.[68] This modified approach is attractive as it minimizes the burden and cost for women and the healthcare system. In addition, this approach provides diagnostic efficacy. In the above-mentioned comparative study of different screening approaches for GDM, the prevalence of GDM was 3.7% in both the modified approach (50-g glucose

Table 8-1   **CRITERIA FOR SCREENING AND DIAGNOSING GDM***

Criteria	Approach	Screen 1st step in 2-step approaches	Diagnosis Glucose dose	Fasting glucose, mg/dL (mmol/L)	OGTT 1-h, mg/dL (mmol/L)	OGTT 2-h, mg/dL (mmol/L)	OGTT 3-h, mg/dL (mmol/L)	Diagnostic criteria
				The numbers are representing cutoff for normal				
C&C[66]	2 step	50 g OGTT, 140 mg/dL cutoff	100 g	<95 (5.3)	<180 (10.0)	<155 (8.6)	<140 (7.8)	2 or more
NDDG[65]	2 step	50 g OGTT, 140 mg/dL cutoff	100 g	<105 (5.8)	<190 (10.6)	<165 (9.2)	<145 (8.0)	2 or more
CDA[68]	2 step	50g OGTT, 140 mg/dL cutoff	75 g	<95 (5.33)	<191 (10.6)	<160 (8.9)	–	1 or more
IADPSG[69]	1 step	N/A	75 g	<92 (5.1)	<180 (10)	<153 (8.5)	–	1 or more
WHO[70]	1 step	N/A	75 g	<126 (7.0)	–	<140 (7.8)	–	1 or more
EASD[161]	1 step	N/A	75 g	<108 (6.0)	–	<162 (9.0)	–	2

*OGTT, oral glucose tolerance test; N/A, not applicable; C&C, Carpenter and Coustan; NDDG, National Diabetes Data Group; CDA, Canadian Diabetes Association; IADPSG, International Association of Diabetes and Pregnancy Study Groups; WHO, World Health Organization; EASD, European Association for the Study of Diabetes.

screen ± 2-hour, 75-g OGTT) and the original 2-step approach (1-hour, 50-g glucose screen ± 3-hour, 100-g OGTT).[68]

Based on the results of the HAPO study, which demonstrated associations between hyperglycemia and an increased risk of obstetric and perinatal morbidities at glucose concentrations below the cutoff for diagnosis of GDM,[63] the International Association of Diabetes and Pregnancy Study Groups (IADPSG) recently proposed new diagnostic criteria.[69] The new approach requires the administration of a 75-g oral glucose load while fasting, and measuring the serum glucose at fasting and 2 hours post-load according to the WHO protocol.[69,70] An additional measurement of glucose at 1 hour post-load is required by the IADPSG protocol (Table 8-1).

The IADPSG criteria are the only criteria aimed at identifying pregnancies with increased risk of adverse perinatal outcomes. Nevertheless, the IADPSG criteria have been criticized,[71,72] and have not been adopted as standard recommendations by many organizations including the ACOG. If the IADPSG criteria were applied retrospectively to the HAPO cohort, it would result in approximately 18% of women meeting the criteria for GDM. The main reasons for not switching to the IADPSG criteria are that there are no properly conducted randomized controlled trials with a sufficient number of patients examining the benefits and risks of screening and treatment on health outcomes.

It should be noted that GTT, especially when performed on fasting pregnant patients, can cause nausea or dizziness in a small percentage of women. For this reason, physicians occasionally ask if other forms of sugar can be used, such as jelly beans, soda, or candy. The proper interpretation of any GTT is dependent on a standard amount of glucose (not sucrose or fructose) in a standard amount of liquid. Substitutes should not be made as results cannot be interpreted.

The American Diabetes Association has recommended the use of hemoglobin A1c (HbA1c) to diagnose DM and to identify subjects at risk for developing diabetes.[73] Because A1c reflects the level of glycemia for a period of 3-4 months, and pregnancy is a relatively short-term state, A1c is not a good reflection of glucose status during pregnancy. In a study from India evaluating the utility of HbA1c in diagnosing GDM, HbA1c was inferior to OGTT as reflected in the area under ROC curve: at a cutoff of ≥5.95% HbA1c had a sensitivity of 28.6% and a specificity of 97.2% in diagnosing GDM, while a cutoff of ≥5.45% had a sensitivity of 85.7% and a specificity of 61.1%.[74] In addition, the HAPO study showed that associations with adverse outcome were significantly stronger with serum glucose than with HbA1c.[75] This was also supported by the US Preventive Services Task Force (USPSTF) in their latest recommendations.[46] Instead, markers that reflect shorter time periods, such as glycated albumin have been suggested.[76] However, currently these markers are not recommended for routine use in pregnancy by the ADA or ACOG.

SCREENING FOR FETAL ANOMALIES

In the last three decades, prenatal screening has witnessed tremendous improvements in detecting fetal genetic disorders. Prior to 1970, physicians identified women at risk for aneuploidy based solely on maternal age. The development of cytogenetic testing of cultured amniocytes allowed prenatal diagnosis of cytogenetic disorders, and then maternal serum testing allowed screening for neural tube defects and trisomies. Today, screening for trisomies can be performed by detecting fetal DNA in maternal serum.

Maternal Serum Screening

Second Trimester Screening

In 1975, maternal serum α-fetoprotein (AFP) measured during the second trimester was found to be elevated in pregnancies which resulted in infants with neural tube defects.[77] In 1984, Cuckle and colleagues suggested maternal serum AFP as a screening test for Down syndrome in the second trimester.[78] After this observation, other maternal serum analytes were investigated and these included human chorionic gonadotropin (β-hCG),[79,80] unconjugated estriol (uE$_3$),[81] and inhibin A.[82] The maternal serum markers of β-hCG, AFP, and uE$_3$ were combined with maternal age in the "triple screen"[83] which was used for many years (Table 8-2). Dimeric inhibin A (DIA) was added as another marker to the triple screen in the late 1990s, which constituted the "quadruple screen" (Table 8-2).[84] The concentrations of these analytes are expressed as multiples of the median (MoM), which is the ratio of the patient's concentration to the median concentration for the given

Table 8-2	**FIRST AND SECOND TRIMESTER SCREENING METHODS***						
Test Name	AFP	hCG	uE3	DIA	PAPP-A	NT	Trimester
Triple	X	X	X				2nd
Quadruple	X	X	X	X			2nd
Integrated					X	X	1st
	X	X	X	X			2nd
Sequential		X			X	X	1st
	X	X	X	X			2nd

*AFP, α-fetoprotein; hCG, human chorionic gonadotropin; uE3, unconjugated estriol; DIA, dimeric inhibin A; PAPP-A, pregnancy-associated plasma protein A; NT, nuchal translucency.

gestational age. Second trimester screening is generally carried out at 15-18 weeks of gestational age but the testing is considered valid up to 22 weeks.

A very recent meta-analysis evaluated the accuracy of different second trimester serum markers in detecting Down syndrome.[85] All studies assessing single serum markers, whether AFP, free β-hCG, or total hCG, combined with maternal age gave low sensitivity of detection ranging between 41% and 56%. The use of double test (AFP and free β-hCG, or AFP and total β-hCG) with maternal age gave a sensitivity range of 69-76%, with a specificity of 91-95%. Better results were obtained when triple or quadruple tests combined with maternal age were implemented with respective sensitivities of 81.5% and 73.9%, and respective specificities of 97.9% and 94.8%.[85] Other studies have also reported that detection rates for the triple screen are inferior to those of the quadruple test.[86,87] According to ACOG guidelines, Down syndrome screening for pregnant women who are first seen during the second trimester should be limited to quadruple test.[88]

Second trimester maternal serum screening is limited by its high false positive rate which necessitates invasive cytogenetic follow-up testing. It is also limited by the fact that testing is not performed until later in gestation. Earlier screening would allow earlier diagnostic testing and allow women to make decisions about pregnancy termination.

First Trimester Screening

The approach of combining maternal age with second trimester quadruple testing and first trimester measurement of maternal serum pregnancy-associated plasma protein A (PAPP-A) with or without free β-hCG or total β-hCG, and ultrasound nuchal translucency to assess the risk of chromosomal abnormalities is now widely available. The first reliable study on nuchal translucency in the prediction of fetal chromosomal defects came in 1992 by Nicolaides et al.[89] This group prospectively examined 827 pregnant women who underwent transabdominal ultrasound at 10-14 weeks of gestation to evaluate the fluid behind the neck in their fetuses. Visualizing a sagittal section of the crown–rump length, the maximum thickness of subcutaneous translucency between the skin and soft tissue overlying the cervical spine was measured. Karyotyping by amniocentesis or chorionic villus sampling was also performed. The incidence of chromosomal defects was 3% (28 of 827 cases). In the 51 (6%) fetuses with nuchal translucency measuring 3-8 mm the incidence of chromosomal defects was 35% (18 cases). In contrast, only 10 of the remaining 776 (1%) fetuses with smaller measurements were chromosomally abnormal. Therefore, increased fetal nuchal translucency of ≥3 mm was a useful first trimester marker for an increased risk of fetal chromosomal defects. This group of investigators altered the concept of prenatal screening, and they were the first to introduce the term "nuchal translucency" into the vocabulary of maternal fetal medicine. It is recommended that the fetal neck be measured in a neutral position, as this was found to be the most reproducible and accurate.[90]

The "integrated" approach uses first trimester PAPP-A and nuchal translucency combined with second trimester quadruple screen to adjust a woman's age-related risk of having a child with chromosomal abnormalities (Table 8-2).[91] The patient is given a single risk assessment after this two-step process is completed. However, many feel that waiting for second trimester results delays diagnosis. Therefore, in the "sequential" screening approach, first trimester hCG is added to the integrated screen and the patient is informed if the first-trimester screening result are found to be abnormal (Table 8-2). Note that the threshold for abnormal is purposefully set high. Those at highest risk can opt for an early diagnostic procedure and those at lower risk continue to have second-trimester screening and a new risk assessment is determined based on the combined results of both steps.

The combination of maternal serum biomarkers and nuchal translucency for prenatal diagnosis was the subject of a number of studies.[92-98] These studies showed an increase in the detection rate of Down syndrome to 85-89% at a false positive rate of 5% with the combination testing. The most sensitive screening tests are the ones that incorporate first and second trimester biochemical tests with ultrasound measurements. Integrated screening provides the highest sensitivity with the lowest false positive rate, thus fewer invasive tests.[87,91] In the FASTER trial, the detection rate was 94-96% using the integrated approach, while it was 85-88% using the serum integrated screen (without incorporating a nuchal translucency measurement).[87] Similar results were achieved in the SURUSS trial.[91]

Studies have shown that the detection rate of stepwise sequential screening is 91-95% for Down syndrome and 91-96% for trisomy 18.[87,99] The other strategy is the "contingent sequential screening" follows the same first step as with stepwise sequential screening. However, patients are divided into low, moderate, and high risk groups. High risk patients are offered diagnostic testing, the moderate risk patients to the second step of serum biomarkers screening, and the low risk patients are not offered further serum testing. Moderate risk patients are again stratified into low or high risk based on the results of the second step screening. The detection rate for this strategy is 91% for Down syndrome and 91-96% for trisomy 18.[99,100]

Cell-Free Fetal DNA From Maternal Blood

In the last 7 years, several studies have reported on the implementation of testing cell-free fetal DNA (cffDNA) in maternal blood to screen for fetal chromosomal abnormalities. Circulating cffDNA in maternal blood was first reported by Lo et al. in 1997.[101] Maternal plasma DNA is a mixture of maternal and fetal DNA. Circulating cffDNA comprises 3-6% of cell-free maternal DNA, and it can be detected as early as day 18 of gestation.[102,103] It is believed that cffDNA is derived from the placenta and is rapidly cleared from the circulation after delivery.

Several large trials have been conducted to validate fetal aneuploidy screening with cffDNA in high-risk populations using massive parallel sequencing (MPS).[104-107] Bianchi et al. conducted a prospective study on 2,882 high-risk women undergoing prenatal testing.[104] Chromosome classifications were made by MPS and compared with fetal karyotype. The sensitivity for the detection of trisomies 21, 18, 13, and monosomy X were 100%, 97.2%, 78.6%, and 93.8%, respectively. Another study by Palomaki and colleagues evaluated the efficacy of cffDNA testing in detecting Down syndrome in high-risk pregnancies.[105] Down syndrome detection rate was 98.6% (209/212), the false-positive rate was 0.20% (3/1471). According to ACOG, high risk patients can be offered testing with cffDNA, with an expected detection rate of 98% of cases of Down syndrome.[108] A patient with a positive test result should be referred for genetic counseling and offered confirmatory invasive prenatal diagnostic testing.

Recently, Bianchi et al. conducted a study on a population of 1914 general obstetric patients using MPS on cffDNA.[109] They reported that the false positive rate for detecting trisomy 2 and 18 was significantly lower than with standard screening (0.3% vs 3.6% for trisomy 21 and 0.2% vs 0.6% for trisomy 18). Furthermore, the positive predictive value was also greater for cffDNA than standard screening (45.5% vs 4.2 % for trisomy 21 and 40% vs 8.3% for trisomy 18), suggesting MPS on cffDNA can be used in a lower risk population.

Diagnostic Tests

The traditional gold standard for diagnosing fetal chromosomal abnormalities involves analyzing the banded chromosomes obtained from cultured amniotic fluid or chorionic villus cells. Chromosomal studies are most commonly done by conventional metaphase cytogenetics or FISH (fluorescence in-situ hybridization). Another recent prenatal cytogenetic testing is chromosomal microarray analysis (CMA) which provides a better detection rate of fetal chromosomal abnormalities.[110]

Chorionic Villus Sampling

Chorionic villus sampling (CVS) is an invasive procedure that was introduced in the early 1980s to allow for early prenatal diagnosis in the first trimester.[111] A sample of the chorionic villi is removed from the placenta for testing; sampling can be performed either transabdominally or transcervically. The accuracy for detecting fetal chromosome abnormalities by CVS is estimated to be more than

98%.[112] It is the only invasive diagnostic procedure prior to 14th week of gestation, allowing for earlier decision-making and intervention.[113] The risk of miscarriage due to CVS is estimated to be approximately 0.5-2.0%.[114,115] Data supports an increased risk of transverse limb deficiencies whose rate and severity are associated with the timing of CVS, specifically prior to 10 weeks of gestation.[114,116]

Amniocentesis

Amniocentesis is used for the detection of fetal chromosomal aneuploidy in the second and third trimester of pregnancy. Under aseptic conditions, a needle is inserted through the abdominal wall, through the uterine wall, and finally into the amniotic sac. Amniotic fluid is collected and amniocytes are cultured for fetal karyotyping. Amniocentesis has a high accuracy rate for detection that is estimated to be 99.8-99.9%.[88] Data from the FASTER trial showed that the miscarriage risk associated with amniocentesis was less than 0.1 %.[117] According to ACOG amniocentesis is associated with 0.2-0.3% risk for miscarriage.[88] Although amniocentesis is associated with a lower risk for miscarriage than CVS, it is limited in that it cannot be performed as early in gestation as CVS.

THYROID TESTING DURING PREGNANCY

The normal physiologic changes associated with pregnancy have profound effects on maternal thyroid function including: 1) an increase in the thyroid hormone transport protein thyroxine-binding globulin (TBG), 2) chorionic gonadotropin (hCG)-mediated stimulation of the thyroid stimulating hormone (TSH) receptor, and 3) increased iodine demand due to increased renal iodide clearance, the need to provide iodine for the fetus, and increased maternal thyroid hormone synthesis (Table 8-3). These changes make the interpretation of thyroid function tests during pregnancy difficult.

Increased concentrations of TBG are caused by elevated estrogen concentrations which: 1) stimulates hepatic TBG synthesis; and 2) reduces TBG metabolic clearance due to enhanced TBG sialylation. Overall, TBG concentrations are increased approximately 2- to 3-fold, which results in a corresponding 1.5-fold increase in total thyroxine (TT4) and total triiodothyronine (TT3).[118]

A second physiologic change that occurs in early pregnancy stems from the ability of hCG to directly stimulate the thyroid receptor. There is significant homology between hCG and TSH as well as between the LH/hCG receptor and the TSH receptor. Therefore, when hCG concentrations peak in the first trimester, negative feedback transiently suppresses TSH concentrations.[119] In the majority of patients, the TSH concentration remains within the non-pregnant reference interval.

Table 8-3 **EFFECTS OF PREGNANCY ON THYROID FUNCTION**[118,126]	
Physiologic change	**Thyroid-related consequences**
↑ serum estrogens	↑ serum TBG
↑ serum TBG	↑ demand for T_4 and T_3 ↑ in total T_4 and T_3
↑ hCG	↓ TSH (1st trimester, within reference interval unless hCG > 400,000 IU/L) transient ↑ in free T_4 (1st trimester, within reference interval)
↑ renal iodine clearance	↑ dietary requirement for I^- ↑ 24-h RAIU ↓ in hormone production in I^- deficient areas
↑ type III deiodinase	↑ in T_4 and T_3 degradation and production ↑ demand for T_4 and T_3
↑ demand for TT_4 and TT_3	↑ serum thyroglobulin ↑ thyroid volume ↑ goiter in I^- deficient areas
↑ plasma volume	↑ in T_4 and T_3 pool size

Finally, pregnancy is associated with an increase in the glomerular filtration rate which causes an increase in the renal clearance of iodide. Maternal iodine losses are also amplified by fetal requirements for iodide as the fetus produces thyroid hormones in the second half of gestation. The maternal 1.5-fold increase in total T3 and T4 also necessitates additional iodine. Provided that maternal iodine intake is sufficient, the additional iodine requirement can easily be supplied by diet. However, in regions of borderline or low iodine intake, the increased iodine demands of pregnancy may lead to iodine deficiency, hypothyroidism, and goiter.[120]

Hyperthyroidism in Pregnancy

Thyroid function tests are particularly valuable in differentiating hyperthyroidism from normal pregnancy. In overt hyperthyroidism, TSH is suppressed while fT4 is increased. TSH measurement is the first line for initial assessment of thyroid dysfunction. However, TSH may be transiently suppressed during the first trimester due to elevated hCG concentrations. Thus, gestational age should be considered when measuring TSH. The American Thyroid Association has recommended trimester-specific reference intervals. If laboratory-specific TSH reference intervals are not available, then the following ranges are recommended: first trimester 0.1-2.5 mIU/L; second trimester 0.2-3.0 mIU/L; and third trimester 0.3-3.0 mIU/L.[121]

The diagnostic accuracy of fT4 immunoassays in pregnant women has been questioned as some immunoassay methods show an unexpected decrease in fT4 the second and third trimesters that has not been observed with reference methods.[122,123] Reference methods (equilibrium dialysis and tandem mass spectrophotometry) for fT4 measurement directly assess the free thyroxine component and are therefore unaffected by altered binding protein concentrations. Therefore, during pregnancy, fT4 should be measured using immunoassay with gestational age-specific reference intervals or a reference method.

In normal pregnancy, TSH suppression is a transient phenomenon and TSH concentrations generally remain within normal, non-pregnant reference intervals. Up to 18% of women may have TSH below the non-pregnant reference interval during the period of highest hCG concentrations.[124] This condition is *not* associated with adverse obstetrical outcome and thyroid function tests typically return to normal without treatment as hCG concentrations decrease in the second trimester. Haddow et al. examined the relationship between hCG and the thyroid hormones TSH and hCG in 9562 women being screened for aneuploidy.[125] They found that TSH was suppressed when the ratio of hCG to TSH was ≥200,000. Lockwood et al. found that TSH was consistently suppressed only when hCG concentrations exceeded 400,000 IU/L and that, despite biochemical evidence of hyperthyroidism, 94% of subjects did not have overt signs or symptoms of hyperthyroidism.[126]

The pregnancy-specific conditions hyperemesis gravidarum and gestational trophoblastic disease can also lead to hyperthyroidism. Both conditions are associated with elevated hCG concentrations and their prompt identification is important because treatment of the underlying disease resolves the hyperthyroidism.

Although Graves' disease is the major cause of hyperthyroidism during pregnancy, it is an uncommon overall pregnancy complication because hyperthyroidism is associated with reduced fertility and increased pregnancy loss. Distinctive symptoms that may accompany Graves disease include ophthalmopathy and localized dermopathy or myxedema.[127]

Graves disease is caused by thyroid-stimulating antibodies that bind to and activate the TSH receptor.[128] Thyrotropin-receptor antibody (TRAbs) can cross the placenta and, at high enough concentrations, can stimulate the fetal thyroid. Hyperthyroidism is present in the fetuses and neonates of 1-5% of women with Graves disease during pregnancy. High titers of TRAbs in maternal serum during the third trimester are predictive of fetal or neonatal dysfunction. Therefore, it has been suggested that TRAbs be measured early in pregnancy and again in the last trimester in women with hyperthyroidism. Values >500% of baseline are considered high and are a predictor of fetal or neonatal disease.[129] In addition, a study by Glinoer et al.[130] demonstrated that women with anti-TPO antibodies or anti-thyroglobulin antibodies were fourfold more likely to have spontaneous abortions than healthy controls (13.3% vs 3.3%).

Hypothyroidism in Pregnancy

Hypothyroidism in pregnant women is frequently unsuspected, unless symptoms are very obvious, because a goiter may not be palpable. Measurement of serum TSH is particularly valuable because it can detect very early primary hypothyroidism, before clinical signs are present. Generally, overt hypothyroidism in pregnancy is associated with elevated TSH and low fT4 concentrations. An elevated TSH with fT4 concentrations within the normal reference interval indicates subclinical hypothyroidism and management is controversial. Subclinical hypothyroidism is diagnosed in asymptomatic women when TSH concentrations are elevated (>5.5 mIU/L) and fT4 is within the reference interval (0.9-1.8 ng/dL). It is unclear whether subclinical hypothyroidism is associated with significant adverse clinical consequences.[131] While T4 supplementation during pregnancy has been associated with improved pregnancy outcomes in overt hypothyroidism, data indicating fetal benefit from T4 supplementation in pregnant women with subclinical hypothyroidism are not currently available.[132] During the early weeks of pregnancy, a normal, transient decrease in TSH, and increase in fT4 can be observed that may delay the diagnosis.

Overt hypothyroidism in pregnancy is infrequent because hypothyroid women are often anovulatory and have a high rate of first trimester spontaneous abortion. Worldwide, iodine deficiency is responsible for the majority of hypothyroidism, with 500 million people living in areas of overt iodine deficiency.[133] In contrast, iodine deficiency is an uncommon cause of hypothyroidism in developed countries where iodine fortification is widespread. In developed countries, common causes of hypothyroidism are: hypothyroidism secondary to radical or surgical treatment of Graves disease and chronic autoimmune thyroiditis (Hashimoto thyroiditis), which occurs in 1-2% of pregnant women.

The association between severe maternal hypothyroidism and neurocognitive impairment in offspring has been recognized for many years. Thyroid hormones are solely supplied by the mother before the fetus begins to synthesize significant concentrations of thyroid hormones at approximately mid-gestation.

The first half of gestation is a critical period for fetal brain development, and this process is particularly sensitive to maternally provided thyroid hormone concentrations.[134] There has been renewed interest in the relationship between insufficient maternal thyroid function and potential risks for progeny following publication of several important studies showing that children of thyroid deficient mothers are more likely to have lower IQ scores.[135,136]

These publications have prompted debate regarding whether screening should be implemented for hypothyroidism in pregnant women.[137] Guidelines from the American Association of Clinical Endocrinologists indicate that TSH screening should be routine before pregnancy or during the first trimester. If the TSH is greater than 10 mIU/L or if the TSH is 5-10 mIU/L and the patient has goiter or positive anti-thyroid peroxidase antibodies, then thyroid hormone replacement therapy should be initiated.[138] The American Thyroid Association and the Endocrine Society agree that there are not enough data for or against universal screening but also acknowledge that lack of evidence of benefit doesn't mean that there is no benefit.[139] They recommend only the screening of pregnant women who are at high risk of overt hypothyroidism (eg, history of thyroid dysfunction, TPO antibody positive, goiter, etc.). However, the ACOG has recommended against screening all pregnant women for hypothyroidism. They argue that there is lack of clear evidence that the identification and treatment of women with subclinical hypothyroidism will improve maternal or infant outcomes and will not cause harm.[132]

Surveying pregnant women for overt hypothyroidism is much less controversial than subclinical hypothyroidism, predominantly because overt hypothyroidism has been more thoroughly studied. Current evidence suggests that TSH should be measured before or early in pregnancy to allow adequate treatment of the mother; however, additional studies are needed before consensus guidelines can be reached.[134,140] Further research is required to determine when screening should occur, what testing algorithm should be employed, and what the optimal treatment regimen is for prevention of neurodevelopmental complications in the infants of thyroid deficient women.

UMBILICAL CORD BLOOD GASES

Neonatal hypoxia/asphyxia has three main etiologies: 1) Maternal oxygen is compromised; 2) Maternal perfusion of the placenta is reduced for reasons, such as preeclampsia, chronic hypertension, hypotension/hypovolemia, or cyanotic heart disease; and 3) Delivery of blood from placenta to fetus is impaired due to placental abruption, cord prolapse, or repetitive cord occlusion. Umbilical cord blood gas and acid-base assessment are the most accurate way of assessing the fetal metabolic condition at the moment of birth and can help give insight into causes of intrapartum fetal distress.

The ACOG recommends that venous and arterial cord blood samples should be obtained in circumstances of Cesarean delivery for fetal compromise, low 5-minute Apgar score, severe growth restriction, abnormal fetal heart rate tracing, maternal thyroid disease, intrapartum fever, and multifetal gestations.[141]

Immediately after delivery, 10-20 cm of umbilical cord should be clamped at both ends, thus isolating it from both the placenta and the environment. The clamped segment is stable for pH and blood gas measurement at room temperature for at least 60 minutes. Blood can be drawn using a 1-2 mL syringe flushed with heparin. Blood should be placed on ice and transported to the laboratory as soon as possible. Samples from the umbilical cord artery provide the most accurate information, however the umbilical vein is larger and easier to sample than the umbilical artery. ACOG recommends obtaining paired venous and arterial samples when possible; however, in practice this is often not done. Samples should be labeled as venous or arterial as reference intervals are different for each.

The pH, PCO_2, PO_2, CO_2 and hemoglobin concentration of the blood can be measured. Bicarbonate concentration, percent oxygen saturation, and base excess (or deficiency) can be calculated. Common calculations used include:

$$Base\,excess = 0.93 \times ([HCO_3^-] - 24.4 + 14.8 \times (pH - 7.4))$$

$$HCO_3 = 0.03 \times PCO_2 \times 10^{\,(pH-6.1)}$$

Base excess and base deficit have the same numerical value; however, a positive value is used for base deficit and a negative value for base excess. The most clinically useful values are pH and bases excess (or deficit).

Lactate is also measured by many blood gas analyzers and can be used as a marker of fetal metabolic acidosis. Umbilical cord lactate has been shown to correlate with both pH and base excess but is less clinically useful.

Fetal pH is normally 0.1 unit lower than maternal pH. Median acid-base and blood gas values from umbilical arterial and venous cord blood in fetuses with Apgar score ≥7 at 5 minutes is shown in Table 8-4.[142] Other studies reporting umbilical cord values for term and preterm infants can be found in a review by Armstrong.[143] Restriction of umbilical blood flow causes a progressive widening of the difference between umbilical vein and artery blood gas values. Impairment of maternal perfusion of the placenta, as in placental abruption, will result in small venous to arterial differences. Evidence of a metabolic acidosis in fetal umbilical cord arterial blood obtained at delivery, that is, pH <7 and base deficit >12 mmol/L, is sufficient to cause cerebral palsy.[141] A normal umbilical artery blood pH virtually excludes "birth asphyxia."

Table 8-4	MEDIAN VALUES OF ACID-BASE AND BLOOD GAS VALUES IN UMBILICAL ARTERIAL AND VENOUS CORD BLOOD IN FETUSES WITH APGAR SCORE ≥ 7 AT 5 MINUTES[†]	
	Median (2.5th-97.5th percentile)	
	Artery	Vein
pH	7.27 (7.10-7.38)	7.35 (7.2-7.46)
pCO_2	52 (35-74)	41 (28-57)
pO_2	17 (6-30)	29 (16-43)
BE	−4 (−11-1)	−3 (−8 to +2)
HCO_3[*]	23.1	21.9

*Calculated based on above median data. $N = 15,073$.
[†]From Helwig et al. 1996.[142]

FETAL LUNG MATURITY TESTING

Respiratory distress syndrome (RDS) is a major cause of neonatal morbidity and mortality that is most commonly caused by a deficiency in lung surfactant in premature infants. Laboratory tests were developed to measure lung surfactant in amniotic fluid and therefore estimate fetal lung maturity (FLM) in utero. These tests include the lecithin to sphingomyelin (L/S) ratio, the detection of phosphatidylglycerol, and the lamellar body count. Specifics of these FLM tests have been reviewed extensively elsewhere.[144-146] They all exhibit high sensitivity for immaturity and an excellent predictive value of a mature result. Of these, the lamellar body count (LBC) offers distinct advantages such as ease of performance, the wide availability of instrumentation, and low cost. A meta-analysis comparing the ability of the LBC and the L/S ratio to predict RDS concluded that both tests performed almost equally, but the LBC was preferred due to the advantages described.[147] Another study by Zhao et al. demonstrated that the sensitivity and specificity of the LBC were further improved through stratification of LBC cutoffs by gestational age.[148]

Despite the excellent performance of the FLM tests, there has been a recent decline in their use.[149-151] The 2008 ACOG practice bulletin on fetal lung maturity does not recommend FLM testing before 32 weeks of gestation or when delivery is mandated due to fetal or maternal indications.[152] FLM testing is only recommended to demonstrate fetal lung maturity before a scheduled delivery at less than 39 weeks of gestation. However, the practice of scheduled deliveries at less than 39 weeks of gestation is now strongly discouraged by ACOG unless delivery is justified by medical or obstetric complications.[153]

Delivery of infants before 39 weeks of gestation is associated with increased risk of neonatal respiratory complications, including RDS, transient tachypnea of the newborn, pneumonia, respiratory failure, and fetal death.[153-155] Interestingly, several studies also demonstrate increased risk of adverse outcomes in neonates *despite demonstration of fetal lung maturity* with antenatal testing.[156-158] These studies provide strong and compelling evidence that decreased respiratory and non-respiratory morbidities are associated with increasing gestational age, regardless of the status of fetal pulmonary maturity. In addition, advancements in antenatal treatment with corticosteroids and postnatal treatment with surfactant have led to increases in the ability of physicians to treat RDS, further limiting the clinical utility of FLM testing.[159,160] Instead, physicians guide decisions by gestational age, which is the greatest predictor of neonatal outcomes.

TRAINING MODULE

1. Which of the following statements is true about hemolytic disease of the newborn (HDN)?
   a. HDN can be caused by maternal IgA alloantibodies
   b. HDN is usually seen with the first pregnancy of a Rh+ mother with a Rh− baby
   c. HDN can be diagnosed by measuring bilirubin in amniotic fluid
   d. The severity of HDN does not correlate with the degree of fetomaternal hemorrhage
   e. HDN is routinely assessed by ΔOD_{450}.

2. Currently, the American College of Obstetrics and Gynecology recommends that all pregnant women be screened for gestational diabetes using which of the following?
   a. A two-step method with a 50 g OGTT screen and 100 g OGTT diagnostic test.
   b. A two-step method with a 100 g OGTT screen and 50 g OGTT diagnostic test.
   c. A one-step 75 g OGTT diagnostic test.
   d. HbA1c in the 2nd trimester
   e. The same method as that recommended by the ADA

3. Which is true about maternal serum screening for Down syndrome?
   a. Triple screen requires measuring AFP, β-hCG, and uE3 during the 1st trimester
   b. Nuchal translucency is a non-invasive screening test that should be done during the 2nd trimester
   c. Sensitivity is highest when 1st and 2nd trimester biochemical tests are incorporated with ultrasound measurements
   d. Amniocentesis is the only invasive diagnostic procedure prior to 14th week of gestation
   e. Has lower sensitivity and specificity than methods using cffDNA.

4. Which of the following changes to thyroid function occur during pregnancy?

   a. The thyroid is not affected by hCG
   b. Total T4 and T3 decrease
   c. Thyroglobulin decreases
   d. Renal iodine clearance decreases
   e. TSH decreases in the 1st trimester

5. Abnormal fetal heart patterns, intrapartum fever, severe fetal growth restriction and C-section for fetal compromise are indications for measuring which of the following:

   a. Fetal lung maturity
   b. Cord blood gases
   c. Maternal TSH and fT4
   d. Maternal AFP
   e. HgbA1c

REFERENCES

1. Urbaniak SJ, Greiss MA. RhD haemolytic disease of the fetus and the newborn. *Blood Rev.* 2000;14(1):44-61.
2. Queenan JT. Current management of the Rh-sensitized patient. *Clin Obstet Gynecol.* 1982;25(2):293-301.
3. Moise KJ. Red blood cell alloimmunization in pregnancy. *Semin Hematol.* 2005;42(3):169-178.
4. Cacciatore A, Rapiti S, Carrara S, et al. Obstetric management in Rh alloimmunized pregnancy. *J Prenatal Med.* 2009;3(2):25-27.
5. Bowman JM. The management of Rh-Isoimmunization. *Obs Gynecol.* 1978;52(1): 1-16.
6. Kennedy MS. Perinatal issues in transfusion practice. In: Roback JD, Grossman BJ, Harris T, Hillyer CD, ed. *Technical Manual.* 17th ed: Bethesda, MD: American Association of Blood Banks; 2011:636-639.
7. Luban NL. Hemolytic disease of the newborn: progenitor cells and late effects. *N Engl J Med.* 1998;338(12):830-831.
8. Pollack W, Ascari WQ, Kochesky RJ, O'Connor RR, Ho TY, Tripodi D. Studies on Rh prophylaxis. 1. Relationship between doses of anti-Rh and size of antigenic stimulus. *Transfusion.* 1971;11(6):333-339.
9. Urbaniak SJ, Robertson AE. A successful program of immunizing Rh-negative male volunteers for anti-D production using frozen/thawed blood. *Transfusion.* 1981;21(1): 64-69.
10. Bowman JM. The prevention of Rh immunization. *Trans Med Rev.* 1988;2(3):129-150.
11. Lee D, Contreras M, Robson SC, Rodeck CH, Whittle MJ. Recommendations for the use of anti-D immunoglobulin for Rh prophylaxis. British Blood Transfusion Society and the Royal College of Obstetricians and Gynaecologists. *Trans Med.* 1999; 9(1):93-97.

12. Fung Kee Fung K, Eason E, Crane J, et al. Prevention of Rh alloimmunization. *J Obstet Gynaecol*. 2003;25(9):765-773.

13. Moise KJ, Jr. Management of rhesus alloimmunization in pregnancy. *Obstet Gynecol*. 2008;112(1):164-176.

14. Robson SC, Lee D, Urbaniak S. Anti-D immunoglobulin in RhD prophylaxis. *Br J Obstet Gynaecol*. 1998;105(2):129-134.

15. Contreras M. The prevention of Rh haemolytic disease of the fetus and newborn–general background. *Br J Obstet Gynaecol*. 1998;105 suppl 18:7-10.

16. MacKenzie IZ, Bowell P, Gregory H, Pratt G, Guest C, Entwistle CC. Routine antenatal Rhesus D immunoglobulin prophylaxis: the results of a prospective 10 year study. *Br J Obstet Gynaecol*. 1999;106(5):492-497.

17. *Standards for Blood Banks and Transfusion Services* 29th ed: AABB, Bethesda, MD 2014.

18. American College of O, Gynecologists. ACOG Practice Bulletin No. 75: Management of alloimmunization during pregnancy. *Obstet Gynecol*. 2006;108(2):457-464.

19. Heddle NM, Klama L, Frassetto R, O'Hoski P, Leaman B. A retrospective study to determine the risk of red cell alloimmunization and transfusion during pregnancy. *Transfusion*. 1993;33(3):217-220.

20. Koelewijn JM, Vrijkotte TG, de Haas M, van der Schoot CE, Bonsel GJ. Risk factors for the presence of non-rhesus D red blood cell antibodies in pregnancy. *BJOG*. 2009;116(5):655-664.

21. Bruce M, Chapman JF, Duguid J, et al. Addendum for guidelines for blood grouping and red cell antibody testing during pregnancy. BCSH Transfusion Task Force. *Trans Med*. 1999;9(1):99.

22. Kim YA, Makar RS. Detection of fetomaternal hemorrhage. *Am J Hematol*. 2012; 87(4):417-423.

23. Sandler SG, Gottschall JL. Postpartum Rh immunoprophylaxis. *Obstetr Gynecol*. 2012;120(6):1428-1438.

24. Nelson M, Popp H, Horky K, Forsyth C, Gibson J. Development of a flow cytometric test for the detection of D-positive fetal cells after fetomaternal hemorrhage and a survey of the prevalence in D-negative women. *Immunohematology*. 1994;10(2):55-59.

25. Kumpel BM. Quantification of anti-D and fetomaternal hemorrhage by flow cytometry. *Transfusion*. 2000;40(1):6-9.

26. Mundee Y, Bigelow NC, Davis BH, Porter JB. Simplified flow cytometric method for fetal hemoglobin containing red blood cells. *Cytometry*. 2000;42(6):389-393.

27. Dziegiel MH, Nielsen LK, Berkowicz A. Detecting fetomaternal hemorrhage by flow cytometry. *Curr Opin Hematol*. 2006;13(6):490-495.

28. Chen JC, Davis BH, Wood B, Warzynski MJ. Multicenter clinical experience with flow cytometric method for fetomaternal hemorrhage detection. *Cytometry*. 2002; 50(6):285-290.

29. Pretlove SJ, Fox CE, Khan KS, Kilby MD. Noninvasive methods of detecting fetal anaemia: a systematic review and meta-analysis. *BJOG*. 2009;116(12):1558-1567.

30. Society for Maternal-Fetal M, Berry SM, Stone J, Norton ME, Johnson D, Berghella V. Fetal blood sampling. *Am J Obstet Gynecol*. 2013;209(3):170-180.

31. van Kamp IL, Klumper FJ, Bakkum RS, et al. The severity of immune fetal hydrops is predictive of fetal outcome after intrauterine treatment. *Am J Obstet Gynecol*. 2001;185(3):668-673.

32. Oepkes D, Adama van Scheltema P. Intrauterine fetal transfusions in the management of fetal anemia and fetal thrombocytopenia. *Semin Fetal Neonatal Med.* 2007;12(6):432-438.

33. Mari G, Hanif F. Fetal Doppler: umbilical artery, middle cerebral artery, and venous system. *Semin Perinatol.* 2008;32(4):253-257.

34. Mari G, Deter RL, Carpenter RL, et al. Noninvasive diagnosis by Doppler ultrasonography of fetal anemia due to maternal red-cell alloimmunization. Collaborative Group for Doppler Assessment of the Blood Velocity in Anemic Fetuses. *N Engl J Med.* 2000;342(1):9-14.

35. Weiner CP. Human fetal bilirubin levels and fetal hemolytic disease. *Am J Obstet Gynecol.* 1992;166(5):1449-1454.

36. Bartsch FK. Bilirubin in the amniotic fluid. A review. *Annali di ostetricia, ginecologia, medicina perinatale.* 1970;92(8):482-492.

37. Oepkes D. Invasive versus non-invasive testing in red-cell alloimmunized pregnancies. *Eur J Obstet Gynecol Reprod Biol.* 2000;92(1):83-89.

38. Liley AW. Liquor amnil analysis in the management of the pregnancy complicated by resus sensitization. *Am J Obstet Gynecol.* 1961;82:1359-1370.

39. Queenan JT, Tomai TP, Ural SH, King JC. Deviation in amniotic fluid optical density at a wavelength of 450 nm in Rh-immunized pregnancies from 14 to 40 weeks' gestation: a proposal for clinical management. *Am J Obstet Gynecol.* 1993;168(5):1370-1376.

40. Oepkes D, Seaward PG, Vandenbussche FP, et al. Doppler ultrasonography versus amniocentesis to predict fetal anemia. *N Engl J Med.* 2006;355(2):156-164.

41. Weissgerber TL, Wolfe LA. Physiological adaptation in early human pregnancy: adaptation to balance maternal-fetal demands. *Appl Physiol Nutr Metab.* 2006;31(1):1-11.

42. Butte NF. Carbohydrate and lipid metabolism in pregnancy: normal compared with gestational diabetes mellitus. *Am J Clin Nutr.* 2000;71(5 suppl):1256S-1261S.

43. Staat BC, Galan HL, Harwood JE, et al. Transplacental supply of mannose and inositol in uncomplicated pregnancies using stable isotopes. *J Clin Endocrinol Metab.* 2012;97(7):2497-2502.

44. Sacks DB, Arnold M, Bakris GL, et al. Guidelines and recommendations for laboratory analysis in the diagnosis and management of diabetes mellitus. *Clin Chem.* 2011;57(6):e1-e47.

45. American Diabetes A. Gestational diabetes mellitus. *Diabetes Care.* 2004;27 suppl 1:S88-S90.

46. Moyer VA, Force USPST. Screening for gestational diabetes mellitus: U.S. Preventive Services Task Force recommendation statement. *Ann Int Med.* 2014;160(6):414-420.

47. Ferrara A. Increasing prevalence of gestational diabetes mellitus: a public health perspective. *Diabetes Care.* 2007;30 suppl 2:S141-S146.

48. Dabelea D, Snell-Bergeon JK, Hartsfield CL, et al. Increasing prevalence of gestational diabetes mellitus (GDM) over time and by birth cohort: Kaiser Permanente of Colorado GDM Screening Program. *Diabetes Care.* 2005;28(3):579-584.

49. Getahun D, Nath C, Ananth CV, Chavez MR, Smulian JC. Gestational diabetes in the United States: temporal trends 1989 through 2004. *Am J Obstet Gynecol.* 2008;198(5):525 e521-e525.

50. Kim SY, Saraiva C, Curtis M, Wilson HG, Troyan J, Sharma AJ. Fraction of gestational diabetes mellitus attributable to overweight and obesity by race/ethnicity, California, 2007-2009. *Am J Public Health.* 2013;103(10):e65-e72.

51. Kim C, Liu T, Valdez R, Beckles GL. Does frank diabetes in first-degree relatives of a pregnant woman affect the likelihood of her developing gestational diabetes mellitus or nongestational diabetes? *Am J Obstet Gynecol.* 2009;201(6):576 e571-e576.

52. Hedderson MM, Williams MA, Holt VL, Weiss NS, Ferrara A. Body mass index and weight gain prior to pregnancy and risk of gestational diabetes mellitus. *Am J Obstet Gynecol.* 2008;198(4):409 e401-e407.

53. Gibson KS, Waters TP, Catalano PM. Maternal weight gain in women who develop gestational diabetes mellitus. *Obstet Gynecol.* 2012;119(3):560-565.

54. Reyes-Munoz E, Castellanos-Barroso G, Ramirez-Eugenio BY, et al. The risk of gestational diabetes mellitus among Mexican women with a history of infertility and polycystic ovary syndrome. *Fertil Steril.* 2012;97(6):1467-1471.

55. Boomsma CM, Eijkemans MJ, Hughes EG, Visser GH, Fauser BC, Macklon NS. A meta-analysis of pregnancy outcomes in women with polycystic ovary syndrome. *Hum Reprod Update.* 2006;12(6):673-683.

56. Buchanan TA, Xiang AH. Gestational diabetes mellitus. *J Clin Invest.* 2005; 115(3):485-491.

57. Kim C, Newton KM, Knopp RH. Gestational diabetes and the incidence of type 2 diabetes: a systematic review. *Diabetes Care.* 2002;25(10):1862-1868.

58. Kjos SL, Buchanan TA. Gestational diabetes mellitus. *N Engl J Med.* 1999;341(23): 1749-1756.

59. MacNeill S, Dodds L, Hamilton DC, Armson BA, VandenHof M. Rates and risk factors for recurrence of gestational diabetes. *Diabetes Care.* 2001;24(4):659-662.

60. Philipson EH, Super DM. Gestational diabetes mellitus: does it recur in subsequent pregnancy? *Am J Obstet Gynecol.* 1989;160(6):1324-1329; discussion 1329-1331.

61. Foster-Powell KA, Cheung NW. Recurrence of gestational diabetes. *Aust N Z J Obstet Gynaecol.* 1998;38(4):384-387.

62. Kim C, Berger DK, Chamany S. Recurrence of gestational diabetes mellitus: a systematic review. *Diabetes Care.* 2007;30(5):1314-1319.

63. Group HSCR, Metzger BE, Lowe LP, et al. Hyperglycemia and adverse pregnancy outcomes. *N Engl J Med.* 2008;358(19):1991-2002.

64. Greuter MJ, van Emmerik NM, Wouters MG, van Tulder MW. Quality of guidelines on the management of diabetes in pregnancy: a systematic review. *BMC Pregnancy Childb.* 2012;12:58.

65. Classification and diagnosis of diabetes mellitus and other categories of glucose intolerance. National Diabetes Data Group. *Diabetes.* 1979;28(12):1039-1057.

66. Carpenter MW, Coustan DR. Criteria for screening tests for gestational diabetes. *Am J Obstet Gynecol.* 1982;144(7):768-773.

67. Prutsky GJ, Domecq JP, Sundaresh V, et al. Screening for gestational diabetes: a systematic review and meta-analysis. *J Clin Endocrinol Metab.* 2013;98(11):4311-4318.

68. Meltzer SJ, Snyder J, Penrod JR, Nudi M, Morin L. Gestational diabetes mellitus screening and diagnosis: a prospective randomised controlled trial comparing costs of one-step and two-step methods. *BJOG Int J Obstet Gynaecol.* 2010;117(4):407-415.

69. Sacks DA, Hadden DR, Maresh M, et al. Frequency of gestational diabetes mellitus at collaborating centers based on IADPSG consensus panel-recommended criteria: the Hyperglycemia and Adverse Pregnancy Outcome (HAPO) Study. *Diabetes Care.* 2012;35(3):526-528.

70. Alberti KG, Zimmet PZ. Definition, diagnosis and classification of diabetes mellitus and its complications. Part 1: diagnosis and classification of diabetes mellitus provisional report of a WHO consultation. *Diabetic Med.* 1998;15(7):539-553.

71. Long H. Diagnosing gestational diabetes: can expert opinions replace scientific evidence? *Diabetologia.* 2011;54(9):2211-2213.

72. Ryan EA. Diagnosing gestational diabetes. *Diabetologia.* 2011;54(3):480-486.

73. American Diabetes A. Diagnosis and classification of diabetes mellitus. *Diabetes Care.* 2010;33 Suppl 1:S62-69.

74. Rajput R, Yogesh Y, Rajput M, Nanda S. Utility of HbA1c for diagnosis of gestational diabetes mellitus. *Diabetes Res Clin Pract.* 2012;98(1):104-107.

75. Lowe LP, Metzger BE, Dyer AR, et al. Hyperglycemia and Adverse Pregnancy Outcome (HAPO) Study: associations of maternal A1C and glucose with pregnancy outcomes. *Diabetes Care.* 2012;35(3):574-580.

76. Pan J, Zhang F, Zhang L, Bao Y, Tao M, Jia W. Influence of insulin sensitivity and secretion on glycated albumin and hemoglobin A1c in pregnant women with gestational diabetes mellitus. *Int J Gynaecol Obstet.* 2013;121(3):252-256.

77. Brock DJ, Scrimgeour JB, Bolton AE, Wald N, Peto R, Barker S. Effect of gestational age on screening for neural-tube defects by maternal plasma-A.F.P. measurement. *Lancet.* 1975;2(7927):195-196.

78. Cuckle HS, Wald NJ, Lindenbaum RH. Maternal serum alpha-fetoprotein measurement: a screening test for Down syndrome. *Lancet.* 1984;1(8383):926-929.

79. Bogart MH, Pandian MR, Jones OW. Abnormal maternal serum chorionic gonadotropin levels in pregnancies with fetal chromosome abnormalities. *Prenat Diagn.* 1987;7(9):623-630.

80. Macri JN, Kasturi RV, Krantz DA, et al. Maternal serum Down syndrome screening: free beta-protein is a more effective marker than human chorionic gonadotropin. *Am J Obstet Gynecol.* 1990;163(4 Pt 1):1248-1253.

81. Canick JA, Knight GJ, Palomaki GE, Haddow JE, Cuckle HS, Wald NJ. Low second trimester maternal serum unconjugated oestriol in pregnancies with Down's syndrome. *Br J Obstet Gynaecol.* 1988;95(4):330-333.

82. Spencer K, Wood PJ, Anthony FW. Elevated levels of maternal serum inhibin immunoreactivity in second trimester pregnancies affected by Down's syndrome. *Ann Clin Biochem.* 1993;30 (Pt 2):219-220.

83. Wald NJ, Cuckle HS, Densem JW, et al. Maternal serum screening for Down's syndrome in early pregnancy. *BMJ.* 1988;297(6653):883-887.

84. Haddow JE, Palomaki GE, Knight GJ, Foster DL, Neveux LM. Second trimester screening for Down's syndrome using maternal serum dimeric inhibin A. *J Med Screen.* 1998;5(3):115-119.

85. Alldred SK, Deeks JJ, Guo B, Neilson JP, Alfirevic Z. Second trimester serum tests for Down's Syndrome screening. *Cochrane Database System Rev.* 2012;6: CD009925.

86. Wald NJ, Rodeck C, Hackshaw AK, Walters J, Chitty L, Mackinson AM. First and second trimester antenatal screening for Down's syndrome: the results of the Serum, Urine and Ultrasound Screening Study (SURUSS). *J Med Screen.* 2003;10(2):56-104.

87. Malone FD, Canick JA, Ball RH, et al. First-trimester or second-trimester screening, or both, for Down's syndrome. *N Engl J Med.* 2005;353(19):2001-2011.

88. Bulletins ACoP. ACOG Practice Bulletin No. 77: screening for fetal chromosomal abnormalities. *Obstet Gynecol.* 2007;109(1):217-227.

89. Nicolaides KH, Azar G, Byrne D, Mansur C, Marks K. Fetal nuchal translucency: ultrasound screening for chromosomal defects in first trimester of pregnancy. *BMJ.* 1992;304(6831):867-869.

90. Whitlow BJ, Chatzipapas IK, Economides DL. The effect of fetal neck position on nuchal translucency measurement. *British J Obstet Gynaecol.* 1998;105(8):872-876.

91. Wald NJ, Watt HC, Hackshaw AK. Integrated screening for Down's syndrome on the basis of tests performed during the first and second trimesters. *N Engl J Med.* 1999;341(7):461-467.

92. Noble PL, Abraha HD, Snijders RJ, Sherwood R, Nicolaides KH. Screening for fetal trisomy 21 in the first trimester of pregnancy: maternal serum free beta-hCG and fetal nuchal translucency thickness. *Ultrasound Obstet Gynecol.* 1995;6(6):390-395.

93. Orlandi F, Damiani G, Hallahan TW, Krantz DA, Macri JN. First-trimester screening for fetal aneuploidy: biochemistry and nuchal translucency. *Ultrasound Obstet Gynecol.* 1997;10(6):381-386.

94. Spencer K, Souter V, Tul N, Snijders R, Nicolaides KH. A screening program for trisomy 21 at 10-14 weeks using fetal nuchal translucency, maternal serum free beta-human chorionic gonadotropin and pregnancy-associated plasma protein-A. *Ultrasound Obstet Gynecol.* 1999;13(4):231-237.

95. Canick JA, Lambert-Messerlian GM, Palomaki GE, et al. Comparison of serum markers in first-trimester down syndrome screening. *Obstetrics Gynecol.* 2006;108(5):1192-1199.

96. Palomaki GE, Lambert-Messerlian GM, Canick JA. A summary analysis of Down syndrome markers in the late first trimester. *Adv Clin Chem.* 2007;43:177-210.

97. Avgidou K, Papageorghiou A, Bindra R, Spencer K, Nicolaides KH. Prospective first-trimester screening for trisomy 21 in 30,564 pregnancies. *Am J Obstet Gynecol.* 2005;192(6):1761-1767.

98. Nicolaides KH. Nuchal translucency and other first-trimester sonographic markers of chromosomal abnormalities. *Am J Obstet Gynecol.* 2004;191(1):45-67.

99. Palomaki GE, Steinort K, Knight GJ, Haddow JE. Comparing three screening strategies for combining first- and second-trimester Down syndrome markers. *Obstet Gynecol.* 2006;107(2 Pt 1):367-375.

100. Cuckle HS, Malone FD, Wright D, et al. Contingent screening for Down syndrome–results from the FaSTER trial. *Prenat Diagn.* 2008;28(2):89-94.

101. Lo YM, Corbetta N, Chamberlain PF, et al. Presence of fetal DNA in maternal plasma and serum. *Lancet.* 1997;350(9076):485-487.

102. Lo YM, Tein MS, Lau TK, et al. Quantitative analysis of fetal DNA in maternal plasma and serum: implications for noninvasive prenatal diagnosis. *Am J Hum Genet.* 1998;62(4):768-775.

103. Guibert J, Benachi A, Grebille AG, Ernault P, Zorn JR, Costa JM. Kinetics of SRY gene appearance in maternal serum: detection by real time PCR in early pregnancy after assisted reproductive technique. *Hum Reprod.* 2003;18(8):1733-1736.

104. Bianchi DW, Platt LD, Goldberg JD, et al. Genome-wide fetal aneuploidy detection by maternal plasma DNA sequencing. *Obstet Gynecol.* 2012;119(5):890-901.

105. Palomaki GE, Kloza EM, Lambert-Messerlian GM, et al. DNA sequencing of maternal plasma to detect Down syndrome: an international clinical validation study. *Genetics Med.* 2011;13(11):913-920.

106. Chiu RW, Akolekar R, Zheng YW, et al. Non-invasive prenatal assessment of trisomy 21 by multiplexed maternal plasma DNA sequencing: large scale validity study. *BMJ.* 2011;342:c7401.

107. Song Y, Liu C, Qi H, Zhang Y, Bian X, Liu J. Noninvasive prenatal testing of fetal aneuploidies by massively parallel sequencing in a prospective Chinese population. *Prenat Diagn.* 2013;33(7):700-706.

108. American College of O, Gynecologists Committee on G. Committee Opinion No. 545: Noninvasive prenatal testing for fetal aneuploidy. *Obstet Gynecol.* 2012;120(6): 1532-1534.

109. Bianchi DW, Parker RL, Wentworth J, et al. DNA sequencing versus standard prenatal aneuploidy screening. *N Engl J Med.* 2014;370(9):799-808.

110. Dhillon RK, Hillman SC, Morris RK, et al. Additional information from chromosomal microarray analysis (CMA) over conventional karyotyping when diagnosing chromosomal abnormalities in miscarriage: a systematic review and meta-analysis. *BJOG Int J Obstet Gynaecol.* 2014;121(1):11-21.

111. Niazi M, Coleman DV, Loeffler FE. Trophoblast sampling in early pregnancy. Culture of rapidly dividing cells from immature placental villi. *Br J Obstet Gynaecol.* 1981;88(11):1081-1085.

112. Ledbetter DH, Zachary JM, Simpson JL, et al. Cytogenetic results from the U.S. Collaborative Study on CVS. *Prenat Diagn.* 1992;12(5):317-345.

113. Wapner RJ. Invasive prenatal diagnostic techniques. *Semin Perinatol.* 2005;29(6): 401-404.

114. Chorionic villus sampling and amniocentesis: recommendations for prenatal counseling. Centers for Disease Control and Prevention. *MMWR.* 1995;44(RR-9):1-12.

115. Mujezinovic F, Alfirevic Z. Procedure-related complications of amniocentesis and chorionic villous sampling: a systematic review. *Obstet Gynecol.* 2007;110(3): 687-694.

116. Brambati B, Simoni G, Travi M, et al. Genetic diagnosis by chorionic villus sampling before 8 gestational weeks: efficiency, reliability, and risks on 317 completed pregnancies. *Prenat Diagn.* 1992;12(10):789-799.

117. Eddleman KA, Malone FD, Sullivan L, et al. Pregnancy loss rates after midtrimester amniocentesis. *Obstet Gynecol.* 2006;108(5):1067-1072.

118. Fantz CR, Dagogo-Jack S, Ladenson JH, Gronowski AM. Thyroid function during pregnancy. *Clin Chem.* 1999;45(12):2250-2258.

119. Hershman JM. Physiological and pathological aspects of the effect of human chorionic gonadotropin on the thyroid. *Best Pract Res Clin Endocrinol Metab.* 2004;18(2): 249-265.

120. Glinoer D. The regulation of thyroid function in pregnancy: pathways of endocrine adaptation from physiology to pathology. *Endocr Rev.* 1997;18(3):404-433.

121. Stagnaro-Green A, Abalovich M, Alexander E, et al. Guidelines of the American Thyroid Association for the diagnosis and management of thyroid disease during pregnancy and postpartum. *Thyroid.* 2011;21(10):1081-1125.

122. Roti E, Gardini E, Minelli R, Bianconi L, Flisi M. Thyroid function evaluation by different commercially available free thyroid hormone measurement kits in term pregnant women and their newborns. *J Endocrinol Invest.* 1991;14(1):1-9.

123. Lee RH, Spencer CA, Mestman JH, et al. Free T4 immunoassays are flawed during pregnancy. *Am J Obstet Gynecol.* 2009;200(3):260 e261-e266.

124. Glinoer D, De Nayer P, Robyn C, Lejeune B, Kinthaert J, Meuris S. Serum levels of intact human chorionic gonadotropin (HCG) and its free alpha and beta subunits, in relation to maternal thyroid stimulation during normal pregnancy. *J Endocrinol Invest.* 1993;16(11):881-888.

125. Haddow JE, McClain MR, Lambert-Messerlian G, et al. Variability in thyroid-stimulating hormone suppression by human chorionic [corrected] gonadotropin during early pregnancy. *J Clin Endocrinol Metab.* 2008;93(9):3341-3347.

126. Lockwood CM, Grenache DG, Gronowski AM. Serum human chorionic gonadotropin concentrations greater than 400,000 IU/L are invariably associated with suppressed serum thyrotropin concentrations. *Thyroid.* 2009;19(8):863-868.

127. Weetman AP. Graves' disease. *N Engl J Med.* 2000;343(17):1236-1248.

128. Rodien P, Jordan N, Lefevre A, et al. Abnormal stimulation of the thyrotrophin receptor during gestation. *Hum Reprod Update.* 2004;10(2):95-105.

129. Mestman JH, Goodwin TM, Montoro MM. Thyroid disorders of pregnancy. *Endocrinol Metab Clin N Am.* 1995;24(1):41-71.

130. Glinoer D, Soto MF, Bourdoux P, et al. Pregnancy in patients with mild thyroid abnormalities: maternal and neonatal repercussions. *J Clin Endocrinol Metab.* 1991;73(2): 421-427.

131. Wartofsky L, Van Nostrand D, Burman KD. Overt and 'subclinical' hypothyroidism in women. *Obstet Gynecol Survey.* 2006;61(8):535-542.

132. Committee on Patient S, Quality I, Committee on Professional L. ACOG Committee Opinion No. 381: subclinical hypothyroidism in pregnancy. *Obstet Gynecol.* 2007;110(4):959-960.

133. Neale DM, Cootauco AC, Burrow G. Thyroid disease in pregnancy. *Clin Perinatol.* 2007;34(4):543-557, v-vi.

134. Smallridge RC, Ladenson PW. Hypothyroidism in pregnancy: consequences to neonatal health. *J Clin Endocrinol Metab.* 2001;86(6):2349-2353.

135. Haddow JE, Palomaki GE, Allan WC, et al. Maternal thyroid deficiency during pregnancy and subsequent neuropsychological development of the child. *N Engl J Med.* 1999;341(8):549-555.

136. Pop VJ, Brouwers EP, Vader HL, Vulsma T, van Baar AL, de Vijlder JJ. Maternal hypothyroxinaemia during early pregnancy and subsequent child development: a 3-year follow-up study. *Clin Endocrinol.* 2003;59(3):282-288.

137. Gronowski AM, Haddow J, Kilpatrick S, Lazarus JH, Negro R. Thyroid function during pregnancy: who and how should we screen? *Clin Chem.* 2012;58(10):1397-1401.

138. Baskin HJ, Cobin RH, Duick DS, et al. American Association of Clinical Endocrinologists medical guidelines for clinical practice for the evaluation and treatment of hyperthyroidism and hypothyroidism. *Endocr Pract.* 2002;8(6):457-469.

139. Abalovich M, Amino N, Barbour LA, et al. Management of thyroid dysfunction during pregnancy and postpartum: an Endocrine Society Clinical Practice Guideline. *J Clin Endocrinol Metab.* 2007;92(8 Suppl):S1-S47.

140. Gyamfi C, Wapner RJ, D'Alton ME. Thyroid dysfunction in pregnancy: the basic science and clinical evidence surrounding the controversy in management. *Obstet Gynecol.* 2009;113(3):702-707.

141. Practice ACoO. ACOG Committee Opinion No. 348, November 2006: umbilical cord blood gas and acid-base analysis. *Obstet Gynecol.* 2006;108(5):1319-1322.

142. Helwig JT, Parer JT, Kilpatrick SJ, Laros RK, Jr. Umbilical cord blood acid-base state: what is normal? *Am J Obstet Gynecol.* 1996;174(6):1807-1812; discussion 1812-1804.

143. Armstrong L, Stenson BJ. Use of umbilical cord blood gas analysis in the assessment of the newborn. *Arch Dis Child Fetal Neonat Ed.* 2007;92(6):F430-F434.

144. Grenache DG, Gronowski AM. Fetal lung maturity. *Clin Biochem.* 2006;39(1):1-10.

145. Leung-Pineda V, Gronowski AM. Biomarker tests for fetal lung maturity. *Biomark Med.* 2010;4(6):849-857.

146. Szallasi A, Gronowski AM, Eby CS. Lamellar body count in amniotic fluid: a comparative study of four different hematology analyzers. *Clin Chem.* 2003;49(6 Pt 1):994-997.

147. Besnard AE, Wirjosoekarto SA, Broeze KA, Opmeer BC, Mol BW. Lecithin/sphingomyelin ratio and lamellar body count for fetal lung maturity: a meta-analysis. *Eur J Obstet Gynecol Reprod Biol.* 2013;169(2):177-183.

148. Zhao Q, Zhao Z, Leung-Pineda V, et al. Predicting respiratory distress syndrome using gestational age and lamellar body count. *Clin Biochem.* 2013;46(13-14):1228-1232.

149. Grenache DG, Wilson AR, Gross GA, Gronowski AM. Clinical and laboratory trends in fetal lung maturity testing. *Clin Chim Acta.* 2010;411(21-22):1746-1749.

150. McGinnis KT, Brown JA, Morrison JC. Changing patterns of fetal lung maturity testing. *J Perinatol.* 2008;28(1):20-23.

151. Yarbrough ML, Grenache DG, Gronowski AM. Fetal lung maturity testing: the end of an era. *Biomark Med.* 2014;8(4):509-515.

152. Gottwein E, Cullen BR. Viral and cellular microRNAs as determinants of viral pathogenesis and immunity. *Cell Host Microbe.* 2008;3(6):375-387.

153. American College of O, Gynecologists. ACOG committee opinion no. 561: Nonmedically indicated early-term deliveries. *Obstet Gynecol.* 2013;121(4):911-915.

154. Tita AT, Landon MB, Spong CY, et al. Timing of elective repeat cesarean delivery at term and neonatal outcomes. *N Engl J Med.* 2009;360(2):111-120.

155. Reddy UM, Ko CW, Raju TN, Willinger M. Delivery indications at late-preterm gestations and infant mortality rates in the United States. *Pediatrics.* 2009;124(1):234-240.

156. Bates E, Rouse DJ, Mann ML, Chapman V, Carlo WA, Tita AT. Neonatal outcomes after demonstrated fetal lung maturity before 39 weeks of gestation. *Obstet Gynecol.* 2010;116(6):1288-1295.

157. Kamath BD, Marcotte MP, DeFranco EA. Neonatal morbidity after documented fetal lung maturity in late preterm and early term infants. *Am J Obstet Gynecol.* 2011;204(6):518 e511-e518.

158. Fang YM, Guirguis P, Borgida A, Feldman D, Ingardia C, Herson V. *J Matern Fetal Neonat Med.* 2013;26(1):79-82.

159. Bahadue FL, Soll R. Early versus delayed selective surfactant treatment for neonatal respiratory distress syndrome. *Cochrane Database System Rev.* 2012;11:CD001456.

160. Rojas-Reyes MX, Morley CJ, Soll R. Prophylactic versus selective use of surfactant in preventing morbidity and mortality in preterm infants. *Cochrane Database System Rev.* 2012;3:CD000510.

161. Lind T, Phillips PR. Influence of pregnancy on the 75-g OGTT. A prospective multi-center study. The Diabetic Pregnancy Study Group of the European Association for the Study of Diabetes. *Diabetes.* 1991;40 suppl 2:8-13.

PEDIATRIC TOXICOLOGY AND THERAPEUTIC DRUG MONITORING | 9

Uttam Garg and Jennifer Lowry

LEARNING OBJECTIVES

1. Explain the unique aspects of toxicology theory and practice in children compared to adults.
2. List requirements for proper specimen selection for toxicology and therapeutic drug monitoring.
3. Discuss various techniques involved in drug screening and confirmation.
4. Explain advantages and disadvantages of immunoassays and chromatographic techniques.
5. List both laboratory and clinical aspects of commonly identified toxins and drugs in pediatric patients.
6. Discuss principles of therapeutic drug monitoring and basics of pharmacokinetics.

INTRODUCTION

Poisonings are recognized as a public health concern as exposures affect individuals across their lifespan. Developmental and behavioral changes throughout childhood result in different exposures, with unintentional exposures occurring in toddlers and young children due to their curious natures versus intentional exposures in adolescents due to drug abuse and suicidal intents. Causes range from overdoses to illicit drugs, environmental exposures, suicides and suicide attempts, homicides, unintended medication misuse, and unintended ingestion of household products. In fact, poisoning is a leading mechanism of injury and mortality. According to the Centers for Disease

Control and Prevention, the drug poisoning death rate in 2008 was 4 times the rate that it was in 1999 and the leading cause of injury deaths in 2008. In addition, unintentional poisoning is the tenth leading cause of nonfatal injuries seen in Emergency Departments (ED). However, it is the second leading cause of injuries seen in EDs in 1-4 year olds.[1,2]

Current and past efforts have focused on preventing unintentional ingestions in young children. The emergence and increased utilization of poison control centers (PCCs), as well as the development of child-resistant closures on pill bottles resulted in a rapid decline of morbidity and mortality in young children attributed to poisoning over the past decades. Since that time, pediatric toxicology has evolved to include additional issues including law enforcement and environmental/public health.

In 2012, 57 PCCs submitted data to the American Association of Poison Control Centers (AAPCC). PCCs cared for 2,275,141 human exposures with 1,402,937 (61%) occurring in children 19 years of age and under.[3] This is a gross underestimation as poison control centers rely on volunteer reporting. By far, the majority of calls and exposures occurred in residences. Approximately 20% of calls to PCCs were from health care professionals, as patients may present to health care facilities due to lack of knowledge of the PCC or the severity of the exposure. Ingestions account for the majority (83%) of exposures while dermal and inhalation exposures occur at a lesser frequency (7% and 6%, respectively).

Management largely occurs at the site of exposure (69%) with the primary site occurring at the patient's residence. Approximately 27% of patients were seen in a healthcare facility; however, this number is largely due to those patients who present to emergency departments prior to calling PCCs. Thus, many of these patients may not have required emergency care. Of those patients seen in the ED, the majority were treated and released with approximately one quarter of those patients admitted for hospitalization.

Exposures during pregnancy that were called to PCCs occurred in over 7000 women in 2012, with exposures occurring equally in the first, second, and third trimesters. The majority (74.1%) were due to unintentional exposures and 20% were intentional exposures. There were four deaths in pregnant women in 2012. The substances most commonly involved in exposures to pregnant women are similar to those in other adults including analgesics (12%), cleaning substances (9%), pesticides (7%), fumes or gases (6%), and envenomations (6%) among other substances to a lesser extent. Unfortunately, poison center surveillance does not include the outcome of the fetus after exposures in pregnancy.

Children under the age of 5 years are more likely to be poisoned by substances that are readily available. The most common categories of substances resulting in exposures are cosmetics/personal care products (13.95%), analgesics (9.93%), household cleaning substances (9.68%), foreign bodies (6.95%), and topical preparations (6.33%). While these products, with the exception of analgesics, are not likely to result in significant toxicity, significant effects have been seen with those pharmaceutical substances that are less likely to be ingested in the younger age group.

Children younger than 4 years of age were involved in 42.8% of exposures, and children younger than 6 years accounted for approximately half of all human exposures (48%) called to PCCs. Of the pediatric exposures, approximately 80% occur in children under the age of 6 years with the majority resulting from unintentional exposures. Ingestions in young children are secondary to development of exploration behaviors and a tendency for hand to mouth activity. Many drugs in a small dose can cause significant toxicity in an infant (Table 9-1).

As children age, the reason for their exposures shifts from unintentional to intentional exposures. Children over the age of 12 are more likely to intentionally ingest drugs for abuse and/or suicide. While the most recent

Table 9-1   **DRUGS THAT IN SMALL DOSES CAN CAUSE SEVERE TOXICITY IN AN INFANT**
Benzocaine
β-Adrenergics
β-Blockers
Calcium channel blockers
Camphor
Chlorpromazine
Clonidine and other imidazolines
Diphenoxylate and atropine
Ethylene glycol
Hydrocarbons
Iron
Lomotil (diphenoxylate/atropine)
Lindane
Methanol
Methylsalicylate
Monamine oxidase inhibitors
Opioids
Phenothiazines
Quinine or chloroquine
Sulfonylurea
Theophylline
Thioridazine
Tricyclic antidepressants

data suggests decreased drug use among high school teenagers, there is concern for persistently high rates of marijuana and nonmedical prescription drug use.[4] Specifically, use of non-medically prescribed opiates is at high levels (eg, hydrocodone use in 7.5% among high school seniors). The use of prescription stimulants is also a cause for concern. The nonmedical use of prescription stimulants such as Adderall (d-amphetamine) in 12th graders has increased from 5.4% in 2009 to 7.6% in 2012. In addition, approximately 68% of 12th graders admit to obtaining prescription pain relievers from friends and family.

Other exposures in adolescents may occur from their environment in school, work and play.[5] While home exposures in this age group are similar to those in the younger child, adolescents tend to spend less time in the home environment and more time in school, work, and play activities. More than 30% of high school aged children work during the school year and summer. These jobs commonly include janitorial jobs, grocery stores, restaurants, landscaping services, and construction jobs where chemicals are used by these untrained workers. Injuries and poisonings are not uncommon and may be higher than in adults with more experience. Adolescents are less likely to wear personal protective gear which increases their risk for exposure.

Specimen Selection for Toxicological Analysis

Various samples are used for toxicological analysis. Urine is the most commonly used specimen for broad-spectrum comprehensive drug screening, and drugs of abuse screening. It is the specimen of choice because it is easy to obtain and most drugs and/or their metabolites accumulate in urine and can be detected from a few hours to several days after drug exposure. Urine is also an easy specimen to work with as most toxicological analytical methods are optimized for urine testing. At times, urine collection from pediatric patients may be challenging and the patient may need catheterization for sample collection. The major drawback of urine as a specimen is that it provides results that cannot be related to blood concentrations of the drugs. 2-10 mL of urine is generally collected to allow initial screening and confirmation testing if needed.

Blood is the specimen of choice when quantification of a particular drug and/or metabolite is needed. Concentration of a drug in the blood generally correlates better to the patient's symptoms as compared to any other matrix. 3-5 mL of whole blood is generally collected for toxicological analyses. Other specimens that may be used for toxicology testing include oral fluid, gastric lavage, hair, nails, cord blood, and meconium.[6,7] Meconium is a frequently used specimen for the detection of in-utero drug exposure. It is easy to collect and provides a wider gestational window for drug detection than fetal or maternal urine as it starts forming between the 12th and 16th week of gestation and accumulates until after birth. If meconium is not available, a newborn's hair can be tested to detect intrauterine drug exposure. Hair and nails are good specimens for evaluating chronic arsenic toxicity.

Analytical Methods in Toxicological Analyses

Commonly used techniques in chemistry/toxicology laboratory are spectrophotometry, immunoassays, and chromatographic methods coupled with detection systems, such as mass spectrometers. Drug and toxin assays that are generally available in a typical hospital laboratory are listed in Table 9-2.

Table 9-2 **DRUGS AND TOXINS ASSAYS THOSE ARE GENERALLY AVAILABLE IN A TYPICAL HOSPITAL LABORATORY**	
Quantitative	Qualitative
Acetaminophen	Amphetamines
Aminoglycosides (Amikacin, Gentamicin, Tobramycin)	Barbiturates
Caffeine	Benzodiazepines
Carbamazepine	Cannabinoids
Carboxyhemoglobin	Cocaine
Digoxin	Ketones
Ethanol	Methadone
Iron	Opiates
Lead	Phencyclidine
Lithium	Propoxyphene
Methemoglobin	Tricyclic antidepressants
Phenobarbital	
Phenytoin	
Salicylate	
Theophylline	
Valproic acid	
Vancomycin	

Immunoassays are rapid and available on automated chemistry analyzers. These methods provide fast turn-around time, but are available for only a limited number of drugs and toxins. Many immunoassays are prone to interferences. Chromatographic methods are more specific and can simultaneously screen for a large number of drugs (>200). The most commonly used chromatographic method for drug screening is gas-chromatography-mass spectrometry (GC-MS). Drugs that can be detected by GC-MS are listed in Table 9-3. In recent years, liquid-chromatography methods involving UV detection or mass spectrometry have become available. Chromatographic methods are technically demanding and the majority of clinical laboratories are not equipped with these methods.

Immunoassays are the most commonly used methods in drug screening. They come in various formats, the two formats that are commonly used being enzymatic and fluorescent. Immunoassays for drugs are usually based on the principle of competitive binding, where a drug in a patient sample competes with the labeled drug for specific binding sites on the antibody. The proportion of labeled drug bound to antibody is either directly or inversely proportional to the concentration of the drug in a patient sample. There are two major types of immunoassays. One type, called homogeneous immunoassays, does not require separation of free and bound drug before the measurement is conducted. The other type, called heterogeneous immunoassays, requires a separation step. Homogenous immunoassays are commonly used and include EMIT (enzyme multiplied immunoassay technique), CEDIA (cloned enzyme donor immunoassay), and FPIA (fluorescence polarization immunoassay). Nowadays, heterogeneous immunoassays, such as RIA (radioimmunoassay) and ELISA (enzyme-linked immunosorbent assay) are less frequently used.

The advantages of immunoassays include that they are fast, automated, and need very small sample volume. Major limitations of immunoassays include lack of specificity and limited menu. Results of immunoassays for drugs of abuse should always be considered presumptive and not evidential of drug abuse. If clinically or legally indicated, presumptive positive results must be confirmed by a more specific method other than immunoassay.

Chromatographic methods are also frequently employed in toxicological analysis or therapeutic drug monitoring. The technique is based on the principle that compounds with different chemical and/or physical properties can be separated by their different interactions with two different media/phases, one being stationary and other mobile. Chromatography methods include thin layer chromatography (TLC), high performance liquid chromatography (HPLC), and gas chromatography (GC). Once the drugs are separated, they are detected by ultraviolet (UV) absorbance, fluorescence, flame ionization, and mass-spectrometry. Chromatographic techniques coupled with mass

Table 9-3	**DRUGS AND/OR METABOLITES THAT CAN BE DETECTED BY GC-MS**	
Acetaminophen	Guaifenesin	Pentobarbital
Amantadine	Ibuprofen	Phencyclidine
Amitriptyline	Imipramine	Phenobarbital
Amphetamine	Ketamine	Phentermine
Benztropine	Levamisole	Phenylpropanolamine
Bupivacaine	Levetiracetam	Phenyltoloxamine
Bupropion	Lidocaine	Phenytoin
Butalbital	Meperidine	Procainamide
Carbamazepine	Mephenytoin	Promethazine
Carisoprodol	Mephobarbital	Propofol
Chlorpheniramine	Mepivacaine	Propoxyphene
Chlorpromazine	Meprobamate	Propranolol
Chlorprothixene	Methadone	Protriptyline
Citalopram	Methamphetamine	Pseudoephedrine
Clomipramine	3,4-Methylenedioxyamphetamine	Quinidine
Cocaethylene	3,4-methylenedioxy-N-ethylamphetamine	Quinine
Cocaine	3,4-methylenedioxy-N-methylamphetamine	Secobarbital
Codeine	Methylenedioxypyrovalerone	Sertraline
Cyclobenzaprine	Methsuximide	Tapentadol
Desipramine	Methylone	Thiopental
Dextromethorphan	Methylphenidate	Thioridazine
Diphenhydramine	Mirtazepine	Timolol
Disopyramide	Morphine	Tramadol
Doxepin	Nicotine	Trazodone
Doxylamine	Norfluoxetine	Trimethobenzamide
Ecgonine Methyl Ester	Normeperidine	Trimethoprim
Ethotoin	Norpropoxyphene	Trimipramine
Fenfluramine	Nortriptyline	Valproic Acid
Flecainide	Olanzapine	Venlafaxine
Fluoxetine	Orphenadrine	Verapamil
Fluvoxamine	Paroxetine	Zolpidem

spectrometers are widely accepted for confirmation of drugs of abuse. To confirm the presence of a drug in a patient sample, the mass spectrum of the unknown drug is compared to the known drug spectrum. Unlike immunoassays, chromatography techniques do not need drug specific reagents and can detect multiple drugs (>200) in a single analysis.

SPECIFIC DRUGS AND TOXINS

Non-Narcotic Analgesics and Antipyretics

Acetaminophen and salicylate are the most commonly encountered drugs in this category. They are used alone or in a variety of combination with other drugs, such as sedatives, antitussives, antihistamines, expectorants, and decongestants.

Acetaminophen

Acetaminophen (*N*-acetyl-p-aminophenol, APAP) is an analgesic and antipyretic drug. It also has weak peripheral anti-inflammatory and anti-platelet aggregation properties. Use of acetaminophen in children gained popularity after the concern about the association between salicylate and Reye's syndrome. Generally, acetaminophen is a safe drug when taken as prescribed. Toxicity in young children is normally due to unintentional ingestions or inappropriate dosing. In adolescents, acetaminophen overdose may be unintentional or intentional. A single dose of 7.5 g in adults or 150 mg/kg in children is considered significant risk for liver damage.[8]

At therapeutic doses, acetaminophen is rapidly and almost completely absorbed from the gastrointestinal tract with bioavailability of 80-90%. The bioavailability decreases with increased doses, such as in overdose situations. Peak levels are seen at ~1 hour with therapeutic doses. In toxic doses, gastric emptying is slow and the peak concentrations are not reached until several hours later. The drug has low volume of distribution of 1 L/kg and is approximately 50% protein bound. At therapeutic doses, its half-life is 1-3 hours. In overdose, the half-life may be significantly prolonged, up to 12 hours. The drug is extensively metabolized in the liver with only 2% excreted unchanged in the urine. The major metabolites, sulfates, and glucuronides, are inactive, and excreted in the urine. Five to ten percent is metabolized by cytochrome P-450 mixed function oxidase system into a highly reactive and hepatotoxic intermediate N-acetyl-p-benzoquinoneimine (NAPQI). Certain medications such as isoniazid, rifampin, and carbamazepine can induce cytochrome P-450 enzymes leading to increased formation of NAPQI. At normal therapeutic doses, NAPQI is rapidly converted to non-toxic cysteine and mercapturic acid glutathione conjugates. In overdose situation, glutathione stores are depleted and free NAPQI binds to hepatocyte proteins and may cause fulminant liver necrosis. Although rare, acetaminophen can cause injury to other organs, such as kidneys and pancreas. Young children are less prone to acetaminophen toxicity as they tend to vomit and have lower cytochrome P-450 mixed function oxidase activity.

Clinical presentation in acetaminophen overdose can be divided into four stages:

Stage 1: 0-24 hour: Patients may be asymptomatic and young children frequently vomit. The patients exhibit gastrointestinal irritation and nausea. Some patients may develop anion gap metabolic acidosis and cardiac arrhythmias.

Stage 2 (latent period): 1-2 days: As nausea and vomiting resolves, patients may appear to improve but hepatic necrosis and renal insufficiency develop. This is evident by increased circulating transaminase activities.

Stage 3 (hepatic failure): 3-5 days: Severe hepatotoxicity and necrosis leading to jaundice, nausea, vomiting, right upper quadrant pain, coagulopathy, and encephalopathy. Laboratory findings include markedly elevated transaminases and bilirubin, and increased prothrombin time. Liver enzymes levels may be over 20,000 IU/L. Young children are less prone to fulminant liver failure.

Stage 4 (recovery or death): 5-14 days: In some untreated patients and most well-treated patients recovery occurs with improved liver function. Other patients may progress to encephalopathy, renal failure, hyperammonemia, bleeding diatheses, and finally death. Fatality can be avoided by a liver transplant.

A glutathione precursor, *N*-acetyl-cysteine (NAC), is an effective antidote used for the treatment of acetaminophen overdose. It enhances the production of glutathione and prevents hepatonecrosis. The Rumack-Matthew nomogram (Figure 9-1) that provides the relationship between acetaminophen blood concentrations and time following the acute ingestion provides a probability of hepatic injury.[9] The patients who have acetaminophen blood concentrations higher than the line of "possible or potential" liver toxicity are candidates for NAC treatment. The nomogram is most useful in a single acute overdose and cannot be used for sustained-released preparations or chronic ingestions. NAC is most effective if given within 10 hours of overdose. However, its benefits have been shown even if given very late. NAC can be administered orally or intravenously. Previously, the standard oral, 72 hour, NAC treatment consisted of 140 mg/kg loading dose followed by 17 doses of 70 mg/kg every four hours. However, current practice allows for individualization of the treatment in order to treat the patient for the duration needed to prevent or treat hepatotoxicity. Patients, who develop intractable vomiting or have medical conditions that preclude them from enteral use of NAC, are given the intravenous treatment. A dose of 300 mg/kg of

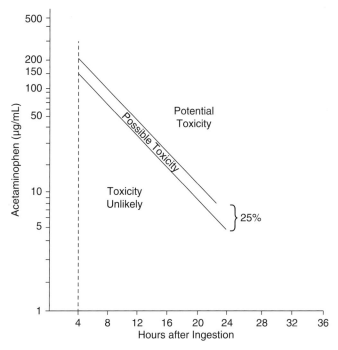

Figure 9-1 ▪ Nomogram for predicting acetaminophen toxicity. Adapted from Rumack,[9] and reprinted with permission from Garg.[30]

NAC is administered intravenously over 21 hours[10] in divided doses. This includes a 150 mg/kg loading dose followed by a continuous infusion. As per the oral dose protocol, treatment is individualized and may result in the need for additional treatment with NAC. The FDA protocol is dependent on the time of initiation of therapy compared to the time of ingestion as the 21-hour course should only be used if the initiation of treatment is within 8 hours of the ingestion and laboratory values (acetaminophen level and liver function tests) are normal at the time of discontinuation.

Although chromatographic methods are available for the analysis of acetaminophen, enzymatic, and immunoassay are routinely used. In enzymatic assay, p-aminophenol produced by the hydrolysis of acetaminophen by aryl enzyme acylamidase is measured. Various kinds of immunoassays including enzyme-multiplied immunoassay technique (EMIT), fluorescence polarization immunoassay (FPIA), and turbidimetric are available. These assays measure free unconjugated but not conjugated drug. Most clinical laboratories use enzymatic or immunoassays on automated chemistry analyzers because they provide rapid (< 20 minutes) and accurate results. Blood sample should be drawn after > 4 hour following acute ingestion.

Salicylate

Acetylsalicylic acid (aspirin) is a widely used analgesic and antipyretic agent. It also has anti-inflammatory and anti-platelet aggregation properties. These properties are attributed to its ability to inhibit the synthesis of prostaglandins and thromboxane via inactivation of cyclooxygenases 1 and 2. Each aspirin tablet contains 325-600 mg acetylsalicylic acid. Therapeutic concentrations are 2-10 mg/dL for analgesia and 10-25 mg/dL for anti-inflammation. Aetylsalicylic acid is rapidly absorbed after oral administration and reaches the peak concentration in 1-2 hours. In overdose, the aspirin tablets may form a tightly packed mass called a bezoar and delay gastric emptying. This results in delayed peak concentration. Acetylsalicylic acid is rapidly and almost completely hydrolyzed to salicylic acid, the active form of the drug. At therapeutic concentrations, the half-life of salicylic acid is 2-3 hours. In overdose, the half-life may be as high as 19 hours because its clearance changes from first-order to zero-order kinetics. The drug is > 90% protein bound and has a low volume of distribution of 0.20 L/kg. Most of the drug is eliminated in the urine as salicyluric acid (80%), salicyl phenolic glucuronide (10%), and salicyl acyl glucuronide (5%).

In overdose, salicylates irritate gastric mucosa and cause nausea and vomiting by stimulating chemoreceptors. Initially respiratory alkalosis results from stimulation of the respiratory center. This is followed by metabolic acidosis due to compensatory renal loss of bicarbonate, uncoupling of oxidative phosphorylation, and inhibition of Krebs cycle.[11] Children may not exhibit a respiratory alkalosis before developing metabolic acidosis. Toxic effects of salicylate overdose include nausea, gastritis, tinnitus, hyperpnea, sweating, and dehydration. Very high blood levels of salicylate, >100 mg/dL, can cause convulsions, respiratory failure, coma, and death. The goals of treatment of salicylate overdose include prevention of further absorption, enhancing elimination and correction of electrolytes, and acid-base imbalance. Most of the patients are severely dehydrated and require fluid treatment. Hypokalemic patients require potassium replacement. Urinary alkalization is used to enhance salicylate excretion. Severity of salicylate intoxication is based on the serum concentration and the clinical status of the patient. The Done nomogram for the workup of salicylate overdose has been recommended in the past to assess for toxicity and need for treatment, but it has not been found to be clinically useful in predicting toxicity in the majority of salicylate exposures.

Although urine can be used for screening, blood is the preferred sample for salicylate measurement. Immunoassays and enzymatic methods are commonly used for the quantitation of salicylate. Colorimetric methods involving Trinder's reagent (mercuric chloride, HCl, and ferric nitrate) are also frequently used. Trinder's method is prone to interferences from bilirubin and ketones. Immunoassays, enzymatic, and colorimetric methods are available on automated chemistry analyzers and provide rapid and reliable results. Gas and liquid chromatographic techniques are used as reference methods, and are too slow for routine use.

Metals

Metals of clinical importance include lead, iron, arsenic, cadmium, and mercury.

Lead

Lead is a non-essential metal with well-known toxic effects. Children are at a higher risk of lead toxicity as lead interferes in the development of the rapidly growing nervous system. In addition to its effect on the nervous system, lead affects bones, kidneys, and the hematopoietic system. Lead crosses the placenta and accumulates in the fetus. Fetal lead exposure results in low birth weight and has adverse effects on neurodevelopment. Children are at higher risk of lead toxicity as they absorb up to 50% of dietary lead as compared to only 5-10% in adults. Calcium and iron deficiency, which are more common in children, also results in increased lead absorption through the intestine.[12] Once absorbed, lead distributes in blood, soft tissues, and bones. During acute exposure, most of the lead (>99%) is found in red blood cells. In chronic exposure, lead stored in bones is released back into the blood and soft-tissues over time prolonging the exposure. Mineralization of the lead into the bones can be seen radiographically. Elimination of lead is triphasic and depends on the depot in the body such that the half-life in blood is faster (one week) than that of soft tissues (one month) and bone (10-20 years).

In the United States, ingestion of lead paint or dust contaminated with lead during renovation of old houses are the common causes of lead toxicity in children. The majority of the houses built before 1970 have lead-based paint. Ingestion of a small lead paint chip containing 50% lead can produce acute lead poisoning in a toddler. Other sources of lead are lead-glazed pottery, water from lead-soldered plumbing, some folk remedies, lead containing batteries, bullets, and occupational exposure. Before the 1970s, leaded gasoline was another significant source of lead. Since the 1970s, lead has been removed from gasoline and paint resulting in a drop of mean lead levels from 16 µg/dL to less than 2 µg/dL in children.[13-15] While the number of children with elevated lead levels is declining, the CDC recently decreased the reference level for action to 5 µg/dL as lower levels are attributable to adverse effects on children's attention and cognition.[14] The effects of lead and updated guidelines from the Pediatric Environmental Health Specialty Units for follow up and actions at different blood concentrations are shown in Tables 9-4 and 9-5.

Table 9-4	CLINICAL MANIFESTATIONS OF LEAD TOXICITY IN CHILDREN
Blood Lead Level (µg/dL)	**Effect (s)**
5-10	Decreased IQ and cognitive deficit, renal dysfunction, neurodevelopment
10-20	Impaired cognition and behavior, fine motor coordination, hearing, growth, hypertension, cardiovascular disease
20-40	Reduced nerve conduction velocity, impaired vitamin D metabolism, decreased hemoglobin synthesis, increased erythrocyte protoporphyrin, peripheral neuropathy
40-90	Colic, frank anemia, nephropathy, encephalopathy
90-150	Encephalopathy (coma, seizure, ataxia, incoordination, bizarre behavior), persistent vomiting, death

Lead exerts its effect by binding to sulfhydryl groups of essential enzymes and other functional and structural proteins. The major organs that are affected include central and peripheral nervous systems, bone marrow, kidneys, and cardiovascular system. CNS effects are exerted through inhibition of calcium-dependent channels and disruption in cell membrane integrity. Heme synthesis is affected by inhibition of delta-aminolevulinic dehyratase, coproporphyrinogen decarboxylase, and ferrochelatase (Figure 9-2).

Measurement of venous whole blood lead is the most important test in assessing lead toxicity. Abdominal x-ray is used to reveal lead paint chips. Bone densitometry and X-ray may also be useful in assessing chronic lead exposure. Common methods for blood lead analysis include atomic absorption spectrometry, inductively-coupled plasma mass spectrometry (ICP-MS), and anodic stripping voltammetry. The methods should have a limit of quantitation of at least 2 µg/dL. Other biomarkers of lead toxicity are zinc protoporphyrin, free erythrocyte protoporphyrin, and delta-aminolevulinic acid. Increase in these markers is due to inhibition of heme synthesis by lead as described earlier. Zinc protoporphyrin can be directly measured by hematofluorometry. It is important to keep in mind that these markers lack sensitivity and specificity, and are not recommended, particularly in children, for the diagnosis of lead exposure. For example, erythrocyte protoporphyrin is not elevated until the blood lead level is >25-35 µg/dL.

Table 9-5	**RECOMMENDED ACTIONS BASED ON BLOOD LEAD LEVEL**
<5 µg/dL	Lead education • Dietary • Environmental Environmental assessment* for pre-1978 housing Follow-up blood lead monitoring
≥5 to ≤45 µg/dL	Lead education • Dietary • Environmental Follow-up blood lead monitoring Complete history and physical exam Lab work: • Iron status • Consider Hemoglobin or hematocrit Environmental investigation Lead hazard reduction Neurodevelopmental monitoring Abdominal X-ray (if particulate lead ingestion is suspected) with bowel decontamination if indicated
≥45 to ≤69 µg/dL	Lead education • Dietary • Environmental Follow-up blood lead monitoring Complete history and physical exam Lab work: • Hemoglobin or hematocrit • Iron status • Free erythrocyte protoporphyrin Environmental investigation Lead hazard reduction Neurodevelopmental monitoring

≥70 µg/dL	Hospitalize and commence chelation therapy (following
	   confirmatory venous blood lead test) in conjunction with
	   consultation from a medical toxicologist or a pediatric
	   environmental health specialty unit
	Proceed according to actions for 45-69 µg/dL

*The scope of an "environmental assessment" will vary based on local resources and site conditions. However, this would include at a minimum a visual assessment of paint and housing conditions, but may also include testing of paint, soil, dust, and water and other lead sources. This may also include looking for exposure from imported cosmetics, folk remedies, pottery, food, toys, etc. which may be more important with low level lead exposure.

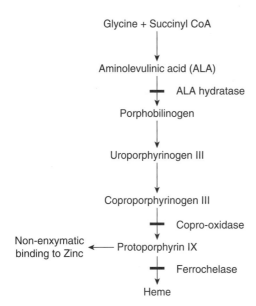

Glycine + Succinyl CoA

↓

Aminolevulinic acid (ALA)

━ ALA hydratase
↓

Porphobilinogen

↓

Uroporphyrinogen III

↓

Coproporphyrinogen III

━ Copro-oxidase
↓

Non-enxymatic ← — Protoporphyrin IX
binding to Zinc

━ Ferrochelase
↓

Heme

Figure 9-2 ▪ Heme synthesis pathways. Lead interference is indicated by black bars for enzymes ALA hydratase, copro-oxidase and ferrochelase, reprinted with permission from Garg.[30]

In children, often there are no symptoms associated with elevated lead levels. However, lethargy, vomiting, irritability, developmental delay, and failure to thrive are symptoms that can be seen. Ataxia, altered consciousness, and seizures have been reported in children with blood lead concentrations higher than 100 µg/dL, although predicting which children will develop these symptoms is impossible. Long term cognitive effects such as ADHD, developmental delay, and decreased IQ have been linked to lead poisoning in childhood. Clinical effects of lead at different blood concentrations are given in Table 9-4.

Diagnosis of lead toxicity is made by obtaining blood lead levels. At levels below 45 µg/dL, children are managed by environmental abatement without medications. At blood lead levels between 45-69 µg/dL, treatment is done with environmental abatement and oral chelation therapy may be given. At levels above 70 µg/dL, children must be admitted to a hospital for inpatient therapy with intravenous and oral chelation therapy. Pediatric Environmental Health Specialty Units (PEHSU) guidelines for recommended actions based on blood lead level are given in Table 9-5, and the recommended schedule for obtaining a confirmatory venous sample is given in Table 9-6. Children who are discharged on oral chelation therapy cannot go to a home with elevated lead levels in the home as this therapy in the presence of lead can increase the absorption of lead in the body. Thus, care must be taken at discharge to ensure that the child returns to a lead safe home.

Table 9-6 RECOMMENDED SCHEDULE FOR OBTAINING A CONFIRMA-TORY VENOUS SAMPLE	
Blood Lead (µg/dL)	Time to Confirmation Testing[*]
≥ 5-9	1-3 months
10-44	1 week to 1 month
45-59	48 hours
60-69	24 hours
≥70	Urgently as emergency test

*The higher the BLL on the screening test, the more urgent the need for confirmatory testing

Iron

Iron toxicity in children, particularly toddlers, generally results from accidental overdose. Iron containing tablets are often bright colored and appear like candy to young children. Iron supplements come in multiple formulations. Iron sulfate tablets contain approximately 65 mg elemental iron per tablet compared to most children's formulations that have approximately 18 mg elemental iron per tablet. Total elemental iron ingested determines the severity of toxicity. Ingestion of only few adult strength iron tablets (> 40 mg/kg) can cause a serious toxicity in a toddler. Iron is corrosive to the gastrointestinal mucosa and produces vomiting, diarrhea, and abdominal pain. Once absorbed, ferrous iron is converted to ferric iron and releases free hydrogen ions. It causes mitochondrial dysfunction resulting in metabolic acidosis.

Serum iron levels are useful in evaluating the severity of toxicity. Iron levels above 500 µg/dL are likely to cause mild to moderate toxicity. Iron levels of more than 800-1000 µg/dL can cause severe toxicity and death. Total iron binding capacity (TIBC) is not useful in the management of iron overdose as it may be falsely elevated and is not a valid indicator of chelation therapy.[16]

Treatment involves good supportive care with intravenous fluid treatment. Whole bowel irrigation with polyethylene glycol solution can be considered especially in cases where tablets are visualized on abdominal X-ray. Serum iron levels are helpful and should ideally be obtained between 2-6 hours following ingestion. After 8 hours iron begins to distribute into the tissues and the iron level will fall making it less helpful in predicting toxicity. Total iron binding capacity and transferrin measurements are not helpful and will be falsely elevated in the setting of toxicity.

Deferoxamine is the preferred antidote for acute iron poisoning and should be considered with any of the following: toxic appearance, shock, metabolic acidosis, coagulopathy, or iron level over 500 µg/dL. Deferoxamine has been associated with hypotension, and acute lung injury. Acute lung injury is seen most often in those that receive it longer than 24 hours. It may be discontinued when the patient is well appearing, and vital signs and labs are normal. Deferoxamine can falsely lower iron concentrations unless atomic absorption is used for measurement. Given iron distribution into tissues after 8 hours and interference by deferoxamine, further iron levels should not be followed.

Arsenic, Cadmium, and Mercury

Arsenic exists in various forms: As^{+3} (inorganic), As^{+5} (organic), and arsine gas. Arsine gas is the most toxic form of arsenic whereas the organic form is the least toxic of the three forms. Major sources of arsenic exposure in humans are food grown in contaminated soil treated with arsenic containing insecticides or pesticides or contaminated well water. Acute toxic effects include abdominal pain, hypotension, tachycardia, rhabdomyolysis, bloody diarrhea, pulmonary edema, and hemolytic anemia. Chronic toxicity manifests as neuropathy, hair loss, hyperkeratosis, and hyperpigmentation. For children, an arsenic dose of 2 mg/kg can cause serious toxicity or death.

Cadmium is used in alloys, electroplating, mining, smelting, and soldering. It is also frequently used in batteries. Acute cadmium exposure causes hepatic injury that appears to be caused by the binding of the Cd^{+2} to sulfhydryl groups. Inactivation of thiol groups in mitochondria leads to oxidative stress and mitochondrial dysfunction. Chronic cadmium toxicity leads to progressive renal failure leading to proteinuria.

Major sources of mercury are occupational (mining and manufacturing), thermometers and seafood. Mercury exists in three major forms: elemental form (Hg^0) that is volatile at room temperature and is less toxic. Elemental mercury is poorly absorbed from the intestinal tract but can enter the body through airborne exposure. Inorganic form (Hg^{+2}) is absorbed through the intestinal tract and causes toxicity by inhibiting metabolism by avidly binding to sulfhydryl groups. Organic forms of mercury (methylmercury and dimethylmercury) are the most toxic forms and are formed from inorganic mercury by biological conversion. Order of toxicity of various forms of mercury is $Hg^0 <$ $Hg^{+2} <$ methylmercury $<$ dimethylmercury. Acute mercury poisoning can result in nausea, vomiting, metallic taste, tremors, and convulsions. Chronic exposure causes peripheral neuropathy, numbness, and tremors.

Blood and urine are tested for arsenic, mercury, and cadmium exposure. Hair and nail are also good specimens for evaluating chronic arsenic exposure. Samples for measurement of heavy metals must be collected in specific metal free tubes and heavy metals are generally measured using atomic absorption spectrometry or inductively coupled plasma.

Alcohols

Ethanol is the most commonly encountered alcohol in children. Mothers who consume ethanol during pregnancy expose their fetuses to ethanol. Ethanol-exposed newborns develop sequelae frequently defined as fetal alcohol syndrome. Infants show irritability, jitteriness, sleeping, and arousal problems. Later in life these children may develop CNS manifestations including hyperactivity, developmental delay, hypotonia, and intellectual disability. Young children accidentally ingest ethanol from unsecured alcoholic beverages or other ethanol containing household products, such as perfumes, colognes, and mouthwashes. More than 10,000 ethanol exposures to children under 6 years of age are reported annually to poison control centers.[3] Ethanol abuse among adolescents is a common problem. It is estimated that almost half of the US high school students drink and one quarter binge drink (ingest 4 or more drinks on one occasion) ethanol.[17] Underage drinking is associated with increased motor vehicle accidents, emergency department visits and violence. Ethanol causes CNS depression in a dose dependent manner. Initially ethanol causes euphoria and a decrease in inhibition. This progresses to lack of coordination, slurred speech, drowsiness, and ataxia. At very high concentrations, > 400 mg/dL, ethanol leads to hypoglycemia, hypotension, respiratory depression, seizures, coma, and potentially death. Young children are prone to these effects at lower ethanol concentrations.

Once consumed orally, ethanol is completely absorbed through the stomach and small intestine. The peak blood concentration occurs between 20-40 minutes. Ethanol is metabolized to acetaldehyde in the liver by alcohol dehydrogenase. Acetaldehyde is further metabolized to acetate via aldehyde dehydrogenase. Children under 5 years of age have reduced ability to metabolize ethanol due to immaturity of hepatic dehydrogenase activity. The microsomal ethanol-oxidizing system comprises a secondary and inducible pathway for ethanol elimination in chronic alcohol use. This pathway is less important in children and adolescents. Above 20 mg/dL, ethanol follows zero order kinetics with metabolism of 10-20 mg/dL/h.

Methanol, ethylene glycol, and isopropanol exposure are common in children due to their presence in a variety of household products. Methanol is widely found in paint thinners, gasoline additives, and windshield washer fluids. Isopropanol is frequently used as disinfectant, and ethylene glycol is found in antifreeze products, coolants, and preservatives. When consumed orally, like ethanol, these alcohols are rapidly and completely absorbed. These alcohols are also metabolized by alcohol dehydrogenase system. Methanol and ethylene glycol are not very toxic by themselves and mainly cause sedation, but their metabolites are toxic. Methanol is metabolized to formic acid which is responsible for metabolic acidosis and may cause blindness. Ethylene glycol is metabolized to glycolaldehyde, glycolic acid, and oxalic acid. These metabolites cause metabolic acidosis. Oxalic acid binds to calcium. This leads to hypocalcemia and precipitation of calcium oxalate crystals in the kidneys resulting in renal failure. Unlike methanol and ethylene glycol, isopropanol is not metabolized to an acidic end product. Like ethanol, it causes CNS depression. Additionally, it is metabolized to acetone which adds to its CNS depressant affects.

Treatments of alcohol toxicities include supportive care including management of hypoglycemia and acidosis. Fomepizole (4-methylpyrazole), an alcohol dehydrogenase inhibitor, can be utilized for the treatment of methanol and ethylene glycol overdose. This drug inhibits the formation of toxic metabolites. Ethanol, although less frequently used since the availability of fomepizole, is also used in the treatment of methanol and ethylene glycol overdose. Ethanol prevents the formation of toxic metabolites by acting as a competitive substrate for alcohol dehydrogenase. Hemodialysis is indicated in severe intoxication.

Commonly used methods for the measurement of alcohols are enzymatic and gas chromatography with flame ionization detector. Enzymatic methods are available on chemistry analyzers but lack specificity. For example, in some enzymatic methods, isopropanol causes falsely elevated concentrations. In certain gas chromatographic methods other volatiles such as acetonitrile, chloroform, difluoroethane, ether, and methyl ethyl ketone may co-elute with ethanol. Headspace gas chromatographic methods are less prone to interference as compared to liquid injection methods.

Drugs of Abuse

Substance abuse among adolescents is a serious problem and is associated with increased motor vehicle accidents, homicides, suicide, and other unintentional injuries. Individuals who start drug use as children are at higher risk of developing addiction as compared to those who begin drug use as adults. In 2013, in the United States, ~50% of young people had used an illicit drug by the time they left high school.[4] Commonly abused drugs include alcohol, amphetamines, cannabinoids, cocaine, opioids, phencyclidine, and sedatives. In children, cannabinoids are the most abused drugs. Immunoassays are commonly used for initial screening of these drugs. Target compounds and detection time window for common drugs of abuse are given in Table 9-7. Positive immunoassays results, if indicated, should be confirmed by definitive methods such as mass spectrometry. In recent years, use of prescription drugs and synthetic drugs such as synthetic cannabinoids, cathinone derivatives (commonly called bath salts), and NBOMe (N-methoxybenzyl derivatives of known 2C phenylethylamines) are gaining popularity. Use of these drugs is increasing and has been attributed to emergency department admissions and deaths.[4,18-20]

Marijuana is often called as a gateway drug that leads to abuse of more potent drugs such as amphetamines, cocaine and heroin. Cannabinoids are

Table 9-7	TARGET COMPOUNDS AND DETECTION TIME WINDOW FOR DRUGS OF ABUSE	
Drug/Drug Class	Typical Target	Window of Detection
Amphetamine	D-amphetamine/ D-Methamphetamine	1-3 days
Barbiturates	Secobarbital	2-14 days, depending on short or long-acting drug
Benzodiazepines	Oxazepam	2-14 days, depending on short or long-acting drug
Cannabinoids	Carboxy-Tetrahydrocannabinol	1-3 days in light use, up to 6 weeks in chronic use
Cocaine	Benzoylecgonine	2-4 Days
Opiates	Morphine/ Codeine	2-4 days
Phencyclidine	Phencyclidine	3-7 days

C_{21} compounds that are found in the plant Cannabis sativa. More than 30 cannabinoids have been identified. The major psychoactive cannabinoid is delta-9-tetrahydrocannabinol (THC). The major metabolite of THC is 11-nor-delta 9-carboxy-tetrahydrocannabinol (THC-COOH). Immunoassays for detecting marijuana use are designed to detect THC-COOH. Since THC is deposited in fat tissues, urine may be positive for THC-COOH for 3-7 days after light to moderate use, and for up to 6 weeks after heavy use. In many states in the United States, selling of marijuana is legal. Passive inhalation of marijuana is unlikely to result in a positive urine test unless the exposure has been extreme (eg, prolonged period of time in an enclosed space).

Amphetamine and methamphetamine are stimulants that can cause hypertension, hyperthermia, tachypnea, diaphoresis, mydriasis, and tachycardia. Their street names include "crystal," "speed," and "ice." They are used in the management of attention-deficit/hyperactivity disorder, narcolepsy, and obesity. Optical isomers of amphetamines exhibit different pharmacological properties. The D-isoforms have much higher CNS activity as compared to L-forms. L-methamphetamine is used as decongestant and may be found in some inhalers. Immunoassays are more sensitive to D-isoforms as compared to L-isoforms. Certain drugs, such as selegiline, benzphetamine, and Adderall, contain amphetamine or methamphetamine or are metabolized to these drugs. Therefore, positive drug screen for amphetamine may truly be positive due to a prescription drug. Sympathomimetic amines (eg, pseudoephedrine, phenylephrine) can cause false positive immunoassays results.

Cocaine is a CNS stimulant that is snorted, smoked, or injected intravenously. The freebase form of cocaine called "crack" volatilizes at lower temperatures and can be easily inhaled by smoking. Its mechanism of action is through inhibition of dopamine and norepinephrine reuptake. Cocaine produces an increase in heart rate and blood pressure, and is associated with arterial vasoconstriction and thrombus formation. The major metabolites of cocaine are benzoylecgonine (BE) and ecgonine methyl ester (EME). When cocaine and ethanol are co-ingested, another metabolite of cocaine called cocaethylene (benzoylecgonine ethyl ester) is produced. Cocaethylene is more toxic than either of the parent compounds. Cocaine use is detected by measurement of BE. Immunoassays for BE are fairly specific and false positive results are rare.

Opioids/opiates are among the most commonly used analgesics for the treatment of severe pain. Opioid is a term used for drugs with morphine-like properties. The term opiates is used for natural occurring opioids. Morphine and codeine (3-methylmorphine) are the most commonly used opioids. Other opioids that are therapeutically used include fentanyl, hydrocodone, hydromorphone, oxycodone, methadone, and tramadol. Heroin, diacetylmorphine, is a synthetic illicit opioid. Opioids have high potential of abuse and addiction. Their toxic effects include nausea, constipation, hypotension, bradycardia, and respiratory depression. Severe overdose can result in coma and death. Naloxone is an effective antidote for the treatment of opioid overdose. Commonly used immunoassays for opioids have cut-off of 300 or 2000 ng/mL. In clinical setting, particularly pediatrics, a cut-off of 300 ng/mL is recommended to avoid false negative results. It is important to note that immunoassays are generally designed to detect morphine and codeine. Therefore, other opioids will not be reliably detected. Additional immunoassays or chromatographic methods are used to detect other opiates/opioids.

Use of synthetic drugs is gaining popularity as these drugs are not easily detected through common drug screens. These drugs are available online or from street retailers commonly known as "C-store," "head," "smart" or "coffee" shops. Synthetic cannabinoids, commonly known as "synthetic marijuana," "K2" or "Spice," are synthetic compounds that mimic the effects of delta-9-tetrahydrocannabinol (THC). Their use in recent years has increased dramatically. According to the 2012 Monitoring the Future survey of youth drug-use trends, one in nine 12th graders in the United States reported using synthetic cannabinoids in the past year.[4] This makes the use of synthetic cannabinoids the second highest after marijuana use. More than 50 synthetic cannabinoids have been identified from illegal markets. Synthetic cathinones, commonly known as "bath salts," are derivatives of cathinones with sympathomimetic effects similar to amphetamines. More than 30 synthetic illegal cathinones have been identified. Another class of drugs called NBOMe has appeared in the illegal market in the last few years.[21] They are psychedelic, derivative of the substituted phenethylamine drugs with sympathomimetic and halluci-nogenic properties. Deaths from the use of these synthetic drugs have been reported.[18-20]

Carbon Monoxide

Carbon Monoxide or CO is a product of incomplete carbon combustion and is colorless, odorless, and non-irritating. CO is a product of normal heme catabolism and thus patients with high red cell turnover, such as sickle cell disease often have elevated carboxyhemoglobin levels. Common exogenous sources of CO include smoke, exhaust, indoor heating/furnaces, generators, stoves, and grills.

CO results in toxicity by binding to hemoglobin and decreasing the oxygen carrying capacity of the red blood cell. It has an affinity for hemoglobin that is 240 times that of oxygen. CO also acts as a direct cellular toxin through inhibition of cytochrome oxidase. This results in a cascade of events that cause free radical formation, leukocyte activation, and lipid peroxidation.

CO poisoning often produces symptoms that are non-specific and can be easily confused with other illnesses. It has been estimated that up to 20% of patients presenting to Emergency Departments (EDs) with viral symptoms in the winter have elevated CO levels.[22] Thus, it is important to maintain a high index of suspicion, especially when the patient is afebrile and if there are other family members with similar symptoms. The early symptoms are mild and can include headache, dizziness, and fatigue. With more severe poisoning patients can exhibit seizures, syncope, altered mental status, or coma. Severe poisoning may also result in cardiac arrhythmias and lactic acidosis.

Obtaining carboxyhemoglobin levels can be helpful in the diagnosis. Co-oximetry, available on most blood gas analyzers, is generally used for the measurement of carboxyhemoglobin. A normal carboxyhemoglobin level does not rule out a significant exposure (depending on the timing of the labs in relation to the time of exposure). Because of this levels do not also correlate with clinical symptoms. Normal levels are 1-3%, but children exposed to second hand smoke could have levels around 5-10%.

Treatment is supportive care and administration of 100% oxygen. High flow oxygen is able to decrease the half-life of CO from 4 hours to 90 minutes. Hyperbaric oxygen is another therapy that has traditionally been recommended, however the exact utility and benefit are debated. Generally accepted indications to consider hyperbaric oxygen include: syncope, altered mental status, pregnancy with CO level >15%.

As a general rule patients that have a relatively quick recovery from an exposure do well and have little risk of chronic sequelae. Patients with severe, acute poisoning or significant symptoms with chronic, significant exposures are at risk for developing persistent neurologic sequelae but this is reported more commonly in adults.

THERAPEUTIC DRUG MONITORING

International Association of Therapeutic Drug Monitoring and Toxicology defines therapeutic drug monitoring as "The measurement made in the laboratory of a parameter which, with appropriate interpretation, will directly influence prescribing procedures. Commonly, the measurement is in a biological matrix of a prescribed xenobiotic, but it may also be of an endogenous compound prescribed as replacement therapy in an individual who is physiologically or pathologically deficient in that compound."[23] It is a multi-disciplinary approach involving correct sample collection, analysis of drug concentrations in the body fluids and interpretation of results to achieve maximum efficacy of drug therapy. The purpose of TDM is to keep the concentration of a particular drug in a specific range called the therapeutic range to achieve the maximum efficacy and minimal adverse reactions.

Once the drug enters the body, it exerts its effects through interactions with receptors or other cellular targets. Though increase in blood drug concentration may not parallel the concentration of the drug at receptor, up to a certain point there is a good relationship between drug concentration and response. Drug disposition is generally studied as drug liberation, absorption, distribution, metabolism, and elimination. In pediatric patients due to growth and development these parameters may be significantly different as compared to adults. For example, growth is very rapid after birth: body weight doubles in the first 5 months of life and triples in 1 year, body length increases by 50%, body surface area doubles and caloric intake increases 3-4 times in the first year of life.[24]

For TDM, plasma and serum are the most commonly used specimens. Whole blood is used for certain drugs which sequester in red blood cells, such as the immunosuppressant drugs cyclosporine, sirolimus, and tacrolimus. Cerebrospinal fluid may also be useful for TDM of some drugs. In most cases, samples are drawn at steady state concentration that is reached after 5-7 drug half-lives. Once the steady state is reached, the drug concentration ideally varies between the minimum effective concentration and minimum toxic concentration (Figure 9-3). For most drugs trough levels correlate better with the clinical outcome, however, for some drugs clinical correlation is better with peak concentrations. Both trough and peak levels are generally measured for these drugs (eg, aminoglycosides). Although samples can be drawn in gel separator tubes for certain drugs, for many drugs (such as tricyclic antidepressants, benzodiazepines etc.) gel separator tubes are not recommended as these drugs

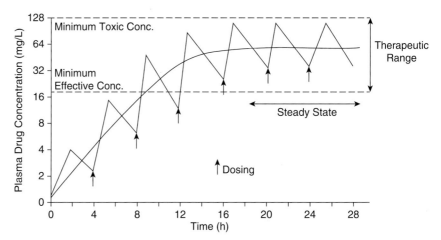

Figure 9-3 ▪ Plasma concentrations of a drug given in multiple doses. Minimum effective concentration and minimum toxic concentrations are also shown. It takes 5-7 drug half-lives to reach a steady state concentration, reprinted with permission from Garg.[30]

bind to the gels. Another frequently encountered issue in TDM is an inappropriate blood drawn from IV site that was used for drug administration. It is recommended that samples should not be drawn from the same lines through which the drug was given. If samples must be collected through the infusion line, the lines should be thoroughly flushed.

Immunoassays and chromatographic techniques are most commonly used for the assay of drugs. Immunoassays are rapid, need small sample volume, and are generally available on automated chemistry analyzers. However, there are only a limited number of immunoassays, and they are prone to interferences from other structurally similar drugs or their metabolites. Commonly used immunoassay techniques are enzymatic or fluorescent. Chromatographic methods are more flexible and unlike immunoassays do not require specific reagents. These tests are technically demanding and not available in most clinical laboratories. Commonly used chromatographic techniques are gas chromatography and high performance liquid chromatography.[25] Gas chromatography is a rugged technique that can be used for quantification of a large number of drugs on the same column under similar conditions. Although, many types of detectors can be used with gas chromatography, in recent years a mass spectrometer has become the detector of choice. The disadvantages of gas chromatography include the need for a large sample volume and complex sample preparation. High performance liquid chromatography (HPLC) is another chromatographic technique widely used in the measurement of drugs. For HPLC, the sample preparation is generally less involved as compared to gas chromatography. The most commonly used detector in HPLC is an UV detector. However, in recent years, HPLC linked to tandem mass spectrometry (LC-MS-MS) has been gaining popularity and is widely used in TDM. Like other methods in clinical chemistry, methods used for measurement of drugs must be validated for accuracy, precision, specificity, limit of detection, linearity, and robustness.

Some pharmacokinetic properties of frequently monitored drugs are given in Table 9-8.[26-30]

Table 9-8	**PHARMACOKINETIC PROPERTIES OF COMMONLY MONITORED DRUGS**[30]			
Drug	~Half-Life (h)	Therapeutic Range	Toxic Concentration	Units
Anticonvulsants:				
Carbamazepine	10-20	4-12	>15	µg/mL
Ethosuximide	25-40	40-100	>150	µg/mL
Gabapentin	4-6	12-20	>85	µg/mL
Lamotrigine	30	3-15	>20	µg/mL
Levetiracetam	5-7	10-60	NA	µg/mL
Oxcarbazepine	5-15	12-35	NA	µg/mL
Phenobarbital	40-120	15-40	>50	µg/mL
Phenytoin	7-30	10-20	>20	µg/mL
Primidone	4-6	5-12	>15	µg/mL
Valproic acid	8-12	50-100	>100	µg/mL
Immunosuppressants:				
Cyclosporine A	6-24	100-400, variable with type and duration of transplant	Variable with type and duration of transplant	ng/mL
Everolimus	18-35	3-10	Variable	ng/mL
Mycophenolic Acid	8-18	1.0-3.5	Variable	µg/mL
Sirolimus	8-20	5-20	>30	ng/mL
Tacrolimus	8-16	5-15	>20	ng/mL
Antibiotics:				
Amikacin	2-3	Peak: 20-30; Trough: <10	Peak: >35; Trough: >10	µg/mL
Gentamicin	2-3	Peak: 5-10; Trough: <2	Peak: >12; Trough: >2	µg/mL
Tobramycin	2-4	Peak: 5-10; Trough: <2	Peak: >12; Trough: >2	µg/mL
Vancomycin	3-10	Peak: 20-40; Trough: 5-15	Peak: >80; Trough: >20	µg/mL

(Continued)

Table 9-8 **PHARMACOKINETIC PROPERTIES OF COMMONLY MONITORED DRUGS**[30] *(Continued)*				
Drug	~Half-Life (h)	Therapeutic Range	Toxic Concentration	Units
Antidepressants:				
Amitriptyline*	21	120-250[†]	>500[†]	ng/mL
Citalopram	30	40-100	>250	ng/mL
Desipramine	20	75-300	>500	ng/mL
Fluoxetine*	60	300-1000[†]	>2000[†]	ng/mL
Fluvoxamine	23	50-900	NA	ng/mL
Imipramine*	12	150-250[†]	>500[†]	ng/mL
Paroxetine	22	20-200	>800	ng/mL
Sertraline	28	30-200	>500	ng/mL
Cardiac Drugs:				
Digoxin	12-48	0.5-2.0	>2.2	ng/mL
Disopyramide	2.5-3.8	2.0-6.0	>7	μg/mL
Lidocaine	1-3	1.5-5.0	>6	μg/mL
Procainamide and N-acetylprocainamide	1.5-2.0	4.0-8.0	>10	μg/mL
Propranolol	3.9-6.4	50-100	NA	ng/mL
Quinidine	2.5-6.7	2-7	>8	μg/mL
Other Drugs:				
Caffeine	40-100 (neonates); 3-5 (older children)	5-20	>50	μg/mL
Methotrexate	8-15 (high dose) 3-10 (low dose)	Variable, depends on therapeutic approach	Variable, See text	μg/mL
Theophylline	1-8	10-20	>25	μg/mL

*Metabolized to active N-demethylated metabolite.

[†]Total concentrations of parent drug and active metabolite.

Specific Drug Classes

Anticonvulsant (Antiepileptic) Drugs

Broadly, anticonvulsants are divided into two categories: first and second generation drugs. The first generation drugs are the older drugs and include phenytoin, carbamazepine, primidone, phenobarbital, ethosuximide and valproic acid. Due to their narrow therapeutic index and high intra and inter-individual variability in drug metabolism, these drugs are good candidates for TDM.[31] Also many first generation anticonvulsants, such as phenobarbital, phenytoin, and carbamazepine stimulate various P450 enzymes and increase their own metabolism making TDM of these drugs more important.[32] Relatively new, clinically used after 1990s, are called second generation anticonvulsants, and include gabapentin, lamotrigine, levetiracetam, and oxcarbazapine.[27,31,33] The newer anticonvulsants do not induce P450 enzymes.[32]

TDM consideration of anticonvulsants in children can be significantly different as compared to adults. For example, neonates will have a higher free fraction of phenytoin compared to adults due to lower plasma protein concentration and reduced protein binding. Therefore, infants require lower dose of phenytoin than adults for the same therapeutic effect. Young children (2-3 years of age) have very high phenytoin metabolic capacity and may require up to 4 times higher dose than adults.[26]

Immunoassays and chromatographic techniques are used for the determination of anticonvulsants. First generation anticonvulsants including phenobarbital, phenytoin, carbamazepine, primidone, ethosuximide, and valproic acid are generally measured by immunoassays. Although, immunoassays provide fast and accurate results, they are prone to interferences due to cross-reactivity of antibody with metabolites or other drugs.[25,34,35] For example, 5-(p-hydroxyphenyl)-5-phenylhydantoin (HPPH), a major phenytoin metabolite cross reacts with many commercial immunoassays. Uremic patients accumulate significant amount of HPPH leading to false positive phenytoin values by immunoassays.[25,36] Hydroxyzine and its metabolite cetirizine are known to interfere with a particle enhance turbidimetric inhibition immunoassay.[34] Carbamazepine is metabolized to an active metabolite carbamazepine 10,11-epoxide. Different immunoassays cross-react differently with 10,11-epoxide. Immunoassays for phenobarbital cross-react with other barbiturates. Chromatographic techniques can provide accurate information in such situations. Immunoassays are not available for most newer second generation anticonvulsants. They are measured by gas and liquid chromatographic techniques.[25,37]

Immunosuppressive Drugs

Immunosuppressive drugs are widely used in organ transplant to prevent acute transplant rejection and improve long-term graft survival. They are also used in the treatment of autoimmune diseases and allergic reactions. Availability of cyclosporine A (CSA) in the 1970s was a major breakthrough in the long-term allograft transplant and survival. Since then many other immunosuppressants including tacrolimus, sirolimus, everolimus, and mycophenolic acid have been discovered and are widely used in organ transplant.[38,39]

CSA, tacrolimus and mycophenolic acid are given orally or intravenously, whereas sirolimus is administered orally. Like many other drugs, disposition of immunosuppressants in children can be significantly different as compared to adults. For example, metabolism of CSA and tacrolimus is 2-3 times greater in younger children as compared to older children and adults resulting in the need for higher doses on mg/kg basis. Immunosuppressants absorption is highly food and intestinal bile concentration dependent, and these parameters are more variable in children.

Due to narrow therapeutic windows, and significant intra-individual and inter-individual variability, TDM of immunosuppressants is warranted. Since significant amount of drug resides in RBCs, whole blood is the specimen of choice for TDM of cyclosporine A, tacrolimus, sirolimus, and everolimus. Plasma is a specimen of choice for the assay of mycophenolic acid. Immunosuppressants are measured by immunoassays or chromatographic methods. Immunoassays are available for cyclosporine A, tacrolimus, sirolimus, and everolimus. Immunoassays are convenient and fast but have issues with cross-reactivity.[39,40] Commonly used chromatographic methods are HPLC with ultraviolet detector and tandem mass spectrometry. Tandem mass spectrometry assays are preferred and are in wide use.[41,42] As compared to HPLC with UV detection, tandem mass spectrometry assays are reproducible, accurate, and sensitive.

Antibiotics

Antibiotics are widely used drugs particularly in hospital settings. Treatment with most antibiotics is empirical and does not require TDM. However, certain antibiotics, such as aminoglycosides and vancomycin require frequent monitoring.[43] Aminoglycosides include amikacin, gentamicin, neomycin, streptomycin, and tobramycin. They are used alone or in combination with other antibiotics in the treatment of aerobic Gram-negative bacteria. They inhibit bacterial protein synthesis by binding to the 30S ribosomal subunit of bacterial mRNA.[44] Aminoglycosides are very polar, do not cross intestinal membranes, and are therefore administered intravenously. They are nephrotoxic and ototoxic. In addition to TDM, renal functions should be monitored through urine output and creatinine clearance. Aminoglycosides can damage vestibular and cochlear cells resulting in auditory loss and vestibular dysfunction. Ototoxicity caused by aminoglycosides may be irreversible. Both trough and peak levels are monitored. Samples for trough levels are drawn just before the next dose, and samples for peak levels are drawn 30 to 60 minutes after completion of intravenous infusion.

Vancomycin is a glycopeptide antibiotic used in the treatment of Gram-positive bacteria. It is most commonly used in the treatment of methicillin-resistant *Staphylococcus aureus* or beta-lactam resistant coagulase negative *Staphylococcus.* It is also used in the treatment of C. difficile-associated diarrhea and enterocolitis caused by *S aureus.* Vancomycin inhibits bacterial growth by inhibiting bacterial cell wall synthesis. Vancomycin is very polar and does not cross intestinal membranes, and is thus given intravenously. Earlier impure forms of vancomycin caused nephrotoxicity and ototoxicity. With improved manufacturing practices these side effects are rare. Like aminoglycosides, both trough and peak levels of vancomycin are monitored. Samples for trough levels are drawn just before the next dose, and samples for peak levels are drawn 30 minutes after completion of 60 or 120 minutes intravenous infusion.

Automated immunoassays that are available on most chemistry analyzers are frequently used for the analysis of aminoglycosides and vancomycin. In general, immunoassays are satisfactory, but may have interferences in some situations. For example, in renal failure, crystalline degradation products of vancomycin (CDP-1) accumulate and may interfere in certain immunoassays.

In children, TDM considerations for aminoglycosides and vancomycin may be significantly different as compared to adults. Volume of distribution (Vd) of gentamicin, in a neonate with gestational age of 32 weeks, is approximately 0.70 L/kg as compared to 0.32 L/kg in older children.[45] On the other hand, due to lower GFR, clearance of these drugs in infants is lower as compared to adults.[45] Also, the incidence of aminoglycoside nephrotoxicity and ototoxicity is lower in infants and children as compared to adults.[45]

Antidepressants

Antidepressants are categorized into tricyclic antidepressants (TCAs) and non-TCAs, such as monoamine oxidase and selective serotonin reuptake inhibitors. Due to their narrow therapeutic window and significant side effects, TCAs are frequently monitored. In children, TCAs are also used for the treatment of enuresis and obsessive-compulsive disorder. They include amitriptyline, nortriptyline, imipramine, desipramine, and doxepin. When tertiary amines TCAs are administered, their corresponding active metabolites are also monitored. When given orally, TCAs are well absorbed in the intestine and reach peak plasma levels in 2-12 hours. Their toxic effects include hypotension, cardiac arrhythmias, seizures, and respiratory depression.

Non-TCAs antidepressants include monoamine reuptake inhibitors (amoxapine and maprotiline), serotonin reuptake inhibitors (trazodone), nor-epinephrine, and serotonin reuptake inhibitors (venlafaxine and mirtazapine) and selective serotonin reuptake inhibitors (citalopram, escitalopram, fluoxetine, fluvoxamine, paroxetine, and sertraline).[46,47] Selective serotonin reuptake inhibitors (SSRIs) are the most commonly used antidepressants.[47,48] In addition, SSRIs are also used in the treatment of obsessive-compulsive disorder, panic disorder, bulimia, and many other conditions.[49] Compared to TCAs, SSRIs have fewer side effects. Overdose with SSRIs is associated with serotonin syndrome that is characterized by mental status changes, agitation, myoclonus, hyperreflexia, incoordination, diaphoresis, shivering, tremor, and fever. It was thought that SSRIs may cause or worsen suicidal thinking or behavior in children and adolescents. However, recent literature does not support this notion.[50]

Tubes without gels are preferred for sample collection as most antidepressants are lipophilic and bind to gels. Immunoassays are frequently used for the assay of TCAs. They provide quantitative or semi-quantitative results. Many drugs including carbamazepine, quetiapine, phenothiazines, diphenhydramine, cyproheptadine, and cyclobenzaprine have been shown to interfere with certain TCAs immunoassays.[46,51-54] HPLC with UV detector or mass spectrometry are frequently used for the assay of non-TCAs.[55]

Cardioactive Drugs

Frequently monitored cardioactive drugs include digoxin, disopyramide, lidocaine, procainamide, and quinidine.[56] The most commonly monitored cardioactive drug in children is digoxin. It is a glycoside isolated from digitalis plant, and is used in the treatment of heart failure, chronic atrial fibrillation, and supraventricular arrhythmias. Immunoassays are commonly used for the determination of digoxin. In several clinical conditions, such as renal insufficiency, complicated third-trimester pregnancy, and infancy, there is accumulation of digoxin-like endogenous substances. These compounds cross-react with many digoxin assays and give falsely high digoxin concentrations.[35]

Toxic effects of digoxin include nausea, vomiting, anorexia, and visual disturbances. Digoxin overdose is treated with Fab fragment of anti-digoxin antibodies. The Fab antibody fragments interfere with most of the immunoassays and results are misleading.[57,58] If needed, free digoxin can be measured after ultrafiltration of the sample. Potassium, calcium, and magnesium should also be monitored in digoxin overdose as abnormalities in these electrolytes are associated with exacerbation of digoxin toxicity.

Lidocaine is used in the treatment of ventricular arrhythmias and ventricular fibrillation. Due to significant first by-pass metabolism, lidocaine is administered intravenously. Quinidine, another antiarrhythmic drug when co-administered with digoxin, can reduce renal clearance and cause significant increase in digoxin concentration. Procainamide is metabolized to active metabolite *N*-acetyl procainamide (NAPA). NAPA can accumulate to significant concentrations in renal dysfunction and fast acetylators. Therefore, both procainamide and NAPA should be monitored. Rarely monitored cardioactive drugs include calcium channel blockers, β-blockers, and catecholamines.

Respiratory Stimulants

Caffeine and theophylline are methylxanthines and commonly used bronchodilators in the management of neonatal apnea. In infants, caffeine is preferred over theophylline for the treatment of apnea due to its longer half-life of 40-100 hours, more consistent intestinal absorption, and lower toxicity. In neonates theophylline is rapidly metabolized to caffeine, and both caffeine and theophylline should be measured. Toxic effects of these drugs include tachycardia, hypotension, vomiting, and seizures. Immunoassays are commonly used for the assay of caffeine and theophylline.

Antineoplastic Drugs

With the exception of a few drugs including methotrexate and busulfan, antineoplastic drugs are generally not monitored.[59] Methotrexate, a folic acid antagonist, is used in the treatment of various neoplasms including acute lymphocytic leukemia, lymphoma, and choriocarcinoma. In low doses, methotrexate is used in the management of autoimmune diseases, such as rheumatoid arthritis, Crohn's disease, and psoriasis. Methotrexate inhibits DNA synthesis in rapidly growing cells by interference through folate metabolism, by inhibiting dihydrofolate reductase (DHFR). The drug can be administered orally, intramuscularly, intravenously, or intrathecally. TDM is most useful in patients receiving high dose methotrexate (exceeding 50 mg/m^2). After high dose methotrexate administration, drug concentrations are measured every 24 hour for 3 days. Toxic concentrations of methotrexate are: >5 μmol/L after 24 hour, >0.5 μmol/L after 48 hour, or >0.05 μmol/L after 72 hour of drug administration.[59] Since methotrexate is toxic to normal cells, leucovorin rescue is initiated if the drug concentrations are in the toxic range. Toxic effects of methotrexate include bone marrow suppression leading to anemia and neutropenia, nausea, vomiting, and diarrhea. Methotrexate is generally analyzed by immunoassays.[59]

Busulfan is an alkylating agent that inhibits DNA replication and transcription of RNA by reacting with the N-7 position of guanosine. It is used in the treatment of chronic myelogenous leukemia (CML). In conjunction with cyclophosphamide, busulfan is used in the conditioning regimen prior to allogeneic hematopoietic progenitor cell transplantation.[59] Toxic effects of busulfan include nausea, vomiting, anorexia, anemia, hyperpigmentation, seizures, and infertility. Busulfan is administered orally or intravenously. It binds to albumin and RBCs and is extensively metabolized in the liver. Immunoassays and liquid chromatography involving UV detection or mass-spectrometry are used for the measurement of busulfan. Therapeutic effect of busulfan correlates with area under the plasma concentration–time curve (AUC) or the average plasma concentrations at steady state.

SUMMARY

Toxicological and therapeutic drug monitoring considerations in children, particularly neonates, are significantly different as compared to adults. Many factors including toxin/drug absorption, distribution, metabolism, elimination, and environment contribute of these differences.

TRAINING MODULE

1. The antidote for acetaminophen toxicity is:
    a. Deferoxamine
    b. *N*-acetylcysteine
    c. Naloxone
    d. Leucovorin

2. The current (2014), CDC, reference level for action for lead is:
    a. 5 µg/dL
    b. 10 µg/dL
    c. 15 µg/dL
    d. 25 µg/dL

3. The most commonly used specimen for drug screening is:
    a. Blood
    b. Plasma
    c. Urine
    d. Saliva

4. Approximately, how many half-lives are needed for a drug to reach steady-state concentration?
    a. 5
    b. 7
    c. 9
    d. 11

5. Benzoylecgonine is measured to detect the use of:
    a. Morphine
    b. Cannabinoids
    c. Phencyclidine
    d. Cocaine

REFERENCES

1. Morbidity and Mortality Weekly Report. Vital Signs: Unintentional injury deaths among persons aged 0-19 years of age in the United States, 2000-2009. 2012;61:1-7.

2. Warner M, Chen LH, Makuc DM, Anderson RN, Minino AM. Drug poisoning deaths in the United States, 1980-2008. NCHS Data Brief 2011;81:1-8.

3. Mowry JB, Spyker DA, Cantilena LR, Jr., Bailey JE, Ford M. 2012 Annual Report of the American Association of Poison Control Centers' National Poison Data System (NPDS): 30th Annual Report. *Clin Toxicol (Phila)*. 2013;51:949-1229.

4. http://www.monitoringthefuture.org/ Accessed 6/30/2014.

5. Anderson ME, Bogdan GM. Environments, indoor air quality, and children. *Pediatr Clin North Am*. 2007;54:295-307.

6. Garg U. Hair, oral fluid, sweat and meconium testing for drugs of abuse: Advantages and pitfalls. In: Dasgupta A, ed. *Handbook of Drug Monitoring Methods: Therapeutics and Drugs of Abuse*. Totowa: Humana Press, 2008:337-364.

7. Garg U, Ferguson AM. Alternate specimens for drugs-of-abuse testing:preanalytical and interpretative considerations. In: M Barbarajean M, MG Bissell MG, TC Kwong TC, Wu AHB, eds. *Clinical Toxicology Testing: A Guide for laboratory Professionals*. CAP Press, 2012:71-80.

8. Lewis RK, Paloucek FP. Assessment and treatment of acetaminophen overdose. *Clin Pharm*. 1991;10:765-774.

9. Rumack BH, Matthew H. Acetaminophen poisoning and toxicity. *Pediatrics* 1975;55:871-876.

10. Dyer KS, Ewald MB, Wiley JF. Acetaminophen (paracetamol) poisoning in children and adolescents. In: Basow MA, ed. *UpToDate Online*. Waltham, MA: UpToDate Inc., 2009.

11. Kim S. Salicylates. In: Olson KR, ed. *Poisoning and Drug Overdoes*. 5th ed. New York: McGraw-Hill, 2007:333-335.

12. Bruening K, Kemp FW, Simone N, Holding Y, Louria DB, Bogden JD. Dietary calcium intakes of urban children at risk of lead poisoning. *Environ Health Perspect*. 1999;107:431-435.

13. Hurwitz RL, Lee DA. *Childhood lead poisoning: Clinical manifestations and diagnosis*. *UpToDate Online*, 2009.

14. Morbidity and Mortality Weekly Report. Blood lead levels in children aged 1-5 years – United States, 1999-2010. *Morb Mortal Wkly Rep*. 2013;62:245-248.

15. Muntner P, Menke A, DeSalvo KB, Rabito FA, Batuman V. Continued decline in blood lead levels among adults in the United States: the National Health and Nutrition Examination Surveys. *Arch Intern Med*. 2005;165:2155-2161.

16. Manoguerra AS. Iron. In: Olson KR, ed. *Poisoning and Drug Overdoes*. 5th ed. New York: McGraw-Hill, 2007:230-232.

17. Baum CR. Ethanol intoxication in children: epidemiology, estimation of toxicity, and toxic effects. In: Ewald MB, ed. *UpToDate Online*. Waltham, MA: UpToDate Inc., 2009.

18. Hassen GW, Ghobadi F, Kalantari H. Synthetic drugs: a new trend and the hidden danger. *Am J Emerg Med*. 2013;31:1413-1415.

19. Gunderson EW. Synthetic cannabinoids: a new frontier of designer drugs. *Ann Intern Med*. 2013;159:563-564.

20. Arnold C. The new danger of synthetic drugs. *Lancet*. 2013;382:15-16.

21. Lawn W, Barratt M, Williams M, Horne A, Winstock A. The NBOMe hallucinogenic drug series: patterns of use, characteristics of users and self-reported effects in a large international sample. *J Psychopharmacol*. 2014:1-9.

22. Zorbalar N, Yesilaras M, Aksay E. Carbon monoxide poisoning in patients presenting to the emergency department with a headache in winter months. *Emerg Med J*. 2014;31(e1):e66-e70.

23. Watson I, Potter J, Yatscoff R, Fraser A, Himberg JJ, Wenk M. Therapeutic Drug Monitoring. *Ther Drug Monit*. 1997;19:125.

24. Kauffman RE. Drug action and therapy in the infant and child. In: Yaffe SJ, Aranda JV, eds. *Neonatal and Pediatric Pharmacology: Therapeutic Principles in Practice*. 3rd ed. Philadelphia: Lippincott Williams and Wilkins, 2005:20-31.

25. Dasgupta A. Introduction to therapeutic drug monitoring and chromatography. In: Dasgupta A, ed. *Advances in Chromatographic Techniques for Therapeutic Drug Monitoring*. Boca Raton: CRC Press, 2010:1-38.

26. Broussard LA. Monitoring anticonvulsant concentrations - General considerations. In: Hammett-Stabler CA, Dasgupta A, eds. *Therapeutic Drug Monitoring Data*. 3rd ed. Washington, DC: AACC Press, 2007:41-75.

27. Garg U, Jacobs DS, Grady HJ, Foxworth J, Gorodetzky CW. Therapeutic drug monitoring. In: Jacobs DS, DeMott WR, Oxley DK, eds. *Jacobs and DeMott Laboratory Test Handbook*. 5th ed. Hudson: Lexi-Comp, 2001:731-771.

28. Lexi. Pediatric Lexi-Drugs Online. http://online.lexi.com/crlsql/servlet/crlonline,. Lexi-Comp, Inc., 2009.

29. Moyer TP, Shaw LM. Therapeutic drugs and their management. In: Burtis CA, Ashwood ER, Bruns DE, eds. *Tietz Textbook of Clinical Chemistry and Molecular Diagnostics*. 4th ed. St. Louis: Elsevier-Saunders, 2006:1237-1285.

30. Garg U, Sandritter TL, Leeder JS. Pediatric therapeutic drug monitoring, toxicology and pharmacogenetics. In: DJ Dietzen MBaEW, ed. *Biochemical and Molecular Basis of Pediatric Disease*. Washington DC: AACC Press, 2010:531-560.

31. Patsalos PN, Berry DJ, Bourgeois BF, Cloyd JC, Glauser TA, Johannessen SI, et al. Antiepileptic drugs–best practice guidelines for therapeutic drug monitoring: a position paper by the subcommission on therapeutic drug monitoring, ILAE Commission on Therapeutic Strategies. *Epilepsia*. 2008;49:1239-1276.

32. Perucca E. Clinically relevant drug interactions with antiepileptic drugs. *Br J Clin Pharmacol*. 2006;61:246-255.

33. Hitiris N, Brodie MJ. Modern antiepileptic drugs: guidelines and beyond. *Curr Opin Neurol*. 2006;19:175-180.

34. Parant F, Moulsma M, Gagnieu MC, Lardet G. Hydroxyzine and metabolites as a source of interference in carbamazepine particle-enhanced turbidimetric inhibition immunoassay (PETINIA). *Ther Drug Monit*. 2005;27:457-462.

35. Datta P, Dasgupta A. Immunoassays for therapeutic drug monitoring: Pitfalls and limitations. In: Dasgupta A, ed. *Advances in Chromatographic Techniques for Therapeutic Drug Monitoring*. Boca Raton: CRC Press, 2010:53-68.

36. Roberts WL, Rainey PM. Interference in immunoassay measurements of total and free phenytoin in uremic patients: a reappraisal. *Clin Chem*. 1993;39:1872-1877.

37. Subramanian M, Birnbaum AK, Remmel RP. High-speed simultaneous determination of nine antiepileptic drugs using liquid chromatography-mass spectrometry. *Ther Drug Monit*. 2008;30:347-356.

38. Gummert JF, Ikonen T, Morris RE. Newer immunosuppressive drugs: a review. *J Am Soc Nephrol*. 1999;10:1366-1380.

39. Butch AW. Introduction to immunosupressive drug monitoring. In: Hammett-Stabler CA, Dasgupta A, eds. *Therapeutic Drug Monitoring Data*. 3rd ed. Washington, DC: AACC Press, 2007:129-161.

40. Kelly KA. Pharmacokinetics and therapeutic drug monitoring of immunosuppressants. In: Dasgupta A, ed. *Advances in Chromatographic Techniques for Therapeutic Drug Monitoring*. Boca Raton: CRC Press, 2010:209-238.

41. Taylor PJ. Therapeutic drug monitoring of immunosuppressant drugs by high-performance liquid chromatography-mass spectrometry. *Ther Drug Monit*. 2004;26:215-219.

42. Deters M, Kirchner G, Resch K, Kaever V. Simultaneous quantification of sirolimus, everolimus, tacrolimus and cyclosporine by liquid chromatography-mass spectrometry (LC-MS). *Clin Chem Lab Med*. 2002;40:285-292.

43. Dasgupta A, Hammett-Stabler CA, Broussard LA. Therapeutic drug monitoring of antimicrobial and antiviral agents. In: Hammett-Stabler CA, Dasgupta A, eds. *Therapeutic Drug Monitoring Data*. 3rd ed. Washington, DC: AACC Press, 2007:163-192.

44. Nagai J, Takano M. Molecular aspects of renal handling of aminoglycosides and strategies for preventing the nephrotoxicity. *Drug Metab Pharmacokinet*. 2004;19:159-170.

45. Hoog MD, vandenAnker JN. Drug metabolism and disposition in infants and children. In: Yaffe SJ, Aranda JV, eds. *Neonatal and Pediatric Pharmacology: Therapeutic Principles in Practice*. 3rd ed. Philadelphia: Lippincott Williams and Wilkins, 2005: 377-401.

46. Garg U. Therapeutic drug monitoring of antidepressants. In: Hammett-Stabler CA, Dasgupta A, eds. *Therapeutic Drug Monitoring Data*. 3rd ed. Washington, DC: AACC Press, 2007:107-128.

47. Ables AZ, Baughman OL, 3rd. Antidepressants: update on new agents and indications. *Am Fam Physician*. 2003;67:547-554.

48. Pacher P, Kecskemeti V. Trends in the development of new antidepressants. Is there a light at the end of the tunnel? *Curr Med Chem*. 2004;11:925-943.

49. Schatzberg AF. New indications for antidepressants. *J Clin Psychiatry*. 2000;61 Suppl 11:9-17.

50. Cooper WO, Callahan ST, Shintani A, Fuchs DC, Shelton RC, Dudley JA, et al. Antidepressants and suicide attempts in children. *Pediatrics*. 2014;133:204-210.

51. Caravati EM, Juenke JM, Crouch BI, Anderson KT. Quetiapine cross-reactivity with plasma tricyclic antidepressant immunoassays. *Ann Pharmacother*. 2005;39: 1446-1449.

52. Hendrickson RG, Morocco AP. Quetiapine cross-reactivity among three tricyclic antidepressant immunoassays. *J Toxicol Clin Toxicol*. 2003;41:105-108.

53. Dasgupta A, McNeese C, Wells A. Interference of carbamazepine and carbamazepine 10,11-epoxide in the fluorescence polarization immunoassay for tricyclic antidepressants: estimation of the true tricyclic antidepressant concentration in the presence of carbamazepine using a mathematical model. *Am J Clin Pathol*. 2004;121:418-425.

54. Chattergoon DS, Verjee Z, Anderson M, Johnson D, McGuigan MA, Koren G, et al. Carbamazepine interference with an immune assay for tricyclic antidepressants in plasma. *J Toxicol Clin Toxicol.* 1998;36:109-113.

55. Garg U. Chromatographic techniques for the analysis of antidepressants. In: Dasgupta A, ed. *Advances in Chromatographic Techniques for Therapeutic Drug Monitoring.* Boca Raton: CRC Press, 2010:191-207.

56. Zalzstein E, Gorodischer R. Cardiovascular drugs. In: Yaffe SJ, Aranda JV, eds. *Neonatal and Pediatric Pharmacology: Therapeutic Principles in Practice.* 3rd ed. Philadelphia: Lippincott Williams and Wilkins, 2005:574-594.

57. McMillin GA, Owen WE, Lambert TL, De BK, Frank EL, Bach PR, et al. Comparable effects of DIGIBIND and DigiFab in thirteen digoxin immunoassays. *Clin Chem.* 2002;48:1580-1584.

58. Dasgupta A, McCudden CR. Therapeutic drug monitoring of cardiac drugs. In: Hammett-Stabler CA, Dasgupta A, eds. *Therapeutic Drug Monitoring Data.* 3rd ed. Washington, DC: AACC Press, 2007:77-106.

59. Dasgupta A, Hammett-Stabler CA, McCudden CR. Therapeutic drug monitoring of antineoplastic drugs. In: Hammett-Stabler CA, Dasgupta A, eds. *Therapeutic Drug Monitoring Data.* 3rd ed. Washington, DC: AACC Press, 2007:209-220.

LIPIDS AND LIPOPROTEINS | 10

Shannon Haymond

LEARNING OBJECTIVES

1. List and describe the three major pathways of lipoprotein metabolism.
2. Recognize clinically relevant hyperlipidemias and their laboratory correlates when presented with patient data.
3. Discuss methods for measurement of routine lipid tests, noting limitations with each.
4. Compare pediatric reference and target ranges for lipids with those in adults.
5. Discuss current recommendations for laboratory lipid screening in children and adolescents.

INTRODUCTION

Laboratory investigation of lipids plays an important role in risk assessment, screening, and management of cardiovascular disease (CVD) and in the diagnosis of dyslipidemias. CVD is the leading cause of death in men and women in developed countries and it is well-established that elevated atherogenic lipids are an independent risk factor for CVD. This has led to routine testing of lipids as part of public health awareness and improvement initiatives, such as various 'Know Your Numbers' campaigns and incorporation of lipid values into cardiovascular risk prediction tools, such as the Framingham Risk Score[1] and calculators published in the associated NCEP and ACC/AHA guidelines.[2,3] According to these guidelines, lipid measurements are also recognized in therapeutic decision-making algorithms. Lipid testing is widely utilized in pediatrics, as evidence indicates that dyslipidemias often begin in childhood or adolescence and contribute to early atherosclerosis with extrapolation to premature CVD, if not treated. Current

237

recommendations call for universal lipid screening in children of specified age ranges.[4] Once identified, children with dyslipidemias may be effectively managed by diet and lifestyle changes and with pharmaceutical interventions, in specific cases. This chapter will review the basics of lipid biochemistry and metabolism with associated pathophysiology, describe methods for lipid measurement and summarize current recommendations for lipid screening in pediatrics.

BIOCHEMISTRY

Structure

Lipids are a structurally heterogeneous class of compounds that are relatively insoluble in water. The main types of lipids include fatty acids, phospholipids, triglycerides (TG), and cholesterol (cholesterol esters). Lipids are vital to normal metabolism and development as they are components of cell membranes, sources of energy, and precursor molecules for synthesis of other compounds, such as steroid hormones and bile acids. Because of their insolubility, lipids are transported in circulation as water-soluble lipoproteins. Lipoproteins are spherical structures comprised of two layers: an amphiphilic surface and a hydrophobic core. Cholesterol esters, free fatty acids, and TG form the inner core and the surface layer contains proteins (apolipoproteins), cholesterol, and a single layer of phospholipid. Lipoproteins are commonly classified, based on their hydrated density (in order of increasing density), as: chylomicrons (CM), very-low-density lipoprotein (VLDL), intermediate density lipoprotein (IDL), low-density lipoprotein (LDL), and high-density lipoprotein (HDL). Lipoprotein particle density is determined primarily by its protein and TG content. Figure 10-1 illustrates that particles with higher lipid content are less dense; therefore, they migrate closer to the top of the tube when centrifuged. These have also been categorized based on their electrophoretic mobility and apolipoprotein content, as both of these characteristics also differ among the classes of lipoproteins.

Metabolism

There are three major pathways for lipoprotein metabolism. The exogenous pathway describes how dietary lipids, primarily as TG, are processed and transported to cells for use or storage as a source of energy. Similarly, the endogenous pathway is the mechanism by which liver-produced TG and phospholipids are packaged and delivered to extra-hepatic cells for energy or storage. In contrast, the reverse cholesterol transport pathway is focused on eliminating excess cellular cholesterol.

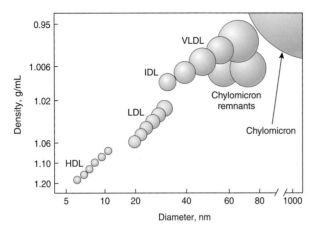

Figure 10-1 ▪ The density and size-distribution of the major classes of lipoprotein particles. Lipoproteins are classified by density and size, which are inversely related. VLDL, very low-density lipoprotein; IDL, intermediate-density lipoprotein; LDL, low-density lipoprotein; HDL, high-density lipoprotein. Used with permission from: Part 16. Endocrinology and Metabolism. Harrison's Principles of Internal Medicine, 18e, 2012. Copyright © 2015 McGraw-Hill Education. All rights reserved.

Exogenous (Transport of Dietary Lipids)

A schematic of the exogenous pathway is shown in Figure 10-2. Dietary lipids are absorbed in the small intestine. TG are hydrolyzed in the intestinal lumen by lipases and are emulsified with bile salts. Cholesterol is esterified in the enterocytes to form cholesteryl esters. Fatty acids are reassembled into TG and combine with ApoB-48, cholesterol, phospholipids, and cholesterol esters to form chylomicrons. These nascent chylomicrons bypass the liver circulation, travelling through the intestinal lymph via the thoracic duct directly into the circulation. Circulating HDL interacts with chylomicrons, resulting in transfer of ApoCs and ApoE from HDL to the nascent chylomicron. With these additional apoproteins, the chylomicron is considered "mature" and has the required co-factors to activate endothelial lipoprotein lipase (LPL). The chylomicron particles are extensively processed by LPL to hydrolyze TG. Hydrolysis of TG releases glycerol and fatty acids that can then be absorbed in peripheral tissues, particularly adipose and muscle, for energy and storage. As the hydrophobic core is hydrolyzed and the hydrophilic lipids (cholesterol and phospholipids) and apolipoproteins on the particle surface are transferred to HDL, the chylomicron particle progressively shrinks in size, creating chylomicron remnants. Chylomicron remnants are rapidly removed from the circulation by the liver through a process that requires ApoE as a ligand for receptors in the liver. This uptake is effective,

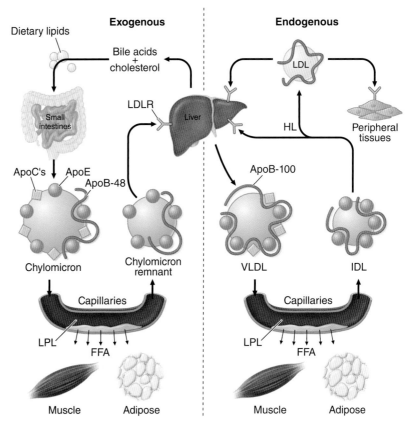

Figure 10-2 ▪ The exogenous and endogenous lipoprotein metabolic pathways. The exogenous pathway transports dietary lipids to the periphery and the liver. The endogenous pathway transports hepatic lipids to the periphery. LPL, lipoprotein lipase; FFA, free fatty acid; VLDL, very low density lipoprotein; IDL, intermediate-density lipoprotein; LDL, low-density lipoprotein; LDLR, low-density lipoprotein receptor; HL, hepatic lipase. Used with permission from Chapter 356. Disorders of Lipoprotein Metabolism. Harrison's Principles of Internal Medicine, 18e, 2012. Copyright © 2015 McGraw-Hill Education. All rights reserved.

resulting in few, if any, chylomicrons or chylomicron remnants present in the blood after a 12-hour fast.

Endogenous (Transport of Hepatic Lipids)

Figure 10-2 also shows an illustration of the endogenous cholesterol pathway, which is focused on the transport and metabolism of lipid particles made in the liver. The liver assembles TG, apoB-100, cholesteryl esters, phospholipids, and vitamin E to form nascent VLDL particles. Similarly to chylomicrons, HDL transfers ApoCs and ApoE to circulating nascent VLDL particles, resulting in "mature" VLDL. ApoC-II containing VLDL activates LPL in endothelial cells, which hydrolyzes the VLDL particle, releasing glycerol and fatty acids for uptake by muscle and adipose tissue. Hydrolyzed VLDL is referred to as VLDL remnants or intermediate-density lipoproteins (IDLs). The liver absorbs 40-60% of IDL via ApoE binding to the LDL receptor. The remaining IDL is further hydrolyzed by hepatic lipase into low-density lipoproteins (LDL). The majority of LDL (~70%) is cleared by LDL receptor-mediated endocytosis in the liver. The remaining LDL is absorbed by peripheral cells and has the potential to accumulate, ultimately resulting in atherosclerotic plaque formation, which forms the basis for the development of atherosclerosis.

Reverse Cholesterol Transport Pathway

The reverse cholesterol transport pathway is shown in Figure 10-3 and describes the process in which HDL facilitates transport of cholesterol from peripheral cells to the liver for excretion. Although all nucleated cells can synthesize

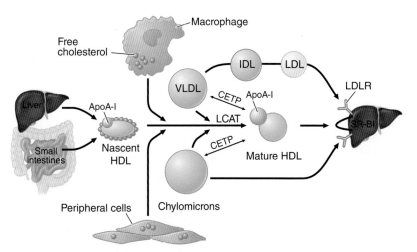

Figure 10-3 ■ HDL metabolism and reverse cholesterol transport. This pathway transports excess cholesterol from the periphery back to the liver for excretion in the bile. The liver and the intestine produce nascent HDLs. Free cholesterol is acquired from macrophages and other peripheral cells and esterified by LCAT, forming mature HDLs. HDL cholesterol can be selectively taken up by the liver via SR-BI (scavenger receptor class BI). Alternatively, HDL cholesteryl ester can be transferred by CETP from HDLs to VLDLs and chylomicrons, which can then be taken up by the liver. LCAT, lecithin-cholesterol acyltransferase; CETP, cholesteryl ester transfer protein; VLDL, very low-density lipoprotein; IDL, intermediate-density lipoprotein; LDL, low-density lipoprotein; HDL, high-density lipoprotein; LDLR, low-density lipoprotein receptor. Used with permission from: Part 16. Endocrinology and Metabolism. Harrison's Principles of Internal Medicine, 18e, 2012. Copyright © 2015 McGraw-Hill Education. All rights reserved.

cholesterol, only hepatocytes and enterocytes can effectively excrete it from the body via the bile or gut lumen, respectively. Nascent HDL particles are synthesized in the liver and the intestine. These particles acquire free cholesterol from macrophages and other peripheral cells. Lecithin-cholesterol acyltransferase (LCAT) within the HDL esterifies the cholesterol, resulting in mature HDL particles. HDL becomes spherical as it acquires more cholesteryl esters and it receives additional apolipoproteins from the surfaces of other particles, such as chylomicrons and VLDL. HDL cholesterol can be transported directly to hepatocytes by SR-BI (scavenger receptor class BI) via selective lipid transfer. Alternatively, HDL cholesteryl ester can be transferred by cholesteryl ester transfer protein (CETP) from HDL to VLDL and chylomicrons, which can then be taken up by the liver via LDL-receptor mediated endocytosis.

PATHOPHYSIOLOGY

Role of Cholesterol in Atherosclerosis

Dyslipidemia is one of the multiple factors that contribute to the pathogenesis of atherosclerosis. Excess LDL cholesterol (LDL-C) may be deposited in the intima of large vessels and is prone to oxidation and other modifications. Oxidized LDL is taken up by scavenger receptors on macrophages, which accelerates their accumulation of cholesterol and converts them to foam cells. Foam cell death leads to mitochondrial dysfunction, apoptosis, and necrosis, promoting inflammatory and immune changes with increased platelet aggregation. Oxidized LDL can also disrupt the endothelial surface and impair endothelial function. Lipid-laden foam cells migrate to the arterial wall just beneath the endothelium and develop into fatty streaks. Fatty streaks are among the first signs of atherosclerosis and over time may develop into atherosclerotic plaques. Plaques with a small lipid pool and thick fibrous cap may grow slowly and stabilize, whereas those with a large lipid pool and thin fibrous cap are prone to rupture. Ruptured plaques lead to clots or occlusion of vessels as the ruptured plaque is repaired.

Several landmark clinical studies have investigated the role of pediatric lipids in atherosclerosis and subsequent CVD risk into adulthood. These include the Bogalusa Heart Study, the Pathobiological Determinants of Atherosclerosis in Youth (PDAY) study, and the Cardiovascular Risk in Young Finns Study. They have been instrumental in showing that atherosclerosis begins in childhood and is associated with elevations in atherogenic lipids and traditional adult CVD risk factors, such as hypertension, insulin resistance, and obesity in children.[5] Additionally these studies have shown that CVD risk factors in childhood/early adolescence, particularly lipids and obesity, predicted clinical manifestations in young adulthood and risk patterns into adulthood, in the absence of intervention.[6-11]

Dyslipidemias

Dyslipidemias often exist in children and young adults without clinical signs or symptoms but can be detected by laboratory tests. As described previously, early recognition and management of lipoprotein disorders can reduce cardiovascular morbidity and mortality. Dyslipidemias have traditionally been categorized using the Fredrickson classification system. This concept originated in a paper by Fredrickson and Lees, published in 1965 and describes dyslipidemias on the basis of which lipids and lipoproteins are elevated.[12] It does not distinguish between primary and secondary hyperlipidemias or the causative etiology and does not include HDL. Therefore, it is more appropriate to see dyslipidemias categorized due to primary and secondary causes and by the type of lipidemia present.

Primary dyslipidemias include genetic disorders that result in defects in the lipoprotein metabolic pathways. Examples of primary dyslipidemias and their associated lipid abnormalities are shown in Table 10-1. Individuals may have pathogenic variants in single or multiple genes that

Table 10-1 **PRIMARY DYSLIPIDEMIAS AND ASSOCIATED LIPID ABNORMALITY***							
	Primary lipid/lipoprotein test(s) elevated						
	HDL	LDL	IDL	VLDL	CR	Chylo	TG
Familial hypercholesterolemia		•					
Familial defective apolipoprotein B		•					
Familial combined hyperlipidemia							
Type IIa		•					
Type IV				•			•
Type IIb		•		•			•
Types IIb and IV	•						
Polygenic hypercholesterolemia		•					
Familial hypertriglyceridemia				•			•
Severe hypertriglyceridemia				•		•	•
Familial hypoalphalipoproteinemia	low						
Dysbetalipoproteinemia			•		•		

*HDL, high-density lipoprotein; LDL, low-density lipoprotein; IDL, intermediate density lipoprotein; VLDL, very low density lipoprotein; CR, chylomicron remnant; Chylo, chylomicron; TG, triglyceride.

contribute to the elevated cholesterol and/or TG. Secondary dyslipidemias are associated with lifestyle and environment, metabolic or endocrine disorders, and medication or co-existing diseases, as listed in Table 10-2. Secondary causes of dyslipidemia must be excluded prior to diagnosis of a primary dyslipidemia.

The most common primary dyslipidemias found in children at increased risk for CVD are familial hypercholesterolemia (FH), familial combined hyperlipidemia (FCHL), polygenic hypercholesterolemia, and hyper-apobetalipoproteinemia (hyper-ApoB). Homozygous FH is a rare disease with

Table 10-2   **CAUSES FOR SECONDARY DYSLIPIDEMIAS**

EXOGENOUS
 • Alcohol
 • Drug therapy:
   ▪ Corticosteroids
   ▪ Isoretinoin
   ▪ Beta-blockers
   ▪ Select oral contraceptives, chemotherapeutic agents, antiretroviral agents

ENDOCRINE/METABOLIC   • Acute intermittent porphyria   • Diabetes mellitus types 1 and 2   • Hypothyroidism/hypopituitarism   • Lipodystrophy   • Pregnancy   • Polycystic ovary syndrome   • Obesity
RENAL   • Chronic renal disease   • Hemolytic uremic syndrome   • Nephrotic syndrome
INFECTIOUS   • Acute viral/bacterial infection   • Hepatitis   • Human immunodeficiency virus infection (HIV)
HEPATIC   • Alagille syndrome   • Biliary cirrhosis   • Obstructive liver disease/cholestatic conditions

(Continued)

Table 10-2   **CAUSES FOR SECONDARY DYSLIPIDEMIAS** *(Continued)*

INFLAMMATORY DISEASE
- Systemic lupus erythematosis
- Juvenile rheumatoid arthritis

STORAGE DISEASE
- Cystine storage disease
- Glycogen storage disease
- Gaucher disease
- Juvenile Tay-Sachs disease
- Niemann-Pick disease

OTHER
- Anorexia nervosa
- Childhood cancer survivor
- Idiopathic hypercalcemia
- Kawasaki disease
- Klinefelter syndrome
- Post solid organ transplantation
- Progeria
- Werner's syndrome

an incidence of 1 in 1,000,000, attributed to inheritance of either 2 pathogenic variants in the same gene or of a combination of single pathogenic variants in two different genes. However, inheritance of a single pathogenic variant in a single gene, causing the heterozygous genotype, has an incidence of 1 in 250-500 in the general population. Mutations in the LDL receptor (LDLR) gene account for ~93% of FH cases. Over 1600 mutations in LDLR have been described and are commonly categorized into one of four alleles that describe the phenotypic outcome of the defective protein. Mutations in apolipoprotein B (APOB) and proprotein convertase subtilisin kexin 9 (PCSK9) genes make up the remaining 3% and 2% of FH cases, respectively. In all cases, mutations disrupt catabolism of LDL-C, resulting in elevations in its plasma concentration and increased risk for CVD. Children with FH (heterozygote or homozygote) will have elevated total cholesterol (TC) and severely elevated LDL-C. Homozygotes present with markedly elevated lipids (LDL-C >500 mg/dL) and physical signs of lipid excess (xanthomas) and can die of atherogenic heart disease during childhood. Heterozygotes have a more varied phenotype in which LDL-C (200-300 mg/dL) and physical signs may not appear until later in life. Children with FH have a strong family history of premature CVD. Early detection of FH is important, as damage to the coronary artery begins early, leading to possibility for severe CVD in the first or second decades of life without intervention.

There is currently great interest in the scientific developments related to the role of PCSK9 in CVD. PCSK9 is a serine protease that binds to an extracellular domain of the LDL receptor on liver cells, preventing LDL receptors from recycling to the cell surface and ultimately accelerating their clearance. Gain of function mutations found in FH result in elevated LDL-C, as fewer LDL receptors results in decreased clearance of LDL-C. However, much of the interest in PCSK9 lies in the loss-of-function mutations, which are much more common and are associated with reduced LDL-C and "protective" effects against CVD. PCSK9 is currently being investigated as both a biomarker and for its role in the effectiveness of lipid-lowering therapies.[13] The US FDA has recently approved the first PCSK9-targeted lipid lowering drugs.

Children with FCHL and hyper-ApoB disorders also present with elevated LDL-C. The elevated LDL-C is often combined with elevated TG in FCHL. The genetic causes for FCHL and hyper-ApoB dyslipidemias are unknown at this time but they appear to be inherited in an autosomal dominant manner and are suspected to be oligogenic in nature in combination with environmental factors. The clinical manifestation of FCHL or hyper-ApoB may not occur in childhood but offspring in families with premature CVD are commonly detected through lipid screening. Polygenic hypercholesterolemia may be difficult to distinguish from heterozygous FH, as children have elevated TC and LDL-C without elevation in TG.

More rare causes of dyslipidemia are related to genetic defects affecting various aspects of LDL catabolism, including those that affect the structure of ApoB100 (familial defective ApoB100) or the disruption of LDL receptor/adaptor protein binding (autosomal-recessive hypercholesterolemia). Children with a rare defect in the absorption of plant sterols (sitosterolemia) may also present with severely elevated TC and LDL-C without a family history of lipid disorders.

A deficiency of HDL cholesterol (HDL-C) may also confer increased CVD risk. Primary dyslipidemias resulting in low HDL-C include familial hypoalphalipoproteinemia, apolipoprotein A-I mutations, variants in the ABCA1 gene resulting in Tangier disease, and lecithin cholesterol acyl transferase (LCAT) deficiency. Hypertriglyceridemias may be due to inherited disorders, such as lipoprotein lipase deficiency and defective ApoC-II. However, elevated TG are most commonly observed due to secondary disorders like obesity and metabolic syndrome. Obesity causes a combined dyslipidemia characterized by elevated TG, low HDL-C, normal to mildly elevated LDL-C with LDL-P profiling showing small, dense particles.[14]

MEASUREMENT METHODS

Measurement of blood lipids and lipoproteins is used in cardiovascular risk assessment, diagnosis of dyslipidemias, and in monitoring effectiveness of lifestyle changes and pharmaceutical lipid lowering therapies. A standard lipid profile contains TC, TG, HDL-C, and calculated LDL-C. Non-HDL-C is also commonly calculated, particularly in non-fasting samples. The National Cholesterol Education Program (NCEP) defines error goals for the standardization of routine lipid testing. Lipids can be significantly affected by pre-analytical variation and have relatively large biological variation. The between day variation in a "healthy" individual can be 10% for TC values and up to 25% for TG. With increased awareness and focus on prevention of cardiovascular disease, routine lipid testing is increasingly performed at the point-of-care. Point-of-care methods are not subject to the NCEP standards since they are considered waived testing and therefore, may not meet the specified error goals. Advanced lipid testing, such as ApoB and LDL-P is used to characterize select patients with dyslipidemias but is not recommended for routine use.

Direct Measurements of Routine Lipids

TC, TG, and HDL-C are measured using enzymatically coupled reactions on automated analyzers (examples shown in Figure 10-4). There may be slight

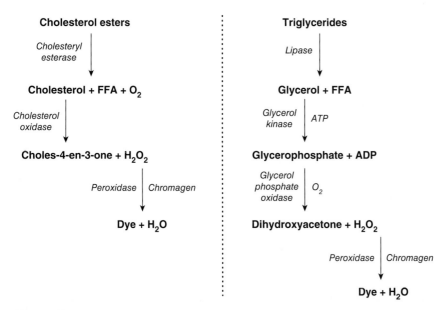

Figure 10-4 ▪ Schematics of enzymatic lipid measurement methods

variation in the configuration used for each assay vendor, but the final reaction uses a substrate generated by previous enzymatic reactions, typically H_2O_2, to generate a detectable change in a colorimetric dye. The specificity for these methods is reasonable but plant sterols and endogenous glycerol are substrates for the cholesterol oxidase and glycerol kinase reactions commonly used in cholesterol and TG assays, respectively. Ascorbic acid and bilirubin may interfere with enzymatic methods, as they consume H_2O_2. The NCEP error goals for TC methods are ≤9% total error, ≤3% bias, and ≤3% CV compared to a reference method. The NCEP error goals for TG methods are ≤15% total error, ≤5% bias and ≤5% CV compared to a reference method.

The HDL-C direct assay works by either shielding other lipoproteins from the enzymatic reaction or by consuming all non-HDL-C cholesterol prior to the specific reaction. Therefore, in some dyslipidemic patients, direct HDL-C assays may not perform as well as traditional, precipitation-based assays.[15] The NCEP error goals for HDL-C methods are ≤13% total error, ≤5% bias, and ≤4% CV compared to a reference method.

Several direct methods for measurement of LDL-C are also available and work similarly to the direct HDL-C assays, including a step to isolate the cholesterol on LDL from that on other lipoproteins. Direct LDL-C assays are also widely available on automated analyzers but given their increased cost and the large body of evidence for cardiovascular risk that is based on calculated LDL-C, their use is limited compared to the practice of calculating LDL-C using the Friedewald equation (described later).

Estimation of Routine Lipids

LDL-C is most commonly estimated from TC, TG, and HDL-C using the Friedewald equation.[16] This formula assumes that LDL-C is comprised of the TC minus the HDL-C and VLDL-C. The measured TG are used to estimate the amount of VLDL-C, as TG/5. This presumes all TG are in VLDL and the VLDL have normal core compositions of 5 times more TG than cholesterol. The Friedewald equation was designed for use in fasting specimens, which should contain little to no chylomicrons or chylomicron remnants. Therefore, it does not work well for non-fasting specimens since it does not include contribution from cholesterol in chylomicrons, which are increased in post-prandial samples. Additionally the calculation fails (compared to the ultracentrifugation reference procedure) when TG > 400 mg/dL. The NCEP error goals for LDL-C methods are ≤12% total error, ≤4% bias, and ≤4% CV compared to a reference method.

Non-HDL-C is also determined by calculation, as the TC minus HDL-C. Since TC and HDL-C are minimally affected by fasting and it does not require TG for calculation, it is suggested as a first line test in non-fasting pediatric lipid screening for children without risk factors.[4] Laboratories should calculate and report non-HDL-C, as its use is increasing, particularly for non-fasting collections and studies in adults suggest that it is a better marker for cardiovascular risk over LDL-C alone.[17]

Advanced Lipid Testing

Advanced lipid testing has been proposed for improving assessment of cardiovascular risk and guidance in lipid-lowering therapies. Such testing is available at lipid testing reference labs and is primarily used in specialty lipid clinics, its use in routine clinical practice and in pediatrics is not well delineated. Current guidelines include some evidence that at risk individuals with low or normal LDL-C may benefit from advanced lipid testing by alternate measurement of atherogenic lipoprotein particle number (eg, ApoB or LDL-P). Utility of other advanced lipid testing remains controversial in cardiovascular risk screening in adults with even less available evidence in children and adolescents.

ApoA-I and ApoB are alternate measurements of HDL and LDL particles, respectively. ApoB is used as a marker of pro-atherogenic lipoproteins, since it exists on non-HDL fractions (particles of LDL, VLDL, and IDL). Adult studies show ApoB is superior to LDL-C for cardiovascular risk assessment but its general use remains controversial as it does not outperform non-HDL-C or TC/HDL-C and there are concerns of its cost-effectiveness. Therefore, although automated methods are available for ApoA-I and ApoB and international reference standards exists for their measurement, their use is limited to specialty cases or research studies. This is also true in children, as current guidelines indicate that there is no benefit of ApoA-I or ApoB in universal screening and that offspring of parents with premature CVD and no other identifiable risk factors may have elevations of ApoA-I, ApoB, or lipoprotein(a).[4]

Determining the number of LDL particles (LDL-P) is an alternate to ApoB measurement, as each lipoprotein particle contains only one ApoB. Although, ApoB is truly a measure of LDL-P, VLDL-P, and IDL-P, concentrations of VLDL and IDL are low compared to LDL; therefore it is most useful as a surrogate marker for LDL-P. Like ApoB, LDL-P, may be useful in higher risk groups to estimate risk not accounted for by LDL-C, including those with hypertriglyceridemia, low HDL-C, insulin resistance, obesity, and metabolic syndrome.[18] LDL-P represents the number of LDL particles of all sizes and is measured by nuclear magnetic resonance spectroscopy (NMR), ultracentrifugation, and staining or ion mobility transfer techniques. Results from the HEALTHY Study showed sixth grade children have as much lipoprotein cholesterol compositional heterogeneity as has been described in adults. Obese 6th graders commonly had a discordant atherogenic phenotype of LDL-P > LDL-C, which may be missed when only LDL-C is considered for risk.[19] Many methods that quantify LDL-P may also provide LDL-P sizing. The utility of LDL-P sizing is more controversial, with some suggesting smaller, dense particles confer increased risk than larger LDL particles. Guidelines do not recommend testing as there is no gold standard and no evidence indicating that changes in LDL size profile impacts disease progression or outcomes or provides benefit over measuring LDL-P.

UTILIZATION OF LAB TESTING

Pediatric Lipid Ranges

Human plasma cholesterol levels are lowest during intrauterine life and at birth with TC and LDL-C increasing rapidly in the first weeks of life and then rising more gradually until age of 2 years, when concentrations remain relatively stable until adolescence. A 10-20% decrease in blood lipid TC and LDL-C concentrations occurs during puberty. With the exception of HDL-C, acceptable concentrations of lipids in children and adolescents are different than those used in adults. It is important that laboratories report lipid results from children using age-specific reference ranges. Pediatric reference cutoffs for children and adolescents (Table 10-3) and young adults (Table 10-4), as per the latest NHLBI guidelines are provided for reference. These values for children 0-19 years were established from the NCEP Expert Panel on Cholesterol Levels in Children. The cut points for high and borderline-high represent approximately the 95th and 75th percentiles in these age groups, respectively. The low cut point for HDL-C represents approximately the 10th percentile.

Similarly for young adults, the NHLBI guidelines refer to data from those 20-24 years old in the Lipid Research Clinics Prevalence Study. The borderline-high and high cut points for TC, LDL-C, and non-HDL-C represent the 75th and 95th percentiles, respectively. The high TG cut point

Table 10-3	**RANGES FOR LIPID CONCENTRATIONS (IN MG/DL) FOR CHILDREN AND ADOLESCENTS***					
	TC	LDL-C	Non-HDL-C	HDL-C	TG 0-9 y	TG 10-19 y
Acceptable	< 170	< 110	< 120	> 45	< 75	< 90
Borderline	170-199	110-129	120-144	40-45	75-99	90-129
High/Low	≥ 200	≥ 130	≥ 145	< 40	≥ 100	≥ 130

*Table created with data from Expert Panel on Integrated Guidelines for Cardiovascular Health and Risk Reduction in Children and Adolescents: Summary Report.[4]

Table 10-4	RANGES FOR LIPID CONCENTRATIONS (IN MG/DL) FOR YOUNG ADULTS (AGED 20-24 YEARS)*				
	TC	LDL-C	Non-HDL-C	HDL-C	TG
Acceptable	<190	<120	<150	>45	<115
Borderline	190-224	120-159	150-189	40-44	115-149
High/Low	≥225	≥160	≥190	<40	≥150

*Table created with data from Expert Panel on Integrated Guidelines for Cardiovascular Health and Risk Reduction in Children and Adolescents: Summary Report.[4]

represents approximately the 90th percentile with borderline high between the 75th and 89th percentile. The low HDL-C cut point represents roughly the 25th percentile with acceptable as greater than the 50th percentile. It is important to note that these differ from the cut points used in the NHLBI adult (ATP III) guidelines, which were derived from combined data of adults of all ages. The Expert Panel recognized this relevant difference and provided these age-specific cut points for use by pediatricians that manage patients in this young adult age group.

Targeted Versus Universal Screening

The National Heart, Lung, and Blood Institute (NHLBI) Expert Panel on Integrated Guidelines for Cardiovascular Health and Risk Reduction in Children and Adolescents, conducted an evidence-based review and released the most current guidelines on pediatric lipid screening.[4] The recommendations were endorsed by the American Academy of Pediatrics (AAP). This release was notable, as for the first time, guidelines recommended universal screening for dyslipidemia in children. Pediatric lipid screening may be performed using a targeted or a universal approach. Targeted screening methods were designed for early detection of children with primary dyslipidemias and were based on family history of premature CVD or lipid disorder. Significant evidence now suggests that reliance on family history as the primary factor in determining eligibility for lipid screening misses approximately 30-60% of children with dyslipidemias. The earliest age recommended for targeted lipid screening is 2 years. Selected or targeted screening, which is based on positive family history and/or high risk factors or conditions in a child, is recommended between 2-8 years and again at 12-16 years, if new knowledge about the child's risk exists. Current recommendations call for universal screening in children 9-11 years and again at 17-21 years. It is known that TC and LDL-C levels fall during puberty and, for most children, the initial screening age range will precede onset of puberty. Children in this age range may also be more accessible for screening (able to fast, visiting pediatrician for school physical) and results are predictive of future adult lipid profiles. Repeat screening between the ages of 17-21 years increases the ability to identify children with false negatives in childhood or those with delayed expression of a primary dyslipidemia. The recommendation for universal screening was met with controversy and recent data shows trends in pediatric screening are lower than expected, even for those with high risk that would be eligible per a targeted screening algorithm.[20-22]

The Expert Panel recommended that non-fasting lipid panels be used as the first line test for universal screening. However, clear recommendations were provided about the need for repeated fasting lipid panels when the atherogenic lipid components of a non-fasting panel are elevated. Selected screening requires repeated fasting lipid panels. When indicated, repeat fasting tests should be collected at least 2 weeks, but within 3 months apart.

MANAGEMENT IN SPECIFIC CONDITIONS

Management in pediatric dyslipidemias is focused on lifestyle modifications, including diet and physical activity. Adherence to a low-fat/low-saturated-fat/low cholesterol diet with increased physical activity is effective at treating children with hypertriglyceridemia. Therefore, lipid-lowering medication is rarely needed in the majority of pediatric patients with dyslipidemia. The NHLBI report on management of pediatric cardiovascular health includes algorithms for TG-focused therapies or LDL-C-focused therapies.[4]

Lipid-lowering drugs, such as bile acid sequestrants or statins, may be used in children after careful assessment of the patient's lipid profile with a complete assessment for CVD risk factors and conditions and in consultation with the patient and family. Decisions related to lipid-lowering therapies should be made using the average of results from at least two fasting lipid panels obtained at least 2 weeks but no more than 3 months apart. Children with an average LDL-C > 250 mg/dL or average TG > 500 mg/dL are referred to lipid specialists for direct care. Medication is not used in children less than 10 years unless they have a severe primary hyperlipidemia (eg, homozygous FH or primary triglyceridemia) or a high-risk condition that is associated with serious medical morbidity and accelerated atherosclerosis (eg, type 1 and type 2 diabetes, kidney disease or transplantation, Kawasaki disease or cardiac transplantation). Use of medication is reserved for children greater than 10 years that continue to have elevated LDL-C after at least 6 months on a physician-supervised or dietician-supervised diet and exercise regimen and in those with a severe primary hyperlipidemia or high risk condition known to accelerate atherosclerosis. LDL apheresis may be effective at lowering LDL-C in children with homozygous FH and extremely elevated LDL-C (ie, >500 mg/dL). The therapeutic target for children and adolescents is LDL-C below the 95th percentile (ie, <130 mg/dL).

SUMMARY

Lipids are necessary for normal cellular metabolism and childhood development but accumulation of excessive "bad" lipids leads to atherosclerosis and CVD risk. Therefore, blood lipid measurements form a routine part of CVD risk assessment and management and are also necessary for the diagnosis of genetic and acquired dyslipidemias. FH is the most severe and common type of primary dyslipidemia, characterized by significant elevations in LDL-C. In its homozygous form, FH presents with early and severe childhood heart disease. Combined dyslipidemias (ie, elevations in TC, LDL-C, and TG) due to secondary etiologies, such as obesity are becoming more common in children and adolescents. TC, HDL-C, and TG are measured directly using automated methods, but LDL-C and non-HDL-C are commonly calculated from other lipid components. Current recommendations call for universal screening in children between 9-11 years and again at 17-21 years. Children with CVD risk factors may be tested as early as 2 years old. Lipid cutoff ranges differ between children and adults, with the exception of HDL-C.

TRAINING MODULE

1. Chylomicrons are formed in which of the lipid metabolism pathways?
   a. Exogenous pathway
   b. Endogenous pathway
   c. Reverse cholesterol transport pathway
   d. Primary pathway
   e. Secondary pathway

2. A well appearing 3 year old male presents for investigation of small, elevated "bumps" on the knees and elbows with lipid profile notable for TC = 752 mg/dL, TG = 97 mg/dL, and LDL-C = 660 mg/dL. Both parents report taking lipid-lowering drugs because their LDL-C >250 mg/dL. Which dyslipidemia is most consistent with this scenario?
   a. Lecithin cholesterol acyl transferase (LCAT) deficiency
   b. Tangier disease
   c. Homozygous familial hypercholesterolemia (FH)
   d. Familial combined hyperlipidemia (FCHL)
   e. Hyper-apobetalipoproteinemia (hyper-ApoB)

3. A 10 year female undergoes lipid screening at the time of a routine well child visit and school physical. She is within normal limits for height and weight for age. History and physical exam are unremarkable. Her non-fasting lipid profile shows: TC = 163 mg/dL; HDL-C = 62 mg/dL; TG = 95 mg/dL. Calculate her non-HDL-C.

   a. 6 mg/dL
   b. 81 mg/dL
   c. 82 mg/dL
   d. 101 mg/dL
   e. 144 mg/dL

REFERENCES

1. Wilson PW, D'Agostino RB, Levy D, Belanger AM, Silbershatz H, Kannel WB. Prediction of coronary heart disease using risk factor categories. *Circulation*. 1998;97: 1837-1847.
2. National Cholesterol Education Program Expert Panel on Detection E, Treatment of High Blood Cholesterol in A. Third Report of the National Cholesterol Education Program (NCEP) Expert Panel on Detection, Evaluation, and Treatment of High Blood Cholesterol in Adults (Adult Treatment Panel III) final report. *Circulation*. 2002;106:3143-3421.
3. Stone NJ, Robinson JG, Lichtenstein AH et al. 2013 ACC/AHA guideline on the treatment of blood cholesterol to reduce atherosclerotic cardiovascular risk in adults: a report of the American College of Cardiology/American Heart Association Task Force on Practice Guidelines. *J Am Coll Cardiol*. 2014;63:2889-2934.
4. Expert Panel on Integrated Guidelines for Cardiovascular H, Risk Reduction in C, Adolescents, National Heart L, Blood I. Expert panel on integrated guidelines for cardiovascular health and risk reduction in children and adolescents: summary report. *Pediatrics*. 2011;128 suppl 5:S213-S256.
5. McGill HC, Jr., McMahan CA, Herderick EE, Malcom GT, Tracy RE, Strong JP. Origin of atherosclerosis in childhood and adolescence. *AM J Clin Nutr*. 2000;72: 1307S-1315S.
6. Berenson GS, Srinivasan SR, Bao W, Newman WP, 3rd, Tracy RE, Wattigney WA. Association between multiple cardiovascular risk factors and atherosclerosis in children and young adults. The Bogalusa Heart Study. *N Engl J Med*. 1998;338: 1650-1656.
7. Berenson GS, Wattigney WA, Tracy RE et al. Atherosclerosis of the aorta and coronary arteries and cardiovascular risk factors in persons aged 6 to 30 years and studied at necropsy (The Bogalusa Heart Study). *Am J Cardiol*. 1992;70:851-858.
8. Davis PH, Dawson JD, Riley WA, Lauer RM. Carotid intimal-medial thickness is related to cardiovascular risk factors measured from childhood through middle age: the Muscatine Study. *Circulation*. 2001;104:2815-2819.
9. Juhola J, Magnussen CG, Viikari JS et al. Tracking of serum lipid levels, blood pressure, and body mass index from childhood to adulthood: the Cardiovascular Risk in Young Finns Study. *J Pediatr*. 2011;159:584-590.

10. McMahan CA, Gidding SS, Malcom GT et al. Pathobiological determinants of athero-sclerosis in youth risk scores are associated with early and advanced atherosclerosis. *Pediatrics.* 2006;118:1447-1455.

11. Webber LS, Srinivasan SR, Wattigney WA, Berenson GS. Tracking of serum lipids and lipoproteins from childhood to adulthood. The Bogalusa Heart Study. *Am J Epidemiol.* 1991;133:884-899.

12. Fredrickson DS, Lees RS. A System for Phenotyping Hyperlipoproteinemia. *Circulation.* 1965;31:321-327.

13. Awan Z, Baass A, Genest J. Proprotein convertase subtilisin/kexin type 9 (PCSK9): lessons learned from patients with hypercholesterolemia. *Clin Chem.* 2014;60:1380-1389.

14. Cook S, Kavey RE. Dyslipidemia and pediatric obesity. *Pediatr Clin North Am.* 2011;58:1363-1373,

15. Warnick GR, Nauck M, Rifai N. Evolution of methods for measurement of HDL-cholesterol: from ultracentrifugation to homogeneous assays. *Clin Chem.* 2001;47: 1579-1596.

16. Friedewald WT, Levy RI, Fredrickson DS. Estimation of the concentration of low-density lipoprotein cholesterol in plasma, without use of the preparative ultracentri-fuge. *Clin Chem.* 1972;18:499-502.

17. Arsenault BJ, Boekholdt SM, Kastelein JJ. Lipid parameters for measuring risk of car-diovascular disease. *Nat Rev Cardiol.* 2011;8:197-206.

18. Davidson MH, Ballantyne CM, Jacobson TA et al. Clinical utility of inflamma-tory markers and advanced lipoprotein testing: advice from an expert panel of lipid specialists. *J Clin Lipidol.* 2011;5:338-367.

19. Mietus-Snyder M, Drews KL, Otvos JD et al. Low-density lipoprotein cholesterol ver-sus particle number in middle school children. *J Pediatr.* 2013;163:355-362.

20. Dixon DB, Kornblum AP, Steffen LM, Zhou X, Steinberger J. Implementation of lipid screening guidelines in children by primary pediatric providers. *J Pediatr.* 2014;164:572-576.

21. Margolis KL, Greenspan LC, Trower NK et al. Lipid screening in children and ado-lescents in community practice: 2007 to 2010. *Circ Cardiovasc Qual Outcomes.* 2014;7:718-726.

22. Vinci SR, Rifas-Shiman SL, Cheng JK, Mannix RC, Gillman MW, de Ferranti SD. Cholesterol testing among children and adolescents during health visits. *JAMA.* 2014;311:1804-1807.

POINT OF CARE TESTING IN THE PEDIATRIC SETTING

11

Khushbu Patel and Sarah Brown

LEARNING OBJECTIVES

1. Define point of care testing and list its advantages in the pediatric setting.
2. Describe the limitations to point of care testing.
3. Define CLIA-waived testing.
4. List important considerations when implementing POCT.
5. List laboratory tests commonly used in critical care.
6. Describe two challenges associated with laboratory testing and the critically ill patient.

INTRODUCTION

Point of care testing (POCT), as the name describes, is testing that can be done at the point of care. It is also referred to as near-patient testing, or bed-side testing. POCT is performed outside of the central laboratory, on small portable devices. There is a significant breadth of technology in POCT, and the field is growing rapidly. Types of technology commonly used in POCT include immunoassay, chemical/enzymatic reactions, electrochemistry, and optical techniques. In general, POCT can be divided into three more or less distinct categories: 1) qualitative, single-use rapid tests, 2) semi-quantitative or quantitative single use cartridges with reader devices, and 3) quantitative multi-use cartridge or benchtop devices.[1] Advantages to POCT include reduced turnaround time (TAT) and sample volume requirement as many POCT devices use small sample volumes. These advantages make POCT particularly useful in pediatric critical care settings. However, there are challenges associated with POCT including inaccuracies and interferences, and poor correlation between POCT devices and the main laboratory analyzers. Co-ordination of POCT programs requires attention to quality control/quality assurance, proficiency testing, validation, cost-benefit analysis, and evidence-based practice.

This chapter will cover all aspects of POCT, focusing on its use in the pediatric environment and especially on POCT use in Critical Care situations.

POINT OF CARE TESTING

Benefits of Point of Care Testing

Benefits of point of care testing include its ease of use, reduced total turnaround time (TTAT), and small sample volume requirement. The TTAT is the time from when the caregiver orders a laboratory test to the time the caregiver acts on the result of the laboratory test. This includes the time to collect supplies, draw, transport, process, and test the specimen as well as the time to review results in the laboratory (see Figure 11-1). In the critical care environment, POCT devices can simplify the process of obtaining lab values at the point of blood collection. It has been described that much less nursing time is involved in POCT versus sending samples to a central laboratory.[2] For example, the steps involved in sending a sample to the central laboratory include ordering

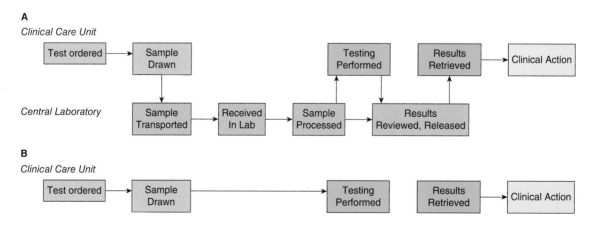

Figure 11-1 ■ Steps involved in (A) central laboratory testing and point of care testing (B). Red boxes highlight additional rate limiting steps in the central laboratory that affect TAT.

the test, drawing and transporting the sample, central lab processing, testing, and reporting, and finally retrieval of the results. When a POCT device is used, the steps can be reduced considerably (Figure 11-1). Policies in the central lab for calling critical value results back to a healthcare provider can add to the TTAT significantly. Turnaround time for critical value call back, in one study, was over 20 minutes.[3] In this study, delays in critical value call back correlated with specimens being obtained from outpatients and testing requisitions lacking name of the ordering physician or ordering location. Decreasing the amount of nursing time spent in obtaining lab values increases nursing time spent in the patient care.

POCT devices are generally easy to use. The operator interface requires little interaction, and the readout requires little interpretation. These features contribute in part to its regulatory status (see Section "Regulatory Considerations of POCT" later). POCT devices can be operated by non-laboratory staff, increasing their availability. The quality control requirements for most POCT devices are simpler to those for central laboratory testing. Single-unit POCT devices often have QC built in to each unit; either the QC appears with the test result (dipsticks/immunostrips), or the QC/calibration is checked after the cartridge is loaded but before the patient sample is delivered. This makes the QC process more streamlined for non-laboratorian users. It should be noted that not all POCT are rapid single use tests; some are smaller bench top devices with multi-use reagent packs. These devices have different QC requirements; QC is generally run more similarly to central lab practices with liquid QC performed at set intervals, and more often are more heavily regulated (see Section "Regulatory Considerations of POCT" later). Most POCT devices are CLIA-waived due to low complexity and ease of use. However, if a POCT device is used outside its FDA cleared/approved use, such as any deviation in collection method or patient population ("off-label" use); it defaults to the high-complexity non-waived category (see later section). With well over 70 waived POCT available, pediatrician offices are expanding their testing capabilities by implementing POCT for a number of tests including influenza, *Streptococcus* Group A, respiratory syncytial virus (RSV), lipids, and transcutaneous bilirubin (TcB).

POCT commonly utilizes very small sample volumes. For example, a whole blood glucose measurement can be obtained from a drop of blood, compared to 600 µL of whole blood for plasma glucose in the central lab. Table 11-1 illustrates differences in volume requirements of common POC and central laboratory tests. One reason for the small volume requirement is POC systems have little to no dead volume (see Chapter 1), and use whole blood. Whole blood assays require less blood overall, since plasma is roughly 40-60% of a whole blood specimen. Due to the small volume requirement, POCT is very attractive especially in pediatrics.

Table 11-1   **BLOOD VOLUME REQUIREMENTS FOR COMMON POCT AND CENTRAL LABORATORY TESTING**

Instrument	Manufacturer	Type	Sample Volume (µL WB)	Test Analytes
i-Stat	Abbott Diagnostics, Bedford, MA	POCT	65 or 95	pO_2, pCO_2, pH, Na^+, K^+, Ca^{++}, Cl^-, Hct, urea nitrogen, glucose, lactate, creatinine.
AVL OPTI	AVL Scientific, Roswell, GA	POCT	125	pO_2, pCO_2, pH, Na^+, K^+, Ca^{++}, Cl^-, Hb
Accu-chek Inform II	Roche Diagnostics, Indianapolis, IN	POCT	1-2	Glucose
StatStrip	Nova Biomedical, Boston, MA	POCT	1-2	Glucose
Piccolo xpress	Abaxis, Inc., Union City, CA	POCT	100	ALT, albumin, ALP, AST, Ca^{++}, Cl^-, creatinine, glucose, K^+, Na^+, total bilirubin, total CO_2, total protein, BUN
ABL800	Radiometer America, Inc., Westlake, OH	Central Lab	300	pO_2, pCO_2, pH, Na^+, K^+, Ca^{++}, Cl^-, Hct, Hb, glucose, lactate, creatinine.
Cobas 6000	Roche Diagnostics, Indianapolis, IN	Central Lab	1000	ALT, albumin, ALP, AST, Ca^{++}, Cl^-, creatinine, glucose, K^+, Na^+, total bilirubin, total CO_2, total protein, BUN
Cobas 6000	Roche Diagnostics, Indianapolis, IN	Central Lab	600	Glucose

Limitations of Point of Care Testing

Historically, POCT have been less accurate than central laboratory testing. Whole blood glucose meter systems (BGMS) can be used to illustrate this point. Table 11-2 lists the accuracy requirements from International Science Institutes (ISI) and Clinical and Laboratory Standards Institute (CLSI) for BGMS. Compare this to central laboratory glucose assays, which typically have accuracy requirements of all values within ± 6 mg/dL or 10%. Due to the imprecision of BGMS, Centers for Medicare and Medicaid Services (CMS) regulates that BGMS cannot be used in critically ill patients,[4] and the American Diabetes Association states that whole blood glucose measurement by POCT glucometers cannot be used for diagnosis of diabetes.

Table 11-2	**ACCURACY REQUIREMENTS OF ISI AND CLSI FOR BGMS**	
Accuracy Criteria	Glucose mg/dL, (mmol/L)	Accuracy specification
ISO 15197:2013	< 100 (5.55)	95% within ± 15 mg/dL (0.83 mmol/L)
	≥ 100 (5.55)	95% within ± 15%
CLSI POCT 12-A3	< 100 (5.55)	95% within ± 12 mg/dL (0.67 mmol/L)
	≥ 100 (5.55)	95% within ± 12.5%
	< 75 (4.2)	98% within ± 15 mg/dL (0.83 mmol/L)
	≥ 75 (4.2)	98% within ± 20%

Capillary blood from a finger or heel stick is often used in POCT. For correct interpretation of laboratory values, it is important to understand the physiological differences in venous, capillary, and arterial specimens. Capillary collections are preferred in pediatrics for a number of reasons, including decreases in iatrogenic anemia and they are perceived as less traumatic for pediatric patients. Capillary collections are more prone to hemolysis; however, causing increased potassium and other intracellular components, and also have an increased risk of clotting. Blood collected by skin puncture (finger or heelstick) is a mixture of arterial and venous blood, as well as interstitial and intracellular fluids. There is a higher proportion of arterial to venous due to arterial pressure. "Arterializing" capillary specimens by warming the skin to 42°C can increase the amount of arterial blood in a capillary specimen up to seven times. Venous samples are suitable for pH and pCO_2, electrolytes. Arterial blood is suitable for the evaluation of gas exchange of the lung (pO_2 and pCO_2) and is required to correctly identify the presence of a respiratory acidosis or alkalosis. pO_2 is generally slightly higher in arterial blood compared to arterialized capillary blood, especially at higher oxygen tension, such as in patients on oxygen supplementation, and the difference can be clinically significant for evaluating hypoxemia. Figure 11-2 illustrates differences in blood gas concentrations across the arterial-venous gradient.

POCT within an institution should be validated against the institution's central laboratory tests. For example, a patient admitted to an ICU may have blood gases and sodium monitored by POCT in the ICU, and sodium checked once a day with a basic metabolic panel in the central laboratory. If there are

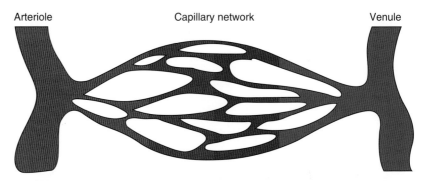

Figure 11-2 ▪ Differences in pH, pCO_2, and pO_2 between arterial and venous blood. Venous samples are suitable for pH, pO_2 and electrolytes; while arterial blood is suitable for evaluation of gas exchange, respiratory acidosis or alkalosis.

significant differences between the two assays, this may cause confusion to the care providers and pose a safety risk to the patient. Due to the methodology, some POCT tests compare more readily to central laboratory assays – for instance the POC devices that measure electrolytes by ion-selective electrodes (ISE) may compare well to ISE methods in the central laboratory, whereas devices that use photometric technology for measuring electrolytes in whole blood may have a more significant bias or lack of correlation. Differences in plasma and whole blood concentrations of different analytes due to water content contributes to the bias between whole blood POCT assays and plasma-based central laboratory assays.

Due to the lack of accuracy of the POCT or to other factors like environmental contamination, POCT is often used as screening and followed up by confirmatory testing, usually in the central laboratory. Two examples pertinent to pediatrics are whole blood lead testing and sweat conductivity. POCT whole blood lead testing can be used to screen for lead exposure in areas with high incidence of lead exposure. The Centers for Disease Control and Prevention (CDC) recommends follow-up on any blood lead level greater than 5 µg/dL.[5,6] The available POCT method for lead quantification is anodic stripping; this method has a range of 3.3 µg/dL to 65 µg/dL and total allowable error of ± 4 µg/dL (LeadSafe II). Thus if POC lead testing is used for screening, positive results should be confirmed with the more sensitive inductively-coupled plasma mass spectrometry or atomic absorption tests. One study showed clinical sensitivity of POC lead testing of 65.6%, using 5 µg/dL as a cutoff.[7] Furthermore, when whole blood collected via fingerstick is tested, false positives can arise from environmental contamination.[8]

Sweat conductivity is sometimes used to screen patients for cystic fibrosis (CF). This POCT measures "electrolyte" (NaCl) concentration in sweat by electrical conductivity.[9] This method is prone to high incidence of both false positives and false negatives, with false positives predominating, and is not accepted by the CF Foundation for diagnosis of CF. Sweat chloride concentration, obtained via iontophoresis, is still required for the diagnosis of CF.[10]

Single-use POC tests are associated with high cost per test due to the high cost of consumables compared to central laboratory testing. Consider a single-use point of care cassette for whole blood gases, sodium, and potassium costs $6.50, while the same panel on a central laboratory blood gas analyzer costs $1.80. Also, CMS reimburses per analyte, not according to the testing modality. Thus reimbursement for POC glucose is the same as reimbursement for central lab glucose, despite the increased POCT cost. Since CMS allows for reimbursement of an analyte once per 24 hours, this cost difference is further increased when multiple POC tests of the same analyte per day are completed, for example, hourly POC whole blood glucose. A cost-benefit analysis should be conducted prior to implementing any new POCT.

Interfacing POC devices to a laboratory information system (LIS) and charting results can be challenging. Many of the devices were made to be portable, and hard-wiring those to a network would remove that advantage. Some devices print out results automatically, and on other devices results are displayed on a screen; there is a risk that the print out or screen result will be used by the care-giver and the results not recorded in the patient chart. Results from unit-use tests that are not connected to a reader device, like a urine dipstick or a rapid flu test, must be entered manually which can lead to transcription error. However, more devices are being made with wireless capabilities that can sync with an LIS.[11]

POCT must adhere to specimen labeling rules. Tests that need more than a drop of blood, for example, blood gas and electrolyte panels, require the specimen to be drawn in to a transfer device (capillary tube or syringe) prior to loading on to the test cartridge. These must be labeled with two patient identifiers in compliance with regulatory standards. For tests that require only a drop of blood, often a transfer device is not required – such as when a drop of blood is loaded directly from the skin puncture to a glucose test strip. To reduce risk of "mislabeled" specimens when no collection/transfer device in used, many POC devices for hospital use are equipped with barcode scanning function that requires the patient armband to be scanned before the device is operable.

It is important to understand the principles of the POCT technology being used, limitations of the device, and possible assay interferences. Four examples of POCT pertinent to pediatric critical care are discussed here.

1. Whole blood glucose meters: Point of care glucose meters utilize reduction/oxidation chemistry for the measurement of glucose in whole blood. Enzymatic oxidation of glucose in whole blood creates an electrical current that is correlated to glucose concentration. For example, glucose oxidase converts glucose to glucuronic acid, or glucose dehydrogenase converts glucose to gluconolactone. These reactions create a DC current that is proportional to the glucose concentration, producing whole blood glucose concentrations that are converted to plasma equivalent values. Because neonates may have lower blood glucose concentrations and higher hematocrit compared to adults, whole blood glucose measurement by POCT in neonates is subject to special consideration. Hypoglycemia is not uncommon in neonates, and it is particularly dangerous in this population because it is difficult to recognize clinical signs of hypoglycemia in infants. Because of the imprecision of POCT glucose meters, which is greatest at the low end of the linear range, POCT whole blood results should be used with caution in the neonatal population. Since the conversion of whole blood glucose to a plasma equivalent is based on estimation of blood water content, hematocrit can interfere with all whole blood methods. Not only do neonates have higher hematocrit (55-65%) compared to adults (35-50%), wide variation in hematocrit can be seen in this population. In one multicenter study, neonatal hematocrit varied from 23% to 70% across three pediatric centers.[12] Thus, it is important to validate POCT glucose meters in the neonatal population prior to putting them to clinical use in that population. Other sugars, like galactose and maltose, can interfere as well. Some assays have eliminated maltose inference by using a modified enzyme that does not recognize maltose. Whole blood glucose meters should not be used in neonates with galactosemia, due to the galactose interference. Furthermore, the inherent imprecision of whole blood glucose meters compared to central laboratory plasma-based assays limits the use of these devices in the care of critically ill patients (see Section Regulatory Considerations of POCT later).

2. Hemoglobin and hematocrit: Hemoglobin can be directly measured or can be estimated from the hematocrit value (hemoglobin (g/dL) = hematocrit (%PCV) × 0.34; hemoglobin (g/dL) = hematocrit (decimal fraction) × 34). In at least one POCT device, hemoglobin is directly measured via an optical technique. More commonly, hemoglobin is calculated from the hematocrit measured by conductance.

Conductance-based measurement of hematocrit may be susceptible to interference from hemodilution and/or volume replacement fluids found in coronary bypass (CBP) and ECMO procedures, which contribute to clinically significant under or over-estimation of hemoglobin. The authors compared hemoglobin results from two POCT devices, an OPTI-CCA TS Blood Gas and Electrolyte Analyzer (OPTI Biomedical) and the epoc POC chemistry analyzer (Alere) in pediatric patients undergoing CPB or ECMO therapy at St. Louis Children's Hospital. The OPTI-CCA TS directly measures hemoglobin by optical fluorescence, while the epoc calculates hemoglobin from hematocrit. Comparisons were made in the operating room on 20 consecutive patients undergoing CBP, and in the central laboratory on 15 consecutive patients on ECMO therapy. The ABL800 (Radiometer) and OPTI-CCA TS had previously been shown to be in agreement and were both were considered standard in this evaluation. Clinically significant bias was seen in results from the epoc compared to the OPTI-CCA TS (and ABL800) in the ECMO population (Figure 11-3). Using just the epoc to monitoring hemoglobin in these patient populations could lead to unnecessary red blood cell transfusions. Thus, different technologies may be more appropriate in specific clinical scenarios.

3. Activated clotting time: ACT, is frequently used to monitor heparin therapy during CPB and ECMO therapy. There are numerous devices that measure ACT, and many different methodologies. For example, some devices warm the sample prior to analysis while some run the sample cold. Devices may use either kaolin or celite to initiate the clotting process. Results from the different methods do not necessarily correlate. In one study authors compared ACT measurement by three different POCT devices in 44 patients less than 6 months old undergoing CPB. ACT was measured immediately after a heparin bolus and immediately prior to termination of CPB on the Hemochron (International Technidyne Corporation), Hepcon (Medtronic), and iStat (kaolin activated assay; Abbott) devices. In this study, ACT results from the Hemochron and Hepcon increased significantly between the two measurements, while no significant increase was seen in results using the iStat device. Also of note, the baseline values differed greatly among the three devices: 600, 700, and 800 seconds for the Hepcon, iStat, and Hemochron, respectively.[13] Another study showed a 26% discrepancy rate between the iStat Kaolin ACT and the Medtronic ACT Plus device in 88 adult patients undergoing cardiac catheterization.[14] Caution should be practiced when using multiple vendor devices within one institution. The end user should be aware that results from one type of device may not compare to results from another version.

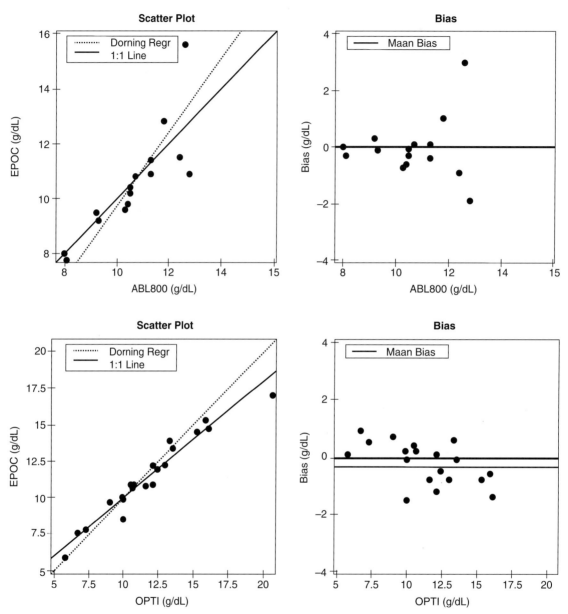

Figure 11-3 ▪ Comparison of **hemoglobin*** results from the epoc® and ABL800® in ECMO patients (*n*=15) (A) and the epoc® and OPTI® in CPB patients (*n*=20) (B). Clinically significant differences were seen in results from the epoc® compared to the ABL800® in the ECMO population. *The epoc® calculates hemoglobin from hematocrit. The ABL800® directly measures hemoglobin via co-oximetry. The OPTI® directly measures hemoglobin by optical fluorescence. Thus in both clinical situations, CPB and ECMO, a calculated value is compared to a direct measurement.

4. Transcutaneous bilirubin (TcB) measurement is an example of a non-invasive POCT. TcB devices use a light meter to measure bilirubin levels in infants. TcB measures total bilirubin and does not differentiate between conjugated (direct) and unconjugated forms. Toxicity from unconjugated bilirubin is a primary concern in neonates and thus serum measurements of conjugated and unconjugated forms are still necessary, if TcB is elevated. Both the American Academy of Pediatrics and the Canadian Pediatric Society recommend either TcB or serum bilirubin as a good screening procedure for neonatal hyperbilirubinemia.[15] Currently insufficient evidence exists to replace serum bilirubin measurements with TcB in neonates; however, it is a good screening tool and can reduce unnecessary skin punctures.[16]

In summary, it is important to understand the technology of each point of care device in use, including accuracy and limitations, and any potential interferences that may be encountered in each clinical setting in which the device will be used. POC devices should be evaluated for potential interferences in all clinical settings in which the device will be used. Ideally, a single POC device should perform similarly in all clinical settings. If multiple devices are used in different areas of the same institution, the users should be aware of how results may differ between devices.

Regulatory Considerations of POCT

All accredited US clinical laboratories are regulated according to Clinical Laboratory Improvement Amendment'88 (CLIA), which classifies tests according to complexity into waived and non-waived categories. Waived status is determined by three criteria: 1) ease of use, 2) insignificant risk of erroneous results, and 3) demonstration of field performance (accuracy and precision). CLIA-waived testing requires the least amount of regulatory oversight and includes most POCT tests. Sites performing waived testing only require a CLIA certificate and must follow manufacturer instructions for performance, quality control, and maintenance of the POC test. Since CLIA-waived devices are not under regulatory oversight, there are no federal requirements for each lab using these devices to perform method/device validation, proficiency testing, or quality control (QC) beyond manufacturer's recommendations; however, it is good laboratory practice to do these things. The College of American Pathologists (CAP) has requirements for waived testing with regard to QC, calibration, and analytical measurement range (Table 11-3). Validation of a new POCT must be performed prior to implementation by comparing the results of the POCT to that of a reference or central hospital laboratory to assure that the methods are comparable. For

Table 11-3	**CLIA CHECKLIST FOR WAIVED AND NON-WAIVED POCT**
Quality Management	Organizational chart with levels of authority responsibility and accountability
	Detection and correctional of unusual laboratory results
	Troubleshooting Responsibilities
	Manufacturer Instructions
Results Reporting	Reporting of results in EMR
	Special precautions in reporting Urine drugs of abuse and Group A *Streptococus* direct antigen
	Testing personnel identification
Instruments and Equipment	Documentation of instrument/equipment approval
Personnel	Section director qualifications
	Authorized POCT personnel
	Initial training
	Competency assessment

- Above applies to waived and non-waived POCT

	Waived	Non-waived
QC	• Documentation of QC results • Evidence of corrective action when QC fails	• Documentation of daily QC • Defined acceptable limits for controls • Documentation of corrective action when QC fails • QC handling procedure same as patient sample • Monthly QC review by lab director
Calibration	• Adherence to manufacturer instructions for calibration, verification, and related functions	• Documentation of established calibration verification criteria • Established criteria for recalibration • Limits of analytical measurement range (AMR) defined for all analytes • Documentation of AMR verification procedure and consistent with manufacturer instructions • Documentation of AMR verification criteria

waived tests, validation can occur as part of proficiency testing. Proficiency testing (PT) is an external quality assurance process required by CLIA for non-waived tests; however, CAP requires PT for both non-waived and waived tests. PT compares a laboratory's test result on an unknown specimen to that of other labs using similar testing methods. If a POCT is enrolled in PT, the same rules that apply to central lab testing apply to the POCT. PT samples should be handled as any patient specimen and analysis should be performed by the usual operator. PT should not be performed by the Point of Care Coordinator (POCC) unless this person is the standard operator.

Not all POCT devices are CLIA-waived. "Off-label" use of a POCT defaults it to the high complexity category. Moderate and high complexity POCT devices are not CLIA waived and require performing laboratories to have a CLIA certificate, be inspected, and meet CLIA quality standards. Quality control must be run on CLIA-waived and non-waived devices. Traditionally QC is used to detect bias and drift in test results over time due to reagent stability and systematic error, as well as failure on the part of the assay. The high-volume automated instruments in the central lab use external liquid QCs that are treated as and batched with patient samples to detect error and bias. The data from QC measurements is used to determine the need for instrumentation recalibration or trouble-shooting. Quality control in POCT is an interesting concept. Many POCT devices have internal electronic QC that runs at a determined frequency. An external QC that is treated in a similar manner as a patient sample is generally not built into these test systems. Internal QCs are built into the system or device and monitor some or all of device's analytic components. Most POC devices rely on single use cartridges with built in QCs and calibrators. The device will check the QC and reject the cartridge if the QC does not pass. These controls do not indicate the performance characteristics of the test before or after it. Internal controls that are performed with each test can be used to detect random errors.

Per CLIA regulations, each laboratory must perform at least two levels of external QC materials each day a non-waived test is performed. Individual Quality Control Plan (IQCP) has been implemented by CMS for CLIA laboratory non-waived testing. This is a risk-based quality control plan that seems particularly suited to POCT. IQCP has three main parts: 1) risk assessment, 2) quality control plan, and 3) quality assessment. The scope of IQCP should include the entire testing phase; the pre-analytical, analytical, and post-analytical processes. Risk assessment could include monitoring failures and errors. The quality control of IQCP allows the individual laboratory to define the optimum frequency of liquid QC in conjunction with manufacturer's control process. As of January 1, 2016, if IQCP is not implemented the lab must follow CLIA QC regulatory requirements as written.[17]

Table 11-4   **ESTABLISHING AND MAINTAINING A POCT**
Considerations for establishing and maintaining a POCT
Establishing the need • Is a faster TAT required? • Will it change the TTAT? • What clinical question is being asked and what actions will be taken based on the POCT result? • What is the anticipated volume of testing? • Why is the core lab not able to meet the clinical need?
Procuring equipment and its evaluation • Will the POCT provide the required accuracy and precision? • What is the medical, operational and/or financial benefit of the POCT? • Are the adequate facilities for test performance and storage of instrumentation and reagents?
Identification, training and certification of operators • Are there personnel available to perform the test? • How many individuals will perform the testing? • Who will supervise the testing on the medical unit? Is there a POCC at the institution?
Establishing a QC, QA and audit policy and ensuring documentation • Are the methods for reporting patient and QC results, error logs and QA data in place?
Establishing POCT testing policy, accountability, accreditation and regulation of POCT policy • Will the end user/medical unit be able to abide by the organization's POCT policy?

Similar to core lab instrumentation, POCT can be purchased outright or can be obtained by reagent rental. Purchasing is fairly straightforward; the instrument is purchased as well as the necessary reagents and quality control material. In a reagent rental, the device is leased based on the amount of reagent that an institution predicts will be used in a determined amount of time. Often a combination is used; the device price can be negotiated based on volumes. Cost and cost savings can differ between institutions and sites within institutions. Institutional practices vary and POCT might be included in the core lab budget, or the costs may be in the budget of the end user, that is, the Emergency Department or PICU. The decision to bring in POCT services are outlined in Table 11-4 and should include consideration of 1) the clinical need, 2) identification and training of operators and supervisor, 3) cost benefit, 4) accuracy and precision of the result, and 5) understanding of why the core lab is not able to meet the clinical need. These considerations should include input from the clinical care team. Some hospitals have POC committees and specific requirements for bringing in POCT. Baystate Health has an institutional website with minutes of the POCT committee, CAP checklists, training checklists, policies and procedures, and contact information of POCC and support staff.[18] Addressing the questions listed in the Table 11-4 can help guide making the decision on whether to bring in a POCT service.

CRITICAL CARE

Critical care encompasses care of patients with clinical instability often associated with multi-organ failure and high risk of decompensation. The care of these patients occurs in intensive care units, such as the neonatal intensive care unit (NICU), pediatric intensive care unit (PICU), or in operating rooms, emergency room trauma bays, and during transport in mobile intensive care units. Critically ill patients are often being treated with vasopressors and diuretics, and are at high risk for acidosis, electrolyte imbalances, bleeding, or thromboembolism. Laboratory values are used frequently in the support of critically ill patients. It has been estimated that laboratory testing comprises over 40% of clinical data used by critical care physicians in the treatment of critically ill patients.[2] Management of these critically ill patients frequently requires the analysis of respiratory function and perfusion, hemostasis, and biomarkers of kidney and liver function. The analytes most often ordered by critical care services generally include arterial and venous blood gases, electrolytes, ionized calcium, magnesium, creatinine, hemoglobin, complete blood counts, and glucose. Lactate is frequently used as a marker of sepsis and to monitor perfusion/reperfusion. Routine coagulation tests, such as PT, aPTT, and fibrinogen are frequently needed in the critical care setting for management of patients on mechanical cardiopulmonary support and anticoagulant therapy. In addition, some laboratory values are required for intensive care unit patient acuity scoring systems (see Table 11-5).

Advantages of POCT in Critical Care

Concerns with laboratory testing in critical care include iatrogenic anemia and TAT. Point of care testing is attractive for use in the critical care setting because POCT devices typically have low sample volume requirements and results are available with a much shorter TTAT. Excessive phlebotomy for laboratory testing has been correlated to iatrogenic anemia in both adult and pediatric ICU populations. Iatrogenic anemia has been associated with greater length of stay in the ICU, more days on mechanical ventilation, and more transfusions. Low

Table 11-5	TESTS COMMONLY ORDERED IN PEDIATRIC CARE AND ACUITY SCORING SYSTEMS*		
Analyte	APACHE III	PRISM III	PIM
Sodium	X		
Potassium		X	
Chloride			
Bicarbonate		X	
Calcium			
Magnesium			
Serum Osmolality			
Total Bilirubin	X		
Hematocrit	X		
BUN	X	X	
RBC			
Hemoglobin			
WBC	X	X	
WBC differential			
PO_2	X	X	X
PCO_2	X	X	
Creatinine	X	X	
PT		X	
Arterial pH	X	X	
Base Excess			X
Glucose	X	X	
PTT		X	
Platelets		X	
Alkaline Phosphatase			
Alanine aminotransferase			
Aspartate Aminotransferase			
Lactate Dehydrogenase			
Albumin			

*APACHE III, Acute Physiology, Age and Chronic Health Evaluation III; PRISM III, Pediatric Risk of Mortality III; PIM, Pediatric Index of Mortality.

hemoglobin (less than 5 g/dL) was the most common reason for transfusion in the PICU. A PICU patient (admitted for greater than 48 hours) typically experiences 3 blood draws per day, with a mean volume of blood loss per draw of 2.7 ± 2.3 mL/draw.[19,20] To put this in perspective, the general guideline for safe volumes of draw in pediatrics is 3-7% of total blood volume in single draw, and no more than 5-10% of total blood volume over 1 month (see Chapter 1). For a 6-pound infant, this mean daily volume of blood loss nearly exceeds the recommendation for the total loss for a month. Not surprisingly, blood loss due to phlebotomy is particularly significant in younger age groups (ie, patients < 2 years). Even so, at least one study showed that a greater percentage of blood volume for requested laboratory tests was drawn from patients admitted to the NICU than to the Intermediate ICU (IICU).[21] There is a clear need to decrease volumes of blood drawn in these patients. In addition to reducing requirement of blood volume, most POCT devices require capillary collections, which work well in critically ill patients with vascular access lines. Capillary collections help reduce the number of times the lines are accessed, reducing the chances of infection. However, capillary blood is not always ideal for testing in critically ill patients, depending on the analyte (see Section "*Limitations of Point of Care Testing*" earlier).

Testing on whole blood also reduces TAT, since no sample preparation is required. The need for a rapid TTAT is also important in critical care. However, implementation of POCT does not always amount to reduced TTAT in critical care settings. One study showed nursing time rather than the perceived central laboratory processes was a rate-limiting step in the TTAT.[2] Additionally, there is limited data demonstrating improved outcomes with the implementation of POC in critical care settings.

SUMMARY

Pediatric critical care requires fast access to reliable laboratory test results. Because the pediatric population is particularly vulnerable to iatrogenic anemia due to excessive phlebotomy, small volume requirements are a priority, POCT is a solution to many of the critical care laboratory testing concerns. POCT is easy to use, fast, and uses small sample volumes. Directors and end users of POCT need to be aware of limitations of POCT, including interferences specific to the type of technology employed by the POCT device, as well as interferences unique to specific clinical situations. While a great number of POCT devices are waived from federal oversight, good laboratory practice as well as some accrediting agencies (eg, the College of American Pathologists) dictates validation and QC programs for POCT. POCT can be relatively costly, and careful evidence-based consideration of costs and benefits of POCT should be carried out prior to bringing POCT in-house.

TRAINING MODULE

1. Which of the following technologies is NOT encountered in POCT devices?
   a. Immunoassay
   b. Electrochemistry
   c. Optical techniques
   d. Chemical/enzymatic reactions
   e. Sequencing/polymerase chain reaction

2. Which of the following is not an advantage of POCT?
   a. Faster TTAT
   b. Reduced blood volume
   c. Cost effectiveness
   d. Accuracy

3. Which of the following statement about capillary blood collection is false?
   a. Capillary collections are preferred in pediatrics for decreases in iatrogenic anemia
   b. "Arterializing" capillary specimens by cooling the skin can increase the amount of arterial blood in a capillary specimen
   c. pO_2 is generally slightly higher in arterial blood compared to arterialized capillary blood
   d. Capillary blood is often collected through a finger or heel stick for POCT

4. Which of the following POCT does not require confirmatory testing?
   a. Sweat electrical conductivity for cystic fibrosis diagnosis
   b. Transcutaneous bilirubin
   c. Lead testing
   d. Glucose
   e. Activated clotting time

5. "Off-label" use of a CLIA-waived POCT device only requires CLIA certification and adherence to manufacturer guidelines
   a. True
   b. False

▌REFERENCES

1. Price CP, St. John A. Point of care testing. In: Burtis CA, Ashwood ER, Bruns E, eds. *Tietz Fundamentals of Clinical Chemistry*. 6th ed. St. Louis, MO: Elsevier Saunders, 2008:189-195.
2. Giuliano KK, Grant ME. Blood analysis at the point of care: issues in application for use in critically ill patients. *AACN Clin Issues*. 2002;13(2):204-220.
3. Dighe AS, Rao A, Coakley A, Lewandrowsi KB. Analysis of laboratory critical value reporting at a large academic medical center. *Am J Clin Pathol*. 2006;125:758-764.

4. CMS Center for Clinical Standards and Quality/Survey & Certification Group. Letter from the Director to State Survey Agency Directors. Directions on the off-label/modified use of waived blood glucose monitoring systems (BGMS); November, 2014. Available at: http://www.cms.gov/Medicare/Provider-Enrollment-and-Certification/SurveyCertificationGenInfo/Downloads/Survey-and-Cert-Letter-15-11.PDF. Accessed March, 2015.

5. Advisory Committee on Childhood Lead Poisoning Prevention. Low level lead exposure harms children: a renewed call for primary prevention. Atlanta, GA: US Department of Health and Human Services, CDC, Advisory Committee on Childhood Lead Poisoning Prevention; 2012. Available at: http://www.cdc.gov/nceh/lead/ACCLPP/Final_Document_030712.pdf. Accessed January, 2015.

6. CDC. CDC response to Advisory Committee on Childhood Lead Poisoning Prevention recommendations in "Low level lead exposure harms children: a renewed call for primary prevention". Atlanta, GA: US Department of Health and Human Services, CDC; 2012. Available at: http://www.cdc.gov.nceh/lead/acclpp/cdc_response_lead_exposure_recs.pdf. Accessed January, 2015.

7. Korpi-Steiner NL, Jenkins AJ. Comparative analysis of lead quantitation via inductively-coupled plasma mass spectrometry and point-of-care LeadCare®II system. *Clin Chem*. 2012;58(10):A166.

8. Parsons PJ, Reilly AA, Esernio-Jenssen D. Screening children exposed to lead: an assessment of the capillary blood lead fingerstick test. *Clin Chem*. 1997;43(2):302-311.

9. Sweat Chek™ sweat conductivity analyzer instruction/service manual (Westcor). Available at: http://westcor.com/translations/Translations/M2672/2A.pdf. Accessed January, 2015.

10. LeGrys VA, Yankaskas JR< Quittell LM, Marshall BC, Mogaqyzel PJ Jr. Cystic Fibrosis Foundation. Diagnostic sweat testing: the Cystic Fibrosis Foundation guidelines. *J Pediatr*. 2007;151:85-89.

11. Louie RF, Tang Z, Shelby D, Kost GJ. Point-of-care testing: millennium technology for critical care. *Lab Med*. 2000;31(7):402-408.

12. Dietzen DJ, Wilhite TR, Rasmussen M, Sheffield M. Point-of-care glucose analysis in neonates using modified quinoprotein glucose dehydrogenase. *Diabetes Technol Ther*. 2013;15(11):923-928.

13. Lewandrowski EL, Van Cott EM, Gregory K, Jang I, Lewandrowski LB. Clinical evaluation of the iStat kaolin activated cloting time (ACT) test in different clinical settings in a large academic urban medical center. *Am J Clin Pathol*. 2011;135:741-748.

14. Guzzetta NA, Monitz HG, Fernandez JD, Fazlollah TM, Knezevic A, Miller BE. Correlations between activated clotting time values and heparin concentration measurements in young infants undergoing cardioplumonay bypass. *Anesth Analg*. 2010;111:173-179.

15. Wainer S, Parmar SM, Allegro D, Rabi Y, Lyon ME. Impact of a transcutaneous bilirubinometry program on resource utilization and severe hyperbilirubinemia. *Pediatrics*. 2012;129:77-86

16. Carceller-Blanchard A, Cousineau J, Delvin EE. Point of care testing: transcutaneous bilirubinometry in neonates. *Clin Biochem*. 2009;42:143-149.

17. Center for Medicare and Medicaid Services. Center for Clinical Standards and Quality/Survey & Certification Group. Re: Individual Quality Control Plan (IQCP) for Clinical Laboratory Improvement Amendments (CLIA) laboratory nonwaived testing. Survey and Cert Letter 13-54 [PDF, 397KB]. Accessed January, 2015.

18. Nichols JH. Point-of-care Testing. In: Clarke W. Ed. *Contemporary Practice in Clinical Chemistry*. Washington DC: AACC Press, 2006. 219-232.

19. Bateman ST, Lacroix J, Boven K, Forbes P, Barton R, Thomas NJ, Jacobs B, Markovitz B, Goldstein B, Hanson JH, Li HA, Randolph AG, for the Pediatric Acute Lung Injury and Sepsis Investigators Network. Anemia, blood loss, and blood transfusions in North American children in the intensive care unit. *Am J Respir Crit Care Med*. 2008;178: 26-33.

20. Valentine SL, Bateman ST. Identifying factors to minimize phlebotomy-induced blood loss in the pediatric intensive care unit. *Pediatr Crit Care Med*. 2012;13(1):22-27.

21. Lin JC, Strauss RG, Kulhavy JC, Johnson KJ, Zimmerman MB, Cress GA, Connolly NW, Widness JA. Phlebotomy overdraw in the neonatal intensive care unit. *Pediatrics*. 2000;106:e19

PEDIATRIC LABORATORY TESTING FOR SPECIFIC ENDOCRINE CONDITIONS

12

Jon Nakamoto

LEARNING OBJECTIVES

1. Explain the basic pathophysiology of congenital adrenal hyperplasia (CAH).
2. Name at least one pre-analytical and one analytical factor that can lead to a false positive diagnosis of 21-hydroxylase deficiency (21OHD) based on measurement of 17-hydroxyprogesterone (17OHP).
3. Discuss the methodologic advantages of steroid assays (immunoassay or mass spectrometry) that involve upfront sample purification by extraction and chromatography.
4. Define the term "gene conversion" and describe its importance in the etiology of 21OHD.
5. State the rationale for newborn screening for classical 21-hydroxylase deficiency (21OHD).
6. Outline the essential steps to the evaluation of a short or poorly-growing child.
7. Understand why random measurement of growth hormone is rarely useful.
8. Explain how biological and analytical variability contribute to both low diagnostic sensitivity and specificity of laboratory testing for growth hormone deficiency.
9. Name at least two reasons why different growth hormone assays can yield widely different results from the same patient sample.
10. Identify the difficulties in establishing reference intervals for insulin-like growth factor I (IGF-I).

INTRODUCTION

Many endocrine disorders are known to affect the pediatric population, beginning from birth and extending throughout childhood, adolescence, and into adulthood. This chapter will focus on the pathophysiology and diagnostic testing for two specific endocrine disorders, congenital adrenal hyperplasia (CAH) and disorders of growth, specifically those related to growth hormone deficiency.

CONGENITAL ADRENAL HYPERPLASIA

Introduction

Understanding the diagnostic approach to congenital adrenal hyperplasia (CAH) is useful for anyone caring for children from birth through adolescence. Although classical forms of CAH are relatively uncommon (world-wide incidence around 1:15,000 live births), the nearly universal screening of infants born in North America and Europe mandates familiarity with the methods used for screening, their limitations, and the proper diagnostic follow-up of the child with an abnormal newborn screen. CAH is also the most common cause of ambiguous genitalia of the newborn, and the one cause that can lead to sudden decompensation and death if not diagnosed in a timely manner. Less severe forms of CAH (so-called non-classical disease, NCCAH) are common (incidence around 1:1000) in the general population and may have a prevalence as high as 5% or more among children presenting for evaluation of early pubic and/or axillary hair appearance (premature pubarche/premature adrenarche) or among adolescent females complaining about excess facial/abdominal hair (hirsutism) or irregular menstrual periods.

Basic Pathophysiology

At its simplest, CAH refers to a group of heritable (autosomal recessive) deficiencies in enzyme activity required for the proper conversion of cholesterol to cortisol (adrenal steroidogenesis, Figure 12-1). The cortisol deficiency can lead to fatigue, hypoglycemia, hyponatremia (due to decreased free water clearance), and hypotension/shock. If the enzyme deficiency also hinders aldosterone production, severe hyperkalemia may also be present. Due to the lack of feedback from cortisol, pituitary ACTH secretion increases, leading to hyperplasia of the adrenal cortex, accumulation of precursor steroids upstream of the enzyme block, and often shunting of steroidogenesis into other pathways, such as those for androgens, which can lead to precocious puberty in young children, or to hirsutism/virilization of females.

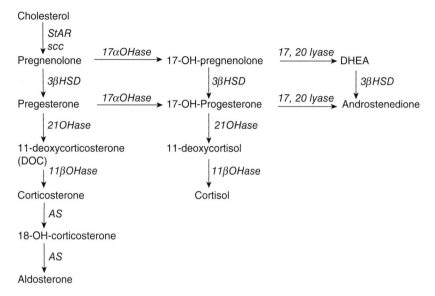

Cholesterol

Pregnenolone

Pregesterone

11-deoxycorticosterone
(DOC)

Corticosterone

18-OH-corticosterone

Aldosterone

17-OH-pregnenolone

17-OH-Progesterone

11-deoxycortisol

Cortisol

DHEA

Androstenedione

Figure 12-1 ■ Adrenal steroidogenesis pathways. Italicized abbreviations (see Legend) indicate enzymes involved in production of the steroids shown in bold text. *StAR*, steroidogenic acute regulatory protein; *scc*, cholesterol side chain cleavage enzyme (P450$_{scc}$, CYP11A1); *3βHSD*, 3-beta-hydroxysteroid dehydrogenase; *11βOHase*, 11-beta-hydroxylase (P450$_{c11}$, CYP11B1); *17αOHase*, 17-alpha-hydroxylase (P450$_{c17}$, CYP17A1); *17,20 lyase* (P450$_{c17,20}$, CYP17); *21OHase*, 21-hydroxylase (P450$_{c21}$, CYP21A2); *AS*, aldosterone synthase (P450$_{c11as}$, CYP11B2).

By far the most common cause (95%) of CAH is a deficiency in 21-hydroxylase activity (21OHD), with 11-hydroxylase deficiency, the next most common (4%). Other enzyme deficiencies are much less often encountered, although there is some ethnic and geographic variability; for example, a significantly higher incidence of 17-hydroxylase deficiency is found in Brazil as compared to the rest of the world. Among those with classic 21OHD, there is a spectrum of disease. In the most severe form, seen in about three-fourth of those with classic 21OHD, the patient is unable to make sufficient amounts of aldosterone as well as cortisol, and therefore has a tendency towards hyperkalemia as well as hyponatremia; this form is termed salt-wasting 21OHD. Females affected by salt-wasting 21OHD are much more likely to present with varying degrees of genital ambiguity at birth due to high levels of androgens during fetal life. The remaining one-fourth of those with classic 21OHD, while still at risk for adrenal insufficiency during times of severe physical stress (such as surgery or severe illness), primarily manifest with clinical signs related to moderate androgen excess, including accelerated growth and appearance of precocious pubertal changes in young children.

Laboratory Diagnostic Approach: An Introduction

By studying the adrenal steroidogenesis pathway shown in Figure 12-1, one can predict which steroid precursors will be elevated—for example, serum 17-hydroxyprogesterone (17OHP) in 21OHD, due to being immediately upstream from the enzymatic block. However, it is often prudent to look at multiple steroid precursors in making a specific diagnosis of CAH, since a single analyte elevation may sometimes be misleading. One may also see an elevated 17OHP in 11β-hydroxylase deficiency, but the difference from 21OHD will be that 11-deoxycortisol will also be high in this condition, versus being low in 21OHD. In many cases, examining the ratio between the precursors (upstream of the enzyme block) and products (downstream from the block) may improve diagnostic discrimination of different CAH forms. To further improve diagnostic sensitivity and specificity, a truncated form of ACTH (cosyntropin) can be administered intravenously for what is often (somewhat inaccurately) termed an "ACTH stimulation test." Since key diagnostic steroids, such as 17OHP in 21OHD will rise substantially higher after cosyntropin stimulation than they will be in unaffected subjects, a stimulated measurement further increases diagnostic accuracy. Drawbacks of cosyntropin stimulation testing include the need for intravenous access and multiple blood draws (at least two: baseline and 60 minutes is typical) that until recently required relatively large volumes of blood relative to the small size of many infants undergoing this testing. An emerging technological improvement is the use of multiplex measurement of adrenal steroids in a single injection onto a mass spectrometer, allowing analysis of multiple serum steroids and ratios in a substantially smaller volume of serum than was previously required for individual steroid assays. An additional alternative is the measurement of urinary steroid metabolites by gas chromatography-mass spectrometry (GC/MS), which offers the ability to study dozens of different metabolites and ratios simultaneously on a random urine sample (less invasive, and no stimulation required). The GC/MS urinary profiling has been used to great advantage in Europe and the United Kingdom,[1,2] although it requires familiarity with a whole different set of steroids (eg, pregnanetriol instead of 17OHP) and is much less often used in the United States at present.

Pre-analytical Considerations: Special Considerations for Neonates/Infants

Accurate analysis of steroids such as 17-OHP in young infants is particularly challenging, due to very high levels in newborns of interfering steroid conjugates, primarily glucuronidated and sulfated forms. For example, in term neonatal plasma, the level of the 17-hydroxypregnenolone sulfate as measured by GC/MS is 2110 nmol/L[3], which far exceeds the molar amount of 17OHP, that is, typically no more than 13 nmol/L (429 ng/dL) in a healthy term newborn. An antibody for 17OHP which had 0.4% cross-reactivity (typical of immunoassays in the late 20th century) with 17-OHpregnenolone-sulfate might therefore produce a result 8.44 nmol/L (279 ng/dL) higher than the actual value based on cross-reactivity from this one steroid conjugate alone—and there are many other conjugates also present in neonatal plasma.

The measurement situation is even worse for premature infants, due to a large and active fetal zone of the adrenal gland, as well as relative immaturity of several enzymes, such as 11β-hydroxylase and 3β-HSD. For these patients, even when using improved 17OHP immunoassays (cross-reactivity for 17-OHpregnenolone reduced to 0.1%), levels of cross-reacting steroid conjugates and steroid precursors may be so high that there remains a substantial chance of a false positive 21OHD diagnosis based on 17OHP measurement alone.

An additional pre-analytical factor to be considered is whether or not the mother has received any corticosteroids prior to delivery or while breastfeeding, since transfer through the placenta or in breast milk may suppress the infant's steroid levels and lead to false negative findings. While it is still worth sending a sample for screening purposes to avoid any delay in diagnosis, in these situations an additional screening test should be sent about a week after the last corticosteroid exposure.

The timing of the blood draw and the clinical status of the patient should also be assessed when interpreting neonatal steroid levels. Even healthy infants have high levels of 17OHP during the first 24-48 hours after birth, so ideally a sample for diagnosis of CAH should be collected after 48 hours of life to avoid false positive results. Physical stress and illness may also elevate 17OHP levels; some authors have proposed also measuring cortisol levels, which tend to be high in sick infants, but low in all forms of CAH, and also an androstenedione level, which is higher in children with 21OHD than in unaffected subjects.

Analytical Considerations: Assay Methodology

Selection of a proper assay for steroid measurement is critical for proper diagnosis when measuring very low analyte concentrations or when interfering/cross-reacting substances are greatly elevated, as in newborns. In the early days of steroid measurement by radioimmunoassay (RIA), it became clear very quickly to clinicians and researchers that additional sample preparation, such as organic solvent extraction (to remove water-soluble steroid conjugates) and chromatography (to isolate the steroid of interest from structurally-related

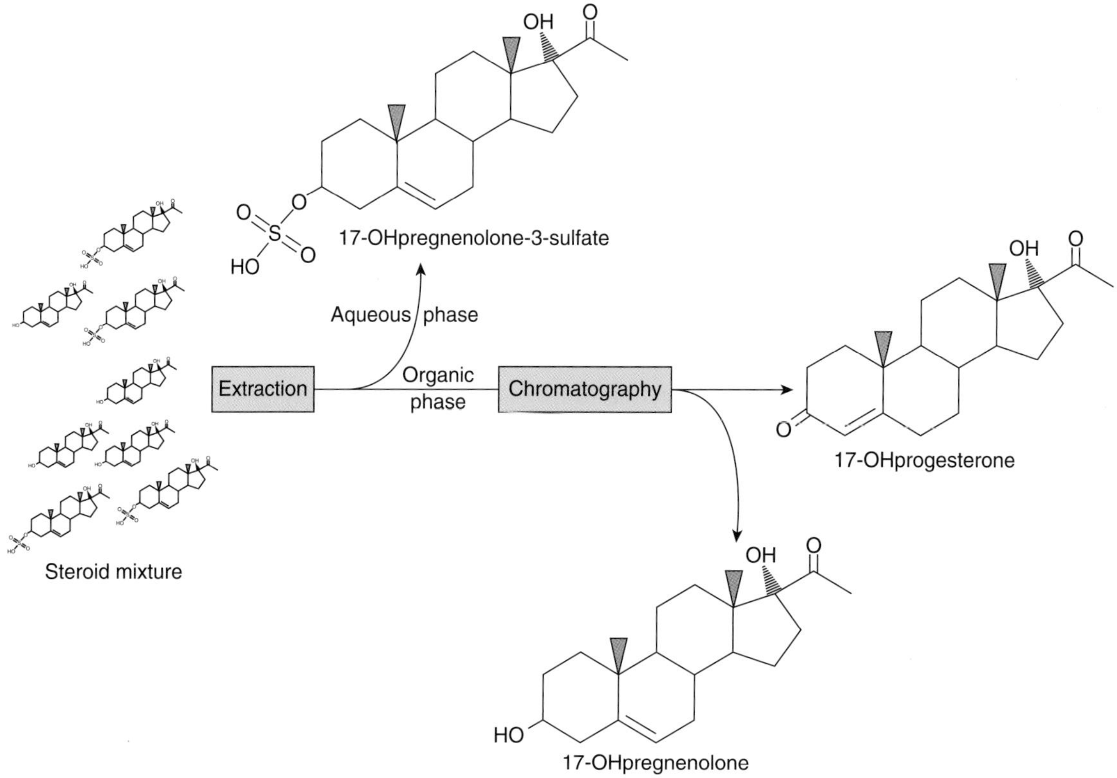

Figure 12-2 ▪ Sample purification by extraction and chromatography.

compounds) were particularly important for accurate results. Figure 12-2 shows schematically how an extraction step can remove water-soluble steroid conjugates and how a chromatography step can separate structurally similar compounds from the analyte of interest. Such sample preparation can greatly aid the accuracy of steroid immunoassays, which are hindered by the inherently low analytical specificity of antibodies developed against steroid molecules. This low specificity reflects the fact that steroid molecules are small and poorly antigenic, with only minor structural difference among steroids of vastly different function.

This extra sample purification has a significant impact on the accuracy of testing. A study on blood spots from healthy newborns[4] showed that the mean values of 17OHP as measured by fluorometric immunoassay went from 578 ng/dL (17.5 nmol/L) down to 106 ng/dL (3.2 nmol/L) after ether extraction. Since the 17OHP +3 SD cutoff used at that time was around 400 ng/dL, the extraction step made a significant diagnostic difference. In premature infants where, for reasons noted earlier, there would be even more issues anticipated, a Japanese study had previously described an infant with a 17OHP value of 11,200 ng/dL on an unextracted sample, versus a value of 210 ng/dL when the ELISA was performed after an extraction step.[5]

Cross-reactions may occur in the other direction as well. The very high levels of 17OHP as well as 21-deoxycortisol or 11-deoxycortisol seen in 21OHD and some other forms of CAH, such as 11βOHase deficiency may falsely elevate cortisol levels measured by immunoassay.[6,7] This could lead to a misinterpretation that cortisol secretion was adequate, when in fact it might be on the low side.

Adoption of tandem mass spectrometry for the measurement of low levels of steroids, or for clinical situations (as in newborns) where concentrations of interfering substances are high, has improved accuracy over direct (ie, not involving extraction or chromatography) immunoassays. In addition, extraction and chromatography steps are part of the mass spectrometry process (ie, high performance liquid chromatography-tandem mass spectrometry, or LC-MS/MS for short) and are typically easier to automate in a mass spectrometry system as compared to most immunoassays. Automation generally allows higher throughput for lower ongoing costs. After the initial high capital cost of purchasing the mass spectrometer and HPLC systems, the reagent and operating costs are also cheaper than most immunoassay platforms. The combination of greater accuracy, faster results and lower ongoing operating costs make LC-MS/MS the current gold standard for measurement of steroids, such as 17OHP.

Post-Analytical Considerations

For the reasons noted earlier, proper interpretation of test results requires knowledge of the patient's age, history, and what methodology was used. In addition, both reference intervals and clinical decision thresholds are important. What may not be well known to many clinicians is how "fuzzy" these cutoffs truly are. For any given method, reference intervals for term and pre-term newborns are generally based on small numbers of study subjects, and in many cases may be based on older methodology, such as RIA after extraction/chromatography versus the more modern method of LC-MS/MS. While in general the method comparisons between older and newer assays show decent overall correlation, there are exceptions for some analytes, such as DHEA; even for analytes with good correlation (see Figure 12-3), there are inevitably individual patients whose results are significantly different when measured by different methodologies. Thus, current reference intervals should be used as general guidelines rather than as clear discriminators between health and disease. Some reference intervals, such as those after a cosyntropin stimulation test, may never be fully replicated for modern

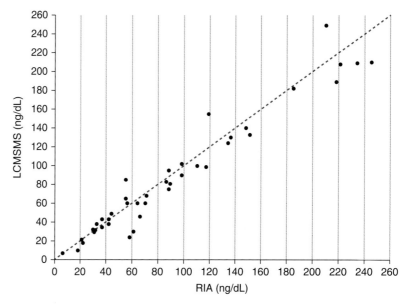

Figure 12-3 ▪ Method comparison of LC-MS/MS versus RIA (after extraction & chromatography) for 11-deoxycortisol.

methodologies, such as LC-MS/MS, due to current Institutional Review Board and other limitations that make stimulation studies in healthy infants nearly impossible to generate.

Molecular Genetic Testing for 21-Hydroxylase Deficiency

The gene locus (CYP2A2) involved in 21-OHD has a number of unique features that make DNA-based testing both highly efficient and tremendously complex. The functional gene (CYP21A2) that produces the 21-hydroxylase enzyme has a closely-related but non-functioning gene (CYP21A1P, a so-called "pseudogene") about 30 kb away on the same chromosome. The two genes are about 98% identical, but the pseudogene has multiple mutations that prevent production of a functional enzyme. Due to the close proximity and sequence similarity between the two genes, during meiosis there is a high frequency of unequal crossing-over recombination events that can produce large deletions (most commonly a 30-kb deletion) or duplications. Additionally, meiotic recombination can lead to replacement of functional gene sequences by mutations from the pseudogene, a so-called gene conversion event. Assays that are able to detect the 30-kb deletion and the 10 (or 12, depending on how a cluster of three closely-associated point mutations is counted) mutations arising from the pseudogene will detect up to 95% of all CYP21A2 mutations

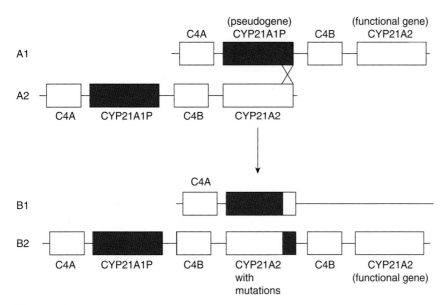

Figure 12-4 ▪ Recombination event that effectively duplicates the CYP21A2 gene on one chromosome.

found in 21-OHD. Thus, genetic analysis of patients with suspected 21-OHD can be conducted efficiently using targeted mutation screening assays, with complete gene sequencing reserved only for unusual cases where a de novo mutation is suspected.

Complexity arises from the many possible variations in recombination events that can occur at the CYP21A2 locus. For example, during meiosis, a crossing-over event may take place between the pseudogene on one chromosome and the functional gene on the other as shown in Figure 12-4. The result is a non-functional chimeric allele on one chromosome that has no intact CYP21A2, nor a CYP21A1P, while the other chromosome carries a non-functional chimeric allele, a pseudogene, and an intact copy of the CYP21A2 gene. The clinical impact of this and similar recombination events is that, depending upon the diagnostic approach used, a potential false positive diagnosis of disease could be made. If an individual carried the alleles shown, and the question is asked, "Is there an inactivating mutation/disruption present in the CYP21A2 alleles on both chromosomes," the answer would be yes, and the prediction would be that the patient would have 21-OHD. On the other hand, if the question asked were "Is there an intact copy of CYP21A2 on either chromosome?" then the answer would also be yes—and since one functional copy of CYP21A2 is sufficient to avoid 21-OHD, the prediction would be that the patient is a carrier, but not affected by 21-OHD.

Newborn Screening for Classical 21-OHD

The rationale for newborn screening for classical 21-OHD revolves around the inability to recognize the condition at birth in many newborns (particularly in males), and the risk in those with salt wasting (SW) 21-OHD, if not detected and treated, of significant electrolyte abnormalities (hyponatremia/hyperkalemia from aldosterone deficiency, with cortisol deficiency/impaired water excretion further contributing to low serum sodium), shock, and death somewhere during the first few weeks of life, typically well after discharge from the newborn nursery.

The analyte of choice for newborn screening has been 17-hydroxyprogesterone (17-OHP), measured from filter paper blood spots. Although measurements of this and other steroids without prior purification steps (eg, organic solvent extraction and chromatography) can lead to false elevations due to interfering mono-sulfated steroids, such as 17-hydroxypregenolone sulfate that are prominent in newborns, particularly premature infants, the small volumes from filter paper samples and the need for high throughput has led to the predominant use worldwide of an automated fluoroimmunoassay (DELFIA) without prior extraction or chromatography on the sample. An additional challenge in the interpretation of 17-OHP levels in newborns is the contribution of physical stress to 17-OHP elevations frequently seen in ill infants who do not have 21-OHD; some newborn screening programs have therefore employed on blood spots from patients with elevated 17-OHP a second tier of testing using HPLC-tandem mass spectrometry to measure not only 17-OHP, but also androstenedione (more likely to be elevated in 21-OHD than with stress) and cortisol (likely to be higher with physical stress and lower with 21-OHD).[8]

Due to the methodological and physiological issues noted earlier, the initial approaches to newborn screening for 21-OHD had very low positive predictive values (typically in the 1-3% range). This led to substantial effort and expense for confirmatory testing. Efforts to improve the PPV of newborn screening have included: 1) adjusting cutoffs for gestational age at birth or birthweight, with the former being more predictive of 17-OHP values, but the latter more often used due to greater objectivity of weight measurements versus gestational age calculations; 2) raising the clinical thresholds for definition of a positive 17-OHP result, understanding that this will reduce sensitivity for detection of some cases of classical 21-OHD, particularly the less severely affected infants with simple virilizing 21-OHD; 3) introduction of second tier testing with tandem mass spectrometry as noted earlier.

Although the false negative rates for 21-OHD screening has previously been reported as being very low, a careful follow-up study of the Minnesota 21-OHD screening program showed a false negative rate for classical 21-OHD newborn screening to be 22%, of which one-third of the false negatives were

SW 21-OHD.[9] This reflects the combination of raising diagnostics thresholds for 17-OHP as noted earlier, plus the significantly delayed rise in 17-OHP exhibited by some infants affected with classical 21-OHD. Therefore, although the negative predictive value of the testing remains excellent (99.998%), newborn screening should not be used to rule out 21-OHD completely when clinical signs and symptoms are suggestive of disease.

GROWTH DISORDERS, WITH A FOCUS ON GROWTH HORMONE DEFICIENCY

Introduction

Evaluation of the short or poorly-growing child is the second most common (after diabetes mellitus) reason for referral to a pediatric endocrinologist.[10] While laboratory testing is an essential part of the diagnostic process, the relatively poor diagnostic performance of available tests for growth hormone deficiency make it essential to screen carefully with a thorough history and physical examination before deciding which patients should progress to the second level of evaluation, such as growth hormone stimulation testing. Even after optimizing the pre-test probability of a condition, such as growth hormone deficiency (GHD), growth hormone stimulation testing has relatively poor diagnostic sensitivity and specificity, for reasons discussed in this chapter.

Basic Physiology

Childhood growth is influenced by many factors, including genetics, hormones, nutrition, a variety of anatomic conditions and chronic diseases, and psychological issues. The most rapid phase of growth occurs during infancy, with the next most rapid growth rates occurring during adolescence in concert with progression through puberty. Because the timing of pubertal onset is so widely variable among different individuals, the timing of the adolescent "growth spurt" is likewise highly variable, leading to an increase in referrals for children who are simply "late bloomers" relative to many of their peers (a condition referred to as constitutional delay of growth and puberty).

Of the many hormones pertinent to growth, the most clinically important are the sex steroids (testosterone and estradiol), thyroid hormone, growth hormone (GH), and growth-hormone associated factors, such as insulin-like growth factor I (IGF-I) and IGF-binding protein-3 (IGFBP-3). With the exception of the early newborn period, growth hormone is secreted in pulsatile fashion and during most of the day is below the limit of assay detection.

Thus, with the possible exception of diagnostic workup for newborns with hypoglycemia, random measurement of GH is not recommended. In the liver, GH from the pituitary gland induces production of both IGF-I and IGFBP-3. GH also induces production of IGF-I directly in target tissues, and in fact this IGF-I (which cannot be effectively measured at present) may be more important than hepatic IGF-I for growth. Most of the time it is likely that the hepatic and locally-produced IGF-I levels parallel one another, so that the circulating IGF-I is a useful proxy indicator of adequate growth hormone action. However, as a caveat, it should be noted that knockout mice with circulating IGF-I levels about 25% of normal due to elimination of hepatic IGF-I production grow normally.[11] This may partially explain a number of situations where a low IGF-I does not actually indicate GH deficiency.

Evaluation of Short Stature/Growth Failure

History, Physical Examination, and Imaging

As noted earlier, there are myriad influences on growth during childhood. Broad laboratory testing for all possible diagnoses affecting growth is neither feasible nor cost effective. In addition, testing for conditions such as GH deficiency (GHD) has inherent limitations on diagnostic sensitivity and specificity. Therefore, before any consideration of a less common diagnosis such as GHD, which comprises only about 5% of all referrals for short stature,[12] a thorough clinical evaluation is important. A thorough medical history and physical examination should include:

1. Birth history: features, such as neonatal hypoglycemia are important clue to GHD.
2. Family history, looking for genetic causes of short stature or chronic diseases affecting growth. In addition, parental heights can be used to calculate a mid-parental target height, with a typically used calculation as follows: for boys, add 5 inches to the mother's height and average with the father's height; for girls, subtract 5 inches from the father's height and average with the mother's height. Four inches below and above this mid-parental target height figure represents approximately –2 to +2 standard deviations [SD] for children born to such parents. While this should be viewed as a rule of thumb calculation only (it will tend to underestimate the child's height for very short parents and overestimate for very tall parents), it can sometimes help distinguish familial short stature from more significant conditions.
3. Past medical history and thorough review of systems, for clues to cryptic chronic disease (eg, chronic abdominal pain suggestive of inflammatory bowel disease or celiac disease) or deficiencies in other

pituitary hormones (central hypothyroidism, gonadotropin deficiency, adrenal insufficiency, diabetes insipidus), which are highly associated with concomitant GHD. Particularly important is to obtain previous accurate height and weight measurements, typically plotted on a standard cross-sectional population growth chart. This also helps distinguish simple short stature from actual growth failure. Short stature is typically defined as height below the 3rd percentile, which is just a bit above –2 SD for the population, although other thresholds are also used (–2.5, –2.67, or –3 SD). Actual growth failure is defined as a growth velocity persistently below the 5th percentile for age on a growth velocity chart, or a height drop across more than two percentile lines on a standard growth chart, with the latter being of greater concern.[13] Two exceptions to this concern about "down-channeling" on the growth chart occur during (a) the first two to three years of life, where many children (often destined to be those late-blooming children with constitutional delay of growth) move down to a lower height percentile, or (b) during the early teenage years, where those with constitutional delay of growth and puberty grow more slowly relative to their peers until they experience their pubertal growth spurt a couple of years later. Recognizing these normal variants of growth and treating them with no more than simple observation can help avoid unnecessary laboratory investigation.

Weight can also provide important clues, since a low weight to height ratio, or crossing down weight percentile lines can be an important clue to sometimes cryptic gastrointestinal disease; a higher weight to height ratio is somewhat more suggestive of endocrine diseases, such as hypothyroidism, growth hormone deficiency, and rare disorders, such as Cushing disease/syndrome (hypercortisolism).

4. Physical examination should include an accurate height measurement (more accurate than is typically performed in most pediatric offices); assessment of weight relative to height; general assessment for dysmorphic features of the face (including teeth, palate, and any indication of midline facial defects associated with pituitary gland abnormalities), trunk, or limbs/digits; fundoscopic exam (looking for optic nerve hypoplasia associated with hypopituitarism); skin (particularly looking for nevi associated with common genetic conditions, such as Turner syndrome); and examination of other systems to screen for renal, cardiac, respiratory, gastrointestinal, metabolic, rheumatologic, or neurologic diseases.

Typically, a radiograph of the left hand is also performed in order to assess the skeletal age (bone age) versus chronological age. If the bone age is younger by about 1-2 years as compared to the chronological age, this suggests that (a) there is more remaining growth potential than typical for this chronological age; and (b) the odds of common variants, such as constitutional delay rise considerably. If the bone age is more substantially delayed, the odds of an endocrinopathy, such as hypothyroidism or growth hormone deficiency rise.

Cranial imaging (typically an MRI scan) is also considered at this step if there is evidence of true growth failure (decreased growth velocity), or if there are any neurological findings, such as recurrent headaches or vision difficulties.

Initial Laboratory Investigations

Many children with short stature need little more than serial height measurements and observation. However, in practice, most of these children get at least the following basic screening tests, which typically include: 1) complete blood count (anemia may indicate cryptic blood loss from conditions, such as inflammatory bowel disease); 2) indicators of chronic inflammation such as C-reactive protein or an erythrocyte sedimentation rate; 3) basic or comprehensive metabolic panel to screen for a variety of conditions such as renal tubular acidosis, renal failure, liver disease, malnutrition, etc.; 4) urinalysis; and 5) thyroid function studies, typically both TSH (looking particularly for elevated levels suggestive of hypothyroidism) and free T4 (to identify those few with hypothalamic-pituitary causes of central hypothyroidism, where TSH is not useful for diagnosis). Additional tests may be prompted by age (eg, sweat chloride testing in infants), weight (eg, tissue transglutaminase IgA antibody, and total IgA level to screen for celiac disease), history of infections (eg, serum immunoglobulin levels), unusual findings (eg, measuring ACTH in a patient with a year-round tan suggestive of primary adrenal insufficiency), or results of other testing (eg, ferritin and other iron-related testing for those found to be anemic). One often overlooked test is a karyotype in short girls, in whom Turner syndrome (estimated incidence 1:2500 live births) may present with features much more subtle than the classic textbook definitions (eg, little more than short stature and a narrow, high-arched palate). Ideally, a karyotype analysis specifically geared towards diagnosis of Turner syndrome should be ordered, so that a minimum of 30 cells are counted as per current American College of Medical Genetics guidelines,[14] and additional appropriate studies are performed based on the initial results.

As noted earlier, random measurement of GH is generally not helpful, since levels will be below the limit of detection most of the time. Therefore, IGF-I, which shows less variability through the day, is often drawn during the initial laboratory work up of short stature, acting as an index of GH sufficiency. IGFBP-3 is often added due to its additional positive predictive value for growth hormone deficiency in children when values are low. If these tests are low, the next step is often measurement of GH after administration of an agent (secretagogue) that induces GH secretion, so-called GH stimulation testing.

Growth Hormone-Related Laboratory Testing

General Issues

Three issues have prevented growth hormone-related testing from achieving the best possible diagnostic performance. First of all was the shift decades ago from diagnosing only the most severe forms of GHD to detection of more subtle forms. When GH was scarce, the focus was solely on the detection of anatomically demonstrable causes of GHD, such as congenital hypopituitarism or pituitary damage due to trauma or surgery. IGF-I levels were profoundly low, and GH responses to stimulation were negligible. As studies revealed that some children with isolated short stature/growth failure showed apparent growth benefit from GH treatment, the emphasis shifted towards detection of idiopathic GHD (IGHD). Unfortunately, no gold standard exists for diagnosis of IGHD. Attempts were made to establish diagnostic thresholds (eg, a peak stimulated GH level of 7 or 10 ng/mL) that best balanced the identification of patients who would respond to GH versus those who would not. There was certainly a correlation between the levels of the growth hormone-related tests and the likelihood of a positive response to GH therapy, with those having very low results more likely to respond to treatment. However, no matter where the diagnostic thresholds were set, it became clear that some patients who exceeded these thresholds (apparently normal results) still showed benefit from GH treatment, while others who "failed" a GH stimulation test (eg, peak stimulated GH <7 ng/mL) continued to grow normally and ultimately achieved a final height fitting their expected genetic potential. Clearly both the diagnostic sensitivity and specificity of these tests was imperfect, likely due to the heterogeneous nature of patients with IGHD. These observations led some groups (eg, the Australian pediatric endocrinologists) to abandon laboratory testing and focus solely upon auxological (observed growth pattern) criteria for justification of growth hormone treatment. Nevertheless, most pediatric endocrinologists continue to use growth hormone-related testing in combination with other criteria to make their best approximate assessment of the odds that a given patient will benefit from GH treatment.

A second issue surrounds the large degree of biological variability of the IGF-I and particularly of GH itself. Combined with the marked analytical differences among different IGF-I and GH tests, measurement variability of the growth hormone-related tests is large, further compromising the diagnostic performance of these assays for detection of GHD. These latter two issues are discussed in more detail in the individual sections later.

IGF-I

IGF-I has proven to be a useful test in the detection of GHD, but with several caveats:

1. IGF-I levels are affected not only by GH, but also by associated conditions, such as hypothyroidism, diabetes mellitus, liver disease, and other chronic diseases;
2. The recent nutritional status can greatly affect IGF-I; even a few days of strict dieting can lead to a significant reduction in IGF-I levels;
3. There is far more individual biological variability than is often appreciated even by endocrinologists—samples from the same individual, taken on different days, may have IGF-I levels that vary anywhere from 5% to 37%[15];
4. IGF-I is inherently a "difficult" analyte to measure reproducibly by immunoassay, in great part due to the need to separate it properly from its binding proteins, of which there are at least eight (seven IGFs, including the low-affinity IGFBP-7, plus a protein called acid-labile subunit, ALS). This separation requires an acidification step to destroy ALS and decrease binding protein affinity, plus an additional purification achieved either by (a) extraction using hydrophobic interaction chromatography (labor intensive and plagued by poor recoveries) or ethanol precipitation (faster and with better recoveries, but not as thorough an extraction technology), or (b) displacement using excess IGF-II to remove the binding proteins. Inadequate separation of binding proteins or alteration in the conformation of the IGF-I molecule can lead to great variability among different immunoassays, and increased risk of large inter-assay variability even for the same assay. Recent developments allowing measurement of IGF-I by mass spectrometry (either after trypsin digestion and quantitation of fingerprint peptides, or by measurement of intact IGF-I using high-resolution mass spectrometry) show promise in reducing inter-laboratory variability from an estimated 33.5% CV down to < 16%.[16]
5. There remain additional variability issues surrounding the use of different standards for immunoassay calibration, with both an older WHO standard, International Reference Reagent (IRR) 87/518, and a newer WHO International Standard (IS) 02/254 in wide use on different IGF-I immunoassay platforms. Results are not transferable between platforms using the different standards.[17] Even among assays using the same 02/254 standard, there remain significant differences among IGF-I immunoassays,[18] similar to the situation well known for GH, as noted in the following section.

6. Because IGF-I levels vary so markedly by age and sex, particularly during childhood and adolescence, good reference interval information to allow proper interpretation of results requires sizeable studies. Such studies are not easily performed, particularly when samples from healthy young children are required. One of the most comprehensive studies was performed over a decade ago,[19] but due to the original assay being discontinued, those results can only be loosely applied to current IGF-I assays. Most IGF-I reference intervals available currently are either based on very small numbers of subjects in certain age groups (eg, in the youngest children, as seen in Figure 12-5) or are hybrids of new primary data for older children, plus reference intervals transferred from older assays. Thus, the reference intervals (typically the −2 to +2 SD range) or z-scores (standard deviation scores) provided should generally be viewed as approximate rather than exact thresholds for clinical decision-making, particularly in the younger patients.

Overall, IGF-I has decent diagnostic sensitivity, but poor diagnostic specificity for GHD. Therefore, an IGF-I value that is not far below −2 SD for age may indicate the need for further testing or at least close follow-up observation, but does not prove GHD. Only if the IGF-I is profoundly low (eg, −5 SD for age) without other issues (severe starvation, liver disease, or rare cases of resistance to GH), is it more definitive for the diagnosis of GHD.

IGFBP-3

IGF-binding protein-3 is produced by the liver upon exposure to GH and is the dominant IGF-binding protein, carrying about 95% of all of the IGF-I and IGF-II present in serum. It has a long serum half-life, is not as strongly affected by acute caloric deprivation as is IGF-I, and due to high concentrations and no requirement for the extraction for accurate quantitation, is relatively easy to measure. Levels rise gradually and continuously during childhood and adolescence before falling just as gradually after age of 30 years in adulthood. Unfortunately, IGFBP-3 has relatively poor diagnostic sensitivity for GHD, with levels often remaining within the reference interval despite a clinical picture, IGF-I and stimulated GH levels all consistent with GHD. The diagnostic sensitivity is so low in adults that it should not be used in most cases beyond childhood. Nevertheless, it can prove useful for its strong positive predictive value: while low (−2 SD) IGF-I levels are commonly seen in otherwise healthy children, if the IGFBP-3 is also below −2 SD for age, the odds of GHD are significantly increased. To this end IGFBP-3 may be particularly useful for assessment of young infants, whose IGF-I levels are normally so low that IGF-I becomes much less useful as a marker for potential GHD.

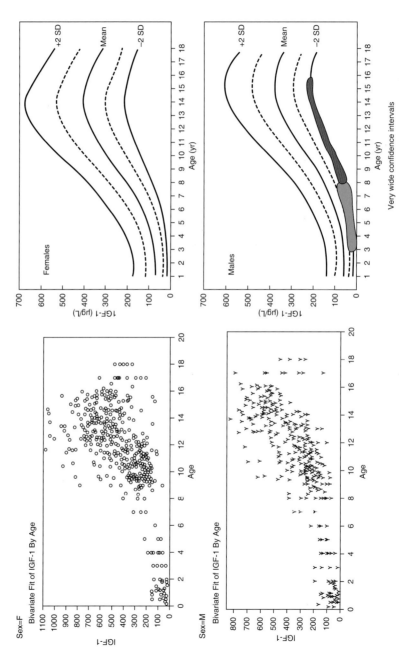

Figure 12-5 ▪ Raw data and derived standard deviation curves for IGF-I.

GH Stimulation Testing

In clinical practice, for the diagnosis of GHD, GH is almost always measured after administration of a secretagogue (GH stimulation test), due to significant limitations of other approaches for the evaluation of GH secretion. Any GH result achieved during the test that is above the chosen clinical cutoff (typically 7 ng/mL or 10 ng/mL) is considered a "passing" (negative) result. Strenuous exercise can also induce a pulse of GH, but since it is difficult to ensure that a child has exercised to the required point of near exhaustion in a typical office setting, any apparently inadequate GH response may be due more to inadequate exertion rather than GHD. As noted previously, the pulsatile nature of GH release renders a random measurement of GH levels useless in most situations. The one exception is in the neonatal period, where GH levels are often tonically elevated to relatively high levels; this may be pertinent during workup of neonatal hypoglycemia, where GHD can be a contributing cause. Extended (eg, 24 hour) sampling of blood using an indwelling cannula and a pump that draws samples at approximately half hour intervals can be used to define 24-hour GH secretion rates, but is unwieldy, and due to biological variability, in a healthy child may look normal one day and abnormal the next. Urine GH shows excessive variability due to variation in renal protein excretion, and has not proven helpful in GHD diagnosis.

There are many GH stimulation test protocols in use, often with widely differing sampling time points, in part dependent upon which secretagogue is used for the stimulus. Among the many different secretagogues, the most commonly used include glucagon, L-arginine, growth hormone releasing hormone, clonidine, L-DOPA, and various combinations of these and other agents. Insulin-induced hypoglycemia (often termed "insulin tolerance test," or ITT) is still viewed as the gold standard for GH stimulation test, although it is much less often used today due to the higher risk it poses to the patient. The main challenge of the ITT is achieving adequate hypoglycemia (serum glucose < 40 mg/dL, or a drop of > 50% from baseline) without lowering blood glucose to the point where seizures and other complications occur. Since insulin sensitivity is highly individual, with some individuals (eg, obese patients) requiring higher doses to achieve the desired low blood sugar goal, ensuring a valid ITT without putting the patient at significant risk is not an easy task.

GH stimulation test challenge #1: Biological variability

One of the greatest challenges surrounding any evaluation of potential GHD is the substantial biological variability in secretion exhibited by any single individual at any given time on any given day, including both spontaneous and stimulated GH levels. This is why even integrated 24-hour measurement of GH was unable to distinguish clearly between healthy and GH-deficient individuals. For GH stimulation testing, the implications are that any single GH test has poor reproducibility, and thus poor diagnostic specificity. In a study of 16 healthy normal adults who underwent two separate insulin-induced hypoglycemia tests at least 3 days apart, the Spearman correlation coefficient between the pairs of test results was only 0.18,[20] which by any interpretation is a very weak correlation. Observational data in a group of 48 children who initially had a subnormal response (defined as < 10 ng/mL peak GH level) to one GH stimulation test showed that 39 of these patients (81.3%) had a level ≥10 ng/mL when tested a second time.[21] Unfortunately, with no absolute gold standard for diagnosis of GHD, an exact diagnostic specificity cannot be calculated. As a result, most clinicians and insurers required that a patient have subnormal responses to two separate GH stimulation tests before making a diagnosis of GHD, unless there were obvious anatomic correlates (eg, absent pituitary gland) or associated findings (eg, profound short stature and growth failure associated with IGF-I levels more than 5 SD below the mean).

GH stimulation test challenge #2: Analytical variability among different GH assays

In the beginning there were only a handful of GH assays, all employing a competitive immunoassay format and relatively similar polyclonal antibodies. However, as immunometric GH assays became available, unquestionably improving both analytical sensitivity and specificity, there was a notable discordance between the older polyclonal competitive immunoassays and one of the most popular immunometric GH assays available at that time (Figure 12-6, lower solid line). While the lower values were ascribed to the use of a more specific monoclonal antibody, it was not necessarily true that all GH assays employing monoclonal antibodies and an immunometric format would give lower values than the competitive RIA, as shown for a second immunometric assay (Figure 12-6, upper solid line). Thus, a competitive GH RIA result right at the clinical threshold of 10 ng/mL might look frankly low (6 ng/mL) on one immunometric GH assay (lower circle), but adequate (13 ng/mL) on a different immunometric GH assay (upper circle). These unpredictable differences persist even when assays are calibrated against the same international standard, and demonstrate that many different factors—antibody specificity, assay format, reference preparation, choice of matrix (ie, animal serum vs. buffered saline/albumin solution) for dilution of standards, to name a few—can lead to very different immunoassay results.

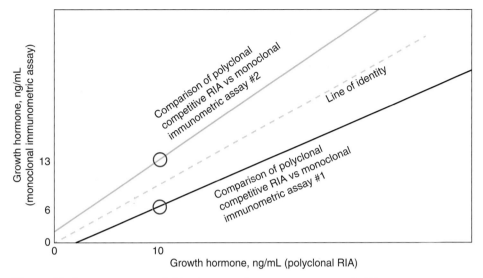

Figure 12-6 ▪ Comparison of older GH RIA with newer immunometric GH assays.

Much of the explanation of differences in GH assay results lies with the heterogeneity of the GH molecule itself. One careful study of GH iso-forms found in circulation after a spontaneous GH pulse showed that 43% was present as the primary 22 kDa form of GH, about 8% was 20 kDa GH derived from a splice variant of the GH gene, and the remainder represented GH oligomers and alternate forms (acetylated or deamidated GH). There is a correlation between antibody cross-reactivity to the 20 kDa form of GH and the total GH results: on the Beckman Access GH assay, which has negligible cross-reactivity to 20 kDa GH, a sample might have results two-thirds of that measured on the Roche Elecsys GH assay, which has substantial cross-reactivity.

Given the issues noted earlier, it is clear that GH stimulation testing has limited diagnostic specificity, and that arbitrary cutoffs, such as 7 ng/mL or 10 ng/mL are only approximate guidelines. Nevertheless, when combined with careful history, physical examination, and appropriate adjunctive test results, GH stimulation testing appears to be clinically helpful. Nevertheless, due to the lack of a gold standard for diagnosis of GHD and the variability issues discussed, plus the difficulty in ascertaining how much incremental height gain has been achieved in GH-treated children who are not part of a large-scale study, no one can be entirely certain of the true diagnostic performance of this testing.

SUMMARY

Proper functioning of the endocrine system is integral to normal growth and development. Diagnosis of endocrine-related diseases states that the monitoring of healthy development in children often requires the use of many different laboratory test results. Thus, pediatric endocrinology is a discipline that relies heavily on laboratory testing and laboratory support. Understanding the basic physiology, as well as the strengths and limitations of the laboratory testing, and assays available to assess that physiology, is particularly important in the pediatric realm. This chapter covers those aspects of pediatric laboratory medicine for CAH and for growth hormone-related disorders.

TRAINING MODULE

1. Using Figure 12-1 (adrenal steroidogenic pathway), androstenedione is not likely to be elevated in which of the following disorders?
   a. 17-hydroxylase deficiency
   b. 21-hydroxylase deficiency
   c. 11-β-hydroxylase deficiency

2. An elevated 17-OHP result on a newborn screen:
   a. Indicates a diagnosis of CAH
   b. Suggests the need for follow-up testing
   c. Rules out CAH
   d. Suggests interferences from other steroid forms

3. Which of the following does not cause variability in IGF-1 measurements?
   a. patient going on a strict diet
   b. pulsatile release of IGF-1
   c. IGF-1 binding to its binding proteins
   d. differences in antibodies in immunoassays

REFERENCES

1. Shackleton CH, Marcos J. 2011 GC/MS steroid profiling: diagnosis of disorders affecting steroid synthesis and metabolism. In: Gross M, Caprioli R, eds. *The Encyclopedia of Mass Spectrometry*. Vol 8. Amsterdam:Elsevier;789-813

2. Krone N, Hughes BA, Lavery GG, Stewart PM, Arlt W, Shackleton CH. Gas chromatography/mass spectrometry (GC/MS) remains a pre-eminent discovery tool in clinical steroid investigations even in the era of fast liquid chromatography tandem mass spectrometry (LC/MS/MS). *J Steroid Biochem Mol Biol*. 2010;121:496-504

3. Wong T, Shackleton CHL, Covey TR, Ellis G. Identification of the steroids in neonatal plasma that interfere with 17alpha-hydroxyprogesterone radioimmunoassays. *Clin Chem*. 1992;38:1830-1837.

4. Fingerhut R. False positive rate in newborn screening for congenital adrenal hyperplasia (CAH) – ether extraction reveals two distinct reasons for elevated 17alpha-hydroxyprogesterone (17-OHP) values. *Steroids.* 2009;74:662-665.

5. Maeda M, Arakawa H, Tsuji, A, et al. Enzyme-linked immunosorbent assay for 17alpha-hydroxyprogesterone in dried blood spotted on filter paper. *Clin Chem.* 1987;33:761-764.

6. Broussaud J, Barat p, Gualde D, Corcuff JB Cross reactions elicited by serum 17-OH progesterone and 11-desoxycortisol in cortisol assays. *Clin Chim Acta.* 2009;407:72-74.

7. Krasowski JD, Drees D, Corris CS, et al. Cross-reactivity of steroid hormone immunoassays: clinical significance and two-dimensional molecular similarity prediction. *BMC Clin Pathol.* 2014;14:33.

8. Lacey JM, Minutti CZ, Magera MJ, et al. Improved specificity of newborn screening for congenital adrenal hyperplasia by second-tier steroid profiling using tandem mass spectrometry. *Clin Chem.* 2004;50:621-625.

9. Sarafoglou K, Banks K, Kyllo J, Pittock S, Thomas W. Cases of congenital adrenal hyperplasia missed by newborn screening in Minnesota. *JAMA.* 2012; 307:2371-2374.

10. Rosenbloom AL, Deeb L, Allen L, Pollock B. Characteristics of pediatric endocrinology practice: a workforce study. *Endocrinologist.* 1998;8:213-218.

11. Yakar S, Liu JL, Stannard B, Butler A, Accilli D, Sauer B, LeRoith D. Normal growth and development in the absence of hepatic insulin-like growth factor I. *Proc Natl Acad Sci USA.* 1999;96:7324-7329.

12. Thomsett MJ. The spectrum of clinical paediatric endocrinology: 28 years of referrals to an individual consultant. *J Paediatr Child Health.* 2010;46:304-309.

13. Haymond M, Kappelgaard A-M, Czernichow P, et al. Early recognition of growth abnormalities permitting early intervention. *Acta Paediatrica.* 2013:102:787-796.

14. Wolff DJ, Van Dyke DL, Powell CM. Laboratory guideline for Turner syndrome. *Genet Med.* 2010;12:52-55.

15. Clemmons DR. Commercial assays available for insulin-like growth factor I and their use in diagnosing growth hormone deficiency. *Horm Res.* 2001;55(suppl 2):73-79.

16. Cox HD, Lopes F, Woldemariam GA, et al. Interlaboratory agreement of insulin-like growth factor 1 concentrations measured by mass spectrometry. *Clin Chem.* 2014;60:541-548

17. Gomez-Gomez C, Iglesias EM, Barallat J, et al. Lack of transferability between two automated immunoassays for serum IGF-I measurement. Clin Lab 2014;60: 1859-1864.

18. Blankenstein O, Pedersen BT, Schlump M, et al. Management and interpretation of heterogeneous observational data: using insulin-like growth factor-I data from the NordiNet International Outcome study. *Growth Horm IGF Res.* 2015;25:41-46.

19. Brabant G, von zur MA, Wuster C, et al. Serum insulin-like growth factor I reference values for an automated chemiluminescence immunoassay system: results from a multicenter study. *Horm Res.* 2003;60:53-60.

20. Vastergaard P, Hoeck HC, Jakobsen PE, Laurberg P. Reproducibility of growth hormone and cortisol responses to the insulin tolerance test and the short ACTH test in normal adults. *Horm Metab Res.* 1997;29:106-110.

21. Lee HS, Hwang JS. Influence of body mass index on growth hormone responses to classic provocative tests in children with short stature. *Neuroendocrinology.* 2011;93:259-264.

MOLECULAR DIAGNOSTIC TESTING | 13

Jason Y. Park and Jason Wang

LEARNING OBJECTIVES

1. Know key technology platforms for performing DNA-based clinical tests
2. Learn specific examples of diseases that are tested by DNA-based technologies
3. Recognize the future potential of DNA technology in the clinical laboratory based on recent historical developments

INTRODUCTION

The discovery of the structure of deoxyribonucleic acid (DNA) by Watson and Crick in 1953 revolutionized the science of genetics.[1] Knowledge of the structure of DNA enabled a basic understanding of how genetic information is encoded and inherited. In addition, this discovery was the starting point of modern molecular diagnostic technology. Examination of the 60 years since the Watson and Crick publication shows an initially slow, but steady pace of innovation, leading to the sequencing of the first human genome (Table 13-1). In the 15 years since the completion of the first human genome draft, there has been an explosion of novel technologies which have been commercialized and implemented in the clinical laboratory. Here, we review the technologies, both old and new, that are utilized in today's clinical laboratory and give examples of their clinical utility in the pediatric population.

Table 13-1	TIMELINE OF KEY EVENTS IN DNA TECHNOLOGY
Year	**Event**
1953	James Watson and Francis Crick's publication of the double helix structure of DNA
1977	Frederick Sanger invents DNA sequencing based on radioactively labeled chain-terminating inhibitors
1983	Kary Mullis invents polymerase chain reaction (PCR)
1986-87	Heat stable DNA polymerase (*Thermus aquaticus*) used for polymerase chain reaction[31,32]
1985-86	Leroy Hood invents DNA sequencing based on fluorescently labeled chain terminating inhibitors; Automated DNA sequencers commercialized by Applied Biosystems
1987	First thermal cycler for automated PCR, DNA Thermal Cycler TC1, commercialized by Perkin Elmer
1989	Carl Wittwer invents automated PCR based on capillary tubes with air-based temperature cycling; basis of the Lightcycler real-time PCR instrument commercialized by Roche[33]
1990	Human Genome Project begins
1991	Stephen Fodor invents photolithographic synthesis of high density peptide arrays; technology commercialized by Affymetrix
1996	ABI PRISM 7700 real-time PCR instrument commercialized by Applied Biosystems
1999	Nucleic acid detection in electrified alpha-hemolysin channels; precursor to synthetic nanopore sequencing
2000	Human Genome Project produces first working draft
2001	Solexa sequences the bacteriophage phiX-174 by massively parallel sequencing (aka sequencing by synthesis, foundation of the current Illumina next-generation sequencing technology)
2005	454 Life Sciences launches GS20, the first next-generation sequencer; 454 acquired by Roche in 2007 – 454 systems planned for discontinuation in 2016
2006	Solexa launches the Genome Analyzer; Solexa acquired by Illumina in 2007
2007	Applied Biosystems launches the SOLiD next generation sequencing system
2009	Pacific Biosciences launches single-molecule real-time sequencing (SMRT) platform, PacBio RS
2010	Ion Torrent Systems launches semiconductor-based DNA sequencing platform, the Ion Personal Genome Machine; Ion Torrent acquired by Life Technologies
2014	Illumina launches the HiSeq X Ten which has the specifications to sequence 18,000 human genomes per year at ~$1,000 per genome

CURRENT LABORATORY WORK FLOW

Before we review the technology used in modern clinical molecular genetic laboratories, it is important to emphasize workflow and the prevention of contamination in laboratories that perform nucleic acid testing.[2] Contamination is a serious hazard in the molecular genetic laboratory and can be costly to troubleshoot and correct, delay important clinical results, and even result in incorrect diagnoses. In order to minimize the risk of contamination, molecular genetic laboratories typically have a unidirectional workflow, which means that specimens and personnel move in only one direction. In general, labs are physically separated into pre-Polymerase Chain Reaction (PCR) and post-PCR areas. In the pre-PCR areas, specimens are received, DNA is extracted, and PCR mixtures are prepared. Even before the pre-PCR area, there is typically another physically separate space where oligonucleotide primers, polymerases, and other necessary reaction components are stored and prepared; this area is kept free of template nucleic acids (specimens and extracted DNA). In the post-PCR area, the thermocyclers and other analyzers are still utilized for routine DNA testing (eg, viral DNA detection) as well as the foundation for complex assays, such as massively parallel sequencing. Reactions, reagents, and materials from the post-PCR area do not cross back into the pre-PCR area. Similarly, specimens and extracted DNA from the pre-PCR area do not enter the area of the laboratory where primers and polymerases are stored and prepared. These space limitations were originally very strict in the early days of exclusively manual processes. However, modern laboratory instrumentation in the molecular diagnostics laboratory may internally combine pre-PCR and post-PCR areas into a single sample cartridge. In addition, rather than having separate rooms for each of these processes, the physically separate areas may be comprised of hooded or dedicated workbenches. Regardless of the instrumentation or physical layout, laboratorians should be cognizant of the need to take precautions to avoid cross-contamination of target or amplified nucleic acids.

TECHNOLOGIES USED IN MOLECULAR GENETICS LABORATORIES

Polymerase Chain Reaction (Figure 13-1)[3,4]

Polymerase chain reaction (PCR) is the workhorse technology for most molecular diagnostic technologies including the detection of point mutations, recognition of viral nucleic acids, and sequencing of human genes. PCR exponentially amplifies DNA through the utilization of a heat-stable DNA

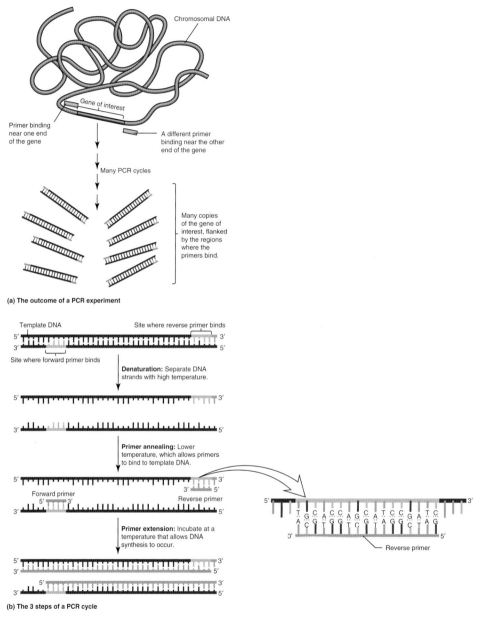

Figure 13-1 ■ Polymerase chain reaction schematic. A. The outcome of a PCR experiment: PCR performed with primers directed at a gene of interest within the chromosomal DNA result in many copies of the gene of interest. B. The three steps of a PCR cycle: First, double stranded DNA template is denatured with heat. Next, the temperature is lowered to allow the forward and reverse primers to anneal to their respective sites. Lastly, the reaction is incubated at a temperature that allows DNA polymerase to synthesize a new double stranded fragment of DNA by extending the primer, producing the complement of the template strand. Reprinted with permission from Brooker RJ, *Genetics: Analysis and Principles*, 4th ed. Figure 18.5.

polymerase and oligonucleotide primers, which are complementary to DNA within or flanking the area of interest. For a PCR reaction with a single target, two primers are required, named the forward and reverse primers. The primers bind to their target sequence and then a heat-stable DNA polymerase, frequently *Taq* polymerase, elongates the primers creating new fragments of DNA composed of one original strand of DNA and its newly synthesized complement. These newly synthesized DNA fragments then serve as templates for the creation of subsequent fragments of DNA. Thus, with each cycle of the reaction, PCR doubles the amount of targeted DNA in the reaction mixture. Twenty cycles of PCR can theoretically multiply a single double-stranded template into over a million copies, 2^{20} to be exact. PCR is a simple but elegant technique, which mimics the biological machinery used for in vivo DNA replication.

A more detailed examination of PCR reveals that the basic components for a reaction are: 1. DNA template, 2. oligonucleotide primers directed at the portion of DNA of interest, 3. heat-stable DNA polymerase, 4. pH buffered solution, 5. deoxynucleotides (dNTP's), and 6. divalent cations (eg, Mg^{2+}). PCR consists of multiple cycles that double the number of DNA fragments targeted by the primers. Each cycle is composed of the following steps: denaturing, annealing, and extension/elongation, and each step is achieved with a change in temperature. In the first step, the reaction mixture is heated to $> 98°C$, denaturing the double stranded DNA template in the reaction mixture; this high temperature requires the polymerase in the reaction to be heat-stable. Next, the temperature is lowered to the annealing temperature; this is the temperature at which complementary oligonucleotide primers bind to the target template. The annealing temperature can be slightly raised or lowered to change the specificity of the reaction. Raising the annealing temperature increases the specificity and lowering the annealing temperature decreases the specificity. The temperature is then changed to the ideal extension temperature of the DNA polymerase ($\sim72°C$ for *Taq* polymerase). The DNA polymerase incorporates the free deoxynucleotides in the reaction mixture and extends the new strand of DNA along the DNA template strand. *Taq* polymerase can replicate DNA at the rate of approximately 35-100 nucleotides per second. The time that the reaction mixture spends at each step can vary by protocols depending on the polymerase used, the concentration of DNA template or primers, or the length of the DNA fragment being targeted for analysis. Typical PCR times for each step are 20-30 seconds for denaturation, 20-40 seconds for annealing, and 1 minute per 1000 bases synthesized for the extension step. After the completion of each cycle, the newly synthesized strand can serve as a template strand in the next cycle, thus allowing for the exponential amplification of the targeted fragment of DNA. Also, PCR protocols typically have a prolonged final extension step to insure all DNA fragments are fully extended. At the completion of the reaction, the products are held at 4°C. In many clinical laboratories, PCR is run on thermocyclers: metal blocks that hold reaction plates which can quickly and accurately change the temperature of the reaction plates based on a programmed protocol. Some PCR assay systems are part of a larger automation apparatus that includes DNA extraction, sample set-up, and detection of amplification. There are even FDA approved molecular assays that combine all of these steps into a single small disposable cartridge no larger than an Apple iPhone.

PCR is a versatile tool in the laboratory that has many different formats. In end-point PCR, the post-PCR amplified DNA is interrogated by gel electrophoresis and the interpretation can be based upon the presence, absence, or size of the PCR product.

Real-time PCR involves a reaction in which the products can be examined during or after every cycle. With real-time PCR, a fluorescent probe is included in the reaction mixture that can either detect a specific sequence of DNA or simply detect the presence of DNA (Figure 13-2). The intensity of the fluorescent signal is proportional to the amount of target in the reaction. Utilization of a set of calibration standards in conjunction with real-time PCR allows for the quantification of the starting material. Reverse-transcription PCR allows for the detection of RNA by adding a reverse transcriptase to the reaction. The reverse transcriptase converts RNA into DNA, which then serves as the template for traditional PCR with one of the detection methods previously mentioned.

A clinical example of the utility of PCR in the clinical lab is the qualitative and quantitative testing of viral nucleic acids. In pediatric hospitals, testing for enterovirus in CSF specimens is qualitative and is a common request for clinical laboratories because enterovirus is the most common cause of viral meningitis, particularly during the summer months. Rapid detection of enterovirus in the CSF of a patient with meningitis can lead to significant cost savings in the health care setting as patients do not typically require further medical therapy. On the other hand, patients with bacterial meningitis require prompt treatment with antibiotics and frequent hospital admission. By using PCR, Enterovirus can be rapidly detected in CSF within several hours.[5] A positive Enterovirus by PCR in the CSF of a patient suspected of having meningitis can spare that patient a hospital admission as well as unnecessary antibiotics and save healthcare dollars.

Testing for Epstein-Barr virus (EBV) is performed by PCR as a quantitative test. In the pediatric transplant population, it can be used to diagnose, monitor, and prevent post-transplant lymphoproliferative disorder (PTLD), a hematologic disorder frequently caused by EBV. EBV remains in a subset of lymphocytes after primary exposure/infection and is normally kept latent by a healthy immune system. However, patients with organ and bone marrow transplants are maintained on immunosuppression that may allow for the

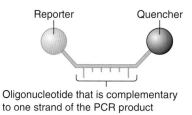

Oligonucleotide that is complementary
to one strand of the PCR product

(a) TaqMan detector

During the primer annealing step, both a primer and TaqMan
detector bind to the template DNA.

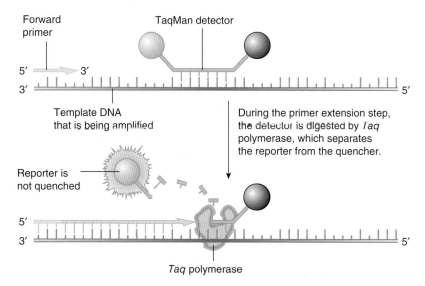

(b) Use of a TaqMan detector in real-time PCR

Figure 13-2 ▪ Real-time PCR utilizes continuously monitoring of the enzymatic reaction and DNA amplification. One method for detection in real-time PCR is the TaqMan chemistry. In this method, an oligonucleotide probe is constructed that is complementary to one strand of the PCR product which is downstream from the primer binding site. The probe is flanked on one end by a reporter fluorophore dye and on the other by a quencher dye. When the probe is intact, the proximity of the quencher to the reporter allows it to quench, or absorb, the energy (light) emitted by the reporter at a specific wavelength. This probe is added to the real-time PCR mixture and binds to its target during the annealing step. During the extension/elongation step, the Taq polymerase (which also has 5'-3' exonuclease activity) digests the oligonucleotide probe, releasing the reporter from the quencher. Now, the energy in the form of light emitted from the reporter can be detected. In the TaqMan method, fluorescence is measured during the extension step before the denaturation step that initiates the next cycle. Reprinted with permission from Brooker RJ, *Genetics: Analysis and Principles*, 4th ed. Figure 18.8.

reactivation of EBV, which can then cause PTLD. EBV viral loads, typically reported in copies/mL, can rise quickly and are usually very high in patients with PTLD caused by EBV and decrease with effective treatment.

Restriction Enzyme-based Assay (Figure 13-3)

Restriction enzymes (RE) are enzymes which were first discovered in bacteria and can cut DNA at specific sequences (recognition sites). In nature, bacteria use RE's as a defense mechanism against bacteriophages.[6] In the laboratory, RE's can be utilized for molecular and genetic testing. RE's recognize and cut at specific sites based on the DNA sequence. The recognition sites (sequence motifs) are usually 4-8 nucleotides in length and are frequently inverted repeat palindromes where the recognition site reads the same forwards as the complementary strand reads backwards. RE's are very specific and a single nucleotide change in the recognition site will typically result in a lack of DNA cleavage. This property of RE's can be utilized in the laboratory to detect single nucleotide mutations, small insertions, and deletions, or differentiate between DNA strands.

Clinical tests based on RE PCR begin by amplifying a fragment of DNA which contains the region of interest using PCR or reverse-transcription PCR. The amplified DNA is then subjected to a specific restriction enzyme digestion. Depending upon the design of the test, a single nucleotide mutation or the insertion or deletion of a small number of nucleotides may introduce or remove a RE recognition or cleavage site. The resulting reaction mixture can then be separated by agarose gel electrophoresis and the products can be visualized. If a mutation/insertion/deletion adds a RE site, two smaller fragments of DNA would indicate the presence of the mutation and a single larger fragment of DNA would indicate the mutation was not present in the original template DNA or RNA. The reverse is true if a mutation/insertion/deletion removes a RE site. The use of RE's is not limited to detecting mutations/insertions/deletions. With the use of a combination of RE's, the fragment size pattern produced can be used to identify specific genes.

An example of the clinical utility of RE's in the pediatric population is in the differentiation of highly homologous genes. The human pulmonary surfactant genes *SFTPA1* and *SFTPA2* are distinct genes with 98% homology in their sequence which encodes the protein.[7] Special PCR reactions tailored to amplifying long sequences can be used to amplify the entire gene (5-10,000 bp). These long sequence fragments can then be RE digested to determine the identity of the amplified fragment. When the RE *EcoRV* is used, fragmentation patterns specific to *SFTPA1* or *SFTPA2* are generated (Figure 13-4). The *SFPTA1* gene product is digested in three fragments of 7883 base pairs (bp), 1243 bp, and 759 bp. In comparison, the *SFTPA2* gene product is digested into three fragments of 5082 bp, 3432 bp, and 1339 bp.

Restriction enzymes frequently used in gene cloning		
Restriction enzyme	**Bacterial source**	**Sequence recognized**
BamHI	Bacillus amyloliquifaciens H	↓ 5′-GGATTC-3′ 3′-CCTAGG-5′ ↑
ClaI	Caryophanon latum	↓ 5′-ATCGAT-3′ 3′-TAGCTA-5′ ↑
EcoRI	E. Coli RY13	↓ 5′-GAATTC-3′ 3′-CTTAAG-5′ ↑
NaeI	Nocardia aerocolonigenes	↓ 5′-GCCGGC-3′ 3′-GACGTC-5′ ↑
PstI	Providencia stuartii	↓ 5′-CTGCAG-3′ 3′-GACGTC-5′ ↑
SacI	Streptomyces achromonogenes	↓ 5′-GAGCTC-3′ 3′-CTCGAG-5′ ↑

Figure 13-3 ■ Restriction enzymes recognize specific DNA motifs. This figure shows the names of the bacteria from which the restriction enzymes were discovered, sequence motifs recognized, and cleavage sites of a select number of restriction enzymes. The DNA sequence motifs are inverted repeat palindromes (ie, the forward strand is the same as the reverse of the complementary strand). The arrows in the far right column indicate the cleavage sites. The cleavage site for *NaeI* results in no overhang between the forward and reverse strands: *blunt end*. The cleavage sites for the other restriction enzymes in the table result in overhangs between the forward and reverse strands: *sticky ends*. Adapted from Table 18.3. Brooker RJ. *Genetics Analysis and Principles*, 4th ed.

The use of RE patterns is helpful in determining not only the identity of the gene, but can also be used to detect the presence of nucleotide variation at the restriction site and the possible presence of deletions or duplications in the gene. Changes to the nucleotides which comprise the RE target size will create different patterns for RE digestion from the wild-type state.

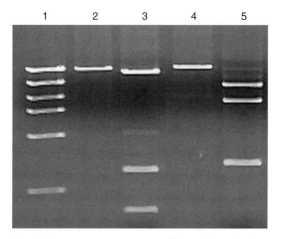

Figure 13-4 ▪ Restriction enzyme assay to differentiate the homologous genes *SFTPA1* and *SFTPA1*. *EcoRV* is used to digest long range PCR products amplifying the *SFTPA1* and *SFTPA2* genes. The genes are 98% identical in their coding DNA regions, but generate restriction enzyme products that are distinct in size. Lane 1: DNA Ladder, the fragment sizes from largest (top) to smallest (bottom) are 10,000 bp, 6,000 bp, 4,000 bp, 3,000 bp, 2,000 bp and 1,000 bp. Lane 2: PCR amplified product of *SFTPA1*. Lane 3: *SFTPA1* amplified product digested into three fragments. Lane 4: PCR amplified product of *SFTPA2*. Lane 5: *SFTPA2* amplified product digested into three fragments.

Hybridization Assay[8]

The complementary nature of DNA can be utilized for molecular testing with hybridization arrays. In this technology, single stranded capture DNA probes are immobilized to a solid surface, such as a nitrocellulose membrane. The capture DNA probes are arranged in bands in a known pattern across the membrane. The assay begins with the selective amplification of certain portions of target DNA or reverse transcription and amplification of certain portions of target RNA with PCR or reverse transcription PCR, respectively. During this amplification, biotin, a B-vitamin with a strong affinity for streptavidin, is incorporated into the newly synthesized fragments of DNA. The specifically amplified DNA is then denatured and incubated with the solid surface which has been coated with DNA capture probes. The incubation allows biotinylated DNA that is complementary to the DNA capture probes to bind to the membrane. The unbound DNA is then washed off of the membrane, leaving behind only the portions of patient DNA complementary to the probes bound to the membrane. In order to visualize which bands of DNA probes have captured complementary DNA targets, the membrane is bathed in a solution containing streptavidin that is bound to alkaline phosphatase. Streptavidin binds to the biotin which has been incorporated in the amplified patient DNA. Alkaline phosphatase is an enzyme commonly used in chromogenic reactions to produce a colored product after dephosphorylation of a substrate. The captured, biotinylated patient DNA binds streptavidin-alkaline phosphatase molecules. The membrane is again washed to remove excess, unbound streptavidin-alkaline phosphatase. The chromogenic reaction substrate is then incubated with the membrane and the bands that captured target DNA, and subsequently captured streptavidin-alkaline phosphatase molecules, will convert the substrate into a colored product which can be visualized. The unbound substrate is again washed away and the pattern of bands is used to interpret the assay. This technology has many applications in the molecular pathology lab, including testing for cystic fibrosis, *Mycobacterium tuberculosis* testing with simultaneous identification of multidrug resistance, and Hepatitis C genotyping. These tests can be time and labor intensive and can only detect known mutations/variants that are targeted by the test. These tests are also known as line probe assays. Cystic fibrosis, a relatively common inherited disorder primarily affecting the lungs and gastrointestinal tract, is an autosomal recessive disease. Most patients are diagnosed in early childhood and genetic testing is important for examining potential carrier status in reproductive planning. Line probe/hybridization is one of many methods of examining the 23 mutations recommended by ACMG/ACOG. The sensitivity of the recommended 23 mutation assays as screening tests is dependent on the ethnicity of the patient: the detection rate may be as low as 49% in Asian Americans or as high as 94% in Ashkenazi Jews.[9] Testing of the 23 mutations for diagnosing cystic fibrosis may also occur in the context of evaluating a patient with a positive sweat chloride screening test.

HLA Testing

Another test that is frequently performed in the pediatric setting, although not unique to pediatric patients, is HLA testing. The human leukocyte antigen (HLA) complex is located on chromosome 6 and plays a vital role in immune system recognition of self versus foreign. Individual HLA alleles are complex multi-single nucleotide polymorphism (SNP) haplotypes, each comprised of up to 60 individual SNPs. Specific HLA alleles can be associated with various diseases or drug hypersensitivity. HLA alleles are also very important in bone marrow and solid organ transplant as matching donor and recipient HLA alleles is important to minimize host rejection of donor tissue.

HLA testing methods vary, but a common technique which is currently widely used in patient and donor HLA genotyping is a bead-based reverse-sequence-specific oligonucleotide assay. This method is similar to the concepts seen in a hybridization assay or DNA microarray. Sample DNA is extracted and HLA loci are amplified with specific primers. The amplified DNA is then hybridized to oligonucleotides which are bound to microscopic beads of various colors. The beads are incorporated with various known proportions of two different dyes. All of the beads of one color (a specific proportion of dyes) are coated with the same oligonucleotide and different colors are coated with different oligonucleotides. Amplified DNA that has hybridized to capture oligonucleotides is then detected with a fluorescent dye. The beads are then run through an analyzer with detectors based on flow cytometric technology. When a fluorescent signal (produced as a result of DNA hybridized to capture oligonucleotides) is detected, the proportions of dyes in the bead can be simultaneously detected and recorded. The proportions of dyes indicates to which oligonucleotide(s) the DNA has hybridized.[10]

HLA testing can also be performed by sequencing, either with traditional Sanger sequencing methods or with next generation techniques. No matter which method is used, the data are then analyzed to assign an HLA genotype. Because a number of SNPs are taken together to categorize a single HLA allele, the analysis of SNP results can be an arduous task, but is now significantly automated.

Melt Curve Assay[11]

DNA is double-stranded and the strands can be separated by heat. The temperature at which 50% of DNA strands are dissociated is named the melting point of DNA. The melting point of DNA is determined by the length of the fragment, the proportion of guanine to cytosine (G-C) base pairs compared to adenine-to thymine (A-T) base pairs within the DNA fragment, and complementarity of the two strands of DNA. G-C base pairings have 3 hydrogen bonds, one more than A-T base pairings, and thus require more energy in the form of heat to dissociate. A fragment of DNA with more G-C base pairings, or a higher G-C content, will require more heat to dissociate. The longer the fragment of DNA, the more hydrogen bonds holding it together and the more heat required to dissociate the two strands. The complementarity, or the appropriateness of the base pairings between complementary strands, is the last factor determining the amount of heat required to dissociate DNA. A double-stranded fragment of DNA that is 100% complementary requires more heat to dissociate than another fragment of DNA of the same length with the same G-C content but with one base pairing that is not complementary, because the non-complementary base pairing does not form stable hydrogen bonds. These properties determining melting point temperatures can be utilized for genetic testing.

Melt curve analysis is accomplished by first amplifying the DNA fragment of interest. Then, a method is employed to visualize DNA, typically a DNA intercalating fluorophore which is fluorescent when intercalated in double stranded DNA. The fluorophore is interrogated as increasing heat is applied and as the two strands are dissociated, there is a decrease in the fluorescent intensity of the reaction mixture. The intensity of the fluorescence is displayed as a graph of the intensity versus temperature. Two reactions with DNA fragments that contain one base pair difference (A-T vs G-C at one locus) will produce characteristic melting curves that differ slightly from one another. A heterogeneous reaction with both of these DNA fragments will produce a melt curve with a characteristic shape that falls between the other curves. This occurs because there is a mixture of double stranded DNA fragments. Some are 100% complementary with an A-T at the variable locus. Other fragments are 100% complementary with a G-C at the variable locus. However, there is a third population of double stranded DNA fragments that are not completely complementary, but instead have a A-C or G-T pairing that fails to produce stable hydrogen bonds, so called heteroduplexes, which impart a characteristic shape to the melting curve. Melting curves can be utilized to detect point mutations and single nucleotide polymorphisms, if the curves are detectably different.

Another utilization of the melting curve is to verify the production of a single specific product in a real time PCR assay that utilizes an intercalating dye for amplification detection. Intercalating dyes are not sequence specific, but will produce a fluorescent signal when bound to any double-stranded DNA. The addition of a melt curve after completion of a real time PCR assay allows for the verification of the production of only one amplicon, based on the number of peaks produced in the melt curve, and can be helpful with the specificity of the amplicon as the expected target should have a characteristic melt curve, both in terms of the melting temperature and the shape of the curve. The FilmArray multiplexed assay system (BioFire, Salt Lake City, UT) utilizes melt curve analysis for the identification of multiple target sequences in parallel. The FilmArray system is a fully automated system that uses multiplex, nested PCR, real time PCR, and a melt curve to rapidly detect multiple pathogens in a single patient sample. The system begins with extraction and purification of nucleic acids. This is followed by a first-stage PCR which is a single, large volume PCR that is massively multiplexed, amplifying many DNA targets at the same time with a mixture of primers. Next is a second-stage PCR which takes the product of the first-stage PCR and separates it into multiple specific individual real-time PCR's which are analyzed to detect specific pathogens. This real-time PCR uses an intercalating dye to detect amplicon production. At the end of the reaction, a melt curve is utilized to verify the production of a single amplicon as well as the expected melting temperature of the specific amplicon. FilmArray offers a number of panels which are FDA-cleared, and are for various purposes including evaluation of respiratory or gastrointestinal illnesses or characterization of positive blood cultures. Respiratory infections are a common disease of pediatric patients, and some severe infections require hospitalization and intravenous antibiotics. The FilmArray respiratory panel is employed in many pediatric settings to allow for rapid detection of 20 viral and bacterial respiratory pathogens to allow for quick and appropriate treatment of acutely ill pediatric patients.

Sanger Sequencing

Sanger sequencing was developed in 1977 by Fredrick Sanger.[12] It takes advantage of the property of dideoxynucleotides (ddNTP's: ddATP, ddGTP, ddCTP, ddTTP) to terminate elongation of DNA when they are incorporated onto a newly synthesized strand. The dideoxynucleotides lack the 3' hydroxyl group, which is essential for the formation of the phosphodiester bond that is required for addition of the next nucleotide. The original assay developed by Fredrick Sanger used dideoxynucleotides labeled with radioactive molecules. These labeled ddNTPs are added, in limited quantities, to a typical PCR reaction with an excess of DNA polymerase, dNTPs, divalent cations, buffer, and one primer. When a ddNTP is incorporated into an elongating, newly synthesized strand of DNA in the PCR reaction, the new strand is terminated. After the PCR is completed, the reaction is run on an electrophoretic gel with a high resolution, separating the fragments which vary in size by as little as 1 base pair. In the radioactive Sanger assay, each of the four types of dideoxynucleotides had the same labeling molecule and therefore had to be run in separate reactions and resolved in separate lanes in a gel.

In the 1980s, Leroy Hood revolutionized two aspects of Sanger sequencing: first, the dideoxynucleotides used fluorescent labels, each ddNTP with a different fluorophore; second, he created the automated DNA sequencer based on loading the fluorescently labeled fragments into single wells of an acrylamide gel. Later, the slab gel was replaced with an array of capillaries for electrophoresis. This allowed for sequencing of one DNA fragment to occur in one high resolution capillary where a DNA ladder is produced, composed of fragments with size variations of 1 base pair that are separated from one another and pass across a fluorescent detector; the color of the fluorescent signal correlating to the specific ddNTP added at that length of DNA. If a patient is heterozygous for a single nucleotide variant, Sanger sequencing will produce less intense peaks of two different colors at the same nucleotide position. The sensitivity for detection of point mutations by Sanger sequencing is approximately 10%; this means that a mutation must be present in 10% of sequenced DNA in order to be detected by Sanger sequencing. Large homozygous deletions and insertions in areas targeted for Sanger sequencing may not produce any sequencing results and large heterozygous deletions and insertions will likely be obscured by the non-deleted allele. Translocations involving a gene targeted for Sanger sequencing will also likely go undetected, as the forward and reverse prim-ers used for the amplification will be on separate chromosomes; too far apart to amplify. Sanger sequencing is a useful methodology for identifying point mutations and small insertions/deletions. It is currently considered the gold-standard method for sequencing, and automated Sanger sequencers provided the vast majority of sequencing capacity for the human genome project.

In the pediatric population, Sanger sequencing remains very effective for testing patients with suspected rare diseases caused by a point mutation or small insertion/deletion in one or a few possible genes. One specific example is Smith-Lemli-Opitz Syndrome, a developmental disorder caused by mutations in the *DHCR7* gene. This gene encodes an enzyme that is involved in choles-terol synthesis. Mutations in the gene cause insufficient cholesterol production and buildup of toxic by-products of the cholesterol synthesis pathway and lead to characteristic facial features, intellectual disability, behavioral problems, microcephaly, and various physical and organ malformations.

Sanger sequencing is also very effective for testing family members of a patient with a known point mutation or small insertion/deletion to deter-mine if those family members are affected with, carriers of, or negative for the disorder. The utility of Sanger sequencing in clinical laboratories has become diminished in recent years with the advent of next-generation DNA sequenc-ing (NGS). The rapid output of high quality sequencing data from NGS has moved the examination of large numbers of genes for a single patient from Sanger sequencing to NGS. Indeed, with gene panels and clinical exome tests, Sanger sequencing is becoming limited to a role as a confirmatory test second-ary to NGS or as a targeted test for the examination of relatives of a proband.

Karyotype[13]

One of the earliest forms of clinical genetic testing in humans is the karyotype. In order to produce a karyotype, living cells are first cultured and then arrested in cell division. A hypotonic solution is introduced to the cells causing red blood cells to lyse and the nucleated white blood cells to swell. The swollen white blood cells are separated from the solution and placed on a slide, dried, and then stained to visualize the chromosome bands. Giemsa and quinacrine are two examples of stains that can be utilized in karyotyping. In modern cyto-genetics laboratories, the slides are digitally analyzed and the chromosomes are arranged based on their sizes and characteristic banding patterns. The res-olution of a karyotype is the number of total bands that can be identified and depends on how condensed the chromosomes are and at what stage of mitosis the cells are arrested. High resolution karyotypes can produce 1200-2000 total bands resulting in bands that have as little as 1.5 megabases (Mb) of DNA, while lower resolution karyotypes typically produce around 300 total bands with 7-10 Mb of DNA per band. Typically, karyotyping can detect changes as small as 5-10 Mb. Analysis of a single patient sample usually involves examining the karyotypes of at least 20 cells from that sample. The traditional karyotype can detect large insertions and deletion, translocations, and absence or addition of chromosomes. Disadvantages of karyotype tests are that the technique is time consuming, labor intensive, requires living cells, and misses deletions, insertions, and translocations that are smaller than 5-10 Mb.

Karyotype can be used effectively and efficiently in the pediatric population. Many inherited conditions are caused by chromosomal changes large enough to be visualized by karyotype, including loss or gain of whole chromosomes like Turner Syndrome (Monosomy X) and Down Syndrome (Trisomy 21). Karyotype is frequently pursued in a variety of pediatric patients with syndromic phenotypes (characteristic facies, developmental abnormalities, constellation of malformations, etc.).

Karyotypes are also performed in pediatric tumors, especially hematologic malignancies, which are frequently characterized or categorized based on specific karyotype abnormalities. Certain changes can also predict behavior of the malignancy or alter the prognosis. One example is the presence of a Philadelphia chromosome, t (9; 22), and a balanced translocation between the long arms of chromosomes 9 and 22, which can often be detected by karyotype of tumor cells. Its presence is a high risk feature when observed in pediatric acute lymphoblastic leukemia and predicts that chemotherapy alone will be insufficient for cure.

Microarrays (Figure 13-5)[14,15]

DNA microarrays allow for the simultaneous interrogation of millions of fragments of DNA. Sequence-specific oligonucleotide probes are bound to a solid surface, such as glass or plastic. The probes are clustered in micro spots, each micro spot contains the same probes, and millions of spots are placed on a single chip in an orderly, known pattern.

The patient DNA is purified and then is minimally amplified. During the amplification, the DNA is labeled with a fluorophore and washed over the chip and hybridizes to probes for which they are complementary. The chip is washed, removing unbound and weakly bound DNA fragments. After completion of the hybridization reaction, the chip is scanned and the strength of the signal of each spot is compared to a reference standard. DNA microarrays are utilized to detect copy number variations (deletions and duplications) and single nucleotide polymorphisms, but cannot identify balanced translocations. The two major types of microarrays currently in clinical use are CGH (Comparative Genomic Hybridization) Arrays and Single Nucleotide Polymorphism (SNP) Arrays. CGH Arrays were originally developed by

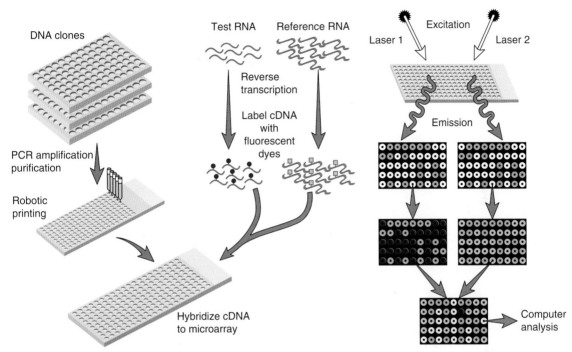

Figure 13-5 ■ Traditional gene expression microarray schematic. DNA oligonucleotide probes are first generated utilizing DNA cloning techniques. These probes are then printed onto a substrate (eg, glass), placing hundreds to millions of microspots on one slide with each microspot composed of the same probe. In this figure, RNA is extracted from the patient sample and a reverse transcription PCR reaction produces amplified cDNA. The figure represents a traditional CGH microarray, so reference RNA is also reverse transcribed and amplified to produce reference cDNA. The cDNA's from the patient and reference are differentially labeled with fluorophores that emit light at different excitation wavelengths and allowed to hybridize to the microarray slide. The slide is washed to remove excess unbound fluorescently labeled cDNA. The slide is then visualized with the two different excitation wavelengths of the fluorophores. The two images are merged and compared by a computer for the intensities of each fluorophore at each microspot. The green spots in this image represent decreased expression in the test sample, the red spots represent increased expression in the test sample, and the yellow spots represent a level of expression similar to the reference sample. In some microarrays, the reference DNA intensities are stored digitally and not physically added to the slide. In these set-ups with digital references, patient samples are hybridized, the fluorescent intensities of the microspots are examined, and the intensities are compared to the digital reference. Reprinted with permission from Willey JM, Sherwood LM, Woolverton CJ. *Prescott's Microbiology*, 8th ed. Figure 16.12.

spotting features comprised not of oligonucleotides, but of fragments from BACs (Bacterial Artificial Chromosomes). Over time, the spotted features became more specific to smaller genomic regions. The CGH Arrays are well suited for determining deletions or duplications in DNA sequence. Currently clinical CGH Arrays are designed to detect not only large structural anomalies, but also small alterations in single exons of a gene. In comparison, SNP arrays target known SNPs within the human genome. These SNP tests are well suited for determining the heterozygosity of a sample and can also detect large deletions. For example, a patient sample can be evaluated for regions of absence of heterozygosity which would identify regions of the genome more vulnerable to genetic disease. Extensive absence of heterozygosity in a single genome is associated with consanguinity.

In 2004, the first microarray system, the AmpliChip Cytochrome P450 Genotyping test was cleared (510k) by the FDA. This assay system by Roche and Affymetrix has over 15,000 oligonucleotide probes to determine 31 DNA variants in two genes (CYP2D6 and CYP2C19). Ten years later (2014), the Cytoscan HD (Affymetrix) was approved for genome wide analysis with the intended use of postnatal detection of copy number variation associated with developmental delay, intellectual disability, congenital anomalies, or dysmorphic features. This device is a high-density SNP array with over 2.7 million probes which can detect deletions as small as 25,000 base pairs. CGH arrays have also evolved and now many clinical CGH arrays are combined with SNP targets; these combined CGH-SNP arrays have not (yet) been submitted for FDA review.

In the pediatric population, microarrays are sometimes used to screen patients with developmental disabilities and/or other neurologic symptoms when the patient does not have a constellation of symptoms or physical findings characteristic for a particular genetic disorder. Various micro-deletions and duplications responsible for disease have complex phenotypes which can manifest with developmental delay or disability as well as congenital malformations. The microarrays can also detect loss of heterozygosity, which, when present throughout the genome, is an indication of consanguinity or parents with high genetic similarity and increases the patient's risk of having inherited an autosomal recessive disorder. The reported diagnostic yield for microarrays is approximately 10-20%.[16,17] Currently, the American College of Medical Genetics and Genomics (ACMG) recommends that microarrays (both array CGH and SNP) are first-line tests for the evaluation of intellectual disability, autism, and multiple congenital anomalies.[18]

Fluorescence in Situ Hybridization[13,19]

Fluorescence in situ hybridization (FISH) is another cytogenetic technique, which is used to investigate the presence or absence of specific sequences of nucleic acid and can be used to identify their locations in relation to other known sequences. The technique uses nucleic acid probes which are specific for the sequence being interrogated. These probes are fluorescently labeled and incubated with cells that have had their DNA denatured. The excess probe is washed off and the cells are visualized to determine if the target DNA is present or absent. FISH is versatile and can be performed on cell cultures, on cells touched onto glass slides, and even on formalin-fixed paraffin embedded (FFPE) tissue.

Not only can FISH detect the presence or absence of specific DNA sequences, but it can also be utilized to detect translocations. In order to accomplish this task, two probes of different colors are used simultaneously and the location of the probes is examined in relation to one another. One specific example of probes used to detect translocations is a break-apart probe. In this design, the two probes, each labeled with a different fluorophore, flank one translocation breakpoint. In a normal cell, the probes are closely approximated next to one another producing two fused signals, one for each homologous chromosome, that are a combination of the two different fluorophores. A translocation at the breakpoint of one chromosome will cause the signals/probes to separate, or break-apart, resulting in two different color signals and one fused signal in the abnormal cell.

FISH testing is critical in pediatric pathology for the evaluation of both solid tumors and hematologic malignancies. Again, some hematologic malignancies are characterized by specific FISH findings (translocations or deletions or duplications), or these changes may represent treatment targets or predict disease behavior. Solid tumors in pediatric patients can also benefit from FISH analysis, as some entities are defined by specific translocations. A specific utilization of FISH in pediatric tumors is the testing of neuroblastomas for *MYCN* amplification. When *MYCN* is amplified in a neuroblastoma, it indicates a high-risk tumor and suggests a poor prognosis for the patient. An example of a disease defining alteration observed in pediatric tumors is a translocation involving the *EWSR1* gene. *EWSR1* rearrangement with certain partner genes defines Ewing sarcoma. However, rearrangement with other partner genes can cause other diseases, such as desmoplastic small round cell tumor, clear cell sarcoma, extraskeletal myxoid chondrosarcoma, and myxoid liposarcomas. A break-apart probe set targeted at the *EWSR1* gene can detect the presence of an *EWSR1* rearrangement in a suspected tumor, however, will not identify the translocation partner. The translocation partner can be detected or sought through additional FISH testing or other molecular techniques like reverse transcription PCR. The DNA product of gene fusions can sometimes be difficult to assess because the exact site of fusion may not be consistent within a region of tens of thousands of bases. Alternatively, the mRNA reverse transcribed from the novel fusion gene arrangement can be reliably assessed by a smaller targeted assay.

Next-generation Sequencing (Figure 13-6)[20-22]

Next Generation Sequencing (NGS) is synonymous with the more descriptive name of massive parallel sequencing, given to the generation of sequencing technologies which became commercially available around 2005. The

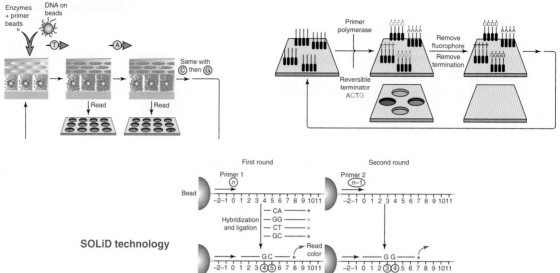

Figure 13-6 ▪ Multiple technologies employed in next-generation sequencing. This figure shows the main chemistry reactions employed by various NGS technologies. In pyrosequencing (Roche 454), a cell composed of hundreds of thousands of microwells are loaded with beads, each bead is coated with many copies of a single DNA target (clonal), enzymes, and primers. Each microwells is only large enough to hold a single bead. dNTPs are sequentially washed across the entire cell and when a nucleotide is incorporated onto the growing strand, a pyrophosphate is released. Enzymes in the microwell convert the pyrophosphate to light. The microwell is monitored by a detector which documents which microwells produce light after addition of specific nucleotides.

Solexa sequencing (Illumina) involves loading fragmented patient DNA onto a glass slide. Through a series of PCR cycles, these fragments generate small clusters of identical and complementary fragments of DNA. The complementary fragments are cleaved and primers, enzymes, and dNTPs with reversible dye terminators are washed across the slide. The slide is then imaged by a charge-coupled device (CCD) to determine the color of the fluorophore that was added to each cluster. Next, a cleavage enzyme is added that cleaves the reversible dye terminator; this is followed by a new cycle of primer, enzyme, and reversible dye terminator dNTP solution which is washed over the slide. These cycles continue for a selected number of times.

SOLiD sequencing technology begins with a set-up similar to pyrosequencing, with the production of clonal beads that have DNA sequencing templates bound by adapter sequences. These clonal beads are deposited onto a glass slide. The actual sequencing reaction begins with hybridization of primers to the adapter sequence. Fluorescently labeled oligonucleotides are added that have specific dinucleotide sequences (CA, GG, CT, etc.) at the 4th and 5th nucleotides and one of four different colored fluorophores. These oligonucleotides compete to bind to the sequencing template strand and those that are complementary to the 4th and 5th position will bind. Next, the newly bound oligonucleotide strand is ligated with a ligase enzyme and the color of the fluorophore is read. The fluorophore is then cleaved and the oligonucleotide mixture is added again, this time binding the complement of the 9th and 10th position. The cycle is repeated for a predetermined number of cycles. Then, the primer with its newly ligated oligonucleotides is melted off of the template and the process is repeated, except with specific dinucleotides at the n-1 (or 3rd and 4th) position. The process is then repeated with n-2, n-3, and n-4 dinucleotides. In this way, each nucleotide is interrogated twice and the color combination at each position indicates the base (since there are 16 dinucleotide combinations and only 4 fluorophores). Reprinted with permission from Willey JM, Sherwood LM, Woolverton CJ. *Prescott's Microbiology*, 8th ed. Figure 16.4.

rapidity and quantity of sequencing accomplished by NGS technologies allow for the sequencing of an entire genome in a single day with a theoretical cost of ~$1,000. In comparison, the Human Genome Project sequenced the first entire human genome in 13 years at a cost of $2.7 billion.

NGS accomplishes this rapid and inexpensive sequencing by simultaneously sequencing billions of short fragments of DNA and using computing power to align the short fragments to a reference genome. There are multiple chemistries which have been developed to achieve massive parallel sequencing. One such method is reversible dye terminator chemistry. In reversible dye terminator chemistry, DNA is fragmented and ligated to two different adapters, one on each end. One of the adapters is used to bind the DNA fragments onto a solid surface with bound oligonucleotides that are complementary to one of the adapters. Primers complementary to the opposite adapter allow sequencing to be initiated. In solution are DNA polymerases and dNTP's which are fluorescently labeled, a different fluorophore for each of the four nucleotides, in a manner which prevents further extension of the newly synthesized DNA. At each cycle, the color of the fluorescent label is collected indicating the base that was added. An enzyme is then added which cleaves the fluorescent label and allows further extension. These steps are repeated and can quickly sequence billions of short fragments of DNA rapidly. After the short fragments of DNA are sequenced, the fragments are compared to a reference genome and aligned to their expected positions within the genome. In this way, aberrations from the genome used for alignment can be identified.

A second major next-generation sequencing technology is based on semiconductor technology. In this method, a semiconductor chip is produced that has an array of millions of microwells. Beneath each microwell is an ion sensitive layer and beneath each ion sensitive layer is an ion sensor. The sensors detect hydrogen ions, which are a by-product that is released when a DNA polymerase adds a nucleotide onto a growing DNA strand. The intensity of the signal detected by the sensor is proportional to the number of nucleotides added to the growing strand. In order to make the reaction massively parallel, microscopic beads, one of which just fits into a microwell, are coated with fragments of a single DNA sequence, each bead covered in one DNA sequence. These beads are then distributed into the microwells on the semiconductor chip. Primers, buffer, polymerase, divalent cations, and nucleotides are washed across the chip with one nucleotide present in solution at a time. The sequential addition of nucleotides and the corresponding release of hydrogen ions indicate the sequence of the DNA fragment coating a bead. Millions of microwells and potentially millions of beads are sequenced at the same time.

A third major NGS technology is single molecule real-time (SMRT) sequencing (Pacific Biosciences, Menlo Park, CA). The advantage of this system is the extraordinarily long single molecules that can be read (>20,000 base pairs). This technology uses microwells that create an extremely small light detection volume at the bottom of the well. In addition, each microwell contains a single DNA polymerase bound to the bottom of the well and a single long strand of DNA template. A solution is introduced that contains dNTP's, each labeled with a different color fluorophore, divalent cations, and buffer. When the appropriate base comes into contact with the polymerase to be integrated into a newly synthesized strand, the color of the light from the fluorophore is recorded. As the dNTP is incorporated into the new strand, the fluorophore is cleaved and released and will diffuse beyond the light detection volume of the well. Thus the sequence of the DNA template is determined by the pattern of light colors observed in the well. The chips that are used for massive parallel sequencing contain thousands of microwells.

A fourth technology that is being developed goes beyond the NGS sequencing by synthesis models previously described. This technology is based on nanopores and is designed to produce DNA sequencing without requiring the synthesis of complementary DNA. Originally based on embedding the biological alpha-hemolysin channel in artificial lipid bilayer membranes, the pores function as coulter counters and measure changes in current as different bases traverse through the pore.[23] Current systems, which have been proposed for commercialization, are based on ion-beam etched holes in silicon nitride membranes. Each ion-beam etched hole is large enough for either single or double-stranded molecules. In theory, the nanopores are a reagentless sequencing system that measures each base by their electrical properties and can rapidly sequence strands of DNA that are hundreds of thousands of base pairs in length. This method is not currently available for clinical testing.

In addition to the variety of analytical technologies available for next-generation sequencing, the amount of data produced from each test can range from 10's to 100's of gigabytes of data. Not only does this present a data storage issue, but it is also computationally burdensome. Finally, the ability to sequence DNA outpaces the ability to interpret the clinical significance of the data generated. For example, of the 22,000+ genes that are known to encode protein in the human genome, less than 7,000 are cataloged and described in relation to human disease in databases, such as the Human Gene Mutation Database (HGMD, www.**hgmd**.cf.ac.uk) and Online Mendelian Inheritance in Man (OMIM, www.omim.org).

CHOOSING THE APPROPRIATE TESTING METHOD

With the development of faster and more powerful sequencing methods in molecular diagnostics, it is important to address the choice of methods for testing when multiple options are available. The most obvious and pressing question is when to choose next-generation sequencing and when to utilize Sanger sequencing.

Next-generation sequencing is appropriate for many sequencing tests and its utilization for constitutional disorders has now become common place. In economic terms, next-generation sequencing will always be more cost effective compared to Sanger sequencing when more than one gene is examined. However, Sanger sequencing remains relevant not only for single gene testing, but remains the gold standard for variant accuracy compared to next-generation sequencing. In addition, next-generation sequencing for panels of genes, exomes, or whole genomes have been shown in multiple studies to have incomplete coverage of coding sequence.[24,25] Thus, when a specific gene or genes are considered clinically, then the best approach may be to perform targeted Sanger sequencing of those genes.[26] If next-generation sequencing is used for panel sequencing, then careful attention needs to be paid to the exact coverage of coding nucleotides or the location of known pathologic variants. Nevertheless, next-generation sequencing is far more sensitive than Sanger sequencing and can detect allele variants that are present in less than 3% of sequenced DNA, making it particularly suitable for interrogating tumor sample which can have significant DNA heterogeneity.

It is also important to recognize the technical limitations of varying testing methods to select the appropriate method for the specific alterations being sought. A pertinent example is for the analysis of deletions and/or duplications. Depending on the clinical syndrome, deletions, duplications, and translocations may be a significant cause of genetic disease. Large deletions and duplications may be detected by microarray analysis, karyotype, or FISH and small deletions and duplications can additionally be detected by sequencing (both NGS and Sanger). Examples of diseases that require testing for deletions and duplications are Fragile X syndrome, DiGeorge syndrome, and some mitochondrial disorders. Balanced translocations, however, which are especially important in cancer genetics, are not detected by DNA microarray. Translocations are best interrogated by karyotype, FISH, PCR, or even by next-generation sequencing assays that have been optimized for translocation detection. Many pediatric sarcomas are defined by specific translocations and various translocations in pediatric hematologic malignancies convey good or bad prognoses and occasionally, even treatment options.

Another determination to be made is whether appropriate testing involves sequencing an entire gene, exome, or genome, or whether targeting hotspot mutation regions of various genes in a 'mutation panel' is a better use of resources. A hotspot mutation region is a segment within a gene where mutations are observed with a high frequency. The use of mutation panels or tests targeted to hotspots is commonplace in oncology. These panels target genes and hotspots within genes that have prognostic or predictive significance.

As an example, a mutation panel might detect a BRAF V600E mutation in a patient with metastatic melanoma, for which there is an FDA approved drug that can lengthen the patient's survival. In oncology testing, it is useful to limit molecular testing to actionable areas with targeted therapeutic options or of prognostic value. As tumors are known to acquire mutations, whole exome and whole genome sequencing may produce many nucleotide variants of which the significance is unknown and may cause confusion or uncertainty in the patient's care.

Not all mutation panels are sequencing-based. Another frequent use of mutation panels occurs with well characterized genes, such as the cystic fibrosis transmembrane receptor (CFTR) gene. Cystic fibrosis is caused by mutations in the CFTR gene. The gene is large (over 250,000 base pairs) and over 1500 mutations have been detected in patients with cystic fibrosis. As mentioned previously, mutation panels targeting the most common disease-causing variants can be a more rapid and cost effective method for confirmation of CFTR mutations than traditional Sanger sequencing at the cost of decreased sensitivity.

The goal of testing should determine whether a mutation panel will be sufficient for gene analysis. In the case of oncology and the testing of tumor samples, mutation panels may be the most efficient route since the goal is to identify specific mutations which are well described and will guide the selection of chemotherapeutic or biologic therapy. In the case of constitutional testing, targeted mutation panels may miss critical pathogenic variants that are novel or recently described. Of particular concern would be a novel variant that results in a frameshift, since these have a higher likelihood of being pathogenic.

Another very relevant question is when to utilize whole exome sequencing. Exome tests have been used in the clinical setting for less than 5 years. These tests have a relatively high diagnostic yield (> 25%). However, careful consideration of the significant percentage of coding nucleotides that are missed by clinical exome and the resultant high percentage of genes that are incompletely analyzed needs to be at the forefront of thought during test selection. Current clinical exome tests are meaningful when they have a positive result, but a negative result cannot be considered a rule-out of any genes unless the sequencing data of that patient is carefully examined to ensure high quality and complete coverage of variant locations related to disease.

Exome tests also have the potential of uncovering incidental pathogenic variants, and thus genetic counseling for patients is of the utmost importance. In the United States, there have been joint policies by the American Academy of Pediatrics and ACMG that children should not have predictive testing for adult-onset diseases.[27] The guiding principle for this practice is children are given the autonomy to decide whether or not they want to know a test result associated with a future adult-onset disease. Clinical exome and whole genome sequencing, by definition, have a high likelihood to uncover incidental pathogenic variants of adult onset diseases. In the case of pediatric patients, issues of patient autonomy and consent for reporting incidental findings need to be discussed with patients and their families prior to testing.

SPECIAL CONSIDERATIONS WITH MOLECULAR GENETIC TESTING

Test Utility

A key problem with current high-throughput methods of sequencing is that many 'incidental' variants may be discovered that are not related to current disease. Furthermore, the penetrance of many genetic variants is not complete. Thus, even a well characterized pathogenic variant may not be disease causing in a particular individual. Phenotypic and functional analyses as well as parental testing are required for the determination of clinical significance of novel DNA variants. For well-established pathogenic DNA variants, careful study is required to determine whether that variant is relevant to the patient's current condition, and whether that variant will be causative of future disease.

Diagnostic Versus Confirmatory Molecular Testing

Some molecular tests confirm the presence of a disease diagnosed by another method. One example is cystic fibrosis. While sequencing and targeted sequencing tests identify specific sequence variants responsible for the disease, the gold-standard test for the diagnosis of CF remains the sweat test. The sweat test is non-invasive and measures the amount of chloride in sweat. However, many molecular tests, both sequencing-based and non-sequencing-based, are diagnostic of disease. As an example, molecular tests that detect and sometimes quantify infectious agents provide diagnostic results.

Privacy

Privacy in the healthcare setting is of the utmost importance to patients and healthcare providers. This concern has become paramount with the advent of whole genome sequencing. A person's DNA is his/her genetic identification and is exquisitely unique, even occasionally between identical twins. The data, however, can be de-identified by removing the link between the DNA sequence data and the patient's common identifying information (ie, name, date of birth, medical record number, address, etc.). The genetic material used to suggest or prove identity in the clinical and forensic fields is the wide variety of short tandem repeats (STR's) dispersed throughout introns of the genome. A number have been well characterized in regards to allele frequencies and have been used internationally for forensic DNA identification. Comparison of an unknown STR profile to a large STR profile database linked to common identifying information can lead to identification of a person or a person's relative(s). The data produced from the majority of clinical molecular tests using the methods discussed in this chapter do not contain STR's. Therefore, without a link to the patient's common identifying information, the results and data are not inherently identifiable. The exception is whole genome sequencing, which may produce enough STR's used for DNA identification to identify the genome's owner or a family member, if the data is linked to common identifiers.[28] Like any other medical information, security of the patient's data and associated common identifiers is of the utmost importance.

Potential Non-Paternity

In certain testing settings, non-paternity may be discovered in the genetic testing of pediatric patients. When only a pediatric patient sample is tested, discovery of non-paternity through the test results will not occur. Suggestions of non-paternity arise only when relatives are tested along with patient samples. DNA microarray can identify loss of heterozygosity (LOH) in patients and significant stretches of copy number neutral LOH may indicate consanguinity. However, even the suggestion of consanguinity does not definitely identify non-paternity, as the parents may be known relatives. Whole genome sequencing also has the potential to uncover a significant number of STR's, used for identity testing. However, the possibility of non-paternity arises only with the knowledge of those same STR's in the patient's parents or sibling(s). HLA genotyping for transplant evaluation may suggest non-paternity if the patient's parents and/or sibling(s) are also typed, which may occur when considering family members as potential donors. Even when testing the patient's parents, the other molecular tests described in this chapter do not have the ability to uncover non-paternity. Genetic counseling is important for tests in which the detection of non-paternity is a possibility.

Utility of Testing Beyond the Patient

Molecular tests involving the constitutional genome performed on pediatric patients can serve dual purposes. It can be used for diagnosis or disease confirmation in the patient, but, coupled with genetic testing of the parent(s), can also be used to inform subsequent pregnancies. When a genetic disorder is found to be inherited in a Mendelian pattern from one or both parents, this can indicate the risk of disease in subsequent pregnancies. Conversely, if a genetic disorder is found to be sporadic and the parent(s) is/are not carriers, the risk of the same disorder in subsequent pregnancies is very low. These results can be used to plan, manage, or avoid future pregnancies.

THE FUTURE OF MOLECULAR DIAGNOSTICS IN PEDIATRIC LABORATORY MEDICINE

In the 21st century, nucleic acid based testing will continue to evolve along three themes: high sensitivity (eg, low concentration of viral load or tumor) testing, diagnosis of genetic diseases, and determination of targeted therapies for chemotherapeutics. Factors that may change the utility of these roles of nucleic acid testing include non-DNA based high sensitivity testing, comprehensive genetic testing in newborn screening, in utero, or in early life, and changes in oncologic therapy.

Molecular testing is relatively new to the clinical laboratory, and until the past 10 years was limited to specialized laboratories. In the 1990s, a molecular testing laboratory had many similarities to the clinical chemistry laboratories of the 1890s. Reagents, assay systems, devices, and protocols were all very manual and truly a *"homebrew."* The role of the molecular laboratorians of the 1990s was to design the gene-specific targeting reagents and determine the appropriate instrumentation and assay conditions. Indeed, a molecular laboratorian needed a strong foundation in chemistry and biology in order to optimize buffers, enzymes, and reproducible procedures. A successful clinical molecular diagnostics laboratory of the 1990s required sophisticated training, experience, and creativity. During the 1990s semi-automated instrumentation became available for extracting nucleic acids, cycling temperatures for PCR, and sequencing DNA. Finally, during the past 10 years (2000-2010), we have seen commercialization of closed DNA analysis systems that have many similarities with automated clinical chemistry instruments. With the introduction of closed DNA analysis systems, there has been an emergence of improved quality control systems for clinical testing. In addition to advances in testing technologies, there have been improvements in laboratory harmonization by the introduction of standardized materials for nucleic acid testing. Beginning in 1997 with Hepatitis C Virus RNA, there are now dozens of molecular reference materials for infectious and genetic diseases that are available as World Health Organization (WHO) international standards.[29] In 2015, the National Institute of Standards and Technology (NIST) released a whole genome reference material (RM 8398; cell line NA12878) which has a corresponding curated data set generated from multiple sequencing centers.[30]

As we look toward the next 10 years of molecular diagnostics, there will be increasing automation and flexibility of testing formats. In addition to providing closed and automated test systems, there will be test systems specific for low volume and high volume laboratories. Based on the progress of molecular diagnostics over the past 20 years, it would not be surprising if some molecular diagnostic testing becomes part of the current trend in clinical laboratories to consolidate testing into the core laboratory. Indeed, 20 years from now, the concept of an independent molecular diagnostics laboratory may seem as quaint as an independent immunology laboratory for hormone testing.

TRAINING MODULE

1. The key components of PCR include:
   a. DNA polymerase
   b. dNTPs
   c. ddNTPs
   d. A and B
   e. All of the above

2. Next-generation sequencing (NGS) is clinically useful in 2015 because:
   a. NGS is always cheaper than Sanger sequencing
   b. NGS is cheaper than Sanger sequencing multiple genes
   c. NGS is highly accurate and considered the gold-standard in sequencing quality
   d. NGS replaces the need to perform microarrays
   e. None of the above

3. Which of the following tests can potentially be used to determine a patient's identity through the identification of short tandem repeats (STRs)?
   a. Whole exome sequencing
   b. Sanger sequencing of the exons of the *DHCR7* gene
   c. Quantitative analysis of EBV by PCR
   d. FISH for *MYCN* amplification
   e. Screen for 23 gene mutations in *CFTR* by hybridization assay

| REFERENCES

1. Watson JD, Crick FH. Molecular structure of nucleic acids; a structure for deoxyribose nucleic acid. *Nature*. 1953;171(4356):737-738.
2. (CDC) CfDCaP. Good laboratory practices for molecular genetic testing for heritable diseases and conditions. *Morb Mortal Wkly Rep*. 2009;58(RR06):1-29.
3. Mullis KB, Erlich HA, Arnheim N, Horn GT, Saiki RK, Scharf SJ, Inventors; Cetus Corporation (Emeryville, CA), assignee. Process for amplifying, detecting, and/or-cloning nucleic acid sequences. US patent 4 965 188 A. 1987.

4. Maurin M. Real-time PCR as a diagnostic tool for bacterial diseases. *Expert Rev Mol Diagn*. 2012;12(7):731-754.

5. Hamilton MS, Jackson MA, Abel D. Clinical utility of polymerase chain reaction testing for enteroviral meningitis. *Pediatr Infect Dis J*. 1999;18(6):533-537.

6. Loenen WA, Dryden DT, Raleigh EA, Wilson GG, Murray NE. Highlights of the DNA cutters: a short history of the restriction enzymes. *Nucleic Acids Res*. 2014;42(1):3-19.

7. Horton CJ, Mitui M, Leos NK, Garcia CK, Park JY. Long-range PCR based sequencing of the highly homologous genes, SFTPA1 and SFTPA2. *Mol Cell Probes*. 2013;27(3-4): 115-117.

8. WHO Expert Group Report. Molecular line probe assays for rapid screening of patients at risk of multi-drug resistant tuberculosis (MDR-TB). Geneva: World Health Organization; 2008.

9. American College of O, Gynecologists Committee on G. ACOG Committee Opinion No. 486: Update on carrier screening for cystic fibrosis. *Obstet Gynecol*. 2011;117(4):1028-1031.

10. Dalva K, Beksac M. HLA typing with sequence-specific oligonucleotide primed PCR (PCR-SSO) and use of the Luminex technology. *Methods Mol Biol*. 2014;1109:87-99.

11. Wittwer CT, Reed GH, Gundry CN, Vandersteen JG, Pryor RJ. High-resolution genotyping by amplicon melting analysis using LCGreen. *Clin Chem*. 2003;49(6 Pt 1): 853-860.

12. Sanger F, Nicklen S, Coulson AR. DNA sequencing with chain-terminating inhibitors. *Proc Natl Acad Sci USA*. 1977;74(12):5463-5467.

13. Smeets DF. Historical prospective of human cytogenetics: from microscope to microarray. *Clin Biochem*. 2004;37(6):439-446.

14. Heller MJ. DNA microarray technology: devices, systems, and applications. *Annu Rev Biomed Eng*. 2002;4:129-153.

15. Fodor SP, Read JL, Pirrung MC, Stryer L, Lu AT, Solas D. Light-directed, spatially addressable parallel chemical synthesis. *Science*. 1991;251(4995):767-773.

16. Henderson LB, Applegate CD, Wohler E, Sheridan MB, Hoover-Fong J, Batista DA. The impact of chromosomal microarray on clinical management: a retrospective analysis. *Genet Med*. 2014;16(9):657-664.

17. Pfundt R, Kwiatkowski K, Roter A, et al. Clinical performance of the CytoScan Dx Assay in diagnosing developmental delay/intellectual disability. *Genet Med*. 2016;18(2): 168-173.

18. South ST, Lee C, Lamb AN, et al. ACMG Standards and Guidelines for constitutional cytogenomic microarray analysis, including postnatal and prenatal applications: revision 2013. *Genet Med*. 2013;15(11):901-909.

19. Langer-Safer PR, Levine M, Ward DC. Immunological method for mapping genes on Drosophila polytene chromosomes. *Proc Natl Acad Sci USA*. 1982;79(14):4381-4385.

20. Mardis ER. The impact of next-generation sequencing technology on genetics. *Trends Genet*. 2008;24(3):133-141.

21. McGinn S, Gut IG. DNA sequencing - spanning the generations. *N Biotechnol*. 2013;30(4):366-372.

22. Voelkerding KV, Dames SA, Durtschi JD. Next-generation sequencing: from basic research to diagnostics. *Clin Chem*. 2009;55(4):641-658.

23. Howorka S, Cheley S, Bayley H. Sequence-specific detection of individual DNA strands using engineered nanopores. *Nat Biotechnol.* 2001;19(7):636-639.

24. Park JY, Clark P, Londin E, Sponziello M, Kricka LJ, Fortina P. Clinical exome performance for reporting secondary genetic findings. *Clin Chem.* 2015;61(1):213-220.

25. Dewey FE, Grove ME, Pan C, et al. Clinical interpretation and implications of whole-genome sequencing. *JAMA.* 2014;311(10):1035-1045.

26. Park JY, Kricka LJ, Clark P, Londin E, Fortina P. Clinical genomics: when whole genome sequencing is like a whole-body CT scan. *Clin Chem.* 2014;60(11):1390-1392.

27. Abdul-Karim R, Berkman BE, Wendler D, et al. Disclosure of incidental findings from next-generation sequencing in pediatric genomic research. *Pediatrics.* 2013;131(3):564-571.

28. Hong C, Wang J, Xing C, Hwang TH, Park JY. Intersection of DNA privacy and whole-genome sequencing. *Clin Chem.* 2015;61(7):900-902.

29. Madej RM, Davis J, Holden MJ, Kwang S, Labourier E, Schneider GJ. International standards and reference materials for quantitative molecular infectious disease testing. *J Mol Diagn.* 2010;12(2):133-143.

30. Zook JM, Chapman B, Wang J, et al. Integrating human sequence data sets provides a resource of benchmark SNP and indel genotype calls. *Nat Biotechnol.* 2014;32(3):246-251.

31. Mullis K, Faloona F, Scharf S, Saiki R, Horn G, Erlich H. Specific enzymatic amplification of DNA in vitro: the polymerase chain reaction. *Cold Spring Harb Symp Quant Biol.* 1986;51 Pt 1:263-273.

32. Scharf SJ, Horn GT, Erlich HA. Direct cloning and sequence analysis of enzymatically amplified genomic sequences. *Science.* 1986;233(4768):1076-1078.

33. Wittwer CT, Fillmore GC, Hillyard DR. Automated polymerase chain reaction in capillary tubes with hot air. *Nucleic Acids Res.* 1989;17(11):4353-4357.

PEDIATRIC MICROBIOLOGY | 14

Christopher D. Doern and Kaede Sullivan

LEARNING OBJECTIVES

1. Understand the importance of specimen collection in the diagnosis of infectious diseases in children.
2. Discuss the most common infectious diseases in children and how their epidemiology differs from that in adults.
3. Discuss the appropriate methods for diagnosing infections in children.
4. Understand the treatment of pediatric infections and the role that laboratory plays in management.

INTRODUCTION

In many ways, the practice of diagnosing infectious diseases in children is very similar to that in adults. The pathogens are largely the same and the methods used to identify them do not typically differ because they originated from a child. Also, inoculum greatly impacts on the sensitivity of the diagnostic method used. However, there are some important areas where diagnosing disease differs in children. While a comprehensive review of all microbiology is outside the scope of this chapter, the focus will instead be on specific areas where working with children requires a unique approach. Complete information regarding all areas of clinical microbiology can be found in many texts. Two of the more commonly used references include the Manual of Clinical Microbiology (ASM Press) as well as Koneman's Color Atlas and Textbook of Diagnostic Microbiology (Lippincott Williams & Wilkins).[1,2]

This chapter will be divided into two general sections. The first will provide a discussion of laboratory methods that should be known to all microbiologists working with pediatric specimens. The second section is organized by clinical presentation. Within each clinical condition discussed will be sections that briefly introduce the disease and the relevant pathogens, pediatric considerations in specimen collection, laboratory diagnosis, treatment, and antimicrobial susceptibility testing. Of note, this chapter will only address the microorganisms that are relevant to each clinical condition and will not include an exhaustive list of all bacterial, viral, fungal, and parasitic infections. Where applicable, important basic considerations in organism identification will be addressed but in-depth discussions about biochemical profiles and antimicrobial resistance mechanisms is outside the scope of this chapter.

▌ THE INDIGENOUS MICROFLORA OF CHILDREN

Proper interpretation of microbiology culture results requires in-depth knowledge of the specimen type and the spectrum of diseases that may be considered when a given specimen is submitted for microbial testing. Knowledge of a patient's medical history, age, gender, and past culture results inform the workup of specimen. With respect to specimen type, there are generally two main categories: sterile and non-sterile. Sterile site specimens are of utmost importance because they may represent life threatening, invasive infections, but culture interpretation is simpler because in most cases, any organism recovered is considered significant. However, microbiological testing results from specimens from non-sterile sites (eg, respiratory tract, genitourinary tract, gastrointestinal tract, etc.) can be more challenging to interpret. These cultures are complicated by the presence of indigenous microbiota otherwise referred to as normal flora, which can exist as harmless colonizers but can also cause infection. Having a detailed understanding of the normal flora from each specimen is critical to interpreting these cultures.

At birth, neonates move from the sterile intrauterine environment to a world of continuous microbe exposure. As a result, the process of bacterial colonization begins immediately and the evolution of an individual's indigenous flora is continuous. What follows is a brief discussion of the primary components of a child's normal flora.

The Newborn

Many factors contribute to the evolution of a neonate's flora. For example, gestational age, duration of ruptured membranes prior to delivery, antibiotic exposure, mode of delivery, and diet have all been shown to impact the development of a neonate's flora. Premature babies with extended hospitalizations have delayed bacterial colonization and when they do become colonized, it is with hospital-associated organisms, such as the *Enterobacteriaceae*[3-5] as well as methicillin-resistant *Staphylococcus aureus*.[6] Maternal intrapartum antibiotics as well as prolonged rupture of membranes (ROM) has also been associated with decreased transmission of *Lactobacillus* during birth.[7] Babies born by cesarean delivery have delayed intestinal colonization with important organisms, such as anaerobes and those who are breastfed have more complex intestinal microbiota than those who are formula fed.[8,9]

Respiratory Tract Flora

The term respiratory tract is too broad to accurately describe all of the small niches within it. Anatomic colonization is dictated by organism/receptor interactions and can lead to some very specific niches. For example, *Streptococcus salivarius* binds to the buccal mucosa while organisms, such as *Streptococcus mutans* have an affinity for tooth enamel. Nonetheless, respiratory tract flora can be described with some generalizations. The dominant organisms in the mouth and throat include the Viridans group streptococci, *Neisseria* spp., *Actinomyces* spp., *Fusobacterium* spp., along with a variety of anaerobic organisms including *Veillonella, Bacteroides, Peptostreptococcus*, among many others.

The nasopharynx has a smaller spectrum of colonizing organisms and commonly includes *Staphylococcus* spp. (including *S aureus*), Viridans group streptococci, and *Corynebacterium*. In addition, children can also be colonized with *Haemophilus influenzae, M catarrhalis, Neisseria meningitidis*, and *Streptococcus pneumoniae*.

Skin

Children generally have similar skin flora as adults including coagulase-negative staphylococci, *Bacillus* spp., *Micrococcus* spp., *Corynebacterium* spp., and *Propionibacterium acnes*. Enterobacteriaceae (*Escherichia coli, Klebsiella* spp., *Citrobacter* spp. etc.) are not considered to be normal skin flora but are known to transiently colonize the skin. Their presence can often complicate the interpretation of certain specimens, such as wounds where they can exist as pathogens or as colonizing flora. This is particularly true in diapered children in which enteric organisms are frequently isolated from anatomic areas distal to the gastrointestinal tract.

Gastrointestinal Tract

The gastrointestinal tract is made up of several distinct anatomic locations including the esophagus, stomach, intestine, and colon. A tremendous amount of research has been dedicated to exploring the human microbiome of the gastrointestinal tract and how it impacts on individual's health. With the use of next generation sequencing as a tool to investigate the microbiome, scientists are discovering numerous organisms that are not cultivatable using routine methods. However, for the purposes of this chapter, we will focus on those organisms commonly isolated in the clinical laboratory.

The stomach is not considered a sterile environment but its acidic environment is not conducive to proliferation of diverse bacterial communities. Among the organisms that can be found in the stomach are *Lactobacillus* spp. and the streptococci. The seroprevalence of *Helicobacter pylori* in children can be high and increases with age but this organism requires special culture conditions and is not typically a confounding factor in culture results. The intestines contain a larger number of organisms including streptococci, lactobacilli, *Enterobacteriaceae* as well as anaerobes, such as *Bacteroides* spp., *Clostridium* spp., *Veillonella* spp., and *Bifidobacterium*. The colon contains the highest burden of organisms and includes all of the bacteria mentioned in the small intestines as well as *Enterococcus* and other anaerobes, such as *Fusobacterium*, *Prevotella, Porphyromonas,* and *Peptostreptococcus.*

Genitourinary Tract

Until recently, urine was thought to be sterile but urine microbiome studies using next generation sequencing suggest that this may not be the case.[10] However, many of the organisms we now know to be present in urine are not cultivatable.[11] In urine specimens submitted to the clinical laboratory, there are organisms that are commonly recovered as both commensals and pathogens. To help differentiate between colonization and infection, laboratories utilize quantitative cultures with thresholds ranging from 10,000 colony forming units (CFU)/mL to 100,000 CFU/mL. Organisms commonly isolated from urine include the *Enterobacteriaceae, Lactobacillus* spp., Viridans group streptococci, and enterococci.

The microbiology of the vagina should also be considered in the context of bacterial vaginosis. Overgrowth of lactobacilli, *Candida* spp., *Gardnerella vaginallis, Mobiluncus* as well as others is associated with bacterial vaginosis. Lastly, between 10% and 30% of women of child-bearing age are colonized with group B *Streptococcus* (GBS). Many laboratories will have protocols in place to identify and report any amount of GBS from female urine specimens in the event that the patient is pregnant.

SUSCEPTIBILITY TESTING AND ANTIMICROBIAL RESISTANCE

One of the most important functions of the microbiology laboratory is to provide information regarding the treatment of infectious diseases. This guidance can be presented through testing of an organism isolated from a patient, by compiling an antibiogram or through a review of the literature.

Susceptibility Testing

Methodologically, antimicrobial susceptibility testing in children is similar to that performed for isolates recovered from adults. There are a variety of strategies that can be used to assess antimicrobial susceptibility. These include using automated systems, such as the Vitek 2 (bioMérieux, Durham, NC), the Phoenix (Becton Dickinson, Sparks, MD), the Microscan (Siemens, Princeton, NJ), and the Sensititre system (ThermoFisher, Waltham, MA). These systems all work in slightly different ways but ultimately generate minimum inhibitory concentration (MIC) for predetermined organism-drug combination. MICs represent the lowest concentration of antibiotic that inhibits the growth of an organism.

There are non-automated mechanisms by which antimicrobial susceptibilities can be assessed as well. These methods include disk diffusion, gradient diffusion, agar dilution, and broth microdilution. Gradient diffusion (most commonly the E-test (bioMérieux)) is a test in which an antibiotic impregnated strip contains an increasing gradient of antibiotic. The strip is placed on an agar plate that has been inoculated with a lawn of organism and the antibiotic then diffuses out into the media and generates a gradient of concentrations. The point at which the organism is able to grow up to the strip is read as the MIC. Disk diffusion works with a similar principal but the disks contain a fixed concentration of antibiotic. As the antibiotic diffuses out into the agar the concentration decreases the further away from the disk it gets. Organisms will grow around the disk at the concentration in which they can survive. This generates a zone of inhibition that is measured in millimeters. These zone sizes correlate with MIC's. Broth microdilution relies on testing organisms in broth containing increasing two-fold concentrations of antibiotic. Organism growth is measured by visually observing turbidity in each well and identifying the point at which growth is inhibited (the MIC).

Ultimately, the methods discussed earlier are used to generate an interpretation, such as susceptible, intermediate, susceptible dose dependent, resistant, or non-susceptible. Guidance for interpretation is provided by several organizations. The Clinical Laboratory Standards Institute (CLSI) and the European Committee for Antimicrobial Susceptibility Testing (EUCAST) both publish documents that provide interpretive criteria and help to standardize testing. These organizations meet on a regular basis to review and update their documents. The Food and Drug Association (FDA) in the United States also includes interpretive criteria in the package insert for antibiotics.

These interpretive criteria are generated based on an analysis of clinical outcome studies, organism population analyses, pharmacokinetic/pharmacodynamics (PK/PD), and knowledge of resistance mechanisms. PK/PD analyses rely heavily on several factors including the MIC of an organism as well as the dose and bioavailability of the antibiotic. These factors are used in modeling analyses that predict the likelihood of achieving successful treatment. It is important to note that there are no pediatric-specific interpretive criteria documents and that the doses used in these modelling studies are almost exclusively based on adult treatment regimens. In some cases, interpretive breakpoints may be based on adult dosing of a given antibiotic. Therefore, while published interpretive criteria generally work well in pediatric medicine, there may be some scenarios in which interpretive breakpoints may be difficult to apply to children when determining optimal antimicrobial treatment.

Antibiograms

Antibiograms are compilations of data that present organism/antibiotic combinations as "percent susceptible." For example, an institution may look at a year's worth of E coli and determine how many isolates were susceptible to meropenem. Resistance to meropenem among E coli (especially in pediatrics) is generally rare and so a common antibiogram report would read 99% susceptible for that combination. In contrast, the proportion of E coli isolates that are susceptible to ampicillin is significantly lower in many areas and an antibiogram might read only 48% susceptible for the E coli-ampicillin combination.

Antibiograms can be helpful to physicians when making empiric treatment choices before definitive susceptibility information is available, but are ultimately tools that can be used to make educated guesses. It is important to note, however, that pediatric antibiograms can look very different than those produced from adult patient isolates. See Tables 14-1 and 14-2 for an antibiogram from a large, United States-based, free-standing pediatric medical center compared to the antibiogram from a separate free-standing hospital located on the same campus as the pediatric hospital. Notice the difference in organisms, such as Acinetobacter baumannii complex, S pneumoniae, as well as the enterococci. The adult isolates are significantly more resistant overall than those found in children. In addition, notice that nearly all of the Gram-negative organisms have >90% susceptibility to the flouroquinolones where the adult isolates are generally more resistant. There are many possible explanations for the differences observed between these patient populations. First, antibiotic exposure is very different in pediatrics. Due to side-effect profiles, antibiotics, such as the flouroquinolones and tetracyclines are avoided whereas they are commonly used in adults.[12,13] This may explain the difference in the fluoroquinolone profiles but it does not explain other differences, such as the enterococci and Acinetobacter. The increased resistance in adults for these organisms is likely due to greater overall antibiotic exposure in adults as well as the nature of their infections.

Table 14-1 **ANTIBIOGRAM FOR PEDIATRIC PATIENTS. (NUMBERS EXPRESSED AS PERCENT SUSCEPTIBLE.)**

Organism	Number Tested	Levofloxacin	Ciprofloxacin	Penicillin	Pip/Tazo	Ceftriaxone	Meropenem	Vancomycin
Acinetobacter baumannii	9		67			55		
Pseudomonas aeruginosa	179		93		97		98	
Escherichia coli	1551		94		97	98	100	
Klebsiella pneumoniae	172		98		95	96	100	
Streptococcus pneumoniae	126	98		87		90		100
Enterococcus faecium	22			0				91

Table 14-2   **ANTIBIOGRAM FOR ADULT PATIENTS. (NUMBERS EXPRESSED AS PERCENT SUSCEPTIBLE.)**

Organism	Number Tested	Levofloxacin	Ciprofloxacin	Penicillin	Pip/Tazo	Ceftriaxone	Meropenem	Vancomycin
Acinetobacter baumannii	60		60			48	60	
Pseudomonas aeruginosa	291		81		93		89	
Escherichia coli	2726		69		96	92	100	
Klebsiella pneumoniae	524		92		96	93	99	
Streptococcus pneumoniae	67	97		90		97		100
Enterococcus faecium	78			0				31

PEDIATRIC INFECTIOUS DISEASES

Pharyngitis

Etiology, Clinical Presentation, and Epidemiology

Pharyngitis can be caused by a wide variety of pathogens with bacteria and viruses being the most common. Fungi such as *Candida* spp. was well as parasites have less commonly been implicated. Common pathogens in children include group A *Streptococcus* (GAS) (also known as *Streptococcus pyogenes*), other beta-hemolytic streptococci (group C and G), *Arcanobacterium* spp. and a variety of viruses including Adenoviruses, Influenza A and B, Parainfluenza virus, Respiratory Syncytial Virus (RSV), and many others. In addition, there is some literature to suggest that *Fusobacterium necrophorum* is as common a cause of pharyngitis as GAS.[14] There is also a large body of evidence suggesting that group C and G beta-hemolytic streptococci are capable of causing pharyngitis that is indistinguishable from that of GAS. Two other important infectious agents to consider are Epstein-Barr virus (EBV) and Cytomegalovirus (CMV), both of which can cause infectious mononucleosis which often includes pharyngitis.[15,16]

The clinical presentation of pharyngitis can vary by pathogen but generally involves acute onset with fever and the complaint of a sore throat. Inspection of the throat will often reveal red tonsils and may be accompanied by exudative lesions. Although some feel that there are clinical signs and symptoms that can help a clinician differentiate between a viral and bacterial process, others have shown that the presentations are indistinguishable from each other. Fortunately, these infections are usually self-limiting but complications including peritonsillar and retropharyngeal abscesses, acute rheumatic fever, and post-streptococcal glomerulonephritis do occur.[17]

Epidemiologically, viral infections tend to occur more frequently in the colder months while enterovirus-associated pharyngitis occurs more frequently in the summer. Viral illnesses seem to have a predilection for younger children while bacterial infection occurs more often in older children.[18]

Laboratory Diagnosis

Diagnosis of bacterial pharyngitis can be accomplished with a variety of methods including culture, rapid antigen detection, and nucleic acid amplification testing. Group A *Streptococcus* antigen detection assays are popular as they offer rapid turn-around times and perform with high specificity (usually > 95%).[19] However, antigen tests can suffer from poor sensitivity and therefore a negative result does not rule-out disease. Consequently, culture is required for confirmation of negative rapid antigen results.

The main bacterial pathogen sought in a pharyngeal culture is group A *Streptococcus*. Typically, a 5% sheep blood agar plate (BAP) is inoculated and incubated. GAS yields a large zone of beta-hemolysis on BAP that is easily identified among other respiratory flora. Beta-hemolysis is a reliable mechanism for GAS screening as non-hemolytic isolates are rare. Once hemolysis is identified, several biochemical tests can be performed to confirm the identification. On Gram stain, GAS is a Gram-positive cocci arranged in pairs and chains; it is catalase-negative, and pyrolidonyl arylamidase (PYR)-positive. These characteristics along with typical colony morphology and beta-hemolysis are sufficient for most laboratories to report the recovery of GAS. However, it should be noted that there are some streptococci that resemble the biochemical profile of GAS such as *Streptococcus porcinus* and *Streptococcus pseudoporcinus* but these are rare in humans. If the identification of a colony is suspect, Lancefield antigen typing can also be performed. *S pyogenes* is termed GAS because it carries the Lancefield A carbohydrate antigen. The Lancefield type of streptococci can be determined through latex agglutination tests that detect the A, B, C, D, F, and G antigens. Bacitracin susceptibility is also a unique characteristic of GAS but that is rarely used as part of routine identification.

One disadvantage of rapid antigen testing is that it does not detect other bacterial pathogens that are capable of causing pharyngitis. Laboratories have adopted several different mechanisms for reporting group C and G *Streptococcus* from throat cultures. Laboratories electing to report these strains can report them by name or simply state "beta-hemolytic streptococci isolated (not GAS)."

An alternative to culture and rapid antigen testing is a nucleic acid amplification testing. A variety of PCR-based assays have now been FDA-approved and have demonstrated high sensitivity and specificity.[20] PCR assays suffer from the same limitation as rapid antigen testing in that they only detect GAS. There is still a paucity of published data suggesting clinical or cost benefits in implementing molecular GAS detection methods.

Treatment and Susceptibility Testing

When treatment of GAS is indicated, routine susceptibility testing is not required as the organism is universally susceptible to penicillin. As a result, penicillin V or amoxicillin are antibiotics of choice for infected patients.[21] In patients with penicillin allergies, a first generation cephalosporin can be used (for those not anaphylactically sensitive), clindamycin or clarithromycin for 10 days, or azithromycin for 5 days. GAS resistance to macrolide antibiotics is generally low (<5%), especially in areas of low macrolide use and as a result routine susceptibility testing for non-serious GAS infections is generally not performed.[22]

Suppurative Pharyngeal Processes

Etiology, Clinical Presentation, and Epidemiology

Suppurative pharyngeal infections are pus forming processes that can result in deep abscesses. These infections begin with a small area of cellulitis in the pharynges but then progress to invade adjacent spaces and lead to major complications. Such infections include abscess formation in the peritonsillar, retropharyngeal, and parapharyngeal spaces with peritonsillar abscesses being the most common.[23] There does appear to be some age association with clinical presentation. Retropharyngeal abscesses occur most commonly in young children with an average presentation at about 4 years of age.[24,25] In contrast, peritonsillar abscesses present later in childhood at an average age of 11 years.[25]

Staphylococcus aureus and *S pyogenes* are the organisms most commonly associated with deep neck infections. Given that these infections typically originate from the oral space it is also not surprising that anaerobes, such as *Fusobacterium*, *Peptostreptococcus*, and *Bacteroides* are frequently recovered. Other aerobic organisms that have been linked to these infections include Viridans group streptococci and *H influenzae*.[26-29]

There is strong evidence that *Fusobacterium necrophorum* is a significant cause of pharyngitis and recurrent tonsillitis.[30] *Fusobacterium* is also associated with Lemierre's Syndrome also known as postanginal septicemia. The original description of the disease included infection arising from the jaw, ear, gut, and genital tract.[31] However, the definition is now limited to infections arising from the oropharynx. Lemierre's Syndrome usually includes thrombophlebitis of the internal jugular vein and can involve septic pulmonary emboli.

Laboratory Diagnosis

Laboratory specimens are usually obtained through incision and drainage procedures. These infections are polymicrobial, and treatment typically requires broad organism coverage. There is therefore little value in performing a full-work up of all organisms recovered. Nevertheless, it can be helpful to know if significant amounts of a pathogen are present and so laboratories will generally limit work up to two or fewer potential predominating pathogens. Exceptions to this work up strategy would be GAS and *S aureus*, which are generally identified and reported if present in any amount.

Anaerobes are frequently associated with these infections. Anaerobic cultures aren't always sought but if they are, special attention should be paid to specimen storage and transport. If tissue is collected, it should be placed underneath the surface of semisolid anaerobic transport media. If abscess material is collected through needle aspiration, all of the air should be expelled from the syringe and then it should be capped and transported to the lab as quickly as possible.

Laboratory detection of *Fusobacterium* in the diagnosis of pharyngitis is rarely performed. *Fusobacterium* is an obligate anaerobe and the abundant anaerobic microflora of the oral cavity makes it difficult to isolate the organism. However, when disease progresses to deep neck spaces, anaerobic cultures are usually included and *Fusobacterium* can be recovered. Not all species of *Fusobacterium* are associated with disease so it is important to identify the organism to the species level. *Fusobacterium nucleatum* is a considered normal flora in the mouth and is generally non-pathogenic whereas *F necrophorum* should usually be considered a pathogen.[32] Thus it is important to differentiate these species and there are a few distinguishing characteristics that can be used for this purpose. First, both organisms are catalase-negative, indole-positive, non-pigmented, anaerobic Gram-negative rods. Both species fluoresce chartreuse when exposed to long-wave UV light. The organisms also differ in Gram stain morphology: *F necrophorum* is a short pleomorphic rod while *F nucleatum* is a long, slender, pointy rod. However, one cannot assume that a *Fusobacterium* demonstrating a short, pleomorphic rod-like shape is *F necrophorum* as *F nucleatum* and *F periodonticum* are the only species to demonstrate the fusiform morphology. In addition, *F necrophorum* is lipase-positive, while *F nucleatum* and most other *Fusobacterium* are negative.[1] Lipase activity can be demonstrated by observing growth on an egg yolk agar plate. Positivity is indicated by observing a characteristic sheen on the surface of the agar.

Treatment and Susceptibility Testing

The treatment of suppurative pharyngeal infections usually involves a combination of incision and drainage as well as antimicrobial therapy. Given the probability that mouth-associated organisms will be present, it is likely that a beta-lactamase producing strain will be present.[33] Even if the predominant pathogen appears to be penicillin susceptible, it has been postulated that beta-lactamase-producing bacteria may provide protection to those susceptible strains if penicillin were used to treat the infection. Therefore, it is recommended that a beta-lactamase stable antibiotic be used for these infections.[34]

The anaerobes associated with deep neck infections rarely warrant susceptibility testing because they are present in mixed cultures. However, significant rates of resistance have been identified in *Bacteroides* spp., *Prevotella* spp., *Peptostreptococcus* spp., and *Fusobacterium* spp. There is guidance on how to perform such testing provided by the CLSI document M11-A8.[35] Currently, broth microdilution standards have only been published for *Bacteroides fragilis* group and agar dilution is the recommended method for all other anaerobic susceptibility testing.[35]

Surprisingly little is known about *Fusobacterium necrophorum* antibiotic susceptibility from human isolates. One study did show that of over 200 isolates collected in the United Kingdom (UK), only 2% were resistant to penicillin. 100% of isolates were metronidazole susceptible while 15% were erythromycin resistant.[36] The 2% of isolates that were penicillin resistant were almost certainly due to beta-lactamase production. However, there is very little literature showing that *F necrophorum* can harbor a beta-lactamase whereas *F nucleatum* have been shown to make produce beta lactamases.[37]

Otitis Media

Etiology, Clinical Presentation, and Epidemiology

Acute otitis media (AOM) is one of the most common childhood diseases and can be caused by bacteria and viruses. The most common bacterial etiologies are *S pneumoniae, H influenzae, M catarrhalis,* and group A *Streptococcus.*[38,39] Viral etiologies include Adenovirus, Influenza, Rhinovirus, Parainfluenzavirus, Respiratory Syncytial Virus (RSV), and Enterovirus.[40,41] A 1991 publication showed that overall about 17% of AOM is viral with the majority of viral AOM being caused by RSV (7%).[41]

Children suffering from AOM often have non-specific symptoms, such as fever, headache, and irritability.[42] Among children who are capable of verbalizing their symptoms, ear pain is the most common complaint while younger children may indicate ear infection by pulling at the affected ear. Rarely, the tympanic membrane will rupture, resulting in otorrhea (discharge from the ear). The rupture provides an almost immediate relief from pain and may lessen the fever if present. Other symptoms and complications of AOM may include dizziness, hearing loss, conjunctivitis, and facial paralysis.

Otitis media is common in children but rare in adults. This is due in part to anatomical differences between them. The Eustachian tube of an adult is longer and extends up, back and laterally to reach the tympanic membrane. In contrast, the Eustachian tube of a child is shorter and less rigid. That along with other anatomical differences helps predispose children to ear infection. It is estimated that by 6 years of age approximately 80% of children will have experienced a middle ear infection.[43]

Laboratory Diagnosis

The diagnosis of middle ear infection is often a clinical one and does not include laboratory diagnostics. When culture is performed, middle ear fluid obtained through tympanocentesis. If any of the earlier-mentioned pathogens are isolated from properly collected middle ear fluid, they should be reported as pathogens.

Routine bacterial culture of middle ear specimens includes inoculation of blood, chocolate, and MacConkey agar. Given that the most common pathogens are (*S pneumoniae, M catarrhalis,* and *H influenzae*) MacConkey agar is not usually helpful. The identification of GAS is discussed elsewhere in this chapter. *M catarrhalis* is a Gram negative diplococci on Gram stain that is oxidase-positive and catalase-positive. It has been described as a "hockey-puck" colony that stays intact when slid around the agar plate. In addition, *M catarrhalis* isolates are nearly all beta-lactamase positive which is a feature that can be used to aid identification of this organism. A hallmark feature of *H influenzae* is that it fails to grow on sheep blood agar but grows on chocolate agar. This growth pattern is a product of two growth factor requirements for *H influenza*, the X factor (hemin) and V factor (NAD). Unfortunately, routinely viral diagnostics are not usually pursued in cases of AOM while a viral diagnosis could be very useful for antimicrobial management. Given the overlap in viral etiologies of upper respiratory tract infection and otitis media, it may be tempting to assume that an NP swab could be used to aid in the etiologic diagnosis of AOM. This however, has been shown not to be the case.[44]

Treatment and Susceptibility Testing

Antimicrobial therapy is a mainstay of otitis media management. Selection of antimicrobial should provide activity against the most likely bacterial etiologies including *H influenzae, S pneumoniae,* and *M catarrhalis.* Effective treatment of AOM should result in resolution of symptoms within 72 hours with no evidence of recurrence. Amoxicillin is the recommended front-line treatment of AOM and it has been suggested that high doses can be used to overcome low-level resistance in *S pneumoniae.*[45] However, amoxicillin would not be an ideal choice for infections caused by *H influenzae* (~30% beta-lactamase positive) or *M catarrhalis* (>95% beta-lactamase positive).[46] Beta-lactamase producing strains can be treated with amoxicillin-clavulanate or with oral second or third generation cephalosporins, such as cefuroxime and cefdinir, respectively.

In most cases AOM is managed without the benefit of culture and susceptibility testing. *H influenzae* from non-sterile sources, such as ear specimens, are usually only tested for beta-lactamase production. Beta-lactamase production is assessed with the use of a chromogenic cephalosporin called Nitrocephin otherwise known as the Cefinase test (BD, Sparks, MD). The principle of this test is that Nitrocephin-impregnated disks are inoculated with the organism of interest. If the test organism is beta-lactamase positive, the chromogenic substrate is hydrolyzed and results in a color change. Beta-lactamase positivity in *H influenzae* confers resistance to penicillin, ampicillin, and amoxicillin. In less than 1% of *H influenzae* isolates a beta-lactamase negative ampicillin resistant phenotype exists. These strains should be considered resistant not only to ampicillin and amoxicillin, but also to ampicillin-sulbactam, amoxicillin-clavulanate, cefuroxime, and piperacillin-tazobactam.[47] For serious infections a third generation cephalosporin is recommended as no *H influenzae* strain has even been found to be resistant. The beta-lactamase produced by nearly all *M catarrhalis* confers resistance to penicillin and amoxicillin however most strains are susceptible to the macrolides.[48]

In rare instances, formal susceptibility testing of *H influenzae* may be warranted. Due to its unique growth requirements a specialized media (Haemophilus test media) is used to perform these tests and can be used to assess the activity of non-beta-lactam antibiotics, such as the fluoroquinolones, trimethoprim-sulfamethoxazole, tetracycline (although rarely used in children), and rifampin.[47] This testing can also be used to determine whether or not a strain is beta-lactamase negative ampicillin resistant (BLNAR).

Otitis Externa

Etiology, Clinical Presentation, and Epidemiology

Otitis externa (OE) can present as acute, chronic, or invasive disease and is an infection of the external auditory canal. Peak incidence is in children between 7 and 12 years of age and happens with equal frequency in males and females.[49] It is rare in children younger than 2 years of age.[50] Acute disease can manifest in a localized or diffuse manner. Localized acute disease results in a pustule or furuncle associated with hair follicles. Pain may be severe in acute OE and is typically present with lymphadenopathy. The two most common organisms for localized acute OE are *Staphylococcus aureus* and *S pyogenes* (group A streptococci (GAS)).

Diffuse OE (swimmer's ear) presents with itching and increasing pain and the most common etiology is *Pseudomonas aeruginosa*. The disease is often associated with swimming and is most common during the warm summer months. Other water-associated organisms have also been implicated in diffuse OE, such as *Achromobacter* spp., *Vibrio* spp. as well as the *Enterobacteriaceae*. Skin flora associated organisms are often associated with these cultures and probably represent colonization rather than disease unless they are the predominating organism.

Chronic otitis externa results from irritation of auditory canal following chronic drainage secondary to rupture of the tympanic membrane. The underlying disease is chronic suppurative otitis media. The primary symptom is itching which may at times be severe.

Invasive or malignant otitis externa is a serious infection that spreads from the ear canal to surrounding tissue and causes severe pain and drainage of pus.

Infection can be life-threatening if the disease spreads to the base of the skull, meninges, and brain. A common manifestation is facial paralysis which can be permanent. The vast majority of malignant OE is caused by *P aeruginosa*.[38]

Laboratory Diagnosis

The diagnosis of OE is primarily clinical; however, cultures can be useful in assessing antibiotic susceptibility of causative organisms. As discussed earlier *S aureus*, GAS, and *P aeruginosa* are the primary etiologies of disease and with the exception of GAS can have variable susceptibility profiles. A swab of the inner ear canal or ear drainage should be collected and processed for aerobic bacterial pathogens. Anaerobic cultures need not be obtained unless there is specific concern for anaerobic infection. Fungus can occasionally cause OE and fungal cultures should be sought in situations where fungal etiologies are suspected. Specifically, *Candida* spp. are a frequent cause of OE in patients with oral candidiasis.[51] Typically, these are monomicrobic infections and overly mixed cultures should receive minimal work-up unless there is a clearly predominant potential pathogen.

Treatment and Susceptibility Testing

Successful treatment of OE should result in complete resolution of signs and symptoms and reduce the recurrence of disease. Acute forms of OE are typically managed with otic drops of either a flouroquinolone or polymyxin B.[52] In some cases, incision and drainage may be necessary. Malignant OE is a much more serious condition that warrants systemic, directed therapy for up to 9 weeks.[53] Typically this therapy will be directed toward *P aeruginosa* and will include an aminoglycoside and a broad-spectrum beta-lactam, such as ceftazidime, cefepime, or a carbapenems. Debridement of devitalized tissue is also an important component of management.[54]

Gastroenteritis

Etiology, Clinical Presentation, and Epidemiology

For the purposes of this section, gastrointestinal (GI) disease will be categorized as two general entities: infectious and toxin-mediated disease. Infectious etiologies of GI disease can be bacterial, viral, or parasitic. The most common bacterial etiologies of GI disease in children are *Salmonella*, *Shigella*, Enterohemorrhagic *E coli*, *Yersinia enterocolitica*, and *Campylobacter*.[55] While these diseases are most common, others such as *Vibrio* spp. (non-Cholera), and *Aeromonas hydrophila* do occur with some regularity. Less common pathogens in the United States include *Plesiomonas shigelloides*, *Vibrio cholera*, and *Edwardsiella*.

There are five forms of *E coli* gastroenteritis: enteroinvasive (EIEC), enterotoxigenic (ETEC), enteropathogenic (EPEC), enteroaggregative (EAEC), and enterohemorrhagic (EHEC). EIEC produce a watery and sometimes bloody diarrhea that is similar to *Shigella* in presentation. ETEC results in the so-called "traveler's diarrhea" and is common in developing countries. ETEC produce a heat-stable toxin and results in a relatively mild diarrheal illness. EPEC has historically been associated with infant diarrhea and is characterized by a prolonged illness with non-bloody diarrhea, vomiting, and fever. EAEC has been associated with children of lower-socioeconomic status and results in non-bloody diarrhea accompanied by mild abdominal cramping and fever. Finally, EHEC are Shiga-toxin producing *E coli* (also known as STEC) that result in a hemorrhagic colitis and hemolytic-uremic syndrome (HUS).

Toxin-mediated disease occurs when an organism proliferates in a food and produces an enterotoxin that is then consumed. There are three primary organisms responsible for this type of disease: *Staphylococcus aureus, Clostridium perfringens,* and *Bacillus cereus.* This form of GI disease is characterized by a relatively short incubation period (<14 hours), lack of fever, diarrhea, and vomiting. This is in contrast to bacterial GI disease that has a longer incubation period (1-4 days), fever, diarrhea, and only occasional vomiting.

Several parasites can also cause GI disease including *Entaemoba histolytica, Cryptosporidium, Giardia intestinalis, Isospora belli,* and *Cyclospora.* These infectious agents usually result in diarrhea but fever is rarely experienced. In addition, the incubation time for parasitic infection is up to 2 weeks.

Viral etiologies of GI disease primarily include Norovirus, Rotavirus, Adenovirus, and Astroviruses. The range of symptoms differs slightly from that of the bacterial GI pathogens. Viral etiologies don't always elicit fever but vomiting is very common as is diarrhea. The typical incubation time for viral causes of GI disease is 1-3 days and results in symptoms that include acute onset of vomiting, diarrhea, and last a relatively short period of time.

Laboratory Diagnosis

The laboratory diagnosis of bacterial gastroenteritis at this time is primarily culture-based although multiplex PCR panels are being used with increased frequency (discussed later). For culture, most laboratories will inoculate several different types of media that optimize the detection of *Salmonella* spp., *Shigella* spp., *Campylobacter* spp., and *E coli* 0157. In addition, a guideline published in 2009 by the CDC recommends that all stools submitted from patients suspected of having acute, community-acquired gastroenteritis should have testing for all Shiga-toxin producing *E coli* (STEC) performed.[56] There are a variety of assays that can be used to detect STEC and they generally involve the inoculation of an overnight MacConkey broth with subsequent testing via an enzyme immunoassay (EIA) for Shiga toxin detection. The recommendation to test all stool specimens in this manner is somewhat controversial as STEC disease is relatively rare and the amount of resources needed to detect a small number of positive results is significant.[57,58] Routine culture media includes a blood agar plate (BAP) which can be useful in screening for oxidase positive pathogens, such as *Aeromonas hydrophila*, *Vibrio* spp., *Plesiomonas* spp., and *Edwardsiella* spp. MacConkey agar can be useful for isolating *Y enterocolitica*, *Salmonella* spp., and *Shigella* spp. which are lactose non-fermenters. MacConkey agar with sorbitol or a chromogenic medium is added for the detection of *E coli* 0157. An important part of any stool culture is optimizing the detection of *Salmonella* spp. and *Shigella* spp. A variety of media can be used for this purpose including *Salmonella/Shigella* media (SS), Xylose-lysine-deoxycholate agar, and Hektoen enteric agar (HE) among several others. Although these media are all based on different biochemical reactions, they all function with the same general principal. Non-pathogenic enteric flora will ferment the sugars present in the media and turn the media a bright color (usually yellow or red) where the pathogenic organisms do not ferment these sugars and remain colorless. In addition, the production of H_2S by *Salmonella* spp. and a few other organisms is detected by the presence of ferric ammonium citrate and manifests as a black center in the bacterial colony. *Campylobacter jejuni* and *C coli* have long been recognized as agents of gastroenteritis and have been strongly linked to Guillain-Barre Syndrome.[59] Due to special growth requirements, *Campylobacter* require selective media to inhibit overgrowth from faster growing organisms as well as elevated incubation temperatures (42°C) and microaerophilic conditions. Isolation of *Y enterocolitica* can be optimized using cefsulodin-irgasan-novobiocin (CIN) agar. This media is selective for *Y enterocolitica* and produces colonies with a deep red center (often described as a "bulls-eye"). A number of *Vibrio* spp. are capable of causing gastroenteritis (primarily *V cholera* and *V parahemolyticus*). *Vibrio* can be isolated from routine media but their recovery is enhanced by using selective media. Both *V cholera* and *V parahemolyticus* will be colorless colonies on MacConkey agar and blood agar plates can be used to perform oxidase screens for these organisms as well. If *Vibrio* spp. disease is specifically suspected, thiosulfate-citrate-bile salts-sucrose agar (TCBS) can be used and is both somewhat selective and differential for *Vibrio* spp. It contains sucrose on which the sucrose fermenting *V cholera* will produce yellow colonies while *V parahemolyticus* (sucrose non-fermenting) produce green colonies.

Diagnostic options for viral etiologies of gastroenteritis have historically been limited to culture, and antigen detection. Culture diagnostics have been limited by the fact that the primary etiologies (Rotavirus, Norovirus, and Adenovirus 40/41) are not cultivatable by routine laboratory methods. As a result, the only diagnostic test routinely used in laboratories has traditionally been antigen detection (either EIA or lateral flow assay) for Rotavirus. The diagnostic test of choice for Norovirus is RT-PCR, however this testing has traditionally been limited to outbreak investigations only or special reference testing.

The diagnosis of infectious gastroenteritis is changing with increasing adoption of multiplex PCR panels that detect commonly encountered pathogens. These panels are capable of detecting bacterial, parasitic, and viral pathogens. In some cases the work-flow of these assays is very simple and involves only basic reagent and specimen manipulation and takes around an hour to complete.

Treatment and Susceptibility Testing

In many cases gastroenteritis is self-limiting and treatment is not necessary. The treatment of viral gastroenteritis is supportive and for bacterial gastroenteritis most infections are self-limiting and treatment can be associated with prolonged carriage. Antibiotic treatment of EHEC is generally discouraged as it can lead to symptom exacerbation. Antimicrobial susceptibility testing can be useful for treatment of some agents of bacterial enteritis. Young infants, children with immune deficiencies or intestinal disorders may qualify for antibiotics if *Salmonella* is recovered. Also, antimicrobials are routinely prescribed for shigellosis.

Tuberculosis in Children

Etiology, Clinical Presentation, and Epidemiology

In 2000, *Mycobacterium tuberculosis* (MTB) caused approximately 8.3 million new infections of which 11% were in children under the age of 15.[60] This figure though is likely an underestimate due to poor diagnostic capacity in endemic areas. Pediatric tuberculosis is most prevalent in poorly developed countries and rates are significantly reduced in developed countries.[61] Despite the perception that children rarely develop serious MTB infection, children under 5 years of age often present with advanced disease with significant morbidity and mortality.[62] Human Immunodeficiency Virus (HIV) infection in adults has had a major impact on the spread of the MTB epidemic and children born into families with HIV-infected parents have a significantly higher MTB exposure rate.[63]

Laboratory Diagnosis

The diagnosis of *Mycobacterium tuberculosis* in children poses some challenges not encountered in adults. The diagnosis of pulmonary tuberculosis relies on the collection of respiratory specimens which are then submitted for analysis (culture or PCR). For most patients this is produced in the form of a sputum specimen. Young children are unable to produce sputum on command and as a result gastric aspirates are collected. These specimens are based on the premise that children cough up the organism and swallow it. Although tuberculosis can be readily cultured from gastric aspirates, it is important that these acidic specimens are neutralized upon receipt in the laboratory to maintain organism viability. Once the specimen has been neutralized laboratories can proceed with their routine culture practices. For a detailed description of mycobacterial culture practices, see the Manual of Clinical Microbiology.[1] Unfortunately, currently available molecular assays have not been approved for use from gastric aspirate specimens and laboratories will likely have to find a reference laboratory that has performed an off-label validation to test this specimen.

Purified protein derivative (PPD) and interferon gamma release assays (IGRA) can be used to diagnose latent tuberculosis infection (LTBI). The CDC produced a summary document in 2012 that summarized the current body of literature regarding the use of these diagnostic tools. Within that document they state that there is not sufficient performance data for IGRA testing in children less than 5 years of age and could not recommend its use in that patient population.[64] For that reason, the PPD is generally preferred in these patients although it is important to note that this recommendation is predicated on an absence of data, not inferior performance. In fact, there is growing evidence that IGRA assays are equivalent to PPDs in young children and it is likely that the assays can be used interchangeably in children of all ages.[65]

Treatment and Susceptibility Testing

As is the case in adults, the goal of treating active MTB infection is to improve clinical symptoms, cure the infection, terminate transmission, and prevent the emergence of drug resistance.[66] The backbone of MTB therapy is a three-drug regimen that includes rifampin (RF), isoniazid (INH), and pyrazinamide (PZA). This therapy is appropriate for susceptible organisms causing low bacterial load infections. Four-drug therapy (which adds ethambutol may be required for high-burden infections, infections with radiographic evidence of advanced disease, in immunocompromised patients, and infections in which drug resistance is present. Where possible, directly observed therapy (DOT) has proven to be an effective mechanism for ensuring patient compliance.

Children are less likely than adults to acquire and/or transmit drug resistant MTB infection. However, there are documented clusters of drug-resistant MTB transmission in children.[67,68] The term multi-drug resistant (MDR) refers to isolates that have acquired resistance to INH and RF. MDR MTB isolates are treated with second-line drugs, which are more toxic but when used appropriately have been shown to have few side-effects in children. Extensive drug-resistant (XDR) MTB infections are defined as MDR plus resistance to fluoroquinolones and at least one second-line injectable drug (ie, kanamycin, amikacin, or capreomycin).[66]

The agar proportion method using Middlebrook 7H10 or 7H11 agar is considered by CLSI to be the gold standard method for defining MTB resistance.[69] This is a method that defines resistance by comparing the growth of a strain on an agar plate which contains a "critical" concentration of anti-tuberculous drug to growth in the absence of drug. The agar proportion method is limited by the slow turnaround time and a more rapid, broth-based test is recommended for routine patient care. It is recommended that susceptibility testing be performed on the first isolate of MTB obtained from every patient and testing should be repeated if cultures fail to convert to negative after three months of therapy. Initial testing should include all first-line MTB drugs including INH, RF, ethambutol, and PZA. If resistance is detected to any one of these drugs additional testing for second-line agents is warranted.[69]

Urinary Tract Infection

Etiology, Clinical Presentation, and Epidemiology

The etiology of urinary tract infection (UTI) in children is similar in spectrum to that seen in adults. The most common causes of infection are Gram-negative enteric organisms, such as *E coli, K pneumoniae,* and *Proteus* spp.[70] Gram-positive UTI is less common but does occur and is usually caused by *Enterococcus* spp. and less commonly, *Aerococcus urinae, Corynebacterium urealyticum,* and *Staphylococcus saprophyticus.*[70] *Candida* may also cause infection, most commonly in the form of hospital acquired infection. *Candida* spp. UTI is typically associated with immunosuppressed patients and those who are receiving broad-spectrum antibiotics.

The symptoms of an uncomplicated UTI in children can be similar to those in adults and include dysuria, urgency, or frequency and patients often complain of abdominal or suprapubic pain. Fever may not always be present and it is usually low-grade if present at all. By contrast, children with pyelonephritis will present with fever, chills, flank pain, vomiting, and diarrhea. In addition, dysuria, urgency, or frequency may or not be present for pyelonephritis.

UTI can occur in any age group and any gender, but certain populations are more prone to infection than others. Infection in uncircumcised infant boys is more common than in infant girls. However, after 6 months and throughout adolescence, girls are more likely than boys to develop infection.[71] When hospitalized, catheters are a major risk factor for the development of infection.[72]

Laboratory Diagnosis

The laboratory diagnosis of UTI in children primarily relies on urinalysis and urine culture. Collection of urine specimens can be challenging in children as the clean catch methodology is often not possible. As a result, providers can use either an in-and-out catheterization technique in which the child is temporarily catheterized for the purposes of urine collection or they can perform a suprapubic aspirate (SPA) in which a needle is inserted directly into the bladder to withdraw urine. Both collection techniques provide high quality specimens although the SPA is rarely performed. A "bag-urine" can also be collected from very young children. This is a technique in which an adhesive bag is attached to a child until the child urinates at which point the urine is retained in the bag and can be submitted for testing. Bag-urine specimens are commonly contaminated by colonizing flora which makes culture interpretation very difficult. Most laboratories do not accept these specimens for culture as recommended by the American Academy of Pediatrics.[73]

Urine cultures are quantitative because the organisms that cause UTI can also be part of the patient's normal flora. Colony count thresholds are applied to the culture results and used to distinguish between colonization and infection. The threshold used to interpret these cultures varies by laboratory and usually falls between 10,000 and 100,000 CFU/mL. A recent American Association of Pediatrics (AAP) guideline suggested that 50,000 CFU/mL be used in children between 2 and 24 months old.[73] One thing that is consistent between laboratories is limiting work-up to two pathogens. Cultures that yield more than two potential pathogens above threshold may represent contamination from a poorly collected specimen and laboratories should request that the specimen be recollected.

The exception to this rule would be the work-up of sterile urine specimens. These are specimens such as SPA's that are not expected to contain any colonizing flora. If a specimen is truly collected in a sterile manner, any organisms isolated may be potential pathogens, regardless of threshold.

An important part of a UTI evaluation is a urinalysis. There are many different results that can be derived from a urinalysis but the most relevant to assessing infection are leukocyte esterase, nitrate, and the visualization of bacteria. The detection of leukocyte esterase in urine is indicative of the presence of white blood cells which can be a marker of infection. Many Gram-negative bacteria can convert nitrate to nitrite, so detection of nitrite in urine may also be indicative of infection. Nitrate positivity results from the presence of Gram-negative organisms in the urine. Gram-positive organisms will not result in a positive nitrite test.[74] When taken together, nitrate and/or leukocyte esterase positivity have a reasonably high sensitivity and specificity for diagnosing infection.[75] This led the AAP in the aforementioned guidelines to suggest that UTI in 2 to 24 month olds could not be diagnosed without a positive urinalysis.[73]

Treatment and Susceptibility Testing

Antimicrobial susceptibility testing for the organisms typically implicated in pediatric UTI is discussed elsewhere in this chapter. Most UTIs in children are managed in the outpatient setting and as a result antibiotics are prescribed empirically and typically includes activity against *Enterobacteriaceae* because these agents are most common. Quinolones are typically avoided in children out of concern for cartilaginous development. For cystitis, oral antimicrobials are typically prescribed according to local antimicrobial susceptibility patterns. Amoxicillin/clavulanate, an oral cephalosporin, such as cefuroxime, cefixime, or cefdinir, or trimethoprim-sulfamethoxazole are frequently used. Pyelonephritis is typically managed with parenteral antibiotics, such as ampicillin-sulbactam, intravenous cefuroxime, a third generation cephalosporin, cefepime, or gentamicin.[76]

Sexually Transmitted Diseases

Etiology, Clinical Presentation, and Epidemiology

Specimens for sexually transmitted infection (STI) testing in children are typically submitted as part of an assessment of symptoms, such as vaginal discharge, or as a part of a sexual abuse investigation. The majority of patients who test positive for an STI are asymptomatic.

In their STD Treatment guidelines, the Centers for Disease Control and Prevention (CDC) in the United States indicates that diagnosis of any of the following in pre-pubertal children are diagnostic for sexual abuse if perinatal acquisition (from mother to child) and rare nonsexual vertical transmission are excluded: *Neisseria gonorrhea*, *Chlamydia trachomatis*, *Treponema pallidum* (syphilis), and human immunodeficiency virus (HIV). *Trichomonas vaginalis* is considered "highly suspicious"; anogenital warts and genital herpes (herpes simplex virus (HSV)) are thought to be "suspicious" for sexual abuse.[77] If a pre-pubertal child is diagnosed with any of the above diagnoses, the CDC recommends reporting to a community agency that has been mandated to receive reports of suspected child abuse.[77] Distinguishing perinatal acquisition versus acquisition through sexual abuse can be challenging and requires consideration of a number of factors including the identity of the pathogen, STI diagnoses in the mother, and the age of the child[78] (Table 14-3). Involvement of seasoned clinical professionals is important to navigate this issue.

Table 14-3 IMPLICATIONS OF A DIAGNOSIS OF STIS FOR A DIAGNOSIS OF SEXUAL ABUSE		
Incubation period of infection	Probability of abuse	Mother-to-child transmission
Gonorrhoea: 2–7 days	Strong; probable if child >1 year	Can be seen in children from 0–6 months of age
Chlamydia: 1–3 weeks, but up to 6 weeks	Probable; strong if child >3 years	Can be seen in children up to 3 years of age
Herpes simplex virus: 2–14 days	Probable	Can be seen in children up to 3 months of age
Trichomoniasis: 1–4 weeks	Strong if child >6 months	Can be seen in children 0–6 months of age
Human papillomavirus: ≥1 month	Possible; probable if >2 years	Can be seen in children from 0–2 years of age
Syphilis: up to 90 days	Strong	Must be excluded
HIV: up to 6 months, but the majority seroconvert within 4–12 weeks	Possible	Must be excluded
Hepatitis B: up to 3 months	Possible	Must be excluded

Laboratory Diagnosis

Diagnosis of an STI in a child can have serious legal, safety, and medical implications. Strategies for specimen collection, testing, reporting, and interpretation of STI test results therefore require collaboration between the laboratory and members of sexual abuse assessment teams. The goal is to ensure complete, timely, and appropriate testing when it is required.

The CDC provides recommendations for initial testing. Viral culture is recommended by the CDC if vesicular or ulcerative lesions are present on the genitals or perianal area and are compatible with genital herpes simplex virus infection. *N gonorrhea* and *C trachomatis* testing requires careful attention. Culture methodologies preceded more sensitive nucleic acid amplification testing (NAAT) but remains "gold standard" methodology in some cases. *C trachomatis* culture is rarely available outside of reference laboratories and has very poor sensitivity compared to NAATs. Due to lack of data supporting the use of NAAT in "extra-genital" sites (pharynx and rectum), and in boys, *C trachomatis* culture is still the preferred diagnostic method for rectal specimens and meatal swabs in boys with urethral discharge.[75] The yield is considered too poor to justify systematically testing the pharynx. The CDC supports the use of NAAT is female urine and vaginal specimens and cites data from a multi-centered pediatric study.[77]

N gonorrhea NAAT testing is complicated by reported cross-reactions with other Neisseria species.[78] Similar to *C trachomatis*, the CDC cites the paucity of data supporting the use of NAAT in "extragenital" sites and in boys to recommend *N gonorrhea* culture in extra-genital specimens and genital specimens submitted from boys. The CDC does support the use of NAAT in female urine and vaginal specimens. All isolates and primary specimens should be retained for possible additional testing.

In addition, vaginal swabs for *T vaginalis* culture and wet mount are recommended. Serum antibody testing for *T pallidum*, HIV, and hepatitis B virus infection should be performed on a "case-by-case" basis.

Treatment

Discussion of the treatment approaches to each of the STI discussed is beyond the scope of this chapter. The CDC provides detailed guidance in their STD Treatment guidelines.[75]

Lower Respiratory Infections

Etiology, Clinical Presentation, and Epidemiology

In children, the clinical presentation and responsible etiologic agents for community-acquired infections of the lower respiratory tract vary considerably by age. Bacterial pneumonia in neonates is caused predominantly by organisms swallowed in the vaginal tract during delivery. *S agalactiae* predominates but *E coli* and other *Enterobacteriaceae*, and rarely, *Listeria* can also be responsible for pneumonia in this population.[79] Infants in the first two months of life are also at highest risk of severe bronchiolitis, a condition that involves inflammation and obstruction of the bronchioles. Bronchiolitis is primarily caused by respiratory syncytial virus, human metapneumovirus, and parainfluenza type 3. Other viruses, including influenza have also been implicated.[80] Viral agents continue to dominate lower respiratory infections until school age. Although uncommon, *C trachomatis* and *Bordetella pertussis*-associated pneumonia present between 1 and 3 months. Organisms that are "typical" in adults with lobar pneumonia—*S pneumoniae, H influenzae,* and less commonly, *S aureus*—tend to emerge at 3 months and continue until school age when *Mycoplasma pneumoniae* and *Chlamydophila pneumoniae* become the predominant causative agents. While the above provides a "classical" progression of the etiologic agents responsible for lower respiratory tract infections in children, epidemiological trends (eg, *B pertussis* outbreaks; emergence of community-acquired methicillin-resistant *S aureus*) can subtly alter the distribution of the causative agents of pneumonia in children in a given geographic region. Finally, the introduction of conjugate *H influenzae* b and polyvalent conjugate *S pneumoniae* vaccines have reduced incidence of severe pneumonia related to this organisms.[81-83] Hospital-acquired pneumonia in children is caused predominantly by *Enterobacteriaceae*, *P aeruginosa*, and *S aureus*. In immunocompromised children (eg, as a result of chemotherapy or stem cell transplantation), *Pneumocystis jiroveci*, *Cryptococcus* and mold should be considered.

Laboratory Diagnosis

Ascertainment of a bacterial etiology of pneumonia is limited by the ability of a child to produce sputum for Gram stain and culture. When a child is appearing unwell and able to produce sputum, a sample should be obtained and submitted for Gram stain and bacterial culture. Results of Gram staining can be used in two ways: for assessment of specimen quality, and provision of an early diagnosis. In adults, sputum cultures are typically assessed for quality by quantifying contaminating oral squamous epithelial cells and/or neutrophils per low power field. Specimens that do not meet minimum criteria (eg, >10 squamous epithelial cells (SECs)/low power field (LPF) or <25 neutrophils/LPF) are typically rejected and clinicians are advised to collect another specimen.[84] Enforcement of this practice varies in pediatrics due to a paucity of pediatric data supporting this approach. Used in a diagnostic capacity, Musher et al reported the sensitivity of Gram stain for diagnosis of *S pneumoniae* pneumonia in children to be 31%.[85] When culture is pursued, at minimum, non-selective media such as 5% sheep's blood agar and chocolate agar should be inoculated and incubated in 3-5% CO_2. The latter is useful for the detection of *H influenzae*. Sensitivity of sputum culture has been reported as 44%.[85] Some cases of bacterial pneumonia are complicated by a parapneumonic effusion or empyema. If pleural fluid is obtained, Gram stain and culture should be performed.

Blood culture should be obtained in neonates with suspected bacterial pneumonia and/or sepsis. Webber et al. reported 46% yield in blood cultures obtained in neonates admitted to a neonatal intensive care unit.[79] In healthy, vaccinated children who are being treated as outpatients, blood culture provides little additional data. Blood culture yield of 2% has been reported in this population.[86] In ill children who require hospital admission, a blood culture is advisable as yield has been reported to be higher.[87] Endotracheal tube aspirates can be cultured in children who have been intubated and are being mechanically ventilated.

Ascertainment of a viral etiology of pneumonia can promote discontinuation of antibiotics. In the case of influenza, detection of a virus may prompt consideration of antiviral use. Detection of "atypical" agents of pneumonia

(*B pertussis, M pneumoniae,* and *C pneumoniae*) requires molecular diagnostics as culture methods are insensitive, labor intensive, and increasingly, unavailable. Until recently, laboratory-developed tests (LDT, also known as "home-brew" tests) were commonly used to detect these organisms. A variety of molecular platforms have now gained FDA clearance. These include the FilmArray Respiratory Panel (BioFire, Salt Lake City, UT), an automated nested multiplex PCR platform that detects all three pathogens in addition to a variety of viral targets. The Verigene Respiratory Pathogens *Flex* Test is an automated microarray panel that also detects a variety of respiratory viruses in addition to *Bordetella* (genus-level) and *B pertussis* (to the species level). The *illumigene* Pertussis assay uses loop-mediated isothermal amplification to detect *B pertussis* (Meridian Biosciences, Cincinnati, OH).

Treatment and antimicrobial susceptibility testing

Suspected neonatal bacterial pneumonia is treated with intravenous antibiotics. A typical first-line empiric antimicrobial regimen is ampicillin and gentamicin to provide activity against *S agalactiae, E coli,* and *Listeria.*[88] Cefotaxime is a reasonable alternative to gentamicin, particularly if meningitis is suspected. In children older than 3 months, the Pediatric Infectious Disease Society and the Infectious Disease Society of America have jointly published recommendations for the management of community acquired pneumonia in children >3 months of age.[83] In well-appearing, healthy, and immunized children, in an outpatient setting, amoxicillin is recommended first-line in infants, preschool, and older children when bacterial pneumonia is suspected, to provide activity against *S pneumoniae,* the most likely bacterial etiology of pneumonia. In school age children, a macrolide (eg, azithromycin) is recommended if an atypical agent of pneumonia is suspected. In children who are unwell and hospitalized, intravenous antimicrobials are recommended and should be tailored according to pneumococcal immunization status and local penicillin susceptibility trends in *S pneumoniae.*

C difficile-associated disease

Etiology, Clinical Presentation, and Epidemiology

C difficile-associated infection (CDI) is the most common cause of antibiotic-associated diarrhea in both adults and in children. *C difficile* toxins A and B bind to cell surface receptors, enter intestinal epithelia through endocytosis, are activated through proteolytic cleavage. They damage intestinal epithelia by destabilizing cytoskeleton structures.[89]

Children with CDI can present with either bloody or non-bloody diarrhea but severe cases can be complicated by intestinal perforation, sepsis, and toxic megacolon.[90] Classically, pseudomembrane is observed in the sigmoid colon on colonoscopic examination.

Longitudinal studies have shown that asymptomatic colonization with *C difficile* (toxin-forming and non-toxin-forming) is common in infants, particularly those younger than 6 months of age.[91] Animal studies have suggested that young mammals lack the toxin receptors required to bind *C difficile* toxin.[92] In a clinical study, Tang et al showed that infants with positive *C difficile* toxin in their stool are clinically no different from those who test toxin-negative and that clinical outcomes are similar whether or not they receive treatment. These findings suggest that the presence of *C difficile* toxin in the stool of infants does not necessarily translate to colonic disease in healthy infants.[93] Nevertheless, a small number of case reports have described histological or colonoscopic evidence of pseudomembranous colitis in infants with Hirshsprung disease and necrotizing enterocolitis, indicating that care is required when developing *C difficile* testing policies in children.[93-95]

Laboratory Diagnosis

Although asymptomatic adults and children can test positive for *C difficile* toxin particularly following therapy for CDI, routine testing of formed stool specimens is not recommended nor is testing for cure.[96] In addition, testing on healthy infants less than 12 months of age is not recommended although it is reasonable to make exceptions in infants with known intestinal disorders as described previously.[97]

Until recently, toxin-A and toxin-B enzyme immunoassays (EIA) were widely used. Evidence demonstrating highly variable sensitivity and specificity in both adults and children has led to consideration of other methods.[98,99] Commercially available nucleic acid amplification tests (NAAT) that exclusively detect the presence of the *tcdA* and/or *tcdB* genes include *illumigene C difficile* (Meridian Biosciences, Cincinnati, OH), the BD GeneOhm Cdiff assay, the BD Max Cdiff (BD Diagnostics Inc., Sparks, MD), ProDesse Pro-Gastro Cd assay (Hologic Gen-Probe Inc., San Diego, CA), the Xpert C. difficile Epi assay (Cepheid Inc., Sunnyvale, CA), the Simplexa *C difficile* Universal Direct assay (Focus Diagnostics Inc, Cypress, CA), the Portrait Toxigenic *C difficile* assay (Great Basin Inc, Salt Lake City, UT), and the AmpliVue *C difficile* assay (Quidel Molecular, San Diego, CA). The Verigene *C difficile* test (Nanosphere Inc., Northbrook, IL) uses a microarray format to detect *tcdA* and *tcdB*. The actual clinical meaning of a positive *toxA* or *toxB* NAAT remains to be determined.[100] Regulatory genes including *tcdA* and *tcdB* impact upon the expression of *toxA* and *toxB*, making actual toxin production difficult to predict.[101] Concomitantly, literature describing "algorithmic" approaches to CDI diagnosis emerged. This approach involves screening with an EIA detecting glutamate dehydrogenase a*nd "confirmation" using an alternative method, such as NAAT,* cell culture cytotoxicity neutralization assay (CCNA), toxigenic culture, or EIA. The advantage of this method is the rapid turnaround time of the screening procedure (15-30 minutes) and cost savings compared to "standalone" use of NAAT; or lower labor demands, if compared to routine use of CCNA.[102] Sensitivity >95% has been reported in adults but appears to be lower, in the range of 70-80% in children.[103-106] Specificity mirrors the confirmatory method used.

Treatment

Recommended first line therapy in children remains oral metronidazole or oral vancomycin. The use of probiotics remains experimental. Fecal transplantation, while still investigational, has gained some traction in adults with refractory CDI, despite repeated courses of medical therapy.[107] Details related to oversight, regulation, and screening for infectious diseases, are still under discussion.

Bloodstream infections

Etiology, Epidemiology, and Clinical Presentation

The etiology of bloodstream infections in children varies greatly by age. In the neonate, *S agalactiae* and *E coli* are the leading pathogens isolated from blood. While universal screening for recto-vaginal *S agalactiae* has greatly reduced invasive *S agalactiae* infections, cases continue to be reported, with premature infants being particularly at high risk. In older infants and children, prior to the introduction of conjugate vaccines that confer protection against *S pneumoniae, H influenzae,* and *N meningitis,* these pathogens dominated sepsis cases in children. While the introduction of these vaccines have greatly reduced incidence of bacteremia involving these pathogens, cases continue to be reported. In addition, central venous catheters are often placed in children who require ongoing and repeated blood testing, intravenous medication administration, or total parenteral nutrition. While clinically necessary, they serve as foreign bodies that can become colonized with normal flora, and in some cases, may progress to central line associated blood stream infections (CLABSI). A wide variety of organisms can be responsible for CLABSI, coagulase-negative *Staphylococcus* spp. predominate in both adults and children. Finally, children who develop neutropenia as a consequence of chemotherapy or stem cell transplantation protocols become highly at risk of *P aeruginosa* bacteremia. Bloodstream infections carry a high risk of mortality in most cases, particularly if a case progresses to septic shock.

Laboratory Diagnosis

In a bacteremic child, the overall likelihood of a blood culture testing positive is greatly dependent on patient factors (bacterial load and the identity of the infecting organism); phlebotomy factors (the volume of blood drawn); and the sensitivity of the blood culture system in use.

There is significant evidence in the literature that suggest that pediatric bacteremia levels (measured in colony forming units per milliliter of blood, or CFU/mL) can vary considerably but low level bacteremia (<10 CFU/mL) is well documented in children. This is an important consideration when implementing blood draw volume policies in pediatric patients. Currently, there are four sets of published recommendations related to blood culture draw volumes in pediatric patients (Figure 14-1). The Clinical Laboratory Standards Institute (CLSI) states that no more than 1% of total blood volume be drawn in children.[108] The joint Infectious Disease Society of America/American Society for Microbiology guidelines for laboratory utilization, the Cumitech Blood Culture document,[109,110] and the Manual of Clinical Microbiology provide weight-based recommendations.[1] The minimum volume of blood required to detect bacteremia at low levels has not been established but increased yield has been associated with incrementally increasing blood draws in children.[111-113]

The benefit of anaerobic blood cultures in children is unclear, in part, because of a lack of studies designed to compare bacterial recovery from aerobic and anaerobic blood cultures where they are both systematically inoculated. Recently, Shoji et al. analyzed blood culture sets that were obtained from children that were hospitalized at a single tertiary pediatric center.[114] To be

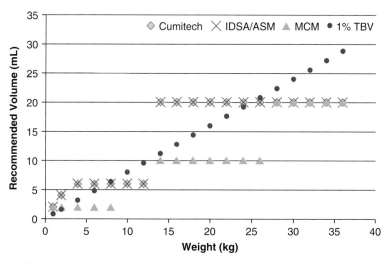

Figure 14-1 ▪ Blood culture volume recommendations by weight.

included, procurement of a blood culture that included both a BacT/ALERT Pediatric FAN or (adult) Aerobic FAN blood culture bottle and a BacT/ALERT Anaerobic FAN bottle was required. They reported an incidence of obligate anaerobic bacteremia of 0.03% but noted that anaerobic bottles detected more cases of bacteremia in which facultative anaerobes were the responsible organism. Similar pediatric studies using the BACTEC Peds Plus/F and Aerobic/F media did not observe a similar effect.

It is advisable to avoid single blood culture draws for a given septic episode. A minimum of 2 blood draws increase the probability of detecting an agent of bacteremia by increasing the blood draw volume and also helps clinicians to discriminate between true bacteremia and blood culture contamination when normal flora is recovered in a single bottle only (eg, *Bacillus* spp., *Corynebacterium* spp., coagulase-negative *Staphylococcus* spp., *Micrococcus* spp.).

In patients with a CVC in place, the practice of drawing blood from both a peripheral vein and from the CVC is advisable but difficult to enforce in children due to discomfort that may be associated with a peripheral venous blood draw. Scheinneman et al showed in an oncology population that when blood is drawn from peripheral and CVC sources, 28% of cases grew non-contaminant bacteria from peripheral blood cultures only. Other adult and pediatric studies have reported similar findings.[115]

BacT/ALERT Pediatric FAN (bioMérieux, Durham, NC) and BACTEC Peds Plus/F (PedsPlus; BD Diagnostics, Sparks MD) are two widely used pediatric blood culture media products. To compensate for smaller blood draw volumes in children, Pediatric FAN bottles contain smaller broth volumes than their adult counterpart. Also, to support the growth of *N meningitidis,* both products contain lower concentrations of sodium polyanetholsulfonate (SPS), an anticoagulant that suppresses growth of *N meningitidis,* than the adult products. Finally, both systems use antibiotic neutralizing agents: an 8.5% charcoal suspension in PF, and antibiotic binding resins in Peds Plus/F. Sullivan et al reported in an in-vitro study that sensitivity and time to detection may be superior in BACTEC Peds Plus/F media compared to Pediatric FAN. They also described higher recovery of bacteria in the presence of antibiotics.[116]

Following the alert of a positive blood culture from a blood culture instrument, subculture to solid media and ascertainment of the identity and antimicrobial susceptibility status of the organism typically follows. Recently, a number of novel methods have been developed and cleared by the FDA to expedite determination of the responsible agent. The Verigene Gram-Positive Blood Culture Nucleic Acid Test (Nanosphere, Northbrook, IL) is a microarray assay with a run time of 2.5 hours and is supported by pediatric performance data.[117] The microarray detects 12 genus-level or species-level targets in positive blood cultures with Gram-positive organisms, and three resistance determinants (*mecA, vanA, vanB*). The FilmArray Blood Culture Identification

Panel (BioFire Diagnostics, Salt Lake City UT) is an automated multiplex PCR platform that requires 1 hour to detect 23 Gram-positive, Gram-negative, and candida targets in addition to *mecA*, *vanA*, *vanB*, and *bla*KPC. By expediting provision of blood culture results to clinicians, the goal of these assays is to optimize clinical outcomes by facilitating earlier clinical decision making about antimicrobial therapy and discharge. Lastly, MALDI-TOF MS has been applied to the identification of organisms directly from positive blood culture bottles. Although this work-flow requires several centrifugation steps, it is an unbiased approach that is in theory capable of identifying any organism present within the MALDI-TOF MS database.

Treatment

Optimal antimicrobial treatment of bacteremia is largely dependent on the responsible organism. Removal of foreign bodies, such as CVCs is advisable where clinically possible and has been shown to expedite clearance of bacteria from blood and improve outcomes in many circumstances.[118]

Upper Respiratory Tract Infections

Etiology, Epidemiology, and Clinical Presentation

There are a wide range of upper respiratory tract infections (URI) in children. Common presentations include the common cold, croup, pharyngitis, herpangina, uvulitis, peritonsillar abscesses, and many others. A few of these infections warrant their own section and are discussed elsewhere in this chapter. A full discussion of all pediatric URIs is outside the scope of this chapter and we will instead focus on the most common URI, viral infection.

Respiratory viral infections can be caused by a wide variety of viruses and with the advancement of rapid, multiplex molecular diagnostics, microbiology laboratories can now detect many of them. The most common causes of viral URI in children are rhinovirus, enterovirus, adenovirus, coronavirus, parainfluenza virus, respiratory syncytial virus (RSV), and influenza A and B.[119] With a few exceptions, the epidemiology in very young children infants does not differ significantly.[120,121] Rhinovirus, although it can be found in infants, is more common in children of advancing age. Conversely, RSV is the dominant virus found in infants with bronchiolitis.[120]

It is important to note that there is seasonal variation for many viral causes of URI, especially influenza and RSV. In the northern hemisphere, RSV typically peaks from December through February.[120] Influenza demonstrates winter seasonality as well but is less predictable than RSV.[120] Other viruses may be present throughout the year but peak at certain times. For example, rhinovirus can usually be detected throughout the year but generally peaks in November.[120]

Viral URI is very common in children and particularly so in those that attend daycare. Wald and colleagues found that children in daycare had on average 7.1 illnesses per year while those that were cared for at home had 4.7 illnesses per year.[122] Among school-aged children, it is not uncommon for one child to come home with an illness and expose other family members to the illness. Hall and colleagues found that older siblings were most likely to introduce an infection to the family and that secondary attack rate for all family members was 27%, but was highest for infants at 45.4%.[123] Generally speaking, boys experience more URI than girls and in the traditional family setting, mothers are more likely to get ill than fathers.[120,124]

Due to the high number of viruses that cause URI, clinical presentation can vary widely. Generally speaking though, URI consists of nasal discharge, nasal obstruction, cough, sneezing, and sore throat. In addition, many will have fever and malaise. Although fever is a relatively common symptom, it is important to note that less than 50% of patients with the common cold will report feeling feverish or having chills.[125] Sinusitis presents most typically with persistent rhinorrhea with purulent discharge and a cough. Fever presents in some, but not all children and is more common in acute sinusitis than in chronic presentations. Croup is a term used to define several different categories of respiratory illness. These categories include laryngitis, laryngotracheitis, laryngotracheobronchitis, bacterial croup, and spasmodic croup.[34] The symptoms for these presentations vary but include cough, fever, hoarseness, dysphagia, and inspiratory stridor. Bronchiolitis presents with predominantly nasal symptoms, and include sore throat and fever. Cough is always present and is initially dry and progresses to become looser, and bark-like. Rhinitis may be present and evaluation of the chest frequently reveals rhonchi and coarse rales.

Laboratory Diagnosis

The primary specimens used for the diagnosis of URI is the nasopharyngeal (NP) swab, nasopharyngeal aspirates, nasal washes, throat swabs, and in some cases nose swabs may be acceptable. For viral etiologies of URI, swab specimens are placed into viral transport media (VTM), which is designed to preserve viral viability and inhibit bacterial overgrowth. Liquid specimens, such as aspirates and washes should be collected in sterile containers and transported to the laboratory as quickly as possible. A common mistake is the collection of NP swabs for bacterial culture in the diagnosis of sinusitis. Unfortunately, the nasopharyngeal space is colonized with the same organisms that cause sinusitis and it is very difficult to differentiate colonization from pathogenicity. As a result, the preferred specimen for the diagnosis of sinusitis is a sinus aspirate.

A number of test methodologies are available for the diagnosis of viral URI. These methods include rapid antigen testing (RAT), polymerase chain reaction (PCR) including microarray technology, direct fluorescence antigen (DFA) testing, and viral culture. Due to the acute and often mild nature of these infections, most patients are cared for as outpatients and physicians must make rapid treatment decisions. As a result, the laboratory is expected to provide timely and inexpensive testing. This has been traditionally achieved through moderate or waived complexity testing in the form of RAT. RATs are typically lateral flow antigen capture assays that require only the mixing of patient specimen with a test buffer and the pipetting of that solution on to the test strip. The test strip includes a line of antibodies that are specific to the pathogen of interest in question as well as a control line that ensures proper migration of specimen across the strip. These tests are simple to perform and can typically be completed in less than 30 minutes. Unfortunately, RAT tests suffer from poor performance for the detection of influenza and RSV. Sensitivities have been reported to be as low as 30% and specificities between 80% and >99%.[126,127] In addition, RATs are only available for influenza and RSV. Due to poor performance and the development of high performance molecular tests many laboratories elect not to perform RAT.

Viral culture and DFA are also available for the detection of respiratory viral infection but are quickly being replaced by molecular methods due to their superior sensitivity and relatively short turnaround time. For an excellent discussion on non-molecular methods of viral detection please refer to the following reference.[128] The advent of PCR revolutionized viral diagnostics; more recently, the development of rapid, automated, walk-away PCR technology has largely replaced viral culture and DFA in many laboratories. There are a variety of platforms and molecular chemistries that are being applied to the diagnosis of URI. However, the field appears to be moving in two general directions, narrow spectrum testing and multiplex testing. Narrow spectrum molecular methods are designed to detect a limited number of analytes (typically influenza and/or RSV) but do so very quickly, with high sensitivity and specificity, and for a lower cost than multiplex methods. Multiplex methods are also available and offer the detection of a wide range of analytes including, but not limited to, influenza A (with subtyping), influenza B, rhinovirus/enterovirus, coronavirus, adenovirus, RSV, and some bacterial pathogens, such as Bordetella pertussis, *M pneumoniae*, and *Chlamydia pneumoniae*. Performance of these assays has been extensively evaluated and they have generally proven to have high specificity and high sensitivity although performance for specific viruses can vary significantly.[129] Adenovirus has proven to be particularly problematic for some manufacturers, probably as a result of the high number of serotypes that must be covered.[130] Although these assays are generally only marketed for detection of pathogens from NP swabs, Ruggiero and colleagues showed that they perform very well from lower respiratory tract specimens as well.[131]

Initially these multiplex assays were performed as traditional PCRs in which nucleic acid extraction, amplification, and detection all took place in distinct steps on separate instrumentation. These steps have now been consolidated onto single platforms and the hands-on-time required of the technologist is typically less than 5 minutes.[132] These assays are powerful in that they have simplified what has traditionally been a very complex process requiring highly skilled technologists. Now, a technologist with minimal experience with molecular techniques can safely perform these assays. This may change the landscape or where these tests can be offered, as one could imagine them being performed outside of the traditional laboratory setting. Currently though, these assays are categorized by CLIA as moderate complexity and as result they are primarily still performed in centralized laboratories. In addition, multiplex assays are very expensive and the resulting patient charges are high. Consequently, many providers will reserve the order of multiplex testing for those patients who are going to be admitted or for those who are at risk for severe infection, such as the immunocompromised.

Treatment and antimicrobial susceptibility testing

Because most URI is viral in nature, antibiotics have very little role in managing these infections. Analgesics can be used but providers are usually encouraged to avoid aspirin in the setting of viral infection due to the risk for developing Reye syndrome. Limited antiviral agents are available and include options for the treatment of influenza and RSV. There are four licensed prescription influenza antivirals available in the United States, which are zanamavir, oseltamivir, amantadine, and rimantadine. Zanamavir and oseltamivir are related in that they are both neuraminidase inhibitors and have activity against both influenza A and B. Amantadine and rimantadine are adamantanes and are only active against influenza B.[133] Resistance to these antivirals can vary depending on the currently circulating influenza viruses. For example, in 2010 influenza A H3N2 and H1N1 were co-circulating and were both resistant to the adamantanes but susceptible to oseltamivir and zanamavir.[133] A yearly vaccine for seasonal influenza is also produced and is recommended by the Centers for Disease Control in Prevention. The vaccine is typically available in the form of an injection or as a nasal spray. While the injectable formulation does not include live virus, the nasal spray does (live attenuated). This virus is cold-adapted so that it only replicates in the relatively cooler temperatures of the nares. Despite being attenuated, it is not recommended that young children or those who are immunocompromised be given the nasal spray form of the vaccine.[134]

Antiviral susceptibility testing for influenza is not performed routinely. Surveillance programs monitor for resistance on a population level but testing on individual isolates is infrequently performed. Resistance to influenza antivirals is typically done through genotypic methods to detect amino acid changes that result in a resistant phenotype. Phenotypic methods can also be used to detect resistance and more often, to confirm resistance identified through genotypic methods. Phenotypic methods measure antiviral activity by exposing cultured virus to neuraminidase enzyme with and without the drug being present. The amount of substrate produced by the enzyme is measured, compared, and reported as a ratio called the 50% inhibitory concentration (IC_{50} value), the higher the IC_{50} value, the more resistant the virus.[135]

For RSV infection, children born prematurely or those with preexisting conditions are at greatest risk for developing severe infection. Although vaccination is not available, palivizumab has been licensed for use in the prevention of severe RSV disease in at-risk children and is not approved for treating active RSV disease.

Malaria

Etiology, Epidemiology, and Clinical Presentation

Malaria is an important cause of infection in children and is caused by *Plasmodium falciparum, P vivax, P ovale, P malariae,* and *P knowlesi.* Approximately half of the world's population lives in a malaria-endemic region and it is estimated that over 200 million cases and over 600,000 deaths occurred in 2010. Many of these cases and deaths were in children less than 5 years old living in sub-Saharan Africa.[136] For those that live in non-endemic locations, most infections occur in returning travelers and a significant percentage of those patients are children. In the United Kingdom between 2005 and 2010, there were 1600 cases of imported malaria, of which 10-15% were in children.[137] Of those children, 90% were acquired by African children who had returned to Africa to visit friends and relatives.[138] These species all have different world-wide distributions and clinical presentations which will be discussed for each organism.

P falciparum causes the most severe form of malaria and reaches much higher levels of parasitemia than other forms of malaria. It frequently causes severe and life threatening disease, which can result in any of the following symptoms: impaired consciousness, prostration, failure to feed, multiple convulsions, circulatory collapse or shock, spontaneous bleeding, pulmonary edema, severe normocytic anemia, among others.

Plasmodium vivax (also known as benign tertian malaria) causes its primary clinical disease 7-10 days following exposure. However in some patients, a more prolonged incubation (weeks to months) can occur. *P vivax* causes a less severe form of disease than *P falciparum* but symptoms can include myalgias, headache, nausea, fever, and anorexia. Complications from *P vivax* infection are rare but coma and sudden death have been reported. Untreated disease can last for several weeks to months and relapses are thought to occur in up to 50% of patients.

Plasmodium ovale and *P vivax* cause very similar forms of diseases but *P ovale* is generally thought to be less severe. Like *P vivax*, *P ovale* infects reticulocytes and results in lower levels of parasitemia than *P falciparum*. *P ovale* also relapses less frequently than *P vivax*. *P malariae* causes less severe disease than *P falciparum* and has a longer incubation period than *P vivax* and *P ovale*. In children, infection can result in proteinuria and a nephrotic syndrome. True relapses do not occur with *P malariae* but recrudescence is well documented and can occur up to 50 years after primary infection. Patients who experience recrudescence will have latent infection and persistent low-levels of parasitemia.

P knowlesi was first recognized as a primate pathogen in Southeast Asia but has since been firmly established as a human pathogen. It causes disease that is mild to moderate in severity with a 9 to 12 day incubation period. Central nervous system manifestations occur infrequently and true relapse does not occur.[139]

Laboratory Diagnosis

Because the course of malaria can evolve quickly and result in severe infection, rapid diagnosis is critical for patient care. The standard of diagnosis is microscopic evaluation of thick and thin blood Giemsa smears. Blood specimens can either be collected by venipuncture or by finger prick. It is essential that blood smears be prepared and stained within an hour of collection. Delays in processing will allow the parasites to continue to mature, which distorts their morphology and can lead to misidentification. The microscopic identification of *Plasmodium* spp. is dependent on the morphology of the parasite. A detailed description of *Plasmodium* spp. morphology is outside the scope of this chapter, please see the following resources for information on the morphologic identification of malaria.[1,140]

A single set of negative blood smears does not rule-out malaria infection and additional blood specimens should be collected and evaluated at 12 hour intervals over the next 36 hours.[1] The thick smear evaluates a greater volume of blood and provides a more sensitive test than the thin smear, which is used primarily for morphologic identification and calculation of percentage parasitemia. Species-level identification can be achieved with a thick smear in some cases, but it typically requires an experienced parasitologist that is capable of differentiating the organism from platelets, leukocyte granules, and other debris.

There are several alternatives to the thick and thin smear when diagnosing malaria. The two most common are antigen detection with an immuochromatographic assay and nucleic acid detection. Antigen detection offers a rapid result in a test format that is easy to perform. The test is relatively inexpensive but suffers from high limits of detection and a correspondingly poor sensitivity for non-*P falciparum* infections.[141,142] Nucleic acid has been shown superior sensitivity to microscopy and its advantage is the ability to detect mixed infections.[142] The disadvantages of nucleic acid detection are that it is not widely available and in most cases, specimens must be sent to reference labs which may contribute to prolonged turnaround-times.

Treatment and Antimicrobial Susceptibility Testing

Treatment of malaria infection is dependent on the epidemiology of resistance for endemic strains, severity of illness, the species of infecting *Plasmodium*, percent parasitemia, and patient-specific factors. For severe malaria, intravenous artesunate or intravenous quinine may be given. If the species of *Plasmodium* is *P vivax* or *P ovale* or unknown, primaquine can also be administered. In addition, exchange transfusions may be considered when parasitemia reaches high levels. There is no firm recommendation for when to consider exchange transfusion, but 5 or 10% parasitemia are frequently used cut-offs. However, due to a lack of data demonstrating improvement in clinical outcome, the CDC no longer recommends exchange transfusion in the treatment of severe malaria infections.

Uncomplicated infection can be treated in a variety of ways once the infecting species has been determined. If the species is *P falciparum*, the treatment of choice is artemether plus lumefantrine with alternatives being atovaquone proguanil or quinine plus clindamycin, doxycycline, or tetracycline. If the infecting species is *P vivax*, *P ovale*, *P malariae*, or *P knowlesi* and the infection did not occur in a chloroquine-resistant area, chloroquine or artemether plus lumefantrine can be used. Primaquine should be used if the species is *P vivax* or *P ovale*. The treatment of choice for organisms likely to be resistant to chloroquine would be artemether plus lumefantrine, atovaquone plus malarone, quinine plus clindamycin or doxycycline, or mefloquine. Primaquine can be used for *P vivax* that are resistant to chloroquine.[136] The CDC has published a treatment algorithm to aid in the treatment of malaria infection.[143]

Susceptibility testing for individual isolates of malaria for the treatment of specific patients is not performed. Surveillance programs run by government agencies such as the CDC and the WHO provided epidemiological data on malarial drug resistance. These organizations and others provide updated surveillance data that is freely accessible on their websites and can be used to guide therapy.

Conjunctivitis

Etiology, Epidemiology, and Clinical Presentation

Infectious conjunctivitis in children manifests as itching, burning, tearing, discharge, photophobia and foreign body sensation. Common bacterial etiologies include *H influenzae, P aeruginosa, S pneumoniae, M catarrhalis,* and *Staphylococcus aureus. N gonorrhea* may cause a hyperacute form of disease while *C trachomatis* causes a distinct form of disease as well. Inpatients may develop infections mediated by *P aeruginosa* and the *Enterobacteriaceae*. The most common viral etiologies of conjunctivitis are adenovirus, enterovirus, and coxsackievirus.

Laboratory Diagnosis

Clinical suspicion for bacterial conjunctivitis is usually sufficient to initiate empiric therapy with Gram stain and culture being the laboratory diagnostic methods of choice for bacterial conjunctivitis. In most laboratories, ocular cultures involve inoculation of sheep blood and chocolate agar followed by incubation at 35-37°C for 48 hours.

In certain circumstances, culture can provide important and actionable information. The identification of *N gonorrhea* in a child beyond the neonatal period should raise concern for sexual abuse. *P aeruginosa* also can cause serious eye infection which should be considered a medical emergency.

Laboratory testing plays a minor role in the diagnosis of viral conjunctivitis. However, the wide-spread adoption of respiratory viral panels, which include adenovirus and enterovirus can be used as a general marker of respiratory tract infection which may point to the etiology of conjunctivitis.

Treatment and Antimicrobial Susceptibility Testing

Bacterial conjunctivitis is usually a self-limited disease. However, topical antimicrobial treatment can be administered and results in faster resolution of symptoms. Such treatments include topical trimethoprim-polymyxin B, tobramycin, gentamicin, erythromycin, or a fluoroquinolone. Systemic treatment is required for *N gonorrhea* and *C trachomatis* infections but susceptibility testing does not play a role in managing these infections. The ability of in vitro susceptibility testing to predict the outcome of topically administered antibiotics is unproven. In addition, isolates of *P aeruginosa* should be tested as they can lead to complicated infections which may require systemic therapy in addition to topical treatment.[144]

Treatment of viral conjunctivitis is usually supportive. However, antiviral therapy may be warranted for Herpes Simplex Virus (HSV) infections or for infections that progress to corneal involvement.[145]

Bone and Joint Infections and Septic Arthritis

Etiology, Epidemiology, and Clinical Presentation

Bone and joint space infections are a significant cause of morbidity in children. The etiologies of these infections vary by presentation. The principal pathogens in pediatric osteomyelitis and septic arthritis are bacterial but vary with the age of the child. For all age groups *Staphylococcus aureus* is the most commonly isolated pathogen. In infants, Group B *Streptococcus* (*Streptococcus agalactiae*) has been shown to cause osteomyelitis and Gram-negative rods, such as the *Enterobacteriaceae* are also commonly encountered. In young children (<5 years old) *Kingella kingae* may be an underappreciated cause of disease. In addition, Group A *Streptococcus* (*S pyogenes*), *P aeruginosa*, *Candida albicans*, and *S pneumoniae* have been reported to cause bone and joint infection with some frequency.[146] In sexually active adolescents, disseminated *N gonorrhea* infection can lead to septic arthritis.

Most children with acute osteomyelitis experience persistent and increasing pain over the affected bone. In infants, this may manifest as irritability or reluctance to move the affected bone. Fever is typically present. Trauma is commonly a predisposing event but hematogenous spread is responsible for a significant amount of bone infection. Septic arthritis often follows trauma but may be preceded in some cases by upper respiratory tract infection. Symptoms include, joint pain, fever, and irritability. Children will complain of pain in the affected joint and will experience restricted range of motion.[147]

Laboratory Diagnosis

Given that most pediatric bone and joint infection is bacterial, Gram stain and culture are the primary laboratory diagnostic techniques utilized. Despite the fact that there is often a high suspicion for infection, culture frequently fails to yield a pathogen. It is estimated that up to 30% of osteomyelitis cases are culture-negative.[148] Identifying a pathogen from a bone aspirate provide conclusive evidence of infection, however, a positive blood culture plus abnormal imaging or physical findings suggestive of osteomyelitis is also considered diagnostic. Broad spectrum molecular assays targeting the 16S rRNA gene has been shown to be a useful diagnostic supplement to culture. Although pediatric specific data evaluating the utility of 16S PCR in the diagnosis of osteomyelitis is sparse, Choi et al. conducted a prospective study in adult patients with vertebral osteomyelitis and found that 16S PCR identified twice as many pathogens as culture.[149]

The diagnosis of septic arthritis should include both blood and joint fluid cultures. Blood cultures are particularly useful because they can yield a pathogen when joint fluid cultures are negative. Joint fluid should be collected and sent for Gram-stain and culture. It is believed that synovial fluid exerts an inhibitory effect on bacterial growth which is why cultures are negative in up to 35% of patients with clinical evidence of joint infection. *Kingella kingae* is notorious for causing culture-negative septic arthritis. As a result, it is recommended that joint fluid be incubated into blood culture media, a maneuver that has been shown to increase the yield of *K kingae*. It has also been shown that molecular methods can increase the diagnostic yield of joint fluid specimens.[150]

Treatment and Susceptibility Testing

Surgical therapy through debridement or drainage is an important component of managing osteomyelitis. These procedures also provide material that can be sent to the lab for culture and susceptibility testing. If culture fails to provide a definitive diagnosis these infections must be managed empirically which should include coverage for *S aureus* and Group A *Streptococcus*. In some areas it may be necessary to empirically cover for methicillin resistant *S aureus* (MRSA). Common choices for MRSA would be vancomycin and clindamycin. Duration of therapy is important for successful management of osteomyelitis and there is strong evidence that longer treatment regimens have higher success rates.[151,152]

Septic arthritis should be treated empirically in much the same way as osteomyelitis. *S pneumoniae* is a common cause of septic arthritis and when isolated, antimicrobial susceptibility testing should be performed. Lemaitre et al conducted a study before and after the introduction of the 7-valent pneumococcal vaccine and found that the epidemiology of osteoarticular infection shifted with serotype 19A replacing vaccine strains as the most common serotype.[153] Unfortunately, the majority of serotype 19A strains also had reduced sensitivity to penicillin. Overall, 46% of the pneumococcal population was intermediate to penicillin with only 12% being resistant. Third generation cephalosporins maintained good activity against *S pneumococcus* with only 12% of isolates being intermediate and no isolates demonstrating resistance. *K kingae* is a relatively common cause of septic arthritis in pediatrics and is generally treated with beta-lactam antibiotics. Patients with *K kingae* infection who are covered empirically with vancomycin or clindamycin will not respond.

Skin Infections, Wounds, and Animal Bites

Etiology, Epidemiology, Clinical Presentation, Diagnosis, and Treatment

Children develop a variety of skin and wound infections and a full discussion of the topic is outside the scope of this chapter. Instead this section will focus on the most common manifestations in children and each clinical presentation will be discussed individually along with its etiology and epidemiology.

1. Impetigo

The most common skin infection encountered by children is non-bullous impetigo. The infection is spread through direct human-to-human contact and is most prevalent in the warmer months. This infection occurs following trauma to the skin which can be as minor as an insect bite. Non-bullous impetigo presents as erythematous macro-papules that start out as small pustules. Common characteristics include the honey-colored crust as well as the frequent spread to adjacent exposed areas. Non-bullous impetigo lesions are slow to develop and have mild symptoms. In the United States these infections are most commonly caused by *S aureus* and Group A *Streptococcus*.

Bullous impetigo starts with small vesicles or pustules but evolves to painless bullae. The infection typically remains localized except in neonates where dissemination occasionally occurs. In infants a severe, toxin-mediated form of disease can develop from bullous impetigo and is known as Ritter disease. These infections are almost always caused by *S aureus*.

The laboratory diagnosis of impetigo involves the collection of vesicle material and evaluating it with Gram stain and bacterial culture. Specimen is obtained by unroofing a crusted vesicle and collecting the exudate. Gram stains performed directly from specimen will commonly show Gram-positive cocci and culture will typically yield either group A *Streptococcus* or *S aureus* or a combination of both.

Non-serious manifestations of impetigo can be managed with topical treatments that cover the affected area. For more severe disease, systemic antibiotics may be required and should include anti-staphylococcal coverage. Community acquired methicillin resistant *S aureus* (CA-MRSA) is a common cause of impetigo and as such, empiric treatments should be selected accordingly. Clindamycin and trimethoprim-sulfamethoxazole are common choices for the treatment of CA-MRSA. Both are highly active against methicillin susceptible *S aureus* as well as MRSA.[154]

2. Perianal cellulitis

Perianal cellulitis (also known as perianal streptococcal dermatitis) is a superficial skin infection that results in perirectal swelling and tenderness but does not result in systemic symptoms. Some patients will experience pain during stooling and bloody stools.[155] These infections are primarily caused by group A *Streptococcus* but there is some evidence that *S aureus* may be an emerging cause of disease.[156] There are reports of *Streptococcus dysgalactiae* causing perianal cellulitis but those are primarily reported in adults and not children.[157]

Surface cultures collected with a swab from the perianal area are the primary diagnostic method employed. These cultures will frequently yield abundant growth of the causative pathogen so despite the presence of contaminating intestinal flora; culture usually provides a clear diagnosis.

The principle pathogen for perianal cellulitis is Group A *Streptococcus* which is uniformly susceptible to beta-lactam antibiotics. Nonetheless, approximately 35% of patients treated with penicillin or amoxicillin experience a recurrence. These rates are higher than what has been reported when a beta-lactamase resistant antibiotic is used, although recurrence still occurs in approximately 30% of these patients.[158]

3. Erysipelas

Erysipelas presents as a bright erythematous plaque with raised borders and a clear line of demarcation. The infection is typically localized to either the face or the lower extremities. Patients are frequently febrile, ill-appearing and the disease has been known to rapidly progress. The primary pathogen of erysipelas is group A *Streptococcus* but there is some evidence that some other non-group A beta-hemolytic streptococci are capable of causing this disease as well.[159]

The diagnosis of erysipelas is primarily made on clinical grounds. However, if culture confirmation is sought it should be pursued with aspiration of the leading edge of the lesion. The etiologies of this disease are bacterial and as such routine aerobic bacterial cultures are the laboratory diagnostic method of choice.

Group A *Streptococcus* is the most common cause of erysipelas and is uniformly susceptible to penicillin. Susceptibility testing is not warranted for individual isolates of GAS and patients with erysipelas generally respond promptly to treatment.

4. Bite Wounds

Bite wounds can be divided into two distinct categories; human and animal. Human bites occur under varying circumstances, such as in child abuse, accidental bites during play, or intentional toddler biting. They may also occur in "clenched-fist" encounters which can lead to severe and rapidly progressive infection. Bites may present as minor abrasions, scratches, or indentations or they may present as lacerations, or contusions. These infections are usually polymicrobic and include a mixture of aerobic and anaerobic organisms from the mouth of the biter and the skin of the victim. The most frequently isolated organisms from human bite wounds include *S aureus, Streptococcus* spp., *Eikenella corrodens, Bacteroides* spp., *Fusobacterium* spp., and anaerobic Gram-positive cocci.[160]

Over 4 million animal bite wounds are reported annually in the United States with children accounting for over half of patients who reported to emergency departments.[161] Cats and dogs combine for the majority of bites and are associated with significant morbidity. Reptiles, rodents, horses, sheep, and pigs are also responsible for a significant percentage of animal bites. Due to their puncture-like nature, cat-bites are more likely than dog bites to become infected. The most common pathogens associated with dog and cat bites are *Pasteurella* spp., *S aureus, Capnocytophaga* spp., streptococci, and anaerobes. Reptiles have different oral flora and their bites frequently result in anaerobic as well as enteric Gram-negative infection. Rabies can be a concern when an animal bite occurs. Up until the 1960s domestic animals accounted for the majority of rabies transmissions, however, the majority of transmissions now result from wild animal bites including raccoons (36.5%), skunks (23.5%), bats (23.2%), and foxes (7.0%) (http://www.cdc.gov/rabies/index.html (accessed 2/16/15)).

Human and animal bite wounds are polymicrobic in nature and swabs of the wound should be collected for both aerobic and anaerobic culture prior to initiation of antibiotic therapy. Not all swab collection devices are appropriate for anaerobic culture so laboratories should be familiar with the recommendations for their collection devices before accepting the specimen for anaerobic culture.[160]

Research has shown that antimicrobial prophylaxis for human bite wounds in children is not necessary as most resolve without complicating infections. When human or animal bite wounds become infected antibiotic therapy should be administered and should include a penicillin or aminopenicillin plus a penicillinase-resistant penicillin or amoxicillin-clavulanate.[160] If rabies is of concern, the vaccine should be administered and has been shown to be highly effective at preventing the development of disease. Lastly, health care providers should ensure that the child is up-to-date on their tetanus vaccine.

5. Viral Skin Infections

There is no treatment for most viral skin infections and care is only supportive. For HSV infections care is usually supportive but acyclovir can be used in cases where therapy is deemed necessary. Chickenpox does not require antiviral therapy in otherwise healthy patients. However, antiviral therapy may be needed for infants and the immunocompromised. In addition, a VZV vaccination program was initiated in 1996 and has drastically reduced the number of chickenpox-related deaths, hospital admissions, and overall cases in the United States (http://www.cdc.gov/chickenpox/vaccine-infographic.html (accessed 2/16/15)).

Children are commonly infected with viruses that result in cutaneous disease. These infections can result in a wide variety of manifestations including rash, warts, lesions, and vesicles. Clinically, some presentations are distinct but many viral exanthems cannot be distinguished accurately by clinical presentation alone.[162]

Molluscum contagiosum is caused by a poxvirus that can infect children of any age with the highest prevalence being seen in children less than 14 years of age.[163] The characteristic lesions of molluscum can measure as large as 5 mm in diameter, and have a dome-shape with a distinct central depression.

Fifth disease is caused by Parvovirus B19 and is also known as erythema infectiosum. This infection results in a classic rash that is termed the "slapped cheek" disease because of its location and appearance on a child's cheeks. The infection can also result in a glove-and-sock eruption as well as a manifestation around the groin area. Children with fifth disease are generally well-appearing and may run a low-grade fever.

Hand, foot, and mouth syndrome presents classically with fever and vesicles on the palms and soles with painful sores in the mouth (herpangina). The rash is typically on the hands and feet but can also appear on the genital area, knees, and elbows.[164] Outbreaks are common and occur frequently within daycare centers, homes, and schools. The disease is most frequently caused by coxsackievirus A16 and less commonly by enterovirus.[71]

The herpesvirus family includes herpes simplex virus types 1 and 2 (HSV1/2), varicella-zoster virus (VZV), Epstein-Barr virus (EBV), cytomegalovirus (CMV), and human herpesviruses. Of those, HSV and VZV frequently cause skin infection in children. HSV causes oral or perioral vesicles that are painful and result in erosions with a "punched-out" appearance. Oral infection is most common but several other HSV manifestations can also occur. These include infection transmitted through close contact during sporting events (herpes gladiatorum), painful vesicles of the finger tips (herpetic whitlow), and HSV spread over abnormal skin barriers (eczema herpeticum). Finally, chickenpox, mediated by VZV, is a common manifestation in children. The characteristic vesicles on erythematous bases are seen over the entire body and commonly involve the mucous membranes. Although the mortality of chickenpox is low, the infection is highly contagious and the implementation of a VZV vaccine in 1996 has reduced mortality by 90%.[165]

Because the management of viral skin infections is often supportive, laboratory confirmation of a diagnosis is not always sought. The diagnosis is based primarily on clinical presentation. Laboratory confirmation of molluscum contagiosum, fifth disease, hand, foot, and mouth syndrome is rare. However, HSV and VZV can both be readily cultured from infected lesions. Direct fluorescent antibody (DFA) assays can also be performed directly from specimen and allow for a more rapid diagnosis than culture. In addition, there are now commercially available PCR assays that can detect HSV and VZV and differentiate between HSV 1 and 2. These assays can be performed quickly and have high sensitivity and specificity.

6. Fungal Skin Infections

Tinea infections are superficial skin infections that are caused by dermatophytes and frequently occur in children. Dermatophytes are capable of infecting the hair, nail, or skin. Tinea infections of the scalp (tinea capitis or scalp ringworm) are caused most commonly by *Trichophyton* spp. which is transmitted through human-to-human contact or by *Microsporum* spp. which is transmitted more commonly through contact with infected cats and dogs. Infection results in scaling of the scalp which may be diffuse or localized and may or may not result in hair loss. Tinea corporis refers to infections of the trunk and/or extremities where rash results in a red-ringed patch of blisters or scaled skin and is often accompanied by severe itching. Tinea pedis is an infection of the feet that afflicts adolescents and specifically targets the instep and the area between the toes.

Candida spp. is one of the more common fungal infections in children and can cause disease in both the immunocompetent and the immunocompromised. *Candida* spp. prefer a warm, moist environment are associated with a wide variety of diseases, such as vulvovaginitis (in adolescents), diaper rash, thrush, and onychomycosis secondary to thumb sucking.

Many fungal skin infections are diagnosed by clinical presentation alone as tinea and *Candida* infections have very characteristic features. In addition, the treatment for these infections is often administered empirically and topically such that culture is rarely useful in guiding treatment. Nevertheless, culture is occasionally sought when the etiology of disease is not clear or patients do not respond to treatment. For dermatophyte infections, skin scrapings from the affected area are commonly collected as are nail clippings and hair specimens. These specimens come from body sites that are colonized with other flora and as a result selective media should be used to reduce contaminating growth while allowing the dermatophytes to grow. Such media include inhibitory mold agar (IMA), dermatophytes test media (DTM), Mycosel, and others. Dermatophytes are generally slow-growing and will be readily overtaken by faster growing organisms. Once isolated, microscopic evaluation of lactophenol cotton blue tape preparations are the key to identification and diagnosis.

The culture-diagnosis of *Candida* spp. presents a different challenge in that it can be normal flora but it can also be a pathogen. In addition, *Candida* spp. grow much faster than dermatophytes and can be readily isolated from routine bacterial cultures on sheep blood agar as well as chocolate agar. Interpretation of these cultures can be difficult though as it may be difficult to distinguish *Candida* colonization from disease. Growth of *Candida* that is abundant or predominant provides strong evidence that it is acting as a pathogen as is a direct-specimen Gram stain that shows the organism with many white blood cells and few squamous epithelial cells.

Tinea infections as a broad category are treated with topical antifungals for several weeks but severe or refractory disease may require oral antifungals.

Griseofulvin is the only oral antifungal that is FDA-cleared for use in children. Nonetheless, other antifungals, such as fluconazole, itraconazole, and terbinifine have all been used off-label.[166]

Superficial *Candida* spp. infections can usually be treated with topical antifungals with nystatin being the drug of choice. However, refractory or serious disease may require systemic treatment, such as oral fluconazole or intravenous amphotericin B. In cases of diaper rash, it is important to keep the affected area clean and dry which can be accomplished with frequent diaper changes and the use of barrier creams.

Pinworm, Lice, and Scabies

Etiology, Epidemiology, Clinical Presentation, Diagnosis, and Treatment

Pinworm, lice, and scabies are parasitic diseases that can infect all ages but children are particularly prone to disease. Each disease will be discussed individually in the sections later.

Pinworm

Pinworm (*Enterobius vermicularis*) is a nematode that may be the world's most common parasitic infection. Although adults can become infected prevalence in children is particularly high. Human infection begins with consumption of infective eggs which then hatch in the intestine and develop into adults. Female worms will migrate to the anus where eggs are deposited. Clinically, patients will present with severe pruritus in the perianal region. In many patients this is the only symptom while some are asymptomatic. Eosinophilia is not always present and cannot be used to exclude disease.

The laboratory diagnosis of pinworm is relatively simple. Scotch tape is applied to the perianal area which will collect the female-deposited eggs. The Scotch tape is then applied to a microscope slide which can then be examined for the presence of the pinworm eggs. The worms themselves are rarely visualized during this procedure but presence of the eggs is diagnostic. Pinworm eggs have a characteristic appearance with a thin shell wall and a distinct flattening of one side. They measure 50-60 μm in length by 20-30 μm in width.

Pyrantel or mebendazole have been shown to be extremely effective in treating pinworm infection. Laboratories do not provide susceptibility testing in pinworm infections with their sole role being diagnostic.

Lice

Children acquire three primary types of louse infection, head louse (*Pediculus humanus capitis*), body louse (*Pediculus humanus corporis*), and pubic louse (*Pthirus pubis*). Lice are parasitic insects that cause infestations of the host with the most common symptom being itching that results from an allergic reaction to the louse bites. These infections are spread through human-to-human contact and are not spread through contact with animals.

Head lice are 2-3 mm in length and infect the head and neck area by laying their eggs at the base of the hair shaft. It is most common in preschool and elementary-age children but reliable prevalence data in the United States are not available. It is estimated though that between 6 and 12 million infestations occur in the United States annually in 3 to 11 year olds. Girls may be more likely to contract disease than boys because of more frequent head-to-head contact.[167]

Body lice are 2.3-3.6 mm in length and live primarily on clothing. Body lice move to the skin to feed only and lay their eggs on clothing. In contrast to the head louse, body lice are capable of transmitting infections, such as relapsing fever, typhus, and trench fever. Infections occur most commonly in individuals who live under crowded conditions and with poor hygiene. Children are less likely to become infected with body louse and most infections occur in the homeless or those who do not have access to regular bathing. Symptoms include intense itching and a rash that results from an allergic reaction to the louse bites. "Vagabond's Disease" occurs on areas of the body with a high density of louse bites that become darkened with skin thickening.[168]

Pubic lice or "crabs" are 1.1 to 1.8 mm in length and attach to hair found in the pubic area. This infection is spread through sexual contact and is exclusively human-to-human. Due to the nature of contact required for transmission, sexually active adolescents are frequently infected. However, in cases of sexual abuse children can develop infection of the head or eyelashes. Pubic lice infection occurs in all ages, races, and socioeconomic levels of society.[169] Symptoms of pubic lice include itching which leads to scratching and the occasional development of sore and secondary bacterial infection.

Head and body louse infestation is diagnosed by finding a live nymph or adult louse on an infected individual. Louse can be seen with the naked eye but must be observed under a microscope in order to appreciate their features and confirm that they are in fact a louse and no other artifacts that may resemble louse when viewed without magnification.[167,168]

Pubic louse infection is similar to head and body louse in that they are diagnosed by visualization of the parasite on the infected host. Pubic lice are different that head and body lice because they are shorter crab-like insects.

Pediculicides are the medicine used to treat head louse infection. Some are able to kill the eggs (ova) while others do not. With treatments that are weakly ovicidal, a retreatment is recommended after all eggs have hatched but before new eggs can be laid.

Body louse infection is managed by improving personal hygiene. This includes regular bathing as well as changing and washing clothing, bedding, and towels in water that is at least 130°F and machine dried with high heat.

Medical treatment can be used to manage these infections but it is generally not necessary. If treatment is sought, the recommendations are exactly the same as those for head lice.

Pubic louse infection can be treated with over-the-counter medications which contain 1% permethrin or piperonyl butoxide. Lindane shampoo is a prescription medication that kills both the louse and its eggs. Due to toxicities these medication should be used as second-line therapy. Malathion lotion and ivermectin have also been used to effectively treat these infections but these are not approved by the Food and Drug Administration (FDA) for the treatment of pubic lice in the United States.[169]

Scabies

Scabies is a skin infestation that is caused by *Sarcoptes scabiei* that results in extreme pruritus. Symptoms develop weeks to month after the initial infestation. In children, the characteristic burrows and linear pustules form on the palms and soles as well as on the head and neck. Humans are the only known reservoir for this infection and it is transmitted by extended, close, human-to-human contact. Outbreaks of scabies have been reported in hospitals or other institutions where close contact occurs and where sanitary conditions are poor.

The diagnosis of scabies is made by observing the characteristic mites and/or their eggs from a skin scraping from the end of one of the burrows or from a skin biopsy. The mites and eggs are small enough that they must be visualized microscopically.

Treatment of scabies involves the topical application of lindane, permethrin 5%, and crotamiton 10% over the entire surface of the skin. In infants and young children permethrin is topical cream.[170] When treating an index patient, all family members and close contacts should also be treated and clothes, bed sheets, and towels should be washed in hot water (130°F) and dried in high heat.

Meningitis

Etiology, Epidemiology, and Clinical Presentation

Bacterial meningitis is considered one of the most devastating medical diagnoses in children due to its association with high rates of mortality and long-term sequelae including hearing loss and mental retardation. The etiology of bacterial meningitis varies with age. *S agalactiae, E coli,* and *L monocytogenes* dominate in newborns. The vaccine-preventable pathogens *S pneumoniae, H influenzae* b, and *N meningitidis* emerge as the leading etiologic agents in mid-infancy. While the third-trimester *S agalactiae* screening in pregnant women has vastly reduced the incidence of invasive *S agalactiae* infections in infants, cases continue to be reported, particularly in premature infants. Similarly, the introduction of conjugate vaccines in the United States has also dramatically reduced the incidence of invasive infections mediated by vaccine preventable pathogens, but cases continue to be reported, particularly in infants who have yet to receive their full vaccination course and in individuals with either primary or acquired immune deficiencies.

Viral meningitis in the United States is predominantly mediated by nonpolio enteroviruses. Other etiologies include the arboviruses (eg, West Nile Virus) and the herpesviridae (eg, Herpes Simplex virus, Varicella Zoster virus), and less commonly, measles, mumps, and other viral agents.

Laboratory Diagnosis

Laboratory diagnosis requires recovery of the responsible pathogen from cerebrospinal fluid (CSF) acquired through a lumbar puncture. Initial rapid diagnostic testing include a cytological "cell count" and Gram stain. Definitive diagnosis requires recovery of the responsible pathogen in culture or detection of its nucleic acid. Recovery from culture can be optimized by collecting CSF prior to administration of antimicrobials, and transport to the laboratory at room temperature within an hour of collection. It is imperative to report positive CSF Gram stains and evidence of growth on culture to the responsible physician immediately to ensure that appropriate antimicrobial therapy is initiated in a timely fashion.

Cytological examination typically involves a white blood cell (WBC) count with differential; glucose and protein concentrations; and is performed on uncentrifuged CSF. In adults, pleocytosis with WBC >10 cells/mm^3 with a predominance of polymorphonuclear (PMNs); decreased glucose (<45 mg/dL); and increased protein concentration (>45 mg/dL) have been considered markers of bacterial meningitis.[171] However, the observation has been made that in healthy, non-infected infants, WBC can range from 10-30 WBC/mm^3 with up to 50% PMNs.[171] Chadwick et al noted that this effect appears to be predominantly seen in the first week of life.[172] Along with Shah et al., they also corroborated data demonstrating a gradual declinc in median CSF protein from 98 to 59 mg/dL over the course of a newborn's first 8 weeks of life.[172,173] CSF protein levels in this population should be interpreted accordingly. Finally, CSF glucose needs to be interpreted in the context of serum glucose level. A ratio of 0.6 has been determined to be normal in children.[174] CSF to serum ratios less than 0.6 can suggest glycolysis by WBC and a bacterial agent of meningitis.

Sedimentation of bacteria through cytocentrifugation (1500 × g for 15 minutes) increases the sensitivity of Gram staining and culture and is typically pursued when CSF volumes of >1 mL are available. Published reports of Gram stain sensitivity for the diagnosis of bacterial meningitis in pediatric populations vary considerably, ranging from 67 to 95%.[175] Also, with declining incidence, positive predictive values have been reported as low as 47%. Therefore, Gram stain results should be used in conjunction with cytology results when making the diagnosis of meningitis in children.

Another direct method of pathogen detection in CSF is the use of latex agglutination to detect capsular polysaccharide bacterial antigen. However, due to problems with sensitivity and specificity, they are not recommended for routine clinical use in the diagnosis bacterial meningitis.[176] Molecular assays have rapidly emerged as an alternative direct method testing on CSF. In the United States, there are currently no FDA-cleared assays designed to detect bacterial agents of meningitis although various monoplex and multiplex laboratory-developed tests have been described. For viral meningitis, the Xpert EV (Cepheid, Sunnyvale, CA) and the NucliSENS EasyQ Enterovirus (bioMérieux, Durham, NC) assays are FDA-cleared and based on real-time PCR and NASBA technology respectively. There are no FDA-cleared assays for detection of HSV1/HSV2 or the arboviruses.

Culture of CSF involves inoculation of either uncentrifuged CSF or sediment on to solid and liquid media. 5% sheep's blood agar is ideal for cultivation of *S pneumoniae*. Requiring both factor X (hemin) and V (NAD), *H influenzae* can be recovered on chocolate agar (NAD is released through heating of and hemolysis of blood agar); 5% sheep's blood agar cross streaked with a *S aureus* "streak" (with organism growth "satelliting" in hemolyzed areas) or sheep's blood agar supplemented with NAD disks. Inoculation of broth media can also be pursued. However, high recovery rates of contaminants have been reported, which can in turn, contribute to diagnostic uncertainty.[176] Inoculated media are incubated for 18-24 hours at 35-37°C in 5% CO_2 to enhance growth of the pathogens of interest. Antimicrobial susceptibility testing reports require additional thought and only antimicrobials that are known to cross the blood brain barrier should be reported (eg, first and second generation cephalosporins; macrolides; and lincosamides do not). The Clinical Laboratory Standards Institute has CSF-specific recommendations for antimicrobial susceptibility interpretation and reporting for *S pneumoniae, H influenzae,* and *Enterobacteriaceae.*[47]

SUMMARY

The laboratory diagnosis of infectious diseases is very different in children than it is adults. The epidemiology of pediatric infectious diseases is unique in that, within the pediatric population, certain age groups are susceptible to different types of infections. For example, the neonate, infants, adolescents, and young adults are all susceptible to different arrays of diseases. Understanding these difference is critical to establish a targeted differential from which the appropriate laboratory testing can be performed. Of particular note is the importance of specimen collection in the pediatric population. Specimen collection in children is complicated by many factors which include small size and low sample volumes (ie, blood), limited bodily function control (ie, incontinence), inability to cooperate for specimen collection, and many other factors. Each of these factors make diagnosing infectious diseases more difficult in children than in adults. Lastly, the treatment of pediatric infectious diseases is complicated by the fact that use of certain antimicrobial agents may be complicated by unique adverse effects (eg, macrolides and pyloric stenosis in infants; sulfonamides, and hyperbilirubinemia in neonates), uncertain dosing, and lack of FDA clearance for use in children. In addition, these treatment decisions are guided by laboratory data that has largely been generated by evidence generated in the adult population.

TRAINING MODULE

1. An 8-year-old child is suspected of having group A *Streptococcus* pharyngitis but rapid antigen testing for this organism is negative. Which of the following statements is correct?
   a. The child does not have group A *Streptococcus* pharyngitis
   b. It is uncertain whether the child has group A *Streptococcus* and confirmatory culture should be performed before concluding that the child does not have disease.
   c. Rapid antigen testing is not the standard of care and a molecular test should have been ordered instead.
   d. Group A *Streptococcus* pharyngitis is not common in children less than 15 years of age and testing should not have been ordered.

2. A neonate is suspected of having early onset sepsis and blood cultures reveal a Gram-negative rod that grows on chocolate, sheep blood, and MacConkey agar. The organism grows on MacConkey as a lactose fermenter, is indole-positive, and oxidase-negative. What is the identity of this organism?
   a. Group B *Streptococcus*
   b. *Kingella kingae*
   c. *Escherichia coli*
   d. *Klebsiella pneumoniae*

3. A child is suspected of having *Kingella kingae* septic arthritis, however, synovial fluid cultures are negative. Which of the following culture techniques can help to improve the yield of *K kingae* from synovial fluid cultures.
   a. Incubate cultures anaerobically
   b. Incubate cultures at 42°C
   c. Add buffered charcoal yeast extract media
   d. Inject some specimen in blood culture bottles and incubate in a standard blood culture system

REFERENCES

1. Versalovic J, Carroll KC, Funke G, Jorgenson JH, Landry ML, Warnock DW, eds. *Manual of Clinical Microbiology*, 10th ed. ASM Press. Washington DC. 2011.

2. Winn WC, Allen SD, Janda WM, Koneman EW, Procop G, Schreckenberger PC, Woods G, eds. *Koneman's Color Atlas and Textbook of Diagnostic Microbiology*. 6th ed. Lippincott, Williams & Wilkins. Baltimore. 2006.

3. Ehrenkranz NJ. Bacterial colonization of newborn infants and subsequent acquisition of hospital bacteria. *J Pediatr*. 1970;76(6):839-847.

4. Fryklund B, Tullus K, Berglund B, Burman LG. Importance of the environment and the faecal flora of infants, nursing staff and parents as sources of gram-negative bacteria colonizing newborns in three neonatal wards. *Infection*. 1992;20(5):253-257.

5. Goldmann DA, Leclair J, Macone A. Bacterial colonization of neonates admitted to an intensive care environment. *J Pediatr*. 1978;93(2):288-293.

6. Zervou FN, Zacharioudakis IM, Ziakas PD, Mylonakis E. MRSA colonization and risk of infection in the neonatal and pediatric ICU: a meta-analysis. *Pediatrics*. 2014;133(4):e1015-e1023.

7. Keski-Nisula L, Kyynarainen HR, Karkkainen U, Karhukorpi J, Heinonen S, Pekkanen J. Maternal intrapartum antibiotics and decreased vertical transmission of Lactobacillus to neonates during birth. *Acta paediatrica*. 2013;102(5):480-485.

8. Benno Y, Sawada K, Mitsuoka T. The intestinal microflora of infants: composition of fecal flora in breast-fed and bottle-fed infants. *Microbiol Immunol*. 1984;28(9):975-986.

9. Gronlund MM, Lehtonen OP, Eerola E, Kero P. Fecal microflora in healthy infants born by different methods of delivery: permanent changes in intestinal flora after cesarean delivery. *J Pediatr Gastroenterol Nutr*. 1999;28(1):19-25.

10. Hilt EE, McKinley K, Pearce MM, et al. Urine is not sterile: use of enhanced urine culture techniques to detect resident bacterial flora in the adult female bladder. *J Clin Microbiol*. 2014;52(3):871-876.

11. Wolfe AJ, Toh E, Shibata N, et al. Evidence of uncultivated bacteria in the adult female bladder. *J Clin Microbiol*. 2012;50(4):1376-1383.

12. Vennila V, Madhu V, Rajesh R, Ealla KK, Velidandla SR, Santoshi S. Tetracycline-induced discoloration of deciduous teeth: case series. *J Int Oral Health*. 2014;6(3):115-119.

13. Liu HH. Safety profile of the fluoroquinolones: focus on levofloxacin. *Drug Safety*. 2010;33(5):353-369.

14. Batty A, Wren MW. Prevalence of Fusobacterium necrophorum and other upper respiratory tract pathogens isolated from throat swabs. *Br J Biomed Sci*. 2005;62(2):66-70.

15. Odumade OA, Hogquist KA, Balfour HH, Jr. Progress and problems in understanding and managing primary Epstein-Barr virus infections. *Clin Microbiol Rev*. 2011;24(1):193-209.

16. Taylor GH. Cytomegalovirus. *Am Family Physician*. 2003;67(3):519-524.

17. Van Brusselen D, Vlieghe E, Schelstraete P, et al. Streptococcal pharyngitis in children: to treat or not to treat? *Eur J Pediatr*. 2014;173(10):1275-1283.

18. Ambrosioni J, Bridevaux PO, Wagner G, Mamin A, Kaiser L. Epidemiology of viral respiratory infections in a tertiary care centre in the era of molecular diagnosis, Geneva, Switzerland, 2011-2012. *Clin Microbiol Infect*. 2014;20(9):O578-O584.

19. Uhl JR, Adamson SC, Vetter EA, et al. Comparison of LightCycler PCR, rapid antigen immunoassay, and culture for detection of group A streptococci from throat swabs. *J Clin Microbiol.* 2003;41(1):242-249.

20. Henson AM, Carter D, Todd K, Shulman ST, Zheng X. Detection of Streptococcus pyogenes by use of Illumigene group A Streptococcus assay. *J Clin Microbiol.* 2013;51(12):4207-4209.

21. Bisno AL, Gerber MA, Gwaltney JM, Jr., Kaplan EL, Schwartz RH. Diagnosis and management of group A streptococcal pharyngitis: a practice guideline. Infectious Diseases Society of America. *Clin Infct Dis.* 1997;25(3):574-583.

22. Richter SS, Heilmann KP, Beekmann SE, et al. Macrolide-resistant Streptococcus pyogenes in the United States, 2002-2003. *Clin Infect Dis.* 2005;41(5):599-608.

23. Ungkanont K, Yellon RF, Weissman JL, Casselbrant ML, Gonzalez-Valdepena H, Bluestone CD. Head and neck space infections in infants and children. *Otolaryngol Head Neck Surg.* 1995;112(3):375-382.

24. Craig FW, Schunk JE. Retropharyngeal abscess in children: clinical presentation, utility of imaging, and current management. *Pediatrics.* 2003;111(6 Pt 1):1394-1398.

25. Thompson JW, Cohen SR, Reddix P. Retropharyngeal abscess in children: a retrospective and historical analysis. *Laryngoscope.* 1988;98(6 Pt 1):589-592.

26. Brook I. Microbiology of retropharyngeal abscesses in children. *Am J Dis Children.* 1987;141(2):202-204.

27. Brook I. Microbiology and management of peritonsillar, retropharyngeal, and parapharyngeal abscesses. *J Oral Maxillofac Surg.* 2004;62(12):1545-1550.

28. Kieff DA, Bhattacharyya N, Siegel NS, Salman SD. Selection of antibiotics after incision and drainage of peritonsillar abscesses. *Otolaryngology Head Neck Surg.* 1999;120(1):57-61.

29. Jokipii AM, Jokipii L, Sipila P, Jokinen K. Semiquantitative culture results and pathogenic significance of obligate anaerobes in peritonsillar abscesses. *J Clin Microbiol.* 1988;26(5):957-961.

30. Jensen A, Fago-Olsen H, Sorensen CH, Kilian M. Molecular mapping to species level of the tonsillar crypt microbiota associated with health and recurrent tonsillitis. *PloS one.* 2013;8(2):e56418.

31. Zheng L, Giri B. Gastrointestinal Variant of Lemierre Syndrome: Fusobacterium nucleatum Bacteremia-Associated Hepatic Vein Thrombosis: a Case Report and Literature Review. *Am J Ther.* 2014.

32. Riordan T. Human infection with Fusobacterium necrophorum (Necrobacillosis), with a focus on Lemierre's syndrome. *Clin Microbiol Rev.* 2007;20(4):622-659.

33. Brook I. Anaerobic bacteria in upper respiratory tract and other head and neck infections. *Ann Otol Rhinol Laryngol.* 2002;111(5 Pt 1):430-440.

34. Feigin R CJ. *Textbook of Pediatric Infectious Diseases.* 6th ed. Elsevier. Philadelphia. 2009.

35. CLSI M11-A8. *Methods for Antimicrobial Susceptibility Testing of Anaerobic Bacteria.* Clinical Laboratory Standards Institute. Wayne, PA. 2013.

36. Brazier JS, Hall V, Yusuf E, Duerden BI. Fusobacterium necrophorum infections in England and Wales 1990-2000. *J Med Microbiol.* 2002;51(3):269-272.

37. Rams TE, Degener JE, van Winkelhoff AJ. Prevalence of beta-lactamase-producing bacteria in human periodontitis. *J Period Res.* 2013;48(4):493-499.

38. Lee H, Kim J, Nguyen V. Ear infections: otitis externa and otitis media. *Primary Care.* 2013;40(3):671-686.

39. Pumarola F, Mares J, Losada I, et al. Microbiology of bacteria causing recurrent acute otitis media (AOM) and AOM treatment failure in young children in Spain: shifting pathogens in the post-pneumococcal conjugate vaccination era. *Int J Pediatr Otorhino-laryngol.* 2013;77(8):1231-1236.

40. Nokso-Koivisto J, Marom T, Chonmaitree T. Importance of viruses in acute otitis media. *Current Opin Pediatr.* 2015;27(1):110-115.

41. Ruuskanen O, Arola M, Heikkinen T, Ziegler T. Viruses in acute otitis media: increasing evidence for clinical significance. *Pediatric Infect Dis J.* 1991;10(6):425-427.

42. Dickson G. Acute otitis media. *Primary Care.* 2014;41(1):11-18.

43. LS G. *Clinical Microbiology Procedures Handbook.* Washington, DC:ASM Press. 2007;1.

44. Gehanno P, Lenoir G, Barry B, Bons J, Boucot I, Berche P. Evaluation of nasopharyngeal cultures for bacteriologic assessment of acute otitis media in children. *Pediatr Infect Dis J.* 1996;15(4):329-332.

45. Thanaviratananich S, Laopaiboon M, Vatanasapt P. Once or twice daily versus three times daily amoxicillin with or without clavulanate for the treatment of acute otitis media. *Cochrane Database System Rev.* 2013;12:CD004975.

46. Tapiainen T, Kujala T, Renko M, et al. Effect of antimicrobial treatment of acute otitis media on the daily disappearance of middle ear effusion: a placebo-controlled trial. *JAMA Pediatr.* 2014;168(7):635-641.

47. Institute CaLS. M100-S24—Performance Standards for Antimicrobial Susceptibility Testing; Twenty-Fourth Informational Supplement. 2014.

48. Flamm RK, Sader HS, Jones RN. Spectrum and potency of ceftaroline against leading pathogens causing community-acquired respiratory tract and skin and soft tissue infections in Latin America, 2010. *Braz J Infect Dis.* 2013;17(5):564-572.

49. Beers SL, Abramo TJ. Otitis externa review. *Pediatr Emergency Care.* 2004;20(4):250-256.

50. Stone KE. Otitis externa. *Pediatr Rev.* 2007;28(2):77-78; discussion 78.

51. Lacovou E, Vlastarakos PV, Papacharalampous G, Kampessis G, Nikolopoulos TP. Diagnosis and treatment of HIV-associated manifestations in otolaryngology. *Infect Dis Rep.* 2012;4(1):e9.

52. Rosenfeld RM, Schwartz SR, Cannon CR, et al. Clinical practice guideline: acute otitis externa. *Otolaryngol Head Neck Surg.* 2014;150(1 Suppl):S1-S24.

53. Hobson CE, Moy JD, Byers KE, Raz Y, Hirsch BE, McCall AA. Malignant Otitis Externa: Evolving Pathogens and Implications for Diagnosis and Treatment. *Otolaryngol Head Neck Surg.* 2014;151(1):112-116.

54. Brook I. Treatment of otitis externa in children. *Paediatr Drugs.* 1999;1(4):283-289.

55. Elliott EJ. Acute gastroenteritis in children. *BMJ.* 2007;334(7583):35-40.

56. Gould LH, Bopp C, Strockbine N, et al. Recommendations for diagnosis of shiga toxin–producing Escherichia coli infections by clinical laboratories. *MMWR.* 2009;58 (RR-12):1-14.

57. Buchan BW, Olson WJ, Pezewski M, et al. Clinical evaluation of a real-time PCR assay for identification of Salmonella, Shigella, Campylobacter (Campylobacter jejuni and C. coli), and shiga toxin-producing Escherichia coli isolates in stool specimens. *J Clin Microbiol.* 2013;51(12):4001-4007.

58. Schindler EI, Sellenriek P, Storch GA, Tarr PI, Burnham CA. Shiga Toxin-Producing Escherichia coli: A Single Center, 11-Year Pediatric Experience. *J Clin Microbiol.* 2014.

59. Zautner AE, Johann C, Strubel A, et al. Seroprevalence of campylobacteriosis and relevant post-infectious sequelae. *European J Clin Microbiol.* 2014;33(6):1019-1027.

60. Nelson LJ, Wells CD. Global epidemiology of childhood tuberculosis. *Int J Tuberc Lung Dis.* 2004;8(5):636-647.

61. Donald PR. Childhood tuberculosis: out of control? *Current Opin Pulm Med.* 2002;8(3):178-182.

62. Chintu C, Mudenda V, Lucas S, et al. Lung diseases at necropsy in African children dying from respiratory illnesses: a descriptive necropsy study. *Lancet.* 2002;360(9338):985-990.

63. Cotton MF, Schaaf HS, Lottering G, et al. Tuberculosis exposure in HIV-exposed infants in a high-prevalence setting. *Int J Tuberc Lung Dis.* 2008;12(2):225-227.

64. Mazurek GH, Jereb J, Vernon A, et al. Updated guidelines for using Interferon Gamma Release Assays to detect Mycobacterium tuberculosis infection – United States, 2010. *MMWR.* 2010;59(RR-5):1-25.

65. Starke JR, Committee On Infectious D. Interferon-gamma release assays for diagnosis of tuberculosis infection and disease in children. *Pediatrics.* 2014;134(6):e1763-e1773.

66. Marais BJ, Schaaf HS. Childhood tuberculosis: an emerging and previously neglected problem. *Infect Dis Clin North Am.* 2010;24(3):727-749.

67. Moss AR, Alland D, Telzak E, et al. A city-wide outbreak of a multiple-drug-resistant strain of Mycobacterium tuberculosis in New York. *Int J Tuberc Lung Dis.* 1997;1(2):115-121.

68. Marais BJ, Victor TC, Hesseling AC, et al. Beijing and Haarlem genotypes are overrepresented among children with drug-resistant tuberculosis in the Western Cape Province of South Africa. *J Clin Microbiol.* 2006;44(10):3539-3543.

69. CLSI M24-A2. *Susceptibility Testing of Mycobacteria, Nocardiae, and Other Aerobic Actinomycetes; Approved Standard.* 2nd ed. Clinical Laboratory Standards Institute. Wayne, PA. 2011; 31(5).

70. Frumkin K. Bacteriology of urinary tract infections in emergency patients aged 0-36 months. *J Emerg Med.* 2014;48(4):405-415.

71. Shaw KN, Gorelick M, McGowan KL, Yakscoe NM, Schwartz JS. Prevalence of urinary tract infection in febrile young children in the emergency department. *Pediatrics.* 1998;102(2):e16.

72. Davis KF, Colebaugh AM, Eithun BL, et al. Reducing catheter-associated urinary tract infections: a quality-improvement initiative. *Pediatrics.* 2014;134(3):e857-e864.

73. Subcommittee on Urinary Tract Infection SCoQI, Management, Roberts KB. Urinary tract infection: clinical practice guideline for the diagnosis and management of the initial UTI in febrile infants and children 2 to 24 months. *Pediatrics.* 2011;128(3):595-610.

74. Holloway J, Joshi N, O'Bryan T. Positive urine nitrite test: an accurate predictor of absence of pure enterococcal bacteriuria. *South Med J.* 2000;93(7):681-682.

75. Deville WL, Yzermans JC, van Duijn NP, Bezemer PD, van der Windt DA, Bouter LM. The urine dipstick test useful to rule out infections. A meta-analysis of the accuracy. *BMC Urol.* 2004;4:4.

76. Mandell B, Dolin. *Principles and Practice of Infectious Diseases.* 6th ed. Elsevier. Philadelphia. 2005

77. Workowski KA, Berman S, Centers for Disease C, Prevention. Sexually transmitted diseases treatment guidelines, 2010. *MMWR.* 2010;59(RR-12):1-110.

78. *Canadian Guidelines on Sexually Transmitted Infections, 2010.* Public Health Agency of Canada. Revised 2013. http://www.phac-aspc.gc.ca/std-mts/sti-its/cgsti-ldcits/index-eng.php. Accessed 12/3/2016.

79. Webber S, Wilkinson AR, Lindsell D, Hope PL, Dobson SR, Isaacs D. Neonatal pneumonia. *Arch Dis Child.* 1990;65(2):207-211.

80. Mansbach JM, McAdam AJ, Clark S, et al. Prospective multicenter study of the viral etiology of bronchiolitis in the emergency department. *Acad Emerg Med.* 2008;15(2):111-118.

81. Centers for Disease C. Pneumococcal disease, Surveillance and Reporting.

82. Livorsi DJ, Macneil JR, Cohn AC, et al. Invasive *Haemophilus influenzae* in the United States, 1999-2008: epidemiology and outcomes. *J Infect.* 2012;65(6):496-504.

83. Sharp SE, A. Robinson, M. Saubolle, M. Santa Cruz, K. Carroll, and V. Baselski. *Cumitech 7B, Lower Respiratory Tract Infections.* Washington, DC; ASM Press, 2004.

84. Musher DM, Montoya R, Wanahita A. Diagnostic value of microscopic examination of Gram-stained sputum and sputum cultures in patients with bacteremic pneumococcal pneumonia. *Clin Infect Dis.* 2004;39(2):165-169.

85. Mendoza-Paredes A, Bastos J, Leber M, Erickson E, Waseem M. Utility of blood culture in uncomplicated pneumonia in children. *Clin Med Insights Pediatr.* 2013;7:1-5.

86. Byington CL, Spencer LY, Johnson TA, et al. An epidemiological investigation of a sustained high rate of pediatric parapneumonic empyema: risk factors and microbiological associations. *Clinical Infect Dis.* 2002;34(4):434-440.

87. Polin RA, Committee on F, Newborn. Management of neonates with suspected or proven early-onset bacterial sepsis. *Pediatrics.* 2012;129(5):1006-1015.

88. Bradley JS, Byington CL, Shah SS, et al. The management of community-acquired pneumonia in infants and children older than 3 months of age: clinical practice guidelines by the Pediatric Infectious Diseases Society and the Infectious Diseases Society of America. *Clinical Infect Dis.* 2011;53(7):e25-e76.

89. Reineke J, Tenzer S, Rupnik M, et al. Autocatalytic cleavage of Clostridium difficile toxin B. *Nature.* 2007;446(7134):415-419.

90. Pokorn M, Radsel A, Cizman M, et al. Severe Clostridium difficile-associated disease in children. *Pediatr Infect Dis J.* 2008;27(10):944-946.

91. Tullus K, Aronsson B, Marcus S, Mollby R. Intestinal colonization with Clostridium difficile in infants up to 18 months of age. *Eur J Clin Microbiol Infect Dis.* 1989;8(5):390-393.

92. Eglow R, Pothoulakis C, Itzkowitz S, et al. Diminished Clostridium difficile toxin A sensitivity in newborn rabbit ileum is associated with decreased toxin A receptor. *J Clin Invest.* 1992;90(3):822-829.

93. Tang P, Roscoe M, Richardson SE. Limited clinical utility of Clostridium difficile toxin testing in infants in a pediatric hospital. *Diagn Microbiol Infect Dis.* 2005;52(2):91-94.

94. Qualman SJ, Petric M, Karmali MA, Smith CR, Hamilton SR. Clostridium difficile invasion and toxin circulation in fatal pediatric pseudomembranous colitis. *Am J Clin Patho.* 1990;94(4):410-416.

95. Pozo F, Soler P, Ladron de Guevara C. Pseudomembranous colitis associated with Hirschsprung's disease. *Clin Infect Dis.* 1994;19(6):1160-1161.

96. Cohen SH, Gerding DN, Johnson S, et al. Clinical practice guidelines for Clostridium difficile infection in adults: 2010 update by the society for healthcare epidemiology of America (SHEA) and the infectious diseases society of America (IDSA). *Infect Control Hospital Epidemiol.* 2010;31(5):431-455.

97. Schutze GE, Willoughby RE, Committee on Infectious D, American Academy of P. Clostridium difficile infection in infants and children. *Pediatrics.* 2013;131(1): 196-200.

98. Toltzis P, Nerandzic MM, Saade E, et al. High proportion of false-positive Clostridium difficile enzyme immunoassays for toxin A and B in pediatric patients. *Infect Control Hospital Epidemiol.* 2012;33(2):175-179.

99. Burnham CA, Carroll KC. Diagnosis of Clostridium difficile infection: an ongoing conundrum for clinicians and for clinical laboratories. *Clin Microbiol Rev.* 2013;26(3):604-630.

100. Wilcox MH, Planche T, Fang FC, Gilligan P. What is the current role of algorithmic approaches for diagnosis of Clostridium difficile infection? *J Clin Microbiol.* 2010;48(12):4347-4353.

101. Dupuy B, Govind R, Antunes A, Matamouros S. Clostridium difficile toxin synthesis is negatively regulated by TcdC. *J Med Microbiol.* 2008;57(Pt 6):685-689.

102. Schroeder LF, Robilotti E, Peterson LR, Banaei N, Dowdy DW. Economic evaluation of laboratory testing strategies for hospital-associated Clostridium difficile infection. *J Clin Microbiol.* 2014;52(2):489-496.

103. Ticehurst JR, Aird DZ, Dam LM, Borek AP, Hargrove JT, Carroll KC. Effective detection of toxigenic Clostridium difficile by a two-step algorithm including tests for antigen and cytotoxin. *J Clin Microbiol.* 2006;44(3):1145-1149.

104. Chapin KC, Dickenson RA, Wu F, Andrea SB. Comparison of five assays for detection of Clostridium difficile toxin. *J Mol Diagn.* 2011;13(4):395-400.

105. Selvaraju SB, Gripka M, Estes K, Nguyen A, Jackson MA, Selvarangan R. Detection of toxigenic Clostridium difficile in pediatric stool samples: an evaluation of Quik Check Complete Antigen assay, BD GeneOhm Cdiff PCR, and ProGastro Cd PCR assays. *Diagn Microbiol Infect Dis.* 2011;71(3):224-229.

106. Ota KV, McGowan KL. Clostridium difficile testing algorithms using glutamate dehydrogenase antigen and C. difficile toxin enzyme immunoassays with C. difficile nucleic acid amplification testing increase diagnostic yield in a tertiary pediatric population. *J Clin Microbiol.* 2012;50(4):1185-1188.

107. van Nood E, Vrieze A, Nieuwdorp M, et al. Duodenal infusion of donor feces for recurrent Clostridium difficile. *N Engl J Med.* 2013;368(5):407-415.

108. Centers for Disease C, Prevention. Perinatal group B streptococcal disease after universal screening recommendations–United States, 2003-2005. *MMWR.* 2007;56(28): 701-705.

109. Baron EJ WM, Dunne WM, Yagupsky P, Welch DF, Wilson DM. *Cumitech 1C, Blood Cultures IV.* Washington, DC; ASM Press, 2005.

110. Baron EJ, Miller JM, Weinstein MP, et al. A guide to utilization of the microbiology laboratory for diagnosis of infectious diseases: 2013 recommendations by the Infectious Diseases Society of America (IDSA) and the American Society for Microbiology (ASM)(a). *Clin Infect Dis.* 2013;57(4):e22-e121.

111. Isaacman DJ, Karasic RB, Reynolds EA, Kost SI. Effect of number of blood cultures and volume of blood on detection of bacteremia in children. *J Pediatr.* 1996;128(2): 190-195.

112. Kellogg JA, Ferrentino FL, Goodstein MH, Liss J, Shapiro SL, Bankert DA. Frequency of low level bacteremia in infants from birth to two months of age. *Pediatr Infect Dis J.* 1997;16(4):381-385.

113. Kaditis AG, O'Marcaigh AS, Rhodes KH, Weaver AL, Henry NK. Yield of positive blood cultures in pediatric oncology patients by a new method of blood culture collection. *Pediatr Infect Dis J.* 1996;15(7):615-620.

114. Shoji K, Komuro H, Watanabe Y, Miyairi I. The utility of anaerobic blood culture in detecting facultative anaerobic bacteremia in children. *Diagn Microbiol Infect Dis.* 2013;76(4):409-412.

115. Scheinemann K, Ethier MC, Dupuis LL, et al. Utility of peripheral blood cultures in bacteremic pediatric cancer patients with a central line. *Support Care Cancer.* 2010;18(8):913-919.

116. Sullivan KV, Turner NN, Lancaster DP, et al. Superior sensitivity and decreased time to detection with the Bactec Peds Plus/F system compared to the BacT/Alert Pediatric FAN blood culture system. *J Clin Microbiol.* 2013;51(12):4083-4086.

117. Sullivan KV, Turner NN, Roundtree SS, et al. Rapid detection of Gram-positive organisms by use of the Verigene Gram-positive blood culture nucleic acid test and the BacT/Alert Pediatric FAN system in a multicenter pediatric evaluation. *J Clin Microbiol.* 2013;51(11):3579-3584.

118. O'Grady NP, Alexander M, Burns LA, et al. Guidelines for the prevention of intravascular catheter-related infections. *Clin Infect Dis.* 2011;52(9):e162-193.

119. Chonmaitree T, Revai K, Grady JJ, et al. Viral upper respiratory tract infection and otitis media complication in young children. *Clin Infect Dis.* 2008;46(6):815-823.

120. Miller EK, Gebretsadik T, Carroll KN, et al. Viral etiologies of infant bronchiolitis, croup and upper respiratory illness during 4 consecutive years. *Pediatr Infect Dis J.* 2013;32(9):950-955.

121. Kalu SU, Loeffelholz M, Beck E, et al. Persistence of adenovirus nucleic acids in nasopharyngeal secretions: a diagnostic conundrum. *Pediatr Infect Dis J.* 2010;29(8):746-750.

122. Wald ER, Dashefsky B, Byers C, Guerra N, Taylor F. Frequency and severity of infections in day care. *J Pediatr.* 1988;112(4):540-546.

123. Hall CB, Geiman JM, Biggar R, Kotok DI, Hogan PM, Douglas GR, Jr. Respiratory syncytial virus infections within families. *New Engl J Med.* 1976;294(8):414-419.

124. Foy HM, Cooney MK, Allan ID, Albrecht JK. Influenza B in households: virus shedding without symptoms or antibody response. *Am J Epidemiol.* 1987;126(3):506-515.

125. Pappas DE, Hendley JO, Hayden FG, Winther B. Symptom profile of common colds in school-aged children. *Pediatr Infect Dis J.* 2008;27(1):8-11.

126. Ginocchio CC, Zhang F, Manji R, et al. Evaluation of multiple test methods for the detection of the novel 2009 influenza A (H1N1) during the New York City outbreak. *J Clin Virol.* 2009;45(3):191-195.

127. Jang JW, Cho CH, Nam MH, et al. Clinical performance evaluation of Sofia(R) RSV FIA rapid antigen test for the diagnosis of respiratory syncytial virus infection. *J Clin Microbiol.* 2014;53(2):684-686.

128. Specter S HR, Young SA. *Clinical Virology Manual*. 3rd ed. Washinton, DC;ASM Press. 2000.

129. Popowitch EB, O'Neill SS, Miller MB. Comparison of the Biofire FilmArray RP, Genmark eSensor RVP, Luminex xTAG RVPv1, and Luminex xTAG RVP fast multiplex assays for detection of respiratory viruses. *J Clin Microbiol.* 2013;51(5):1528-1533.

130. Doern CD, Lacey D, Huang R, Haag C. Evaluation and implementation of FilmArray version 1.7 for improved detection of adenovirus respiratory tract infection. *J Clin Microbiol.* 2013;51(12):4036-4039.

131. Ruggiero P, McMillen T, Tang YW, Babady NE. Evaluation of the BioFire FilmArray respiratory panel and the GenMark eSensor respiratory viral panel on lower respiratory tract specimens. *J Clin Microbiol.* 2014;52(1):288-290.

132. Butt SA, Maceira VP, McCallen ME, Stellrecht KA. Comparison of three commercial RT-PCR systems for the detection of respiratory viruses. *J Clin Virol.* 2014;61(3):406-410.

133. Fiore AE, Fry A, Shay D, et al. Antiviral agents for the treatment and chemoprophylaxis of influenza — recommendations of the Advisory Committee on Immunization Practices (ACIP). *MMWR.* 2011;60(1):1-24.

134. Pickering LK, Baker CJ, Freed GL, et al. Immunization programs for infants, children, adolescents, and adults: clinical practice guidelines by the Infectious Diseases Society of America. *Clin Infect Dis.* 2009;49(6):817-840.

135. Laplante J, St George K. Antiviral resistance in influenza viruses: laboratory testing. *Clin Lab Med.* 2014;34(2):387-408.

136. Kiang KM, Bryant PA, Shingadia D, Ladhani S, Steer AC, Burgner D. The treatment of imported malaria in children: an update. *Arch Dis Child Edu Pract Ed.* 2013;98(1):7-15.

137. Shingadia D, Ladhani S. UK treatment of malaria. *Arch Dis Child Edu Pract Ed.* 2011;96(3):87-90.

138. Mali S, Tan KR, Arguin PM, et al. Malaria surveillance–United States, 2009. *Morb Mortal Week Rep.* 2011;60(3):1-15.

139. Garcia LS. Malaria. *Clin Lab Med.* 2010;30(1):93-129.

140. Garcia L. *Diagnostic Medical Parasitology*. 4th ed. Washington, DC; ASM Press. 2001.

141. Dimaio MA, Pereira IT, George TI, Banaei N. Performance of BinaxNOW for diagnosis of malaria in a U.S. hospital. *J Clin Microbiol.* 2012;50(9):2877-2880.

142. Khairnar K, Martin D, Lau R, Ralevski F, Pillai DR. Multiplex real-time quantitative PCR, microscopy and rapid diagnostic immuno-chromatographic tests for the detection of Plasmodium spp: performance, limit of detection analysis and quality assurance. *Malaria J.* 2009;8:284.

143. Centers for Disease C. Malaria Treatment Algorithm. Last accessed 2/24/15.

144. Chaurasia S, Ramappa M, Ashar J, Sharma S. Neonatal infectious keratitis. *Cornea.* 2014;33(7):673-676.

145. Revere K, Davidson SL. Update on management of herpes keratitis in children. *Curr Opin Ophthalmol.* 2013;24(4):343-347.

146. Gafur OA, Copley LA, Hollmig ST, Browne RH, Thornton LA, Crawford SE. The impact of the current epidemiology of pediatric musculoskeletal infection on evaluation and treatment guidelines. *J Pediatr Orthoped.* 2008;28(7):777-785.

147. Gutierrez K. Bone and joint infections in children. *Pediatr Clin North Am.* 2005;52(3):779-794, vi.

148. Mustafa MM, Saez-Llorens X, McCracken GH, Jr., Nelson JD. Acute hematogenous pelvic osteomyelitis in infants and children. *Pediatr Infect Dis J.* 1990;9(6):416-421.

149. Choi SH, Sung H, Kim SH, et al. Usefulness of a direct 16S rRNA gene PCR assay of percutaneous biopsies or aspirates for etiological diagnosis of vertebral osteomyelitis. *Diagn Microbiol Infect Dis.* 2014;78(1):75-78.

150. Haldar M, Butler M, Quinn CD, Stratton CW, Tang YW, Burnham CA. Evaluation of a real-time PCR assay for simultaneous detection of Kingella kingae and Staphylococcus aureus from synovial fluid in suspected septic arthritis. *Ann Lab Med.* 2014;34(4):313-316.

151. Grimbly C, Odenbach J, Vandermeer B, Forgie S, Curtis S. Parenteral and oral antibiotic duration for treatment of pediatric osteomyelitis: a systematic review protocol. *System Rev.* 2013;2:92.

152. Liu C, Bayer A, Cosgrove SE, et al. Clinical practice guidelines by the infectious diseases society of america for the treatment of methicillin-resistant Staphylococcus aureus infections in adults and children. *Clin Infect Dis.* 2011;52(3):e18-e55.

153. Lemaitre C, Ferroni A, Doit C, et al. Pediatric osteoarticular infections caused by *Streptococcus pneumoniae* before and after the introduction of the heptavalent pneumococcal conjugate vaccine. *Eur J Clin Microbiol Infect Dis.* 2012;31(10): 2773-2781.

154. Talan DA, Krishnadasan A, Gorwitz RJ, et al. Comparison of Staphylococcus aureus from skin and soft-tissue infections in US emergency department patients, 2004 and 2008. *Clin Infect Dis.* 2011;53(2):144-149.

155. Rehder PA, Eliezer ET, Lane AT. Perianal cellulitis. Cutaneous group A streptococcal disease. *Arch Dermatol.* 1988;124(5):702-704.

156. Heath C, Desai N, Silverberg NB. Recent microbiological shifts in perianal bacterial dermatitis: Staphylococcus aureus predominance. *Pediatr Dermatol.* 2009;26(6): 696-700.

157. Abdolrasouli A, Hemmati Y, Amin A, Roushan A, Butler I. Lancefield group G Streptococcus dysgalactiae subsp. equisimilis: an unusual aetiology of perianal streptococcal dermatitis acquired from heterosexual oral-anal intercourse. *Int J STD AIDS.* 2012;23(12):911-912.

158. Olson D, Edmonson MB. Outcomes in children treated for perineal group A beta-hemolytic streptococcal dermatitis. *Pediatr Infect Dis J.* 2011;30(11):933-936.

159. Broyles LN, Van Beneden C, Beall B, et al. Population-based study of invasive disease due to beta-hemolytic streptococci of groups other than A and B. *Clin Infect Dis.* 2009;48(6):706-712.

160. Leung AK, Robson WL. Human bites in children. *Pediatr Energ care.* 1992;8(5): 255-257.

161. Aghababian RV, Conte JE, Jr. Mammalian bite wounds. *Ann Emerg Med.* 1980;9(2): 79-83.

162. Goodyear HM, Laidler PW, Price EH, Kenny PA, Harper JI. Acute infectious erythemas in children: a clinico-microbiological study. *Br J Dermatol.* 1991;124(5):433-438.

163. Olsen JR, Gallacher J, Piguet V, Francis NA. Epidemiology of molluscum contagiosum in children: a systematic review. *Family Pract.* 2014;31(2):130-136.

164. Repass GL, Palmer WC, Stancampiano FF. Hand, foot, and mouth disease: identifying and managing an acute viral syndrome. *Cleve Clin J med.* 2014;81(9):537-543.

165. Papaloukas O, Giannouli G, Papaevangelou V. Successes and challenges in varicella vaccine. *Ther Adv Vaccines.* 2014;2(2):39-55.

166. Hawkins DM, Smidt AC. Superficial fungal infections in children. *Pediatr Clin North Am.* 2014;61(2):443-455.

167. Centers for Disease C. http://www.cdc.gov/parasites/lice/head/epi.html. Accessed February 23, 2015.

168. Centers for Disease C. http://www.cdc.gov/parasites/lice/body/index.html. Accessed February 23, 2015.

169. Centers for Disease C. http://www.cdc.gov/parasites/lice/pubic/index.html. Accessed February 23, 2015.

170. Bethel J. Identification and treatment of scabies in infants. *Emerg Nurse.* 2014;22(4): 24-27.

171. Centers for Disease C. Laboratory Methods for the Diagnosis of Meningitis Caused by *Neisseria meningitidis, Streptococcus pneumoniae,* and *Haemophilus influenzae.* http://www.cdc.gov/meningitis/lab-manual/chpt06-culture-id.html. Accessed February 24, 2015.

172. Chadwick SL, Wilson JW, Levin JE, Martin JM. Cerebrospinal fluid characteristics of infants who present to the emergency department with fever: establishing normal values by week of age. *Pediatr Infect Dis J.* 2011;30(4):e63-e67.

173. Shah SS, Ebberson J, Kestenbaum LA, Hodinka RL, Zorc JJ. Age-specific reference values for cerebrospinal fluid protein concentration in neonates and young infants. *J Hospital Med.* 2011;6(1):22-27.

174. Nigrovic LE, Kimia AA, Shah SS, Neuman MI. Relationship between cerebrospinal fluid glucose and serum glucose. *New Engl J Med.* 2012;366(6):576-578.

175. Brizzi K, Hines EM, McGowan KL, Shah SS. Diagnostic accuracy of cerebrospinal fluid gram stain in children with suspected bacterial meningitis. *Pediatr Infect Dis J.* 2012;31(2):195-197.

176. Perkins MD, Mirrett S, Reller LB. Rapid bacterial antigen detection is not clinically useful. *J Clin Microbiol.* 1995;33(6):1486-1491.

PEDIATRIC HEMATOLOGY AND HEMOGLOBINOPATHIES

15

Hung S. Luu, Charles F. Timmons, and Ayesha Zia

LEARNING OBJECTIVES

1. Describe the general principles behind commonly performed hematology tests and their uses in the pediatric population.
2. Discuss the different components and cellular elements that are evaluated on examination of the peripheral blood smear and bone marrow.
3. List common hematologic conditions in pediatric patients and summarize their expected laboratory findings.
4. Compare and contrast commonly used laboratory methods for the diagnosis of hemoglobinopathies.
5. Describe the pathophysiology of common quantitative and qualitative hemoglobin disorders.

INTRODUCTION

Hematology is the study of blood and its components and encompasses blood cells, hematopoietic precursors in marrow, blood proteins, and mechanisms of coagulation. This chapter deals specifically with the laboratory techniques used in the diagnosis and monitoring of diseases related to the blood with an emphasis on issues specific to the pediatric population. Common hematologic conditions including their clinical presentation, pathophysiology, and laboratory findings are addressed in this chapter. The function of platelets and proteins involved in blood coagulation are described in Chapter 16. Pediatric hematologic malignancies are beyond the scope of this chapter.

HEMATOLOGY PRINCIPLES AND METHODS

The complete blood count (CBC) is performed on whole blood collected in a purple top tube containing ethylenediaminetetraacetic acid (EDTA). The cellular components of blood include red blood cells, white blood cells and platelets and the components of a CBC include red blood cell measurements, white blood cell measurements, platelet measurements, and description of red blood cell morphology. Red blood cell measurements include red blood cell count (RBC), the hemoglobin concentration, hematocrit, the mean corpuscular volume (MCV), the mean cell hemoglobin (MCH), the mean corpuscular hemoglobin concentration (MCHC), and the red cell distribution width (RDW). The reticulocytes count may also be included.

The measurement of red blood cells, white blood cells, and platelets is an automated process performed on an instrument. The CBC is performed by flowing the cellular components through a column toward tubes with apertures through which the cells pass and are counted. Cellular components passing through the smallest aperture are counted as platelets. Red blood cells and white blood cells pass through the large apertures and are analyzed by flow cytometry utilizing forward and side light scattered in the circuit to determine the size of red blood cells and identify white blood cell types by size and granularity. This data allows for the identification of five populations: neutrophils, lymphocytes, monocytes, eosinophils, and basophils. Alternatively, red blood cells may be lysed prior to counting of the white blood cells and the hemoglobin measurement is determined from the lysed red blood cells.

The red blood cell measurements determine the presence of anemia and may provide information on the cause of the anemia. White blood cell measurements include the total number of white blood cells present given by the white blood cell count (WBC) and also a differential including neutrophils, lymphocytes, monocytes, eosinophils, basophils. The WBC and differential count are important in the evaluation of infection, suspected hematologic malignancies, such as leukemia and immunologic disorders. The platelet count provides information on an important component of the patient's coagulative status.

Hemoglobin

The main function of red blood cells is the transportation of oxygen (O_2) to tissues and the return of carbon dioxide (CO_2) from tissues to the lungs. Hemoglobin contains four polypeptide chains, each containing a prosthetic heme group and one atom of iron. The heme groups are located near the surface of the molecule in a pocket of one of the globin chains and reversibly combines with one molecule of O_2 or CO_2. Fractions of hemoglobin may be described based on the oxidation state of the heme iron and the type of molecule bound to the heme iron. Hemoglobin with oxygen bound to the ferrous

Table 15-1	**REFERENCE RANGES FOR HEMATOLOGIC VALUES IN CHILDREN**					
Age	Hemoglobin (g/dL)	Hematocrit (%)	Red Cell Count ($\times 10^6/\mu L$)	MCV (fL)	MCH (pg)	MCHC (g/dL)
1-3 days	14.5-22.5	45.0-67.0	4.0-6.6	88.0-126.0	31.0-37.0	32.0-36.0
3-7 days	13.5-21.5	42.0-66.0	3.9-6.3	88.0-126.0	28.0-40.0	32.0-36.0
1-2 weeks	12.5-20.5	39.0-63.0	3.6-6.2	86.0-124.0	28.0-40.0	32.0-36.0
2-4 weeks	10.0-18.0	31.0-55.0	3.0-5.4	85.0-123.0	28.0-40.0	32.0-36.0
1-3 months	9.5-13.5	29.0-41.0	2.7-4.9	77.0-115.0	25.0-35.0	32.0-36.0
3-6 months	9.8-17.9	30.0-42.0	3.1-4.5	74.0-111.0	25.0-35.0	32.0-36.0
0.5–5 years	11.1-14.2	34.0-43.0	3.7-5.3	70.0-84.0	24.0-31.0	32.0-36.0
5-12 years	11.5-14.9	35.0-45.0	4.5-5.9	75.0-90.0	26.0-34.0	32.0-36.0
12-16 years						
Female	12.0-15.3	36.0-46.0	4.0-5.2	77.0-92.0	26.0-34.0	32.0-36.0
Male	12.1-15.9	38.0-50.0	4.5-5.9	76.0-91.5	26.0-34.0	32.0-36.0
-> 16 years						
Female	12.0-16.0	36.0-46.0	4.0-5.2	78.0-93.0	26.0-34.0	32.0-36.0
Male	13.5-17.5	41.0-53.0	4.5-5.9	80.0-100.0	26.0-34.0	32.0-36.0

heme iron atoms is referred to as oxyhemoglobin (O_2Hb). Hemoglobin containing ferrous iron not bound to oxygen is known as reduced hemoglobin. Methemoglobin (MetHb) is formed when iron is oxidized to the ferric state and the molecule loses its ability to combine with O_2 or CO_2.[1]

The Hb and Hct are highest at birth, but decline rapidly in the first days and weeks of life to a minimum at 2 months of age (Table 15-1). Adult hemoglobin (Hb) A is the dominant hemoglobin in blood after the age 3-6 months (Table 15-2). Blood also contains smaller quantities of two other hemoglobins, Hb F and Hb A_2. The major switch from fetal to adult hemoglobin occurs

Table 15-2	**NORMAL HEMOGLOBIN DISTRIBUTION (AFTER 6 MONTHS OF AGE)**		
	Hb A	Hb F	Hb A_2
Structure	$\alpha_2\beta_2$	$\alpha_2\gamma_2$	$\alpha_2\delta_2$
Normal (%)	> 95	< 2	< 3.5

3-6 months after birth and adult levels of HbA are typically achieved at 6-8 months of age.[2]

Anemia is defined as a decrease below normal of the hemoglobin concentration, erythrocyte count or hematocrit. Anemia is an extremely common condition and is a frequent complication of other diseases. Correct determination of hemoglobin is extremely important and is one of the routine tests performed on practically all patients.

The cyanohemoglobin (hemoglobin cyanide; HiCN) method is the most common method for measuring hemoglobin concentration and involves converting Hb to HiCN, which is then measured by spectrophotometry. This is accomplished by dissolving blood in a solution of potassium ferricyanide ($K_3Fe(CN)_6$) and potassium cyanide (KCN), which oxidizes Hb to Hi and then converts it to HiCN. The absorbance of the solution is measured at 540 nm and compared to that of a standard HiCN solution. This method is capable of detecting all forms of hemoglobin (Hb, HbO_2, HbCO) with the exception of sulfhemoglobin (SHb). The hemoglobin concentration is usually reported as grams per deciliter.[3]

CO-Oximetry utilizes spectrophotometers that are capable of measuring absorbance at 128 wavelengths to measure hemoglobin derivatives by their specific absorbance characteristics. It is performed on arterial blood samples and may report the various hemoglobin fractions (ie, O_2Hb, MetHb, COHb, and SHb) and/or the oxygen saturation.[4] Pulse CO-Oximetry is a non-invasive method for measurement of hemoglobin utilizing multi-wavelength spectrometric sensor that may be an adhesive single use type for continuous monitoring or a reusable finger clip sensor for periodic monitoring. Although, Pulse CO-Oximetry had good correlation with capillary measurements of Hb, the percentage of outliers was higher with non-invasive than with capillary measurement when compared to laboratory CO-Oximetry measurement from arterial blood samples.[5]

Hematocrit (Packed Cell Volume)

The hematocrit (Hct) of a sample of blood is the ratio of the volume of erythrocytes to that of the whole blood. It is typically expressed as a percentage (conventional), but can also be reported as a decimal fraction (SI units). The Hct can be measured directly by centrifugation of a tube of whole blood and determining the ratio of the packed red blood cell column height to the total height. This method has also been adapted for small samples (micromethod) by drawing blood into a microtube by capillary action with subsequent centrifugation of microtube to calculate the hematocrit. In most automated instruments, the hematocrit is measured indirectly as the product of the mean corpuscular volume (MCV) multiplied by red blood cell (RBC) count. Similar to Hb, the hematocrit is highest at birth, but declines rapidly and reaches a low at approximately 2 months of age (Table 15-1).

Red Blood Cell (RBC) Count

Erythrocytes can be counted manually through use of a hemocytometer to give the RBC count or can be counted by automated instruments by impedance, use of optical methods utilizing forward and side light scatter, or a combination of impedance and light scatter. RBC counts may be reported in terms of cells per mm^3 (ie, $4.85 \times 10^6/mm^3$) per µL (conventional units), or per L (SI units). Normal values for RBC are listed in Table 15-1.

When the Hct and RBC count have been determined manually, other information about the RBCs, referred to as the red cell indices, can be calculated. These parameters include mean cell volume (MCV), mean cell hemoglobin (MCH), and mean cell hemoglobin concentration (MCHC).

Red Blood Cell Indices

Red blood cell indices provide information on the size, hemoglobin content, and hemoglobin concentration of red blood cells and are useful for the morphologic characterization of anemias. Normal values for red cell indices are listed in Table 15-1.

Mean Cell Volume (MCV)

The MCV is the average volume of red blood cells. Red blood cells passing through the aperture of an automated instrument come in a range of sizes (volumes) distributed in a roughly Gaussian curve. The mean of this distribution is the MCV. Alternatively, the MCV can be calculated from the hematocrit and the red blood cell count. The MCV is reported in femtoliters (fL). One fL = $1 \, µL^{-3} = 10^{-15}$ L.

$$MCV = Hct \times 1000/RBC$$

Mean Cell Hemoglobin (MCH)

The MCH is the hemoglobin content (weight) of the average red blood cell. It is calculated from the Hb concentration and the red blood cell count. It is reported in pictograms. One pictogram (pg) = 10^{-12} g.

$$MCH = Hb \text{ (in g/L)/RBC (in millions/µL)}$$

Mean Cell Hemoglobin Concentration (MCHC)

The MCHC is the average concentration of Hb in a given volume of packed red blood cells. It is calculated from the Hb concentration and the hematocrit. It is expressed in grams per deciliter.

$$MCHC = Hb \text{ (in g/dL)/Hct}$$

Red Cell Distribution Width (RDW)

The RDW is a measure of the variation of cell volume within a red blood cell population. It is a parameter provided by automated hematology analyzers and is the automated equivalent of anisocytosis or variation in red blood cell size that is assessed by peripheral blood smear examination. It is the coefficient of variation. The normal range for RDW is 11.5-15.0. A high RDW indicates that the red blood cells are more variable in volume than normal.[6]

RDW = (Standard deviation /MCV) × 100

White Blood Cell (WBC) Count

The WBC count is typically provided by automated hematology analyzers. Red blood cells are lysed prior to counting and particles larger than 36 fL are counted as leukocytes. It is typically reported as cells per mm^3 (ie, 10,800/mm^3) per μL (conventional units), or per L (SI units) (Table 15-3).

As previously described, the cells pass through the aperture in the instrument and three simultaneous measurements are performed on each cell including impedance (volume), conductivity (cell complexity) and side-angle light scatter (cytoplasmic granularity). This data is used to generate a 3-dimensional scatter plot that allows for the identification and enumeration of neutrophils, lymphocytes, monocytes, eosinophils, and basophils (Table 15-3). Utilizing only forward and side-angle light scatter can also identify most leukocyte populations with the exception of basophils.[1].

Platelet Count (PLT) and Mean Platelet Volume (MPV)

Platelets are thin discoid cell fragments that are 2-4 μm in greatest dimension. They are fragments of cytoplasm derived from megakaryocytes in the bone marrow and function in hemostastis, maintaining vascular integrity, and in the process of coagulation along with coagulation factors. Methods of counting platelets include impedance, manual counting utilizing a hemocytometer, the immunophenotypic method using monoclonal antibodies and flow cytometry, and the optical method.[6] The impedance method is used in the majority of automated hematology analyzers and is the most common method of platelet estimation.[1] Particles between 2 fL and 20 fL are counted as platelets. The mean platelet volume (MPV) is analogous to the MCV and is determined in a similar manner (Table 15-4).[6] In optical platelet counts, multiangle polarized light scatter separation (MAPSS) is used to estimate the complexity and optical density of the platelets. This is represented as a cystogram of the light intensity at 7- and 90-degree angles. Three moving discrimination lines create a window separating the platelets from other elements such as microcytes. The platelet count (Table 15-4) is reported in terms of platelets per μL (conventional units) or per L (SI units).[7]

		Table 15-3		REFERENCE RANGES FOR LEUKOCYTE COUNTS IN CHILDREN								
Age	WBC	Segmented Neutrophils		Lymphocytes		Monocytes		Eosinophils		Basophils		
	(×10³/µL)	(×10³/µL)	%	(×10³/µL)	%	(×10³/µL)	%	(×10³/µL)	%	(×10³/µL)	%	
<1 day	9.4-34.0	3.00-21.10	32.0-62.0	3.40-15.60	36.0-46.0	0.00-6.10	0.0-18.0	0.00-1.70	0.0-5.0	0.00-0.70	0.0-2.0	
1-7 days	5.0-21.0	1.00-10.30	19.0-49.0	1.80-9.70	36.0-46.0	0.00-3.80	0.0-18.0	0.00-1.10	0.0-5.0	0.00-0.40	0.0-2.0	
1 week to 4 months	5.0-19.5	0.80-6.80	15.0-35.0	2.10-13.80	41.0-71.0	0.00-2.50	0.0-13.0	0.00-1.00	0.0-5.0	0.00-0.40	0.0-2.0	
4 months to 1 year	6.0-17.5	0.80-5.10	23.0-45.0	2.30-10.30	460-76.0	0.00-1.10	0.0-10.0	0.00-0.90	0.0-5.0	0.00-0.40	0.0-2.0	
1-5 years	5.0-14.5	1.20-6.50	32.0-54.0	1.80-9.40	36.0-65.0	0.00-1.10	0.0-10.0	0.00-0.70	0.0-5.0	0.00-0.30	0.0-2.0	
5-10 years	4.5-13.5	1.60-7.30	31.0-61.0	1.40-7.70	27.0-57.0	0.00-1.10	0.0-10.0	0.00-0.70	0.0-5.0	0.00-0.30	0.0-2.0	
10-13 years	4.5-13.0	1.40-8.20	36.0-66.0	1.30-6.50	28.0-48.0	0.00-1.10	0.0-10.0	0.00-0.70	0.0-5.0	0.00-0.30	0.0-2.0	
>13 years	4.5-11.0	1.60-7.30	36.0-66.0	1.10-4.80	24.0-44.0	0.00-1.10	0.0-10.0	0.00-0.60	0.0-5.0	0.00-0.20	0.0-2.0	

Table 15-4	REFERENCE RANGE FOR PLATELET COUNT AND MEAN PLATELET VOLUME		
	Platelet Count	Mean Platelet Volume (fL)	
Age	($\times 10^3/\mu L$)	Female	Male
1-7 days	150-650	10.4-12.0	10.2-11.9
1-4 weeks	150-600	10.0-12.2	10.1-12.1
1-6 months	150-600	9.4-11.1	9.2-10.8
0.5-1 year	150-600	8.8-10.6	8.7-10.5
1-5 years	150-550	8.9-11.0	9.0-10.9
5-10 years	150-475	9.3-11.3	9.2-11.4
>10 years	150-450	9.6-11.7	9.6-11.8

Spuriously low platelet counts can result from clotted specimens, large platelets, or EDTA-antibody induced platelet adherence to neutrophils (platelet satellitism) and platelet agglutination. Falsely elevated platelet counts are rare, but can result from increased fragments of leukocyte cytoplasm in conditions such as leukemias.[6]

Reticulocyte Count

Reticulocytes are immature anucleate red blood cells that contain ribonucleic acid (RNA) and continue to synthesize hemoglobin after expelling the nucleus. The reticulocyte at birth ranges from 3-7% during the first 49 hours of life. After the second day, the reticulocyte count falls rapidly to 1-3% by the seventh day of life (Table 15-5). All methods for differentiating reticulocytes from mature red blood cells rely on the abundance of RNA in the reticulocytes.[6] Methods for enumerating reticulocytes include manual counting by light microscopy, optical light scattered, and flow cytometry. In the first two methods, red blood cells are stained with a supravital dye (new methylene blue or brilliant cresyl blue), which results in precipitation of RNA as a dye-ribonucleoprotein complex. In flow cytometry, the cells are stained with an RNA-specific fluorochrome. The absolute reticulocyte count is determined by multiplying the reticulocyte percentage by the red blood cell count. The corrected reticulocyte count takes into account spuriously increased reticulocyte percentages due to low hematocrit. The reticulocyte production index (RPI) takes into account that in anemia, reticulocytes are released earlier

Table 15-5 **NORMAL RANGE FOR RETICULOCYTE COUNT IN CHILDREN**	
Age	Reticulocytes (%)
<1 day	3.2-7.5
1-3 days	1.2-3.5
3-7 days	0.2-1.5
1-4 weeks	0.4-2.5
4-6 weeks	0.5-4.0
6-8 weeks	0.6-5.3
8-10 weeks	0.5-4.7
10 weeks to 3 months	0.5-4.1
3 months to 1 year	0.4-3.3
>1 year	0.7-2.0

from the bone marrow and therefore have a longer maturation time than normal.

Absolute Reticulocyte Count = % Reticulocytes × RBC count
Corrected Reticulocyte Count = % Reticulocytes × Hct/45
Reticulocyte Production Index = CRC × 1/Correction Factor

The correction factor is 1.0 when the Hct is normal, 2.0 when the Hct is 30, and 3.0 when the Hct is 15.

Conventional automated and manual reticulocyte count methods generally enumerate all RNA stained cells, including both heavy staining (immature) and weakly stained (mature) cells and do not differentiate between immature and mature reticulocytes. Measures of reticulocyte maturity can provide complementary information to the absolute reticulocyte counts for assessing erythropoietic activity. Manual methods are capable of quantifying a maturity fraction, but are labor intensive and suffer from lack of precision. A new automated method available on some hematology analyzers, such as the Sysmex XN-1000 (Sysmex, Kobe, Japan) overcomes these deficiencies and utilizes flow cytometry to quantify the fraction of reticulocytes within low-fluorescence, middle-fluorescence, and high-fluorescence intensity regions.[8] The immature reticulocyte fraction (IRF) is defined as the sum of the fraction of middle-fluorescent intensity and high-fluorescent intensity regions. The IRF is

Table 15-6	REFERENCE RANGE FOR RETICULOCYTE HEMOGLOBIN CONTENT (RET-He) AND IMMATURE RETICULOCYTE FRACTION		
	Immature Reticulocyte Fraction	Reticulocyte Hemoglobin Content (RET-He) (pg)	
Age	(%)	Female	Male
1-3 days	30.5-35.1	23.9-30.9	22.5-31.8
4-30 days	14.5-24.6	23.9-30.9	22.5-31.8
1-2 months	19.1-28.9	23.9-30.9	22.5-31.8
2-6 months	13.4-23.3	23.9-30.9	22.5-31.8
6 months to 2 years	11.4-25.8	23.9-30.9	22.5-31.8
2-6 years	8.4-21.7	26.4-32.1	25.1-32.0
6-12 years	8.9-24.1	25.1-33.3	23.6-33.9
12-18 years	9.0-18.7	28.2-33.9	27.0-33.2
>18 years	9.3-17.4	27.5-34.2	29.0-35.3

most useful as a measure of erythropoietic activity when correlated with the absolute reticulocyte count. These two parameters show a weak positive correlation and provide the similar clinical information as the calculated "corrected reticulocyte count" or the "reticulocyte production index (RPI)." IRF normal ranges are provided in Table 15-6.

Reticulocyte Hemoglobin Content

The reticulocyte hemoglobin content is known by several different names including CHr (Advia) and Retic-He(Sysmex) and is the measure of the amount of hemoglobin in reticulocytes. This is reported in picograms (pg) (Table 15-6). It is a measure of iron available for producing new red blood cells. The reticulocyte hemoglobin content is low in iron deficiency and thalassemia.[6]

Erythrocyte Sedimentation Rate (ESR)

The ESR is a commonly used, but nonspecific marker of underlying inflammation that measures the speed of sedimentation of red cells in plasma measured over a period of one hour (Table 15-7). The speed at which the red blood cells fall to the bottom of the vertical tube is largely dependent on the plasma concentration of large proteins, such as fibrinogen and immunoglobulin.[1] The ESR

Table 15-7	**NORMAL ERYTHROCYTE SEDIMENTATION RATE IN CHILDREN**	
	Erythrocyte Sedimentation Rate	
Age	Female	Male
0-2 days	0-4 mm/h	0-4 mm/h
2-7 days	0-8 mm/h	0-8 mm/h
1-2 weeks	0-18 mm/h	0-18 mm/h
>2 weeks	0-15 mm/h	0-20 mm/h

is elevated in a wide variety of systemic inflammatory and neoplastic diseases.[9] High values (>100 mm/hour) have a 90% predictive value for serious diseases including infections, collagen vascular disease, or malignancy. An elevated ESR is associated with marked rouleaux formation of red blood cells in the peripheral blood smear. Red blood cells with an abnormal or irregular shape, such as sickle cells or spherocytes can hinder rouleaux formation and lower the ESR. Higher than expected ESR values may occur in anemia because the change in the erythrocyte to plasma ratio favors rouleaux formation independent of plasma protein concentration.[1]

Blood Film Examination

For the vast majority of patients, the automated CBC is adequate, but there are instances when supplementation of the automated CBC by manual inspection utilizing light microscopy is required. The automated hematology instruments are screening devices and all abnormalities (eg, high white cell count, low platelet count, blasts identified) must be confirmed by a medical technologist. During the blood film examination, red blood cell morphology is assessed, the white blood cell differential is performed, platelet number and morphology is evaluated, and the presence or absence of abnormal cells, such as normoblasts, granulocytic precursors, or blast cells are noted.

Manual peripheral blood smear analysis is performed by applying a drop of blood to a glass slide and staining it with a stain, such as Wright-Giemsa to visualize the cellular components. Microscopic examination is then performed to detect abnormalities in number (eg, neutropenia or presence of blasts) or in appearance (eg, platelet clumps or schistocytes). Although visual inspection of the peripheral smear can be performed manually by the medical technologists, there is also digital technology currently available that is capable of capturing images of individual white blood cells and representative images of the slide for evaluation of platelet and red blood cell morphology.[10] Microscopic examination of the peripheral blood smear is used to confirm any abnormal findings detected by the automated CBC and is an essential part of the hematologic evaluation and yields valuable information regarding all the formed elements of the blood.

Red Blood Cell Morphology

In the blood film of healthy individuals, the erythrocytes appear as circular, homogenous disks of nearly uniform size, ranging from 6-8 μm in diameter.[11] The center of each cell is somewhat paler than the periphery. In disease processes, erythrocytes can vary in their hemoglobin content, size, shape, staining properties, and structure. In reviewing red blood cell morphology, it is important to evaluate the color (normo- or hypochromic), size (anisocytosis or dual population), shape (dominant cell shape), arrangement (rouleaux formation), number (erythrocytosis or anemia), and inclusions (Howell-Jolly bodies, malaria or nucleated red blood cells).[1] Common red blood cell morphologic findings are listed in Table 15-8.

White Blood Cell Differential

White blood cells (leukocytes) can be divided broadly into phagocytes and immunocytes. The phagocytes are comprised of monocytes and granulocytes, which include neutrophils, eosinophils, and basophils. Lymphocytes, which include B-cells, T-cells, and natural killer (NK) cells, make up the immunocyte population. Phagocytes and immunocytes function to protect the body against infection.

Neutrophils

Neutrophils are typically the most numerous leukocytes present and have nuclei with condensed chromatin divided into 2-5 lobes. Neutrophils have an average diameter of 12 μm.[1] The cytoplasm is pale with many fine pink-blue or gray-blue granules. The granules are divided into primary, which appear at the promyelocyte stage, and secondary (specific) which appear at the myelocyte state and predominate in the mature neutrophil. Both types of granules are lysosomal in nature. The primary granules contain myeloperoxidase, acid phosphatase, and other acid hydrolases. Secondary granules contain collagenase, lactoferrin, and lysozyme. The average lifespan of a non-activated neutrophil is 5.4 days.[12] After leaving the bone marrow, the neutrophils enter either the circulating pool or marginated pool. Neutrophils are believed to live

Table 15-8 **RED BLOOD CELL MORPHOLOGIC FINDINGS**		
RBC Morphology	Morphologic Description	Clinical Association
Acanthocyte (Spur Cell)	RBC has spiked cell membrane, due to irregularly distributed abnormal thorny projections	Liver dysfunction, hyposplenism, malnutrition, malabsortion syndrome, pyruvate kinase deficiency, McLeod syndrome
Agglutination	Clumping of red blood cells forming aggregates	Cold agglutinin, cold autoimmune hemolytic anemia
Anisochromia	Variable coloration and central pallor among a population of RBCs, caused by a non-uniform distribution of hemoglobin	Iron deficiency, hypochromic anemia post transfusion
Anisocytosis	Variation in size among red blood cells	Iron deficiency, thalassemia, megaloblastic anemia, partially treated anemia of various causes, post transfusion. Common nonspecific finding.
Basophilic Stippling (Coarse)	Coarse, dark granular patterns in the erythrocytes; represents spontaneous aggregation of ribosomal RNA	Thalassemia, lead poisoning, myelodysplasia, pyrimidine 5′ nucleotidase deficiency, post chemotherapy
Basophilic Stippling (Fine)	Fine, small punctuate basophilic inclusions in the erythrocyte	Reticulocytosis, normal finding
Dacrocyte (Teardrop Cell)	Type of poikilocyte that is shaped like a teardrop; having squeezed through a reticuloendothelial system with increased connective tissue	Non-specific finding seen in several conditions including myelophthisic anemia
Degmacyte (Blister Cell/Bite Cell)	Abnormally shaped RBC with one or more semicircular portions removed from the cell margin resembling "bites" taken from the cytoplasm of the cell	Oxidative hemolysis
Dimorphism	Two distinct populations of RBCs are present (eg, microcytic and normocytic, hypochromic and normochromic)	Post transfusion, partially treated iron deficiency anemia, myelodysplasia
Echinocyte (Burr Cell)	Numerous small, evenly spaced rounded projections on RBC surface	EDTA induced artifact, renal failure, post transfusion, phosphate deficiency, burns
Elliptocyte	RBC is oval shaped	Iron deficiency, megaloblastic anemia, hereditary elliptocytosis, post chemotherapy

(Continued)

	Table 15-8 **RED BLOOD CELL MORPHOLOGIC FINDINGS** *(Continued)*	
RBC Morphology	**Morphologic Description**	**Clinical Association**
Heinz Body	Small, round inclusions within RBC body composed of denatured hemoglobin, visible only by supravital stains	Oxidative hemolysis, hyposplenism, alpha thalassemia
Howell-Jolly Body	Single, round, basophilic inclusion within cytoplasm of RBC	Hyposplenism, erythroblastosis, myelodysplasia, megaloblastic anemia, post chemotherapy, severe hemolytic anemia, hereditary spherocytosis
Hypochromia	Zone of central pallor is > 1/3 the diameter of the RBC	Iron deficiency anemia, thalassemia, anemia of chronic disease
Pappenheimer Body	Localized small basophilic, granular inclusions within the hemoglobinized portion of the RBC; represent iron deposits in phagosomes	Iron overload, hyposplenism, Sideroblastic anemia, hemolytic anemia
Polychromasia	Subset of RBCs show color variability and are bluish-grey in color	Reticulocytosis, normal neonate
Rouleaux	RBCS aggregate into linear pattern, resembling a "stack of coins"	Normal finding in thick part of smear, hypergammaglobulinemia
Schistocyte	Irregularly shaped, jagged fragments of RBCs, often with two pointed ends, and lacking central pallor	Microangiopathic hemolytic anemia; hemolysis secondary to cardiac valve
Sickle Cell	Abnormally shaped RBCs shaped like a crescent or sickle with two sharply pointed or tapered ends	Sickle Cell Disease
Spherocyte	RBCs that are smaller and darker than normal with perfectly round shape lacking central pallor	Autoimmune hemolytic anemia, alloimmune hemolytic anemia (eg, hemolytic disease of the newborn), hereditary spherocytosis
Stomatocyte	RBC with linear rather than circular zone of central pallor	Artifact, obstructive liver disease, hereditary stomatocytosis, South East Asian ovalocytosis, Rh null syndrome
Target Cell	RBC has central red area within the zone of central pallor resembling a bullseye	Thalassemia, iron deficiency anemia, liver disease, hyposplenism, Hemoglobin C Disease or Hemoglobin SC Disease

only a few hours outside the bone marrow after which they are destroyed in the same rate as produced.[13]

Monocytes

Monocytes are usually larger than other peripheral blood leukocytes and have a large oval or indented nuclei with clumped chromatin. Their average diameter is 14-20 μm. The abundant cytoplasm stains blue and contain many fine vacuoles, giving a "ground-glass" appearance. Cytoplasmic granules are often present. The main function of monocytes in the immune system are phagocytosis, antigen presentation, and cytokine production. Monocytes become larger [20-40 μm] when they transform into a macrophage.[1]

Eosinophils

Eosinophils are characterized by coarse cytoplasmic granules that are refractile and stain deeply red. Unlike neutrophils, they rarely have more than three nuclear lobes. They have an average diameter of 13 μm.[1] Eosinophils enter inflammatory exudates and have a special role in allergic responses, defense against parasites and removal of fibrin during inflammation. They can release a wide array of pro-inflammatory mediators including cytotoxic granule proteins, cytokines, chemokines, and lipid mediators.[14]

Basophils

Basophils are characterized by many darkly staining cytoplasmic granules which overlie the nucleus. The nucleus usually has two lobes. The granules contain heparin and histamine and like eosinophils, basophils play a role in both parasitic infections and allergies. Basophils can be found in tissues where allergic reactions are occurring and likely contribute to the severity of these reactions.[15]

Lymphocytes

Lymphocytes assist the phagocytes in the defense of the body against infection and other foreign invasion. The three major types of lymphocytes are B-cells, T-cells, and NK cells. It is impossible to distinguish between B-cells and T-cells in the peripheral blood smear by morphologic evaluation alone. Identification of and quantification of B-cell and T-cell populations can only be accomplished utilizing flow cytometry and the identification of cell lineage using surface antigen markers specific for B-cells (CD19) and T-cells (CD3). Lymphocytes are variable in size with some appearing approximately the size of a red blood cell (about 6-10 μm in diameter) with dark-staining nucleus and scant cytoplasm. Activated lymphocytes are medium to large in size with clumped chromatin and occasional nucleoli. Some activated lymphocytes show a clear perinuclear halo.[1] NK cells are cytotoxic cells that lack the T-cell receptor (TCR). They are large cells with condensed chromatin, abundant clear cytoplasm, and scattered cytoplasmic granules.

Platelets

Platelets appear as small discoid fragments containing dark purple granules on the peripheral blood smear. Platelets are 2-4 μm in greatest dimension. The peripheral blood smear is used to examine platelets for size, number, granularity, and clumping.[1]

Bone Marrow Examination

The bone marrow examination is performed by aspiration and/or trephine biopsy. During bone marrow aspiration, a needle is inserted into the marrow and a liquid sample of marrow is drawn into a syringe. This aspirated bone marrow can be used for morphologic examination, flow cytometric evaluation, microbiologic culture, and cytogenetic and molecular analysis. The optimal specimen will be the first aspirate or "pull" from the bone marrow. Each subsequent aspirate or pull will increase the chance of dilution of the bone marrow with peripheral blood. The order of collection for the bone marrow aspirate specimens should be 1) sample for morphologic examination, 2) specimen for flow cytometric analysis, 3) cytogenetic and molecular analysis, and 4) microbiologic culture. For morphologic examination, the bone marrow aspirate is spread on a slide and stained with the Romanowsky technique for microscopy.[16] Information that can be obtained from morphologic examination of the bone marrow includes hematolymphoid malignance, the presence of cells foreign to the bone marrow (ie, metastatic neuroblastoma), the proportion of the different cell lines (myeloid:erythroid ratio), and details of the morphology and maturation of the developing cells can be examined (ie, megaloblastic anemia, myelodysplasia, maturational arrest, viral inclusions). The age-related percentages of erythroid precursors, granulocytic precursors, and lymphocytes are provided in Table 15-9. An iron stain can be performed to assess for storage iron in reticuloendothelial stores (macrophages) and for appropriate incorporation of iron into hemoglobin in the form of sideroblastic iron (fine granules in developing erythroblasts).[1,16]

A trephine core biopsy is an essential part of the bone marrow examination and provides a solid core of trabecular bone with marrow and is examined as a histologic specimen after fixation, decalcification, and sectioning. The core

Table 15-9	**AGE-RELATED NORMAL VALUE IN BONE MARROW**			
Age	% Cellularity	% Granulocytes	% Erythroid	% Lymphocytes
Newborn	80-100	50	40	10
1-3 months	80-100	50-60	5-10	30-50
Child	60-80	50-60	20	20-30

biopsy is valuable for assessing cellularity, overall marrow architecture, the presence of fibrosis, and any abnormal cellular infiltrates. It should be collected at all times with the bone marrow aspirate if at all possible. The core biopsy also provides material for histochemical studies that may provide diagnostic or prognostic information. In cases where the bone marrow stroma is fibrotic, the bone marrow aspirate may result in a "dry tap" or only peripheral blood due to lack of shedding of particles due to the fibrosis. In such cases, additional core biopsies may be obtained for flow cytometry, cytogenetic and molecular studies and microbiological culture. Ideally, the core should be 1.5 cm in length and obtained at right angles to the cortical bone to avoid excessive cartilage in the specimen and a subcortical specimen that may not be representative of the bone marrow.[17]

Hematopoiesis

During the first few weeks of gestation, the yolk sac is the main site of hematopoiesis. From 6 weeks until 6-7 months of fetal life, the liver and spleen are the main organs involved and they continue to produce hematopoietic cells until about 2 weeks after birth (Table 15-10). The bone marrow is the most important site of hematopoiesis from 6-7 months of fetal life and serves as the only source of new blood cells in normal childhood and adult life.[18] The developing hematopoietic cells are situated within the marrow space. Mature cells are

Table 15-10	**SITES OF HEMATOPOIESIS**
Fetus	0-2 months (yolk sac) 2-7 months (liver, spleen) 5-9 months (bone marrow)
Infants	Bone marrow (virtually all bones)
Adults	Vertebrae, ribs, sternum, skull, sacrum and pelvis, proximal ends of femur and humerus

released into marrow sinuses where they enter the marrow microcirculation and migrate into the general circulation.[19]

Virtually all bone marrow is hematopoietically active during infancy, but there is progressive fatty replacement of marrow throughout the long bones in childhood into adult life until hematopoietic marrow is largely confined to the central skeleton and proximal ends of the femurs and humeri. Even in the hematopoietically active areas, a certain percentage of the marrow consists of fat, which increases with age (Table 15-9). The remaining fatty marrow is capable of reversion to active hematopoiesis and the liver and spleen is capable of resuming their fetal hematopoietic role (extramedullary hematopoiesis).[16,20]

Erythropoiesis

There are four stages in the development of the erythroid precursor: pronormoblast, basophilic normoblast, polychromatophilic normoblast, and orthochromic normoblast.[21] No matter what stage of development, erythroid precursors are characterized by a relatively round nucleus. The first recognizable erythrocyte precursors in the bone marrow is the pronormoblast. This is a large cell with light blue cytoplasm, a round central nucleus with nucleoli and relatively open to slightly clumped chromatin. The pronormoblast gives rise to a series of progressively smaller normoblasts by a number of cell divisions. The next stage, the basophilic normoblasts, is therefore slightly smaller in size than its predecessor with a central round nucleus with clumped chromatin and dark blue cytoplasm. As the normoblasts progress through the different stages, they acquire progressively more hemoglobin (which stains pink) in the cytoplasm; the cytoplasm stains paler blue as it loses its RNA and protein synthetic apparatus while nuclear chromatin becomes more condensed. The polychromatophilic normoblasts is thus even smaller in size with a round nucleus with condensed chromatin and a gray cytoplasm resulting from increased hemoglobin. The orthochromic normoblast is the last stage before the nucleus is expelled and has cytoplasm that is indistinguishable from reticulocytes with a round dark nucleus. The erythroid precursors mature and differentiate in islands that migrate toward the sinusoids as the cells become more differentiated.[16]. The nucleus is extruded from the late orthochromic normoblast within the bone marrow resulting in a reticulocyte which still contains some ribosomal RNA and is still able to synthesize hemoglobin. The reticulocyte is slightly larger than a mature red blood cell and spends 1-2 days in the marrow before migrating to the peripheral blood where it circulates for another 1-2 days before maturing, mainly in the spleen, when RNA is completely lost. A pronormoblasts usually gives rise to 16 mature red blood cells. Total erythropoiesis is assessed from the marrow cellularity and the myeloid: erythroid ratio (ie, the proportion of granulocyte precursors to red blood cell precursors in the bone marrow. The M:E ratio is normally 2:1 to 4:1.[21]

Granulopoiesis

The earliest recognizable granulocytic precursor in the bone marrow is the myeloblast. This is a variably sized cell with fine chromatin and usually multiple nucleoli. The cytoplasm is basophilic and no cytoplasmic granules are present. The normal pediatric bone marrow can contain up to 4% of myeloblasts.[21] Myeloblasts give rise by cell division to promyelocytes, which are slightly larger and have more abundant cytoplasm with primary (azurophilic) granules. These cells then produce myelocytes, which have specific or secondary granules. Myelocytes are characterized by an accumulation of the secondary granules in the golgi area forming the so called "dawn" of neutrophilia. As the cell matures closer to the metamyelocytes stage, the secondary granules fill the entire cytoplasm. The nuclear chromatin is now more condensed and nucleoli are not visible. Separate myelocytes of the neutrophil, eosinophil, and basophil series can be identified. The myelocytes then give rise to metamyelocytes. Metamyelocytes are non-dividing cells with an indented or horseshoe-shaped nucleus and cytoplasm filled predominantly with secondary granules. Neutrophil forms intermediate between the metamyelocyte and fully mature segmented neutrophils are called "band," "stab," or "juvenile" forms. They do not contain the clear fine filamentous distinction between the lobes which are present in mature neutrophils. The early myeloid precursors are localized in the paratrabecular areas and close to the small arteries. As the cells mature and differentiate, they migrate into the intertrabecular areas.[16] The maturation of the eosinophil and basophil series is analogous to the neutrophils and differ in the color, size, and shape of the secondary granules. The myeloblasts, promyelocytes, and myelocytes form a proliferative or mitotic pool of cells while the metamyelocyte, band and segmented granulocytes make up a postmitotic compartment. The bone marrow normally contains more myeloid cells than erythroid cells in a ratio of 2:1 to 4:1.[21]

Megakaryopoiesis

Megakaryocytes are very large cells in the bone marrow that are usually 10 to 15 times larger than the typical red blood cell. The nucleus is large and lobulated and the cytoplasm of the mature megakaryocytes contains numerous pink-purple granules. Platelets are produced in the bone marrow by fragmentation of the cytoplasm of megakaryocytes. The megakaryocyte matures by endomitotic synchronous nuclear replication, enlarging the cytoplasmic volume as the number of nuclear lobes increase in multiples of two. At a variable stage in development, most commonly at the development of eight nuclear lobes, the cytoplasm becomes granular and platelets are detached.[21] Megakaryocytes are not included in the differential count of bone marrow cells.

Lymphocytes

Following birth, the bone marrow and the thymus are the primary lymphoid organs associated with lymphocyte development. B-cells are derived from bone marrow stem cells. B-cell precursors in the bone marrow are known as hematogones and have been reported in increased numbers in healthy pediatric populations and in a variety of diseases in both children and adults.[22] In contrast to neoplastic lymphoblasts, hematogones usually display a complex spectrum of antigen expression that define the normal antigenic evolution of B-cell precursors and typically lack aberrant expression. B-lymphoblasts usually demonstrate maturational arrest and immunophenotypic aberrancy by flow cytometry. These characteristics are very useful in differentiating hematogones from neoplastic lymphoblasts.[22]

T-cells are also initially derived from bone marrow stem cells, but migrate to the thymus where they differentiate into mature T-cells during passage from the context to the medulla. Self-reactive T-cells are identified and deleted (negative selection) during this process, while T-cells with some specificity for host human leukocyte antigen (HLA) molecules are selected (positive selection).[23] The mature helper cells express CD4 and cytotoxic cells express CD8.

COMMON CLINICAL PEDIATRIC HEMATOLOGIC CONDITIONS

Iron Deficiency Anemia

Iron Deficiency Anemia (IDA) is the most common hematologic condition in the pediatric population and affects 3-7% of young children and up to 9% of adolescent females in the United States.[24] Iron is essential for several vital functions in the human body including the transport of oxygen to tissues from the lungs as a key component of the hemoglobin protein, acting as the transport medium for electrons within cells for energy (ATP) generation in the form of cytochromes, facilitating oxygen use, and storage in the muscles as a component of myoglobin and as an integral component of enzyme reactions in various tissues. Iron deficiency interferes with these vital functions and can lead to morbidity and ultimately to death.

IDA is the most important cause of a microcytic hypochromic anemia, in which all three red cell indices (MCV, MCH, and MCHC) are reduced and the peripheral blood smear shows small (microcytic) and pale (hypochromic) red blood cells. The characteristic appearance of the anemia is caused by an inability to synthesize adequate Hb due to insufficient iron. As previously discussed, each molecule of hemoglobin contains four atoms of ferrous iron, which serve as the ligand for binding of molecular oxygen (O_2) to the porphyrin ring of heme. The amount of iron required each day to compensate for losses from the body and growth varies with age and sex; it is highest in pregnancy, infants, and children at times of rapid growth, adolescent and menstruating females as shown in Table 15-11.[25] These groups therefore are particularly likely to develop iron deficiency if there is additional iron losses or prolonged reduced intake.

An important consideration in the pediatric population is the interaction between, iron and lead. An epidemiologic association has been made between IDA and increased lead concentrations. Human and animal studies have demonstrated that IDA increases intestinal lead absorption. In addition, pre-existing IDA decreases the efficiency of lead chelation therapy. However, iron supplementation in pediatric patients with IDA with concurrent lead poisoning without chelation seems to increase blood lead concentrations and decrease basal lead excretion. In theory, at least, primary prevention of IDA could also serve as primary prevention of lead poisoning, with selective rather than universal iron supplementation being the best approach.[26]

The development of frank anemia, defined as a Hb concentration >2 standard deviations below mean Hb concentration for a normal population of the same gender and age range, is preceded by two preceding stages of iron deficiency.[27] The first stage, iron depletion, occurs when iron requirement exceeds absorption and a negative iron balance is created. Iron is mobilized from stores, storage iron decreases, plasma ferritin decreases, iron absorption increases, and

Table 15-11 **RECOMMENDED DIETARY ALLOWANCES (RDAs) FOR IRON**				
Age	Male	Female	Pregnancy	Lactation
Birth to 6 months	0.27 mg*	0.27 mg*		
7-12 months	11 mg	11 mg		
1-3 years	7 mg	7 mg		
4-8 years	10 mg	10 mg		
9-13 years	8 mg	8 mg		
14-18 years	11 mg	15 mg	27 mg	10 mg

*Adequate Intake (AI)

plasma iron-binding capacity (transferrin) increases (Table 15-12). After iron stores are depleted, iron-deficient erythropoiesis then begins. This stage is characterized by falling plasma iron concentration, decreased saturation of transferrin below 15%, and decreased sideroblasts in the marrow. Even before anemia occurs, the red cell indices fall. The peripheral blood smear shows hypochromic, microcytic cells with occasional target cells and pencil-shaped poikilocytes. In contrast to thalassemia, the RBC is always decreased. The reticulocyte count is low in relation to the degree of anemia due to ineffective erythropoiesis. Serum

Table 15-12 **LABORATORY DIAGNOSIS OF ANEMIA**				
	Iron Deficiency Anemia	Anemia of Inflammation	Sideroblastic Anemia	Thalassemia Trait (α or β)
Red Blood Cell Count	Decreased	Decreased	Decreased	Normal or Increased
Mean Cell Volume (MCV)	Reduced in Relation to Anemia Severity	Normal or Mild Reduction	Usually Low in Congenital Type; Increased MCV in Acquired Type	Decreased; Very Low for Degree of Anemia
Mean Cell Hemoglobin (MCH)	Reduced in Relation to Anemia Severity	Normal or Mild Reduction	Low	Low
Red Cell Distribution Width (RDW)	Increased	Normal	Increased	Normal
Serum Iron	Reduced	Reduced	Increased	Normal
Total Iron-Binding Capacity (TIBC)	Increased	Decreased	Normal	Normal
Serum Transferrin Receptor	Increased	Normal/Low	Normal	Variable
Serum Ferritin	Decreased	Normal or Increased	Increased	Normal
Bone Marrow Iron Stores	Absent	Present	Present	Present
Erythroblastic Iron	Absent	Absent	Ring Forms	Present
Hemoglobin Electrophoresis	Normal	Normal	Normal	Hb A_2 increased in β-thalassemia

ferritin is a sensitive parameter for the assessment of iron stores in healthy subjects. It is widely available and the drop in serum ferritin precedes diminished storage iron in the bone marrow. However, ferritin is an acute phase reactant and may be elevated due to the presence of chronic inflammation, infection, malignancy, or liver disease and concurrent measurement of C-reactive protein (CRP) may be required to rule out inflammation. Reticulocyte Hb concentration (CHr or RET-He) measures the hemoglobin content of reticulocytes and is reported to be an early, direct measurement of available iron for erythropoiesis. CHr concentrations are not affected by inflammation, infection, or malignancy and may be preferable marker for iron status.[26]

Determining and correcting the cause is the most important step in the evaluation and treatment of iron deficiency. The most common causes of increased iron requirements in the pediatric population are growth spurts, poor nutritional intake, menstrual losses, and benign gastrointestinal bleeding. IDA in children due to excessive milk intake is a common finding in the pediatric population. Current screening guidelines by the American Academy of Pediatrics recommends universal screening for anemia should be performed with determination of Hb concentration at one year of age. Universal screening also includes assessment of risk factors associated with IDA, such as history of prematurity or low birth weight, exposure to lead, exclusive breastfeeding beyond 4 months of age without supplemental iron, and weaning to whole milk or complementary foods that do not include iron-fortified cereals or foods rich in iron. Selective screening can be performed at any age when risk factors for IDA have been identified, including risk of inadequate iron intake by dietary history.[26]

Standard therapy for uncomplicated iron deficiency anemia is iron supplementation with ferrous sulfate or other iron salts. Parenteral iron replacement may be necessary under certain circumstances, such as poor tolerance of oral iron, rapid replacement of iron stores is needed, gastrointestinal absorption of iron is compromised, or erythropoietin therapy is necessary, such as in dialysis patients.[28]

Anemia of Inflammation

Anemia of inflammation is a mild to moderate anemia associated with a variety of inflammatory disorders, infection, and malignancy. The pathogenesis of this anemia is related to decreased transport of iron to erythroid precursors, normal or increased iron stores, ineffective erythropoiesis, reduced red blood cell lifespan, and inadequate erythropoietin response to anemia caused by the effects of cytokines, such as interleukin-1, tumor necrosis factor α, interleukin-6, interferon γ, and interleukin-10.[29,30] Hepcidin, an important iron regulatory protein, has been found to play a key role in the development of pathologic iron homeostasis that is a hallmark of anemia of inflammation. Increased levels of lipopolysaccharide and interkeukin-6 up-regulates expression of hepcidin, an acute-phase protein, and leads to decreased release of iron from macrophages, decreased intestinal absorption of iron, and subsequent reduced availability of iron for erythropoiesis. In addition, cytokine-mediated suppression of erythroid proliferation and blunting of the erythropoietin response contribute to the resulting anemia.[30]

The peripheral blood smear typically shows a mild to moderate anemia without increased anisocytosis (normal RDW) or polychromasia. The red blood cells are typically normocytic and normochromic or mildly hypochromic. Both the serum iron and total iron-binding capacity are reduced and the serum transferrin receptor levels are normal. Serum ferritin and bone marrow storage iron are both normal or increased, but erythroblastic iron is reduced (Table 15-12).

The best therapeutic approach for anemia of inflammation is the identification and treatment of the underlying infection, inflammatory disease, or cancer. Blood transfusions may provide short term relief for severe or life-threatening anemia, however, long term blood transfusion therapy is not recommended.[30] Despite the low serum iron, iron therapy in patients with anemia of inflammation is controversial. Specific patient populations, such as those with end-stage renal disease, inflammatory bowel disease, or cancer patients undergoing chemotherapy may benefit from supplemental iron.[30,31]

Sideroblastic Anemias

Sideroblastic anemias are a heterogenous group of congential and acquired bone marrow disorders characterized by pathologic iron deposition in the perinuclear mitochondria of erythroblasts due to impaired iron utilization.[32,33] On a bone marrow stained with Prussian blue, "ringed sideroblasts" can be identified as red blood cell precursors with five or more coarse granules encircling one third or more of the nucleus and forming a halo or "ring."[34] Sideroblasts are not pathognomonic of any one disease but are instead manifestations of several heterogeneous disorders. The bone marrow is typically hypercellular with erytheroid hyperplasia. The anemia is typically microcytic in congenital sideroblastic anemia and can be normocytic or macrocytic in the acquired form (Table 15-12). The congenital and acquired causes of sideroblastic anemias are listed in Table 15-13.[33,35] Treatment of acquired sideroblastic anemia may include removal of toxic agents. Patients with myelodysplastic syndrome may require bone marrow transplantation. Other treatment options depend on the type of sideroblastic anemia and includes administration of pyridoxine, thiamine, or folic acid. In some cases, repeated blood transfusions with iron chelation may be the only method of maintaining an adequate hemoglobin concentration.

Table 15-13 **CAUSES OF CONGENITAL AND ACQUIRED SIDEROBLASTIC ANEMIA**	
Acquired	Congenital
Drugs (Chloramphenicol, Isoniazid and other antituberculous drugs, Penicillamine, Lincomycin)	DIDMOAD Syndrome
	Erythropoietic Protoporphyria (ferrochelatase deficiency)
Ethanol	Glutaredoxin 5 defects
Hypothermia	
	Mitochondrial Myopathy and Sideroblastic
Idiopathic	Anemia (*PUS1* mutation)
Lead Poisoning	Mitochondrial SLC25A38
Myelodysplastic Syndrome	Pearson Marrow Pancreas Syndrome (mitochondrial protein defects)
Nutritional Deficiencies (copper, vitamin B-6)	Thiamine-Responsive Megaloblastic Anemia (*SCL19A2* (thiamine transporter) gene defects)
Zinc Overdose	
	X-linked Sideroblastic Anemia (δ-ALAS mutation)
	X-linked Sideroblastic Anemia with Ataxia (*ABC7* mutation)

Lead Poisoning

Lead poisoning is an insidious environmental threat in the pediatric population. Approximately 35% of inhaled airborne lead is absorbed and 15-18% is retained.[36] Lead inhibits both heme and globin synthesis at a number of points. In addition, it interferes with the breakdown of RNA by inhibiting the enzyme pyrimidine 5'nucleotidase, resulting in accumulation of denatured RNA in red cells. The denatured RNA can be seen as coarse basophilic stippling on the Romanowsky stain. The anemia in lead poisoning can be hypochromic or predominantly hemolytic. The bone marrow may show ring sideroblasts. Free erythrocyte protoporphyrin is usually elevated. The most important step in the treatment of lead poisoning in children is the identification and removal of the source of exposure.[28] Cases of severe lead poisoning may require parenteral chelation treatment.

Hemolytic Anemia

Erythrocyte destruction usually occurs after an average lifespan of 115 days when the red cells are removed from the circulation by the macrophages of the reticuloendothelial system.[37] Iron is liberated for recirculation via plasma transferrin and heme is converted into bilirubin. Bilirubin subsequently circulates to the liver where it is conjugated to glucuronides, which are excreted into the gut via bile and converted to stercobilinogen and stercobilin.[38] Stercobilinogen and stercobilin, excreted into feces, are partially reabsorbed and excreted in urine as urobilinogen and urobilin. Globin chains are broken down into amino acids and reused for protein synthesis in the body. Haptoglobin are acute phase proteins present in normal plasma that bind free Hb released from red cells with high affinity and inhibit oxidative activity.[39] The hemoglobin-haptoglobin complex is removed from plasma by the reticuloendothelial system.[40] Intravascular hemolysis usually plays little or no part in normal red cell destruction. Hemolytic anemia is caused by an increased rate of red cell destruction.

Hemolytic anemia may result from either the breakdown of the red blood cells in the vessels (intravascular hemolysis) or excessive removal of red cells by the reticuloendothelial system. Like sideroblastic anemia, the underlying cause of the hemolytic anemia may either be genetic or acquired (Table 15-14). Laboratory findings associated with hemolytic anemia include features of increased erythrocyte destruction, such as increased serum unconjugated bilirubin, lactate dehydrogenase, alanine aminotransferase, and urine urobilinogen. Haptoglobin is typically decreased because the haptoglobin proteins become saturated with free hemoglobin and the complex is removed by the reticuloendothelial system. Laboratory features of the compensatory increased red cell production include reticulocytosis and bone marrow erythroid hyperplasia. Evidence of damaged red cells may be seen on the peripheral blood smear with microspherocytes and fragments.

Hereditary Spherocytosis

Hereditary Spherocytosis (HS) is the most common cause of inherited hemolytic anemia among Caucasians and affects approximately 1 in 2000 individuals in northern Europe and North America.[41] It is also the most common cause of non-immune hemolytic jaundice in the neonate and the most common hemolytic anemia requiring red blood cell transfusions during the first month of life.[42] HS is characterized by defective vertical linkage between the erythrocyte membrane and the underlying cytoskeleton due to intrinsic defects in the membrane proteins resulting in cytoskeleton instability, loss of membrane surface area, and abnormal osmotic fragility in vitro.[41] This tendency toward loss of membrane surface area gives rise to the spherocytes, which are the morphologic hallmark of the disorder and detectable in 97% of affected patients on the peripheral blood smear.[43] The relative rigidity of the spherocytes slow their passage through the splenic cords and leads to rapid culling of the abnormal cells from the circulation by the frequently enlarged spleen.[41]

Table 15-14 **CAUSES OF HEMOLYTIC ANEMIA**	
Acquired	Inherited
Immune	**Hemoglobinopathies**
Autoimmune	Hemoglobin S, Hemoglobin C,
Warm Antibody Type	Unstable Hemoglobin
Cold Antibody type	
	Red Cell Membrane Defects
Alloimmune	Hereditary Spherocytosis,
Hemolytic Transfusion Reactions	Hereditary Elliptocytosis
Hemolytic Disease of the Newborn	
Allografts (Bone Marrow Transplantation)	**Red Cell Enzyme Disorders**
	Glucose-6-phosphate
Drug Associated	dehydrogenase deficiency
Cephalosporins, Piperacillin	
Infection	
Malaria, Babesia	
Mechanical	
March Hemoglobinuria	
Paroxysmal Nocturnal Hemoglobinuria	
Red Cell Fragmentation Syndromes	
Arterial Grafts, Cardiac Valves	
Microangiopathic	
Disseminated Intravascular Coagulation	
Hemolytic Uremic Syndrome	
Meningococcal Sepsis	
Pre-eclampsia	
Thrombotic Thrombocytopenic Purpura	

The molecular defects associated with HS involve the genes encoding for spectrin, ankyrin, band 3, and protein 4.2 and result in distinct subsets of protein abnormalities including isolated spectrin deficiency, combined spectrin and ankyrin deficiency, band-3 protein deficiency, and protein 4.2 deficiency.[41,43] HS is primarily inherited in an autosomal dominant manner. Recessive inheritance occurs in 20-25% of HS cases and manifests only in individuals who are homozygous or compound heterozygous and is usually associated with severe hemolytic anemia. A small percentage of cases are de novo mutations.[41]

The clinical features of HS include hemolytic anemia, jaundice, reticulocytosis, cholelithiasis, and splenomegaly. HS is clinically highly heterogeneous with the degree of hemolysis varying widely from fully compensated to transfusion dependent anemia.[43] Approximately 20-30% of patients have mild disease with compensated hemolysis and no anemia. The majority of patients (60-70%) have moderate disease that typically presents in childhood with anemia (50% of cases), palpable splenomegaly (50% in young children and 75-95% in older children), and occasional jaundice (50% of patients and usually in association with viral infection). The anemia in these individuals is usually asymptomatic except for pallor or fatigue. About 10% of patients will have moderately severe disease with low hemoglobin concentrations, increased reticulocytes and bilirubin and an intermittent need for red blood cell transfusion. Only about 3-5% of patients will have severe transfusion dependent disease and these patients are almost always autosomal recessive disease.[41]

Laboratory testing for HS includes review of the peripheral smear for microspherocytes and traditional tests that exploit the reduced surface area-to volume ratio in microspherocytes. These include the osmotic fragility test, acid glycerol lysis time (AGLT), and cryohemolysis test.[43] In the osmotic fragility test, fresh and incubated red cells are exposed to various sodium chloride concentrations to determine the concentration that produces 50% cell lysis.[44] The Glycerol Lysis Test (GLT), Acidified Glycerol Lysis Time (AGLT), and the Pink Test, a modified acidified glycerol lysis test, determine the rate or extent of lysis for red cells suspended in buffered glycerol solutions.[45-47] Unfortunately, none of these traditional tests are able to differentiate HS from secondary spherocytes associated with other conditions, such as autoimmune hemolytic anemia.[44] In addition, the traditional laboratory tests for HS are problematic during the newborn period due to the fact that neonatal red cells are physiologically more osmotically resistant than adult cells.[42] It is for this reason that the osmotic fragility test is postponed until the child is at least 6 months of age.[41] The cryohemolysis test is based on the increased susceptibility of the spherocytes to rapid cooling from 37 to 0°C while suspended in hypertonic solutions.[48]

The flow cytometric analysis of eosin-5′-maleimide bound to intact red blood cells (EMA-binding test) has more recently emerged as a highly sensitive and specific screening test for HS.[43,49] The principle behind this flow based assay lies in the fact that the fluorescent probe, eosin-5′-maleimide, binds to the high abundance band 3 and other low abundance transmembrane proteins within the band 3 macro-complex on the surface of the red cells.[49]

The severity of HS is classified as mild, moderate, moderately severe, and severe utilizing common laboratory values (Table 15-15).[41,50] Most cases of HS do not require treatment other than for complications, such as cholelithiasis. Aplastic crisis due to infection with parvovirus B19 is a serious and potentially lethal complication.[41] Patients with severe disease may be considered for splenectomy, however, these patients are at risk for postsplenectomy sepsis.[50]

Table 15-15 **CLASSIFICATION OF HEREDITARY SPHEROCYTOSIS**				
	Mild	Moderate	Moderately Severe	Severe
Hemoglobin (g/dL)	Normal	11-15	8-12	6-8
Reticulocyte (%)	≤3	3.1-6	≥6	≥10
Bilirubin (μmol/L)	≤17	17-34	≥34	≥51
Reticulocyte Production Index	<1.8	1.8-3	>3	
Spectrin per Erythrocyte (% of normal)	100	80-100	50-80	40-60
Osmotic Fragility				
Fresh Blood	Normal	Normal to Slightly Increased	Distinctly Increased	Distinctly Increased
Incubated Blood	Slightly Increased	Distinctly Increased	Distinctly Increased	Distinctly Increased
Transfusions	0-1	0-2	>2	Regular
Splenectomy	Not Necessary	Usually Not Necessary in Childhood or Adolescence	Necessary (at >5 years)	Necessary (at >2-3 years)
Heredity	Autosomal Dominant	Autosomal Dominant, De novo mutation	Autosomal Dominant, De novo mutation	Autosomal Recessive

*Normal (mean ± SD); 226 ± 54 × 10³ molecules per cell.

Glucose-6-Phosphate Dehydrogenase Deficiency

Glucose-6-phosphate dehydrogenase (G6PD) deficiency is the most common enzyme deficiency in the world and is present in approximately 400 million people worldwide.[51] G6PD deficiency occurs with increased frequency in Africa, Asia, the Mediterranean, and the Middle East and geographically correlates with areas historically exposed to endemic malaria.[52] The gene encoding G6PD is located on the long arm of the X chromosome (Xq28) and the condition is therefore inherited as an X-linked recessive disorder.[53] Cases of de novo gene mutations occur in all populations. G6PD deficiency is extremely polymorphic and over 400 mutations have been identified, with the majority being missense mutations.[54]

G6PD is essential in the defense of red blood cells against oxidative stress. G6PD functions to oxidize glucose-6-phosphate to 6-phosphogluconolactone while reducing nicotinamide adenine dinucleotide phosphate (NADP) to its reduced (NADPH) form.[51] In the erythrocyte, this reaction is the only source of NADPH. NADPH in turn is needed to reduce glutathione and stabilize catalase, two compounds with anti-oxidant properties in the erythrocyte.[53] Decreased G6PD activity therefore renders the red blood cells more susceptible to oxidative stress.

The prevalence of neonatal hyperbilirubinemia is twice that of the general population in affected males and homozygous females.[52] A few affected individuals may have a chronic form of hemolysis leading to chronic non-spherocytic hemolytic anemia. All of these cases result from sporadic or de novo *G6PD* gene mutations.[55] Most affected individuals, however, are asymptomatic throughout their life. The disorder usually manifests as acute episodes of hemolysis in response to oxidative stress triggered by causes such drugs, infection, or the ingestion of fava beans. Methylene blue is also known to produce acute hemolysis. The clinical manifestations are fatigue, back pain, anemia, and jaundice.[55]

In individuals with G6PD deficiency, oxidative stress can denature hemoglobin and cause intravascular hemolysis. Laboratory findings for the hemolysis during acute episodes include increased unconjugated bilirubin, lactate dehydrogenase, and reticulocytosis.[55] Heinz bodies are inclusions within red blood cells composed of denatured hemoglobin formed by damage to the hemoglobin component molecules due to oxidant damage and the oxidized, denatured hemoglobin can be visualized on the peripheral smear utilizing supravital stains.[56] The denatured hemoglobin is removed by the reticuloendothelial system and can result in the classic bite cell characterized by semicircular peripheral defects in the red cell margin resembling bites on the peripheral smear.[57] Contracted and fragmented red cells and blister cells may also be present. Diagnostic tests for G6PD deficiency rely on the generation of NADPH from NADP and include the fluorescent spot test and quantitative spectrophotometric assay of G6PD activity.[51] The fluorescent spot test indicates G6PD deficiency when the blood spot fails to fluoresce under ultraviolet light due to lack of production of NADPH.[55] Diagnostic testing should be deferred during acute hemolytic episodes due to the fact that the abnormal G6PD deficient cells have been destroyed and only new cells with normal activity remain during this period.[51]

The hemolytic episodes associated with G6PD are usually short-lived and treatment primarily consists of avoidance of the oxidative stressors.[52] The vast majority of people who harbor the *G6PD* gene mutations are asymptomatic throughout their life and unaware of their status.[55]

Immune Thrombocytopenic Purpura

Immune thrombocytopenic purpura (ITP) is defined as a platelet count less than 100×10^9/L and is an autoimmune disorder characterized by the isolated destruction of otherwise normal platelets in the absence of an identifiable cause.[58] It is estimated to affect 1 in 20,000 children annually in the United States.[59] Most children affected by ITP are healthy prior to disease onset and usually present acutely after a viral infection or insidiously with progressive petechiae, bruising, or purpura.[60] Childhood ITP is associated with an acute onset of thrombocytopenia with disease resolution within 6 months in ~75% of children.[61]

ITP is mediated by autoantibodies to defined platelet antigens with the main antigenic targets for these autoantibodies being the glycoprotein epitopes IIb/IIIa, Ib/IX, Ia/IIa, IV, or V. Most patients have multiple antibodies to multiple platelet antigens at the time of disease presentation and the factors initiating the autoantibody production are unknown.[60] Examination of the peripheral blood smear shows thrombocytopenia with no other characteristic pathologic findings. Bone marrow examination is typically morphologic normal, however, it is mandatory in patients with an atypical presentation, such as lymphadenopathy, hepatosplenomegaly, bone or joint pain, protracted fever, unexplained macrocytosis or neutropenia.[60]

ITP can be classified into acute and chronic classifications based on duration. Acute ITP is defined as complete resolution of thrombocytopenia within 6 months of onset while chronic ITP is defined as persistence of thrombocytopenia for > 6 months. Although ITP is considered to be a self-limited disease few significant complications, it can rarely be associated with life-threatening bleeding including intracranial hemorrhage.[60]

Treatment is generally conservative with current guidelines recommending observation alone regardless of platelet count in children without bleeding or mild bleeding (defined as skin manifestations only, such as bruising or petechiae). Patients with bleeding may require treatment with intravenous immunoglobulin (IVIg) infusion or a short course of corticosteroids. Splenectomy may be required for children with persistent and chronic ITP with significant or persistent bleeding and lack of response or intolerance to other therapies.[58]

HEMOGLOBINOPATHIES

Hemoglobinopathies are the most common recessive disorders in the world and occur as a result of mutations of the globin genes causing defects in the structure and/or expression of the globin protein. The mutations may disrupt gene expression and decrease the production of structurally normal globin chains, causing thalassemia (quantitative hemoglobin disorders), or may alter the structure of the globin gene product, resulting in abnormal hemoglobin variants (qualitative hemoglobin disorders).[62] Approximately 7% of the world's population are thought to be heterozygous carriers of hemoglobin disorders due to α-globin or β-globin gene mutations.[63] There are currently 250 gene defects that are reported to cause different thalassemia phenotypes and more than 1150 mutations reported to cause abnormal hemoglobin variants.[64] The number of reported hemoglobin variants has increased because of the development of more sophisticated laboratory methods, such as high performance liquid chromatography (HPLC) and gene sequencing that can detect subtle changes.[65] Many of these variants occur in the same ethnic populations in areas where falciparum malaria was/is endemic.[63,65] While the vast majority of hemoglobin variants have no clinical significance, some, such as hemoglobins S, C, E, and D can be associated with significant sequelae if inherited in the homozygous state or in combination with other variants.[65] This section deals with inherited diseases caused by reduced or abnormal synthesis of globin.

Hemoglobin Synthesis

Adult hemoglobin (Hb) A is the dominant hemoglobin in blood after the age 3-6 months and consists of two α-chains and two β-chains. Hb F and Hb A_2 are two minor hemoglobin components also present in normal blood and consist of two α-chains with two γ-chains (Hb F) or two δ-chains (Hb A_2) instead of β-chains. In the embryo and fetal stage, Hb Gower 1 ($\zeta_2\varepsilon_2$), Hb Portland ($\zeta_2\gamma_2$), Hb Gower 2 ($\alpha_2\varepsilon_2$), and Hb F dominate at different stages. The genes encoding for the globin chains occur in two clusters on chromosome 11 (ε, γ, δ, and β) and chromosome 16 (ζ and α). There are two forms of the γ-chains, Gγ and Aγ, which have either a glycine or alanine amino acid at position 136 in the polypeptide chain.[62]

Laboratory Methods for the Diagnosis of Hemoglobinopathies

There are many laboratory methods currently available for the diagnosis of hemoglobinopathies including alkaline and acid gel electrophoresis, capillary electrophoresis (CE), globin chain electrophoresis, isoelectric focusing (IEF), high performance liquid chromatography (HPLC) with UV or mass spectrometric detection, and globin gene sequencing.[66] This section will concentrate on the most commonly used methods.

Red Cell Count and Red Cell Morphology

The laboratory evaluation for a possible hemoglobinopathy should begin with an examination of the red cell indices and an assessment of the red blood cell morphology. Thalassemias will often present with microcytic (low MCV) red blood cells with very little anisocytisis (normal RDW) and increased numbers of red blood cells as opposed to IDA which will often have decreased RBCs and increased RDW in addition to microcytosis. The degree of anemia if present will also provide clues to the clinical significance of the possible abnormality of globin chain synthesis. In terms of red cell morphology, pencil cells were reported to be more commonly seen and numerous in IDA compared to thalassemias, however, the number of target cells and basophilic stippling were not found to be helpful in distinguishing IDA from β-thalassemia.[67] Clinical history, if provided, is also useful in distinguishing IDA from thalassemias as thalassemic patients will often have a positive family history.

Hemoglobin Electrophoresis

Alkaline and acidic hemoglobin electrophoresis are still the most widely used methods for the separation and identification of hemoglobin fractions.[68] Hemoglobin electrophoresis is based on the principle that proteins applied to a matrix will separate from each other when exposed to a charge gradient and can be visualized with either a protein stain or a heme stain.[69] The assay can be performed on filter paper, cellulose acetate membrane, starch gel, citrate agar gel or agarose gel. It is best performed using lysed packed red cells to avoid confounding bands from plasma proteins.

Cellulose acetate electrophoresis at alkaline pH

Electrophoresis on cellulose acetate at alkaline pH (8.2-8.4) is commonly employed as the initial test for evaluation of hemoglobin fractions. At this pH, hemoglobin is negatively charged and will migrate toward the positively charged anode. A control sample containing hemoglobins A, F, S, and C should be run with each set of patient samples.[69] This method is inexpensive, rapid, reproducible, and allows for the provisional identification of common hemoglobins, such as A, F, S, C. This technique is limited, however, since hemoglobins C, E, A_2, and O co-migrate as do hemoglobins S, G, D-Los Angeles, and D-Iran.[70] Co-migration of hemoglobins in electrophoresis also occurs with rarer hemoglobin variants. Modification of the matrix and buffer pH alters the migration of hemoglobins and allows for separation of some co-migrating hemoglobin fractions.[70]

Citrate agar electrophoresis at acidic pH

An alternative method is required to confirm the identity of hemoglobin variants detected by alkaline electrophoresis. Citrate agar or agarose gel at acidic pH (6.0-6.2) is often used for this purpose.[69] The separation of the hemoglobins utilizing this technique depends on the electrical charge of the hemoglobin molecule and their interaction with components in the agar or agarose. Agar contains both agarose and agaropectin. While agarose polymerizes and is immobile, agaropectin can complex with some amino acids in hemoglobin. The hemoglobin-agaropectin complex will migrate towards the anode, while any non-complexed hemoglobin will be carried toward the cathode by endosmotic flow.[71] Electrophoresis in citrate agar at pH 6.2 (acidic) is used to separate hemoglobin C from hemoglobins E, A$_2$, and O and to separate hemoglobin S from the G and the D variants. Hemoglobins A, D, G, E, and O co-migrate on acid pH electrophoresis. Electrophoretic methods are nevertheless unable to separate hemoglobin E from O and D from G and many others.[72] This method is useful in distinguishing hemoglobin S from D and G and will separate hemoglobin C from its co-migrating variants, including E, C-Harlem, and O-Arab.[69,71] Citrate agar gel electrophoresis has been reported to be more sensitive than electrophoresis on cellulose acetate for detecting hemoglobins S and F.[73]

Isoelectric Focusing (IEF)

The isoelectric focusing method is based on the principle that the net charge of the protein depends on the pH of the surrounding solution. At low pH, proteins generally have a net positive charge due to the carboxylic group being uncharged and the N-containing basic groups being fully charged (NH$_3$$^+$). Conversely, the carboxylic groups are negatively charged (COO$^-$) and the basic groups are uncharged resulting in a net negative charge at high pH.[69] The polyacrylamide or cellulose acetate media used in isoelectric focusing contain carrier amphoteric molecules that carry both current and pH. When a current is applied to the support media, the ampholytes establish a pH gradient across the plate.[71] When hemoglobin samples are placed on the gel, the hemoglobin molecules will migrate through the plate to the point at which the pH results in a net zero charge for the hemoglobin molecule, known as the isoelectric point (pI). Hemoglobins can therefore be separated on IEF according to their individual isoelectric point.[69] Cellulose acetate electrophoresis at alkaline pH and IEF generally give the same migrational pattern for normal and variant hemoglobins, however, IEF may have better separation of some hemoglobin variants with similar mobilities on alkaline electrophoresis due to minor differences in their pI.[71,74]

Capillary Electrophoresis

In capillary electrophoresis, the specimen is injected into a buffer capillary with a 50-μm inner diameter.[75] The electrophoretic mobility is dependent upon the charge of the hemoglobin molecule, the viscosity, and the atom's radius. The migration times of the separated hemoglobin fractions through the capillary tube are categorized into zones based on the standardizing the location of Hb A and Hb A$_2$ and are compared against a library of known variant migration patterns of genetically confirmed cases.[76] Peaks are assigned position relative to patterns of common variant hemoglobins to give a presumptive hemoglobin identification.[70] The higher surface-to-volume ratios in the capillary tube allows for the use of higher voltage and shorter run times.[69,71] Capillary electrophoresis has the added advantage of being able to cleanly separate hemoglobin A_2 from E, a feat not possible with routine electrophoresis methods and HPLC.[77] Advantages of capillary electrophoresis compared to gel electrophoresis includes small sample size, automation, and precision.[69] As with other electrophoretic methods, capillary electrophoresis is unable to separate hemoglobin E from O and D from G and co-migration of variants remains a problem.

High-Performance Liquid Chromatography (HPLC)

Cation-exchange high-performance liquid chromatography (HPLC) separates hemoglobin fractions by utilizing buffers with increasing ionic strengths to elute hemoglobin molecules from a weak cation exchange column.[66] The cations in the buffer solution compete with the adsorbed proteins in the column for anion binding sites and the adsorbed positively charged hemoglobin molecules are eluted from the column at a rate relative to their affinity for the stationary phase.[69] Elution of the hemoglobin fractions is measured by a photometer and a chromatogram is produced that gives the percentage, retention time, and any distinguishing peak characteristics for each hemoglobin fraction.[66] The retention time is given relative to known normal and abnormal hemoglobins, such as hemoglobin A, F, S, and C.[69] The relative retention time is used to give a presumptive identification of the hemoglobin fraction. Cation-ion HPLC has become the gold standard for population screening for hemoglobinopathies and also for accurate and precise quantitation of Hb A2 and Hb F due to the simplicity of the automated system, excellent resolution, rapid assay time and accurate quantification of hemoglobin fractions.[68,75] Definitive diagnosis of many hemoglobin variants using HPLC is, however, limited by the fact that many variant hemoglobins have retention times that overlap with other variant or normal hemoglobins on HPLC.[69,74] For this reason, definitive diagnosis for hemoglobin variants that cannot be differentiated based on IEF and HPLC characteristics alone may require the use of confirmatory tests, such as DNA analysis or mass spectrometry.[74]

Quantitative Hemoglobin Disorders

Thalassemias are a heterogeneous group of quantitative hemoglobin disorders, resulting from the reduced production of structurally normal α or β globin chains. Thalassemia is caused by large deletions or point mutations in crucial section of globin genes.[62]

α-Thalassemia Syndromes

The genes that encode for the α-globin chains are located on chromosome 16 and are part of the α-globin gene cluster that include one embryonic ζ-globin gene and two α-globin genes ($α_1$ and $α_2$). The α-globin genes contribute to the production of the embryonic hemoglobin Gower 2 ($α_2ε_2$), fetal hemoglobin (Hb F; $α_2γ_2$), and both postnatal Hb A ($α_2β_2$) and Hb A_2 ($α_2δ_2$). α-Thalassemia is most commonly caused by large deletions involving a single gene ($α^+$ thalassemia) or both genes (α°-thalassemia) and much less frequently by point mutations.[62] The degree of decreased α-globin chain production reflects the number of affected α-globin genes.

$α^+$ thalassemia (-α/αα) results from the loss of function of one of the four normal α-globin genes and can be caused by either deletional (-α) or non-deletional (ND) mechanisms ($α^{ND}α$ or $αα^{ND}$). Two common types of deletional $α^+$ thalassemia (previously known as α-thalassemia 2; α-thal 2) have been described and involve either the deletion of 3.7 kb of DNA (rightward type, $-α^{3.7}$) or 4.2 kb of DNA (leftward type, $-α^{4.2}$).[78] These deletions are very common and occur in 30% of African Americans and up to 60-80% of individuals in parts of Saudi Arabia, India, Thailand, Papua New Guinea, and Melanesia [Chui]. Non-deletional $α^+$ thalassemia is rare and 70 different mutations have been described in sporadic families.[78] α°-thalassemia (--/αα or -α/-α) results from loss of two of four normal α-globin genes and there are more than 20 known deletions that result in either removal of both α-globin genes on the same chromosome 16 (in cis) or deletion of the entire ζ–α-globin gene cluster.[79] The majority of mutations resulting in α°-thalassemia occur from deletions of the duplicated α-globin genes from one chromosome (--), previously known as α-thalassemia 1 (α-thal 1).[78]

The α-thalassemia syndromes are classified into four clinical conditions of increasing severity: two carrier states ($α^+$ thalassemia and α°-thalassemia), and two clinical significant forms that include Hb H disease with only one functioning α-globin gene (-α/--) and Hb Barts hydrops fetalis with no functioning α-globin genes (--/--).[80] The carrier states can be further divided into silent carrier and two α-globin gene deletion thalassemia trait. Silent carriers usually have three functioning α-globin genes and may be completely asymptomatic (hematologically normal) or associated with moderate microcytosis, hypochromia, and mild anemia. In contrast to iron deficiency anemia, the RBC is usually normal or elevated.[62] Silent carriers may have mildly increased (1-2%) of Hb Bart, a homotetramer of γ-globin chains ($γ_4$), resulting from a shortage in α-globin chains in the newborn period. Individuals with two residual functioning α-globin genes in either the cis (--/αα) or trans (-α/-α) configuration show a moderate increase in Hb Bart on the newborn screen with moderate microcytosis, hypochromia, and mild anemia with normal Hb A_2 and F (Table 15-7).[80] Hb Bart in these individuals disappears with the transition to adult distributions of hemoglobin and may only be present on new born screen and not on follow-up testing performed after 6 months of age. For this reason, parents of a Hb H patient may appear normal by electrophoresis and HPLC testing despite being carriers for alpha thalassemia trait.

Hemoglobin H disease is the result of having three nonfunctional α-globin genes ($-\alpha/--$ or $\alpha^{ND}\alpha/--$) and is characterized by the presence of Hb H, a nonfunctional and unstable β_2-homotetramer.[80] Individuals with Hemoglobin H disease will have varying degrees of anemia ranging from intermediate to severe with microcytes, target cells, and basophilic stippling on the peripheral smear. There is evidence of hemolysis with hepatosplenomegaly.[62] Reticulocytes range between 5% and 10%.[80] Patients with HbH disease exhibit features of chronic hemolytic anemia, including hepatosplenomegaly, unconjugated hyperbilirubinemia, elevated LDH, and reduced haptoglobin. While hemolysis is generally accepted to be the major cause of anemia, ineffective erythropoiesis also plays a role. The non-deletional ($\alpha^{ND}\alpha/--$) form of Hemoglobin H disease is more severe with affected patients being more symptomatic and more likely to require transfusions.[79]

Hb Constant Spring [α142, Term→ (TAA>CAA in α2)] (α^{CS}) arises from a point mutation in the termination codon of the α_2-globin gene that leads to the production of a variant α-globin chain that has 31 additional amino acids in the protein. The α^{CS} mutation affects only the α_2-globin gene, which normally accounts for 2/3 of normal α-globin chain production for each copy of chromosome 16 and results in poor output (1% of normal) of the variant chain.[81] It is the most common non-deletional α-thalassemic mutation associated Hb H disease. Laboratory diagnosis of Hb Constant Spring can be difficult due to the fact that the messenger RNA is highly unstable and only a very small amount of the protein is produced (less than 1% of a normal α_2-globin gene). If sufficient protein is produced, Hb Constant Spring appears as two bands moving slower than Hb A_2 on alkaline electrophoresis and no separation by acid electrophoresis. By HPLC, Hb Constant Spring migrates as a very small band < 2% in quantity with a retention time close to Hb C in the C window.[66] The phenotype is moderate to severe with a majority of patients requiring repeated transfusions and 50% of patients require splenectomy with an associated risk of portal vein thrombosis. Older patients eventually become transfusion independent, but may still require transfusions during acute illness and increased iron absorption results in iron overload.[82]

Hb Bart hydrops fetalis is the most severe α-thalassemia clinical condition and is associated with no functioning α-globin genes ($--/--$). Due to the inability to produce any α_2-globin chains, the fetal blood contains mainly Hb Bart (γ_4) and small amounts of Hb Gower 1 ($\zeta_2\varepsilon_2$) and Portland ($\zeta_2\gamma_2$).[80] Due to the relatively high prevalence of deletional α° –thalassemia ($--/\alpha\alpha$) in parts of China and Southeast Asia, homozygosity for these deleted alleles ($--/--$) is 2-3 times more common than with β-thalassemia major or intermedia.[79] Most homozygous $\alpha°$ –thalassemia individuals perish in the fetal state and very few survive beyond the third trimester.[78]

β-Thalassemia Syndromes

The β-globin gene cluster is located on chromosome 11 and consists of one embryonic globin (ϵ) gene, two fetal globin (Gγ and Aγ) genes and two post-natal globin genes (one δ-globin gene and one β-globin gene). The β-globin gene contributes to the production of Hb A ($\alpha_2\beta_2$), which normally consti-tutes >95% of hemoglobin after 6 months of age (Table 15-3). In contrast, the δ-globin gene only has 2.5-3% expression.[62] While α-thalassemia is most commonly caused by large deletions affecting one or both α-globin genes, the majority of β-thalassemia syndromes are the result of point mutations and small deletions or insertions in the β-globin gene. These mutations may either reduce (β^+-thalassemia) or eliminate ($\beta°$-thalassemia) the expression of the β-globin gene, resulting in a deficit of β-globin chains.[83]

β-thalassemia has a high prevalence in populations in the Mediterranean, Middle East, Transcaucacus, Central Asia, India, and Far East. It is also relatively common in people of African descent. The clinical severity of β-thalassemia is related to the extent of the imbalance between the α-globin chains and the β-globin-like chains (β-globin, δ-globin, and γ-globin). A reduction or absence of β-globin chains leads to precipitation of the unpaired α-globin chains and ultimately results in apoptosis and ineffective erythropoiesis due to oxidative damage to the cell membrane of red cell precursors. β-thalassemia syndromes can be classified into β-thalassemia carrier state, thalassemia intermedia, and thalassemia major.[84]

The β-thalassemia carrier state, which results from heterozygosity for β-thalassemia is clinically asymptomatic and defined by an elevated Hb A$_2$ level (3.5-6.0%), variable amount of Hb F (0.5-4%), normal or elevated red cell count, markedly decreased MCV (60-75 fL) and reduced MCH (18-24 pg). The red cell morphology shows microcytosis, hypochromia, and anisopoikilocytosis.[75]

Homozygotes for β-thalassemia may develop either thalassemia major or thalassemia intermedia depending on the severity of the inherited β-thalassemia alleles (β^+-thalassemia or $\beta°$-thalassemia).[83] Thalassemia intermedia encompasses a clinically and genotypically heterogeneous group ranging in severity from the asymptomatic carrier state to anemia requiring transfusion.[84] Individual who inherit two mild β-thalassemia mutations (β^+/β^+-thalassemia) generally have mild disease. Compound heterozygosity for a mild and severe allele of β-thalassemia ($\beta°$/β^+-thalassemia) results in variable severity of anemia. In addition, coinheritance of α-thalassemia amelio-rated the severity of disease in individuals who inherited at least one mild β^+-thalassemia allele.[83]

Patients with thalassemia intermedia are clinically heterogeneous. Symptoms may include pallor, jaundice, cholelithiasis, hepatosplenomegaly, moderate to severe skeletal changes, leg ulcers, extramedullary erythropoiesis, osteopenia, and osteoporosis. These patients are at risk for thrombotic complications due to a hypercoagulable state because of the lipid membrane composition of the abnormal red cells. In addition, iron overload often occurs due to increased intestinal absorption of iron caused by ineffective erythropoiesis and mediated by suppression of hepcidin by increased levels of growth differentiation factor 15.[84] Hematologically, these patients show moderate anemia with low MCV, low MCH, and elevated Hb A_2 (3-5.0%). Transfusions are usually not required or only occasionally required.[75,84]

Thalassemia major results from homozygosity for two severe alleles of β-thalassemia (β°/β°-thalassemia) or compound heterozygosity for a mild and severe allele of β-thalassemia (β°/β+-thalassemia) and manifests as severe, transfusion-dependent anemia.[83,84] Co-inheritance of α-thalassemia does not alleviate the severity of the disease.[83] Affected infants with thalassemia fail to thrive and are progressively pale; most patients come to medical attention through abnormalities on the newborn screen or within the first 2 years of life. Complications of the disease are numerous and include feeding problems, diarrhea, recurrent fever, hepatosplenomegaly, complications of iron overload, infectious complications, hypercoagulable state, osteoporosis, hypogonadism, diabetes mellitus, hypothyroidism, hypoparathyroidism, cardiac dysfunction, and pulmonary hypertension. A chronic transfusion program that maintains a minimum hemoglobin concentration of 9.5-10.5 g/dL may help achieve normal growth and development in patients until the age of 10-11 years, after which the patients are at risk for developing complications of iron overload.[84]

Thalassemia major is characterized by severe microcytic and hypochromic anemia with increased red blood cells. The peripheral blood smear shows microcytic and hypochromic red blood cells with marked anisopoikilocytosis including frequent target cells and basophilic stippling.[67] Nucleated red blood cells are increased relative to the degree of anemia. HPLC and electrophoresis findings vary with the degree of β-globin chain suppression.[84] β°-thalassemia, characterized by a complete lack of β-globin chain production, typically presents with absent Hb A, increased Hb F (95-98%), and elevated Hb A_2 (usually >5%). β+-thalassemia is associated with at least some residual β-globin chain synthesis and usually has decreased Hb A (10-30%), elevated Hb F (70-90%), and elevated Hb A_2 (3.5-5.0%) to a lesser extent than the most severe form, β°-thalassemia.[75,84]

δβ-Thalassemia Syndromes

δβ-Thalassemia is an infrequent cause of elevated levels of Hb F after 6 months of age and is usually due to large deletions involving either the δ- and β-globin genes or the Aγ, δ-, and β-globin genes.[85] This disorder results in decreased production of both δ and β-globin chains with intact γ-globin chain production and has been reported in various ethnic groups including individuals of Turkish, German, Japanese, Sicilian, and Spanish descent. The non-deletional form of δβ-thalassemia has also been reported.[86] Heterozygotes for δβ-thalassemia are characterized by 5-20% Hb F on HPLC and hypochromic and microcytic red cell indices.[85] In contrast to β-thalassemia, the clinical presentation is mild in both heterozygous and homozygous δβ-thalassemia. The HPLC findings of elevated Hb F with normal Hb A_2 in heterozygotes and absence of Hb A and Hb A_2 in homozygotes is helpful in making the diagnosis.[86] Deletional hereditary persistence of fetal hemoglobin (HPFH) is the main differential for homozygous δβ-thalassemia since they can both result in100% Hb F. The distinction between δβ-thalassemia and HPFH is subtle and relies on clinical and hematologic findings including lack of thalassemic indices in HPFH.[85] Clinical features, such as mild anemia with hemolytic findings including reticulocytosis, indirect hyperbilirubinemia, and decreased haptoglobin are more consistent with homozygous δβ-thalassemia rather than HPFH.[86]

Hereditary Persistent of Fetal Hemoglobin (HPFH)

Hereditary persistence of fetal hemoglobin is a heterogeneous disorder also characterized by elevated levels of Hb F beyond infancy. HPFH can be divided into non-deletional HPFH in which the β-globin gene cluster are intact and deletional HPFH in which large deletions involving the 3′ end of the β cluster have removed the δ- and β-globin genes. Individuals heterozygous for HPFH usually have higher levels of Hb F (30%) and normal red cell indices compared to heterozygous δβ-thalassemia.[85] Homozygotes for deletional HPFH have 100% HB F with no Hb A or A_2 on HPLC with mildly microcytic and hypochromic red cells with no anemia. The non-deletional form of HPFH is due a mutation in the promoter region of one of the γ-globin genes resulting in increased production of Hb F with concurrent decreased output from the δ- and β-globin genes on the same chromosome. Hb F levels range from 3-31% for the different forms of non-deletional HPFH.[65] Hb F can be homogenously distributed in all cells (pancellular) or limited to some of the cells (heterocellular) depending on the genotypic form.[62] Compound heterozygosity for Hb S and HPFH results in one of the mildest sickling disorder.[87]

Qualitative Hemoglobin Disorders

Qualitative hemoglobin disorders are characterized by the synthesis of abnormal hemoglobin, resulting from amino acid substitutions in any of the globin chains. The vast majority of variant hemoglobins are clinically asymptomatic and are only detectable by laboratory diagnostic tests.[62] Variant hemoglobins that cause sickling disorders are the most clinically significant. The most common of these is sickle cell disease.

Sickle Cell Disease

Sickle Cell Disease (SCD) is a chronic hemolytic anemia that is characterized by the inheritance of a hemoglobin variant (Hb S) with a tendency to polymerize when exposed to low oxygen tension. This results in deformation of the red cell into a sickle (or crescent) shape and causes vaso-occlusive events and hemolysis. The hemoglobin S variant (β6 glu → val) is caused by substitution of valine for glutamic acid in position 6 of the β-globin chain. SCD can result from homozygosity for the HbS (SCD-SS) or as the result of compound heterozygosity for Hb S and another β-globin variant that results in the Sickle Cell phenotype (eg, SCD-SC or SCD-Sβ°).[87]

SCD can be considered both a qualitative and quantitative disorder due to the fact that the disorder is the result of the production of an abnormal hemoglobin, yet the likelihood of sickling is highly dependent on the Hb S concentration in the cell. Individuals heterozygous for Hb S (Hb AS) normally have 30-40% intracellular Hb S and are asymptomatic under normal circumstances. Homozygous Hb S (SCD-SS) is the most common genotype. Other common genotypic causes of SCD include compound heterozygosity for Hb S and C (SCD-SC) and for Hb S and β-thalassemia variants (SCD-Sβ°-thalassemia and SCD-β⁺-thalassemia). SCD-SS and SCD- SCD-Sβ°-thalassemia have the most severe disease due to the fact that almost all of the intracellular hemoglobin is Hb S. Next in severity are SCD-SC and SCD-β⁺-thalassemia.[88] Other rare combinations that are less severe, include Hb S with hereditary persistence of fetal Hb (SCD-S/HPHP), Hb E, Hb D-Los Angeles, Hb O-Arab, Hb Lepore and others.[62]

SCD affects an estimated 90,000 people in the United States, and more than 1,900 new cases are detected annually on newborn screens. Infant screening and early preventive therapy with chronic transfusions, prophylactic antibiotics for hyposplenism and asplenism and hydroxyurea treatment have largely eliminated early childhood mortality from SCD.[89] The most common clinical manifestation of SCD is vaso-occlusive crisis resulting from obstruction of the microcirculation by sickled red cells and resulting in ischemic organ injury and pain. It can involve the bones, abdomen, joints, and soft tissue. Individuals with SCD often have functional asplenia due to progressive autoinfarction of the spleen resulting in increased susceptibility to infection. Other serious clinical sequelae include acute chest syndrome, pulmonary hypertension, avascular necrosis of the femoral or humoral head, priapism, leg ulcers, renal damage, risk of stroke, and aplastic crisis from parvovirus B-19 infection.[87,90]

Identification of Hb S is relatively straightforward on HPLC, citrate electrophoresis and IEF. Laboratory findings for Sickle Cell Trait (Hb AS) include and abnormal pattern of approximately 40% Hb S on HPLC and normal levels of Hb A_2 and F.[62] CBC parameters will be normal and the peripheral blood smear may show microcytosis or target cells.[69] Individuals with SCD-SS and SCD-Sβ°-thalassemia will have 90-95% Hb S on HPLC with 5-15% Hb F and normal or elevated Hb A_2.[69] Hb A_2 may be falsely elevated in the presence of slow eluting hemoglobins, such as Hb S due to the fact that the post-translational modification product of these hemoglobins co-migrate with Hb A_2 on HPLC.[91] The MCV for SCD-SS patients is typically normal in contrast to SCD-Sβ°-thalassemia, which typically has a reduced MCV that can aid in the differentiation of the two genotypes. The reticulocyte count is 5-20% for SCD-SS and 8-9% for SCD-Sβ°-thalassemia.[69] HPLC will typically show 15-30% Hb A, over 50% Hb S, 1-20% Hb F, and 4-6% Hb A2.[65] The peripheral blood smear typically shows sickle cells, target cells, and evidence of hyposplenism including Howell-Jolly bodies and nucleated red blood cells by 1 year of age.[69]

Hb C polymerizes less readily than Hb S. SCD-SC typically has a higher hemoglobin concentration than SCD-SS with a low normal MCV. The reticulocyte count is typically 3-6%. HPLC will show Hb S and C present in similar proportions with normal to slightly elevated Hb F. IEF and citrate electrophoresis will show two dominant bands corresponding to Hb S and C. The peripheral blood smear often shows increased poikilocytes and blunted boat shaped cells rather than classic sickle cells. Occasional cells may show Hb C crystals. Features of hyposplenism, such as Howell-Jolly bodies are less common than in SCD-SS.[69]

Hemoglobin C Disorders

Hb C is characterized by substitution of a glutamic acid residue with a lysine residue at the 6th position if the β-globin chain (β6 glu $\rightarrow$ lys) and is one of the three most prevalent variant hemoglobins.[92] It is found in approximately 2% of African-Americans.[93] Heterozygotes (Hemoglobin C Trait) are hematologically normal with normal hematologic indices and approximately 40% Hb C on HPLC with a corresponding variant band on IEF and citrate electrophoresis.[65] Hb C migrates to the Hb A2 position on alkaline electrophoresis and IEF and has a specific position on HPLC.[62] The homozygous state (Hemoglobin C Disease) is associated with mild hemolytic anemia.[92] Hb C tends to form rhomboidal crystals that can be seen on the peripheral blood smear.[94] The red cells are rigid and less deformable, resulting in increased destruction in the reticuloendothelial system.[65]

Hemoglobin D-Punjab Disorders

Hb D-Punjab (also known as Hb D-Los Angeles) is a variant hemoglobin resulting from the substitution of a glutamic acid for glutamine at the 121st position of the β-globin chain (β121 glu → gln). Heterozygotes and homozygotes for Hb D are clinically asymptomatic. Compound heterozygosity for Hb S and D results in severe SCD (SCD-SD-Punjab) comparable to SCD-SS.[87] HPLC for patients with SCD-SD-Punjab shows 30-40% Hb S and 40-50% Hb D-Punjab. Hb S undergoes polymerization in a two-step process and the substitution of glutamate by glutamine in Hb D-Punjab strengthens the second reaction and accelerates Hb S polymerization in SCD-SD-Punjab.[95] Hb D is indistinguishable from Hb G on acidic and alkaline electrophoresis.[65,72]

Hemoglobin E Disorders

Hb E disorders can be thought of as both qualitative and quantitative hemoglobin disorders. The variant mutation is caused by the substitution of a glutamic acid for lysine at the 26th position of the β-globin chain (β26 glu → lys). The β^E mutation creates an alternate splicing site in the mRNA at codons 25-27 resulting in decreased expression of the gene.[96] Hb E migrates to the Hb A_2 position on alkaline electrophoresis and also elutes to the Hb A_2 position on HPLC.[62] Hemoglobin E Trait (Hb AE) is asymptomatic with borderline microcytosis and approximately 30% Hb E and 65-70% Hb A on HPLC[65] The peripheral blood smear may show microcytosis, hypochromia, target cells, or basophilic stippling, but also may be normal.[69] Homozygous Hb E (Hemoglobin E Disease) is also asymptomatic and resembles thalassemia trait with microcytosis, erythrocytosis, and mild anemia. HPLC typically shows >90% Hb E, 1-10% Hb F and no distinguishable Hb A_2.[65] The peripheral blood smear is similar to thalassemia trait with microcytosis and hypochromia with target cells.[69]

Hb E is frequent in Asian populations and the carrier frequency of the Hb E mutation among California Asians is almost equal to that of the Hb S mutation among African Americans.[82] Compound heterozygosity for Hb S and Hb E (SCD-SE) is relatively uncommon and produces a mild SCD.[87] Compound heterozygosity for HB E and β-thalassemia is exclusive to newborns of Southeast Asian descent with an estimated birth prevalence of 1 in 2600. HB E/β-thalassemia is now more common than classic β-thalassemia in many regions in the United States.[82] Compound heterozygosity of Hb E and β^+-thalassemia results in milder thalassemia intermedia, while compound heterozygosisity for Hb E and β^0-thalassemia produces variably severe anemia with the majority being moderately severe.[83]

Hemoglobin G-Philadelphia Disorders

Hemoglobin G-Philadelphia [α68(E17) asn → lys] is the most common α-globin chain variant in the United States and is present in individuals of African and Mediterranean descent. The point mutation in the alpha globin gene results in replacement of the normal asparagine in the 68th position of the α-globin chain by lysine.[97] Hb G-Philadelphia is associated with deletional α$^+$ thalassemia (-α$^{3.7}$) on the same chromosome (in cis) and the proportion of detectable variant hemoglobin depends on the number of α-globin genes affected by mutation or deleted.[93,97] The variant will be approximately 25% of the hemoglobin on HPLC if no α-globin gene deletion is associated with it. Hb G-Philadelphia will be approximately 35% on HPLC if a single α-globin gene deletion is present (α$^+$ thalassemia trait). Hb G-Philadelphia trait with homozygous α$^+$ thalassemia (two α-globin genes deleted) will produce 45% Hb G-Philadelphia with microcytosis. Homozygous G-Philadelphia with homozygous α$^+$ thalassemia (two α-globin genes deleted) will have approximately 95% Hb G with microcytosis.[93,98] Hb G-Philadelphia migrates to the Hb S on alkaline electrophoresis and cannot be differentiated from Hb S using this method.[93] IEF offers better resolution and is able to separate Hb G-Philadelphia from Hb S, however, IEF is not able to help distinguish Hb G-Philadelphia from Hb D.[72,99]. Hb G-Philadelphia is able to form heterozygous hemoglobins with normal adult Hb A, as well as abnormal β-globin chain variants, such as Hb S and Hb C. When an abnormal α-chain variant, such as Hb G-Philadelphia combines with abnormal β globin chains, it can be difficult to diagnose these patients, as has been reported several times throughout the literature. The difficulty arises because these variants migrate to where Hb C, E, and O are detected on cellulose acetate.[93,99]

TRAINING MODULE

1. A 2-year-old male presents to the hematology clinic for evaluation of persistent microcytic anemia. The peripheral blood smear shows microcytic, hypochromic anemia with frequent target cells and elliptocytes. There is prominent anisopoikilocytosis and no discernable polychromasia. The CBC shows normal WBC and platelets, decreased RBC, MCH, MCHC, and increased RDW. Newborn screen was reportedly normal.

   Based on the earlier scenario, which of the following tests will be most useful in diagnosing the cause for the microcytic anemia?

   a. Evaluation for hemoglobinopathy or thalassemia
   b. Serum Ferritin
   c. Haptoglobin
   d. Serum Iron

2. Which of the following β-globin disorders would be expected to result in the sickling disorder of least severity if inherited in combination with the Hb S mutation?

a. Hb D-Punjab

b. β°-thalassemia

c. Hb C

d. Hb E

3. Which of the following conditions is associated with hemolysis, hyperbilirubinemia, and decreased haptoglobin?

a. Deletional Hereditary Persistence of Fetal Hemoglobin (HPFH)

b. Immune Thrombocytopenic Purpura

c. Hereditary Spherocytosis

d. Anemia of Inflammation

REFERENCES

1. Vajpayee N, Graham SS, Bem S. Basic examination of blood and bone marrow. In: McPherson RA and Pincus MR, ed. *Henry's Clinical Diagnosis and Management by Laboratory Methods*. 21st ed. Philadelphia: Saunders/Elsevier Inc.; 2007. 457-503 pp.

2. Menzel S, Thein SL. Genetic architecture of hemoglobin F control. *Curr Opin Hematol*. 2009;16:179-186.

3. Zijlstra WG. Standardisation of hemoglobinometry: history and new challenges. *Comp Hematol Int*. 1987;1:125-132.

4. Haymond S, Cariappa R, Eby CS, Scott MG. Laboratory assessment of oxygenation in methemoglobinemia. *Clin Chem*. 2005;51(2):434-44.

5. Lindner G, Exadaktylos AK. How noninvasive haemoglobin measurement with pulse co-oximetry can change your practice: an expert review. *Emerg Med Int*. 2013;2013:701529.

6. Buttarello M, Plebani M. Automated blood cell counts: state of the art. *Am J Clin Pathol*. 2008;130:104-116.

7. Pinkowski R. Difference between impedance and optical platelet count methods in patients with microcytosis of red blood cells. *Lab Hematol*. 1999;5:22-27.

8. Chang CC, Kass L. Clinical significance of immature reticulocyte fraction determined by automated reticulocyte counting. *Am J Clin Path*. 1997;108:69-73.

9. Liu S, Ren J, Xia Q, Wu X, Han G, Ren H, Yan D, Wang G, Gu G, Li J. Preliminary case-control study to evaluate diagnostic values of C-reactive protein and erythrocyte sedimentation rate in differentiating active Crohn's disease from intestinal lymphoma, intestinal tuberculosis and Behcet's syndrome. *Am J Med Sci*. 2013;346:467-472.

10. Racsa LD, Gander RM, Southern PM, McElvania TeKippe E, Doern C, Luu HS. Detection of intracellular parasites by use of the cellavision dm96 analyzer during routine screening of peripheral blood smears. *J Clin Microbiol*. 2015;53(1):167-171.

11. Kim YC, Kim KH, YongKeun Park YK (2012). Measurement Techniques for Red Blood Cell Deformability: Recent Advances, Blood Cell—An Overview of Studies in

Hematology, Dr. Terry Moschandreou (Ed.), InTech. Available from: http://www.inte-chopen.com/books/blood-cell-an-overview-of-studies-in-hematology/measurement-techniques-for-red-blood-cell-deformability-recent-advances

12. Pillay J, den Braber I, Vrisekoop N, Kwast LM, de Boer RJ, Borghans JA, Tesselaar K, Koenderman L. In vivo labeling with 2H2O reveals a human neutrophil lifespan of 5.4 days. *Blood.* 2010;116(4):625-627.

13. Bekkering S, Torensma R. Another look at the life of a neutrophil. *World J Hematol.* 2013;2:44-58.

14. Walsh GM. Eosinophil granule proteins and their role in disease. *Curr Opin Hematol.* 2001;8:28-33.

15. Schroeder JT. Basophils beyond effector cells of allergic inflammation. *Adv Immunol.* 2009;101:123-161.

16. Proytcheva M. Bone marrow examination for pediatric patients. *Int J Lab Hematol.* 2013; 35:283-289.

17. Swerdlow SH, Campo E, Harris NL. et al., eds. *WHO Classification Of Tumours And Haematopoietic And Lymphoid Tissues.* Lyon: IARC; 2008:18-30.

18. Bauer DE, Orkin SH. Update on fetal hemoglobin gene regulation in hemoglobinopathies. *Curr Opin Pediatr.* 2011;23:1-8.

19. Wickramasinghe S. Bone marrow. In: Mills S, ed. *Histology for Pathologists.* 3rd ed. Philadelphia:Lippincott Williams & Wilkins; 2007. 799-836 pp.

20. Sieff CA, Zon LI. Anatomy and physiology of hematopoiesis. In: Orkin, SH, Nathan, DG, Ginsburg, D, Look, AT, Fisher, DE, Lux S, eds. *Nathan and Oski's Hematology of Infancy and Childhood.* 7th ed. Philadelphia: Saunders Elsevier; 2009:195-273.

21. Foucar K, Reichard K, Czuchlewski D. eds. *Bone Marrow Pathology.* 3rd ed. Chicago: ASCP Press;2010:3-51.

22. McKenna RW, Washington LT, Aquino DB, Picker LJ, Kroft SH. Immunophenotypic analysis of hematogones (B-lymphocyte precursors) in 662 consecutive bone marrow specimens by 4-color flow cytometry. *Blood.* 2001;98(8):2498-2507.

23. Goldrath AW, Bevan MJ. Selecting and maintaining a diverse T-cell repertoire. *Nature.* 1999;402(6759):255-262.

24. Powers JM, McCavit TL, Buchanan GR. Management of iron deficiency anemia: a survey of pediatric hematology/oncology specialists. *Pediatr Blood Cancer.* 2015;62(5):842-846

25. Institute of Medicine. Food and Nutrition Board. *Dietary Reference Intakes for Vitamin A, Vitamin K, Arsenic, Boron, Chromium, Copper, Iodine, Iron, Manganese, Molybdenum, Nickel, Silicon, Vanadium, and Zinc: A Report of the Panel on Micronutrients.* Washington, DC: National Academy Press; 2001.

26. Baker RD, Greer FR, The Committee on Nutrition. Diagnosis and prevention of iron deficiency and iron-deficiency anemia in infants and young children (0–3 years of age). *Pediatrics.* 2010;126:1040-1050. DOI: 10.1542/peds.2010-2576

27. Hillman RS, Finch CA. *Red Cell Manual.* 7th ed. Philadelphia: FA Davis; 1996.

28. Andrews NC, Ullrich CK, Fleming MD. Disorders of Iron Metabolism and Sideroblastic Anemia. In: Orkin, SH, Nathan, DG, Ginsburg, D, Look, AT, Fisher, DE, Lux S, eds. *Nathan and Oski's Hematology of Infancy and Childhood.* 7th ed. Philadelphia: Saunders Elsevier; 2009:521-570.

29. Means RT, Krantz SB. Progress in understanding the pathogenesis of the anemia of chronic disease. *Blood*. 1992;80:1639-1647.

30. Weiss G, Goodnough LT. Anemia of chronic disease. *N Engl J Med*. 2005;352:1011-1023.

31. Auerbach M, Ballard H, Trout JR, et al. Intravenous iron optimizes the response to recombinant human erythropoietin in cancer patients with chemotherapy-related anemia: a multicenter, open-label, randomized trial. *J Clin Oncol*. 2004;22:1301-1307.

32. Ohba R, Furuyama K, Yoshida K, Fujiwara T, Fukuhara N, Onishi Y, Manabe A, Ito E, Ozawa K, Kojima S, Ogawa S, Harigae H. Clinical and genetic characteristics of congenital sideroblastic anemia: comparison with myelodysplastic syndrome with ring sideroblast (MDS-RS). *Ann Hematol*. 2013;92(1):1-9.

33. Harigae H, Furuyama K. Hereditary sideroblastic anemia: pathophysiology and gene mutations. *Int J Hematol*. 2010;92(3):425-431.

34. Cartwright GE, Deiss A. Sideroblasts, siderocytes, and sideroblastic anemia. *N Engl J Med*. 1975;292:185-193.

35. Ammus S, Yunis AA. Drug-induced red blood cell dyscrasias. *Blood Rev*. 1989;3:71-82.

36. Lin-Fu JS. Vulnerability of children to lead exposure and toxicity (first of two parts). *N Engl J Med*. 1973;289:1229-1233.

37. Franco RS. Measurement of Red Cell Lifespan and Aging. *Transfus Med Hemother*. 2012;39:302–307.

38. Kay IT, Weimer M, Watson CJ. The formation in vitro of stercobilin from bilirubin. *J Biol Chem*. 1963;238:1122-1123.

39. Goldenstein H, Levy N, Levy A. Involvement of haptoglobin in prevention of oxidative stress cause by hemoglobin in preeclampsia. *Adv Biosci Biotechnol*. 2012;3;1037-1042.

40. Wassell J. Haptoglobin: function and polymorphism. *Clin Lab*. 2000;46:547-552.

41. Perrotta S, Gallagher PG, Mohandas N. Hereditary spherocytosis. *Lancet*. 2008; 372:1411-1426.

42. Christensen RD, Agarwal AM, Nussenzveig RH, Heikal N, Liew MA, Yaish HM. Evaluating eosin-5-maleimide binding as a diagnostic test for hereditary spherocytosis in newborn infants. *J Perinatol*. 2015;35(5):357-361.

43. Bianchi P, Fermo E, Vercellati C, Marcello AP, Porretti L, Cortelezzi A, Barcellini W, Zanella A. Diagnostic power of laboratory tests for hereditary spherocytosis: a comparison study in 150 patients grouped according to molecular and clinical characteristics. *Haematologica*. 2012;97(4):516-523.

44. King MJ, Zanella A. Hereditary red cell membrane disorders and laboratory diagnostic testing. *Int J Lab Hem*. 2013;35:237–243.

45. Gottfried EL, Robertson NA. Glycerol lysis time of incubated erythrocytes in the diagnosis of hereditary spherocytosis. *J Lab Clin Med*. 1974;84:746-751.

46. Zanella A, Izzo C, Rebulla P, Zanuso F, Perroni L, Sirchia G. Acidified glycerol lysis test: a screening test for spherocytosis. *Br J Haematol*. 1980;45:481-486.

47. Vettore L, Zanella A, Molaro GL, De Matteis MC, Pavesi M, Mariani M. A new test for the laboratory diagnosis of spherocytosis. *Acta Haematol*. 1984;72:258-263.

48. Streichman S, Gescheidt Y. Cryohemolysis for the detection of hereditary spherocytosis: correlation studies with osmotic fragility and autohemolysis. *Am J Hematol*. 1998;58:206-212.

49. King MJ, Behrens J, Rogers C, Flynn C, Greenwood D, Chambers K. Rapid flow cytometric test for the diagnosis of membrane cytoskeleton-associated haemolytic anaemia. *Br J Haematol*. 2000;111:924-933.

50. Eber SW, Armbrust R, Schröter W. Variable clinical severity of hereditary spherocytosis: relation to erythrocytic spectrin concentration, osmotic fragility, and autohemolysis. *J Pediatr*. 1990;117(3):409-416.

51. Mason PJ, Bautista JM, Gilsanz F. G6PD deficiency: the genotype-phenotype association. *Blood Reviews*. 2007;21:267-283.

52. Frank JE. Diagnosis and Management of G6PD Deficiency. *Am Fam Physician*. 2005;72:1277-1282.

53. Nkhoma ET, Poole C, Vannappagari V, Hall SA, Beutler E. The global prevalence of glucose-6-phosphate dehydrogenase deficiency: a systematic review and meta-analysis. *Blood Cells Mol Dis*. 2009;42:267-278.

54. Beutler E. G6PD deficiency. *Blood*. 1994;84:3613-3636.

55. Cappellini MD, Fiorelli G. Glucose-6-phosphate dehydrogenase deficiency. *Lancet*. 2008;371:64-74.

56. Beutler E. Glucose-6-phosphate dehydrogenase deficiency: a historical perspective. *Blood*. 2008;111:16-24.

57. Yoo D, Lessin LS. Drug-associated "bite cell" hemolytic anemia. *Am J Med*. 1992;92:243-248.

58. Neunert C, Lim W, Crowther M, Cohen A, Solberg L Jr, Crowther MA. The American Society of Hematology 2011 evidence-based practice guideline for immune thrombocytopenia. *Blood*. 2011;117:4190-4207.

59. Schultz CL, Mitra N, Schapira MM, Lambert MP. Influence of the American Society of Hematology guidelines on the management of newly diagnosed childhood immune thrombocytopenia. *JAMA Pediatr*. 2014;168:e142214.

60. Shad AT, Gonzalez CE, Sandler SG. Treatment of immune thrombocytopenic purpura in children : current concepts. *Paediatr Drugs*. 2005;7(5):325-336.

61. Neunert CE, Buchanan GR, Imbach P, Bolton-Maggs PH, Bennett CM, Neufeld E, Vesely SK, Adix L, Blanchette VS, Kühne T; Intercontinental Cooperative ITP Study Group Registry II Participants. Bleeding manifestations and management of children with persistent and chronic immune thrombocytopenia: data from the Intercontinental Cooperative ITP Study Group (ICIS). *Blood*. 2013;121(22):4457-4462.

62. Giordano PC. Strategies for basic laboratory diagnostics of the hemoglobinopathics in multi-ethnic societies: interpretation of the results and pitfalls. *Int J Lab Hem*. 2012;35:465-479.

63. Akl PS, Kutlar F, Patel N et al. Compound heterozygosity for hemoglobin S[β6(A3) Glu6Val] and hemoglobin Korle-Bu [β73(E17)Asp73Asn]. *Lab Hematol*. 2009;15:19-23.

64. Giardine B, van Baal S, Kaimakis P, Riemer C, Miller W, Samara M, Kollia P, Anagnou NP, Chui DH, Wajcman H, Hardison RC, Patrinos GP. HbVar database of human hemoglobin variants and thalassemia mutations: 2007 update. *Hum Mutat*. 2007;28:206.

65. McPherson RA and Pincus MR, editors. *Henry's Clinical Diagnosis and Management by Laboratory Methods*. 21st ed. Philadelphia: Saunders/Elsevier Inc.; 2007:522-532.

66. Szuberski J, Oliveira JL, Hoyer JD. A comprehensive analysis of hemoglobin variants by high-performance liquid chromatography (HPLC). *Int J Lab Hem*. 2012;34:594-604.

67. Harrington AM, Ward PC, Kroft SH. Iron Deficiency Anemia, β-Thalassemia Minor, and Anemia of Chronic Disease: A Morphologic Reappraisal. *Am J Clin Pathol*. 2008;129:466-471.

68. Joutovsky A, Hadzi-Nesic J, Nardi MA. HPLC retention time as a diagnostic tool for hemoglobin variants and hemoglobinopathies: a study of 60000 samples in a clinical diagnostic laboratory. *Clin Chem*. 2004;50(10):1736-1747.

69. Bain BJ. *Hemoglobinopathy Diagnosis*. 2nd ed. Oxford, England: Blackwell Science Ltd.; 2006:26-58, 139-181, 190-227.

70. Higgins T, Mack M, Khajuria A. Comparison of two methods for the quantification and identification of hemoglobin variants. *Clin Biochem*. 2009;42:701-705.

71. Hoyer JD and Kroft SH, eds. *Color Atlas of Hemoglobin Disorders*. College of American Pathologists, Northfield, IL; 2003:3-5.

72. Ou CN, Rognerud CL. Diagnosis of hemoglobinopathies: electrophoresis vs. HPLC. *Clin Chim Acta*. 2001;313:187-194.

73. Hicks EJ, Hughes BJ. Comparison of Electrophoresis on Citrate Agar, Cellulose Acetate, or Starch for Hemoglobin Identification. *Clin Chem*. 1975;21:1072-1076.

74. Racsa L, Luu HS, Park J, Mitui M, Timmons C. Beta-globin gene sequencing of hemoglobin Austin revises the historically reported electrophoretic migration pattern. *Arch Pathol Lab Med*. 2014;138:819-822.

75. Giambona A, Passarello C, Renda D, Maggio A. The significance of the hemoglobin A$_2$ value in screening for hemoglobinopathies. *Clin Biochem*. 2009;42:1786-1796.

76. Keren DF, Shalhoub R, Gulbranson R, Hedstrom D. Expression of hemoglobin variant migration by capillary electrophoresis relative to hemoglobin A2 improves precision. *Am J Clin Pathol*. 2012;137:660-664.

77. Keren DF, Hedstrom D, Gulbranson R, Ou CN, Bak R. Comparison of Sebia Capillarys capillary electrophoresis with the Primus high-pressure liquid chromatography in the evaluation of hemoglobinopathies. *Am J Clin Pathol*. 2008;130:824-831.

78. Fucharoen S, Viprakasit V. Hb H disease: clinical course and disease modifiers. *Hematology Am Soc Hematol Educ Program*. 2009:26-34.

79. Chui DH, Fucharoen S, Chan V. Hemoglobin H disease: not necessarily a benign disorder. *Blood*. 2003;101:791-800.

80. Galanello R, Cao A. Gene test review. alpha-thalassemia. *Genet Med*. 2011;13:83-88.

81. Schrier SL, Bunyaratvej A, Khuhapinant A, Fucharoen S, Aljurf M, Snyder LM, Keifer CR, Ma L, Mohandas N. The unusual pathobiology of hemoglobin constant spring red blood cells. *Blood*. 1997;89(5):1762-1769.

82. Hoppe CC. Newborn screening for non-sickling hemoglobinopathies. *Hematology Am Soc Hematol Educ Program*. 2009;2009(1):19-25.

83. Winichagoon P, Fucharoen S, Chen P, Wasi P. Genetic factors affecting clinical severity in β-thalassemia syndromes. *J Pediatr Hematol Oncol*. 2000;22:573-580.

84. Cao A, Galanello R. Beta-thalassemia. *Genet Med*. 2010;12:61-76.

85. Craig JE, Barnetson RA, Prior J, Raven JL, Thein SL. Rapid detection of deletions causing delta beta thalassemia and hereditary persistence of fetal hemoglobin by enzymatic amplification. *Blood*. 1994;83:1673-1682.

86. Verma S, Bhargava M, Mittal S, Gupta R. Homozygous delta-beta thalassemia in a child: a rare cause of elevated fetal hemoglobin. *Iran J Ped Hematol Oncol.* 2013;3(1):222-227.

87. Rees DC, Williams TN, Gladwin MT. Sickle-cell disease. *Lancet.* 2010;376:2018-2031.

88. Thein SL. Genetic association studies in β-hemoglobinopathies. *Hematology Am Soc Hematol Educ Program.* 2013;2013:354-361.

89. Green NS, Barral S. Emerging science of hydroxyurea therapy for pediatric sickle cell disease. *Pediatr Res.* 2014;75:196-204.

90. Adewoyin AS. Management of sickle cell disease: a review for physician education in Nigeria (Sub-Saharan Africa). *Anemia.* 2015;2015:791498.

91. Zurbriggen K, Schmugge M, Schmid M, Durka S, Kleinert P, Kuster T, Heizmann CW, Troxler H. Analysis of minor hemoglobins by matrix-assisted laser desorption/ionization time-of-flight mass spectrometry. *Clin Chem.* 2005;51(6):989-996.

92. Nagel RL, Fabry ME, Steinberg MH. The paradox of hemoglobin SC disease. *Blood* Rev. 2003;17(3):167-178.

93. Kirk CM, Papadea CN, Lazarchick J. Laboratory recognition of a rare hemoglobinopathy: hemoglobins SS and SG(Philadelphia) associated with alpha-thalassemia-2. *Arch Pathol Lab Med.* 1999;123:963-966.

94. Lawrence C, Hirsch RE, Fataliev NA, Patel S, Fabry ME, Nagel RL. Molecular interactions between Hb alpha-G Philadelphia, HbC, and HbS: phenotypic implications for SC alpha-G Philadelphia disease. *Blood.* 1997;90(7):2819-2825.

95. Patel S, Purohit P, Mashon RS, Dehury S, Meher S, Sahoo S, Dash SS, Das K, Das P, Patel DK. The effect of hydroxyurea on compound heterozygotes for sickle cell-hemoglobin D-Punjab—a single centre experience in eastern India. *Pediatr Blood Cancer.* 2014;61:1341-1346.

96. Chernoff AI, Minnich V, Nanakorn V, Tuchinda S, Kashemsant C, Bangkok, Thailand, Chernoff RR. Studies on hemoglobin E. I. The clinical, hematologic, and genetic characteristics of the hemoglobin E syndromes. *J Lab Clin Med.* 1956;47:455-489.

97. Khalil MS, Timbs A, Henderson S, Schuh A, Hussein MR, Old J. Haemoglobin (Hb) G-Philadelphia, Hb Stanleyville-II, Hb G-Norfolk, Hb Matsue-Oki and Hb Mizushi can form a panel of α-chain variants that overlap in their phenotype: the novel use of StyI to screen for Hb G-Philadelphia. *Int J Lab Hematol.* 2011;33:318-325.

98. Masala B, Musino L, Pirastru M, Manca L. The C→G transition in the alpha 2-globin gene of a normal alpha alpha-chromosome is responsible for the Hb G-Philadelphia variant in Sardinians. *Eur J Haematol.* 2004;72:437-440.

99. Racsa L, Rogers ZR, Mitui M, Park JY, Timmons C, Luu HS. Homozygous hemoglobin S with concomitant hemoglobin G-Philadelphia: a diagnostic challenge. *Pediatr Blood Cancer.* 2014;61(10):1899-1900.

PEDIATRIC COAGULATION | 16

Ayesha Zia, Janna Journeycake, and Hung S. Luu

LEARNING OBJECTIVES

1. Conceptualize that coagulation is a complex but efficient process that culminates in the development of a fibrin clot and subsequent lysis of the clot ensures that the fluidity of blood is maintained.
2. Recognize that the hemostatic system is a dynamic, evolving system in the fetal/neonatal stage that eventually matures into the adult version by the late teenage years.
3. Identify the general principles, including specimen requirements for hemostasis and platelet testing.
4. Identify the general principles, including specimen requirements for thrombophilia and assays related to anticoagulant testing.
5. Recognize various tests of global hemostasis.

OVERVIEW OF THE BASIC COAGULATION AND FIBRINOLYSIS

Coagulation is the process that leads to fibrin formation and involves controlled interactions between protein coagulation factors. *Hemostasis* is coagulation that occurs in a physiological setting and results in sealing of a break in the vasculature by not only forming a fibrin clot but also by subsequent lysis of the clot to ensure that the fluidity of blood is maintained. The components involved in hemostasis consist of vessel walls, platelets, coagulation factors, inhibitors of coagulation, and the fibrinolytic system.

The enzymatic reactions leading to thrombin generation and an eventual fibrin clot were originally described as the waterfall[1] or enzyme[2] cascade, a model that remains conceptually useful today and is able to tie biology with diagnostic laboratory testing. Further insights on the evolution of this process have occurred over the past many decades as proteins have been purified, their function characterized, and additional factors identified. Human coagulation is now known to occur in vivo in the context of a cell-based model of coagulation (Figure 16-1). The cell-based model of hemostasis views the process as having three overlapping phases: initiation, amplification, and propagation, in which a break in the vasculature exposes extracellular matrix to blood and *initiates* the coagulation process. Tissue factor (TF) and factor (F) VIIa are considered the major initiators of coagulation, as opposed to the contact pathway which is now thought to be a key link between coagulation and inflammation. Tissue factor is expressed on vascular smooth muscle cells and on the pericytes that surround blood vessels, the so-called hemostatic envelope. Tissue factor is released upon cell damage or is secreted by cells, such as platelets and monocytes and activates FX, leading to the generation of a small amount of thrombin in the initiation phase of coagulation. Thrombin formed after the initiation phase can promote local fibrin formation, however, it is not sufficient to provide hemostasis throughout the wound area. This minute amount of thrombin then acts as an *amplifier* by activating platelets to facilitate platelet-driven thrombin generation. In addition to platelet processes, plasma concentrations of factors IX and VIII are brought to the

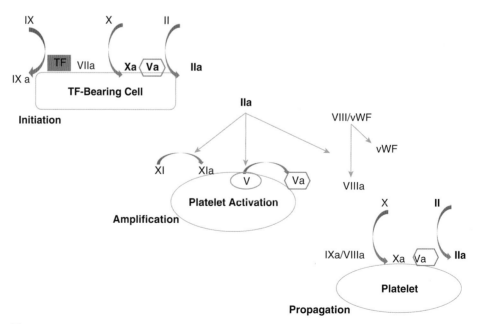

Figure 16-1 ■ Cell-based Model of Coagulation. The Cell-Based Model of Hemostasis views the process as having three overlapping phases: initiation, amplification, and propagation, which culminates in thrombin generation, and an eventual fibrin clot. TF, tissue factor; vWF, von Willebrand factor

preformed FVIIa/TF complexes at the site of injury. The FIXa/VIIIa complex activates factor X on the platelet surface. The platelet surface-generated FXa can move directly into a complex with platelet surface FVa and forms a burst of thrombin. The burst of thrombin during the *propagation* phase leads to cleavage of fibrinopeptides from fibrinogen. Cleavage of these fibrinopeptides exposes new binding sites that fit with complementary sites on other fibrin molecules.[3] These interactions lead to fibrin molecules assembling in long, branched chains thereby stabilizing the initial platelet plug into a consolidated fibrin plug. The nature and stability of the fibrin plug appear to depend on the rate of thrombin generation during the propagation phase.[4] In addition to its role in cleaving fibrinopeptides, thrombin generation participates in a positive feedback loop by activating FXI on the platelet surface; this FXIa can activate FIXa to further enhance FXa generation.[5] High levels of thrombin generated during the propagation phase bind to fibrin and when bound, are protected from inhibition by anti-thrombin. This fibrin-bound thrombin provides an important role in maintaining hemostasis.

It is important to focus on the cellular location of the steps rather than the proteins involved, as protein factors overlap between the steps; for example, thrombin bound to platelets plays a different role than thrombin bound to endothelial cell thrombomodulin. Each of the cellular steps must contribute for the overall process to result in a coordinated hemostatic plug. A defect in initiation means that the coagulation will not start. Tissue factor deficiency is lethal in animal models, and FVII deficiency is associated with bleeding. Hemophilia is a defect of FX activation on the platelet surface, due to lack of FVIII or FIX, during the propagation phase. Factor X activation by FVIIa/TF during initiation cannot substitute for the platelet surface reactions. FXa is confined to the tissue factor-bearing surface where it is formed because, when released from the surface, it is rapidly inhibited by TFPI and anti-thrombin. So for normal hemostasis, a FX-activating complex must be formed on activated platelets. The tie between this model and the standard coagulation assays is that the prothrombin time (PT) and activated partial thromboplastin time (aPTT) assess the initiation and propagation phases, respectively.

Localization and Coagulation Inhibition

Once thrombin is generated, regulation of thrombin occurs either through direct or indirect inhibition by limitation of thrombin generation. Active thrombin is ultimately neutralized over time by *direct* complex formation with either α2 macroglobulin (α2-M),[6] anti-thrombin (catalyzed by heparin),[7] or heparin cofactor II (catalyzed by dermatan sulfate)[8] to form inert 1:1 covalent complexes with thrombin. Although all of the direct inhibitors can neutralize free thrombin effectively, thrombin bound to fibrin is resistant to inactivation.

Clot propagation is due in part to the activity of this clot-bound thrombin.[9] Anti-thrombin–heparin complex is ineffective at inactivating thrombin bound to fibrin and FXa bound to phospholipids.[10,11] In addition, heparin cofactor II-dermatan sulfate has significantly reduced activity against fibrin-bound thrombin.[12]

Alternatively, fibrin formation can be prevented by inhibition of thrombin generation. The two mechanisms by which thrombin formation is *indirectly* shutdown are the protein C (PC) and tissue factor pathway inhibitor (TFPI) pathways. Inhibition of thrombin generation through PC is a pathway in which conversion of PC to activated PC (APC) is cell membrane-mediated. When thrombin is bound to endothelial cell-associated thrombomodulin, it can activate PC. Protein C in its active form, in association with protein S (PS), inactivates FVIIIa and FVa, which quenches thrombin production.[13] The other indirect inhibitor, TFPI can combine with FXa, FVIIa, and TF to form a quaternary complex in which FXa's activity is inhibited.[14] The TFPI–FXa complex inhibits FVIIa, thereby inhibiting the generation of thrombin. However, while TFPI has been shown to exert a significant effect on the inhibition of thrombin generation,[15] the relative involvement of TFPI is somewhat obscured by the fact that elevation in activity requires displacement of vessel wall-bound TFPI (50–80% of total)[16] and in the fluid phase >85% of TFPI is present as lipoprotein complexes with low anticoagulant activity.[17]

The localization process confines platelet deposition and fibrin formation to keep the clot from expanding over healthy endothelium. This is consistent with the observation that defects in anti-thrombin, TFPI, and PC and PS are associated with thrombosis.

Fibrinolysis

Once the fibrin clot has formed in vivo, the fibrinolytic system alters the clot and plays an important role in the dissolution of the clot.[18] Similar to role of thrombin in the coagulation system, plasmin regulation is of central importance in the fibrinolytic system, where it mediates fibrin degradation. A series of serine proteases interact to ultimately cleave insoluble fibrin into fibrin degradation products (FDP). Plasminogen is converted into its active form, plasmin, by tissue-type plasminogen activator (tPA) and urokinase-type plasminogen activator (uPA).

The activators of plasminogen are inhibited by plasminogen activator inhibitor-1 (PAI-1).[19] α2-antiplasmin (α2-AP) and to a lesser extent, α2-M and thrombin activatable fibrinolysis inhibitor (TAFI) are the primary inhibitors of plasmin.[20] TAFI can be activated by thrombin, the thrombin–thrombomodulin complex, or plasmin. The TAFI pathway in vivo likely provides the proper balance between fibrin deposition and fibrin degradation.

DEVELOPMENTAL HEMOSTASIS

Hemostasis is a dynamic, evolving process that is age dependent and begins in utero. The evolution continues throughout life, but the changes are most marked during childhood and are therefore of most clinical relevance during this time. Although evolving, the hemostatic system in healthy fetuses, infants, and children must be considered physiologic. This concept of "developmental hemostasis" was first brought to light by Dr. Maureen Andrew in the late 1980s. Her landmark papers published in 1987, 1988, and 1992, not only demonstrated that the concentrations of the majority of coagulation proteins, as measured by functional assays, changed significantly with age, but also changed the approach to the clinical interpretation of coagulation assays used by many hemostasis laboratories since that time.[21-23]

Compared with adults, children have a number of physiological differences in the functional levels of pro-coagulants, natural inhibitors of coagulation, and fibrinolytic proteins. While the absolute values are reagent and analyzer dependent, the trends in changes observed are consistent across a number of studies:[24]

- Contact factors, FXII, FXI, HMWK, and the vitamin K dependent factors, FII, FVII, FIX, and FX are decreased (about one half of adult values) until about 6 months of age (when they become 80% of normal adult values). They remain decreased throughout childhood.[25]
- Inhibitors of hemostasis are present at nearly half of adult levels at birth and in early childhood. AT reaches adult levels by 6 months of life. Another direct thrombin inhibitor, α2-M is elevated at birth and increases to about twice adult values at 6 months of life. α2-macroglobulin remains elevated throughout childhood and partially compensates for the reduced thrombin inhibition by anti-thrombin in the young until anti-thrombin levels reach adult concentrations. At birth, levels of PC and PS are significantly lower. PC eventually increases to adult levels by adolescence and PS by 1-5 years of age.[26,27]
- The fibrinolytic system is downregulated.[23] At birth, plasminogen (75% and 50% of adult values for the healthy premature and full-term newborns, respectively) and the primary inhibitor of plasmin, α2 anti-plasmin (at 80% of adult values) are decreased. The levels of fibrinolytic activators on the other hand, such as t-PA and u-PA and PAI-1, are elevated at birth compared with adults.[28]
- Fibrinogen exists in a "fetal" form, which is thought to be "dysfunctional" due to increased sialic acid content compared to adult fibrinogen.[29]
- Thrombin generation is decreased 30-50% compared with adult levels.[25] The capacity to generate thrombin increases throughout childhood but remains ~20% less than adults.[22]

- Neonatal platelets are found to be hypo-reactive to thrombin, adenosine diphosphate/epinephrine, and thromboxane A2 due to a defect intrinsic to neonatal platelets.[30]

Some coagulation factors in newborns, such as fibrinogen, FV, FVIII, and FXIII, are similar to adult levels and remain so throughout childhood. In fact, plasma levels of von Willebrand factor (VWF), important in the binding/stabilization of circulating FVIII as well as binding to platelets and endothelial cells, are elevated in fetuses and may contribute to hemostasis in utero.[31] von Willebrand factor levels in newborns are about twice that of adult levels and gradually decrease over the first 6 months of life. The possibilities behind these differences include regulation at the gene level, post-translational modifications affecting protein function, delivery or release of proteins as well as variations in clearance of these proteins. A recent study demonstrated that even with a transplanted liver, children maintained plasma levels of certain coagulation proteins at their expected age-specific levels, which shows that while liver is the major site of synthesis, it is not the regulator of plasma levels.[32] Developmental hemostasis has important biological[33] and clinical implications.

Reference ranges for most hemostatic parameters are age, analyzer, and reagent dependent,[33] and this has critical implications for the definition of healthy children, the diagnosis of disease states and the monitoring of anti-coagulant therapy. Both over diagnosis and missed diagnosis are common when age-appropriate, analyzer-specific and reagent-specific reference ranges are not used. The clinical implications of these types of errors are significant and may lead to multiple investigations, referrals to hematologists, cancellation of surgery, and/or overtreatment of the child during the procedure and misclassification of a child having a bleeding or clotting disorder. The International Society of Thrombosis and Haemostasis (ISTH) recommends that diagnostic laboratories processing pediatric samples should use age-appropriate, analyzer-appropriate, and reagent-appropriate reference ranges. These two factors are essential for making an accurate and physiologically relevant diagnosis. In developing age-appropriate reference ranges, laboratories should strive to standardize age groups (ie, neonates, 1 month to 1 year, 1 to 5, 6 to 10, 11 to 16-year-old children) which have been reported to reflect statistically different groupings. If unable to generate their own reference ranges, laboratories should only use published ranges that were established using the identical analyzer and reagent system to that used in their laboratory. Readers are encouraged to review reference values for coagulation tests in healthy full term infants during the first six months of life with the ACL analyzer,[21] for these values with the STA analyzer and finally to reference values in healthy children aged 1 to 16 years.[23]

LABORATORY MEASURES OF HEMOSTASIS

Results of clotting tests can be affected by the collection and processing of blood samples (pre-analytical factors), by the selection, design, quality control of assays (analytical factors), and finally, by interpretation of screening tests and specific assays (post-analytical factors). General recommendations for sample collection and processing are described in Table 16-1.

Screening Tests

An initial panel of tests to screen for clinically important hemostatic defects includes aPTT, PT, and fibrinogen activity and/or thrombin time. A complete blood count to evaluate platelet number and morphology is just as important and must be a part of initial screening.

Table 16-1 GUIDELINES FOR PEDIATRIC SAMPLE COLLECTION AND PROCESSING

- Veins in the elbow are preferred, when possible. For infants and children, a 22- or 21-gauge needle, respectively, is the preferable gauge.
- Tourniquet should be applied just before sample collection and prolonged application should be avoided.
- A peripheral stick is most preferable. Collection through peripheral venous lines and non-heparinized lines should be avoided but if unavoidable, an adequate amount of blood (5-10 mL in adults) should be discarded (or used for other tests) to avoid contamination or dilution by fluids. A saline flush through a 3-way stopcock prior to collection may help in certain cases.
- After collection, the tubes should be mixed by gentle inversion 4-5 times. Any evidence of clotting or hemolysis should be an indication to discard the sample.
- One volume of the recommended anticoagulant trisodium citrate {0.105 (3.2%)-0.109 (3.8%) mol/L]} should be mixed with nine volumes of blood, and the fill volume must be at least 90% of the target volume to give accurate results. Under filling prolongs screening tests.
- If hematocrit is >55%, adjust anticoagulant: blood ratio to account for altered plasma volume.
- Samples should be tested within 2 hours of collection at room temperature or within 4 hours if kept cold.
- Freezing may affect results depending on the temperature and time of storage. Samples stored at $-24°C$ or lower are stable for up to 3 months and at $-74°C$ for up to 18 months (results within 10% of baseline defined as stable).
- Any deep-frozen plasma should be rapidly thawed at $37°C$ as cryoprecipitation is possible with thawing at lower temperatures.

Prothrombin time

The PT is performed by adding TF (in the form of a thromboplastin reagent) containing calcium chloride to the citrated plasma sample. The time required for clot formation is recorded with an automated instrument that signals the end point, as defined by optical or electromechanical change. The normal (reference) range depends on the instrument/analyzer and the reagent lot of thromboplastin used. The PT measures the activities of FI (fibrinogen), II (prothrombin), V, X (common pathway), and VII (extrinsic pathway). Prolongation of PT beyond the reference range is generally not seen until the functional level of the clotting factors is less than 30% or until fibrinogen is less than 100 mg/dL. Isolated prolongation of the PT may reflect FVII deficiency. Though rare, the PT can also be prolonged by a circulating inhibitor or by the presence of abnormal fibrinogen molecules or fragments in the circulation. Figure 16-2 suggests a pathway for investigation of a patient with prolonged PT.

Activated partial thromboplastin time

The aPTT is performed by adding a "partial thromboplastin" reagent, which is a source of phospholipids (lacking tissue factor, hence the term "partial" thromboplastin) to the patient's citrated plasma sample. Activation of the contact

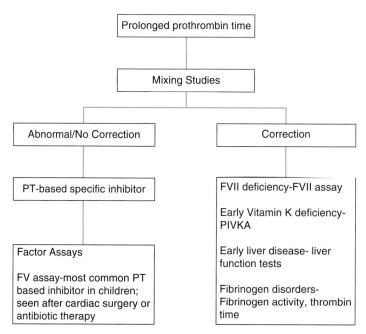

Figure 16-2 ▪ Pathway for investigation of prolonged prothrombin time (PT). PIVKA, proteins induced by vitamin K absence

factors (FXI and XII, prekallikrein and high-molecular-weight-kininogen) is controlled by pre-incubation with a surface activating reagent (such as celite, kaolin, silica or ellagic acid).[34] This mixture is incubated for 2-5 minutes before calcium chloride is added and the time required for clot formation is recorded, generally with an automated instrument. The aPTT measures FI, FII, FV, FX (common pathway), FVIII, FIX, FXI (intrinsic pathway), and FXII; prekallikrein; and high molecular weight kininogen (contact pathway factors). Deficiency of the latter three factors can result in markedly prolonged aPTT in the absence of clinically significant bleeding. Isolated prolongation of the aPTT in a patient with clinical bleeding is likely to result from a deficiency of FVIII, IX, or XI. The sensitivity of the aPTT is highly dependent on the specific reagents used (particularly the activator in the partial thromboplastic reagent). With most aPTT reagents, the aPTT will not be prolonged until the amount of factor VIII is less than 35% (0.35 U/mL). The laboratory should establish a reference range for each new lot of reagent and each new method of clot detection.

The aPTT is somewhat less sensitive than the PT to deficiency of the vitamin K-dependent factors, but it more sensitive to the presence of heparin and circulating anti-coagulants. The aPTT can detect circulating anti-coagulants (such as lupus anti-coagulants (LA) and is often used to monitor heparin therapy.[35] Among hospitalized infants and children, contamination of patient samples with heparin is a very common cause of an unexpected prolongation of the aPTT that does not correct on mixing studies (see later. Figure 16-3 suggests a pathway for investigation of a patient with prolonged aPTT.

Mixing Studies

These are central in the investigation of a prolonged aPTT and PT (Figure 16-4). The prolonged test is essentially repeated, with 50% of the test plasma being replaced by normal pooled plasma (which assumes that this contains normal amounts of all the clotting factors), correcting all the clotting factors to a minimum of 50% in the test plasma. The results are either that the aPTT normalizes if the cause of the prolongation was a deficiency of a clotting factor; or remains prolonged if an inhibitor (either to a specific factor or a lupus anticoagulant) is present.

Thrombin Time

The thrombin time (TT) measures the thrombin-induced conversion of fibrinogen to polymerized fibrin and is performed by adding bovine thrombin to the patient's citrated plasma and recording the clotting time. The TT measures

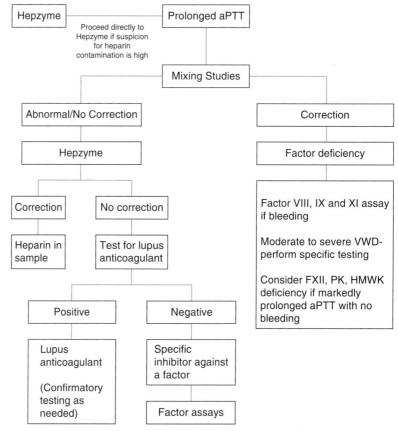

Figure 16-3 ▪ Pathway for investigation of prolonged aPTT.
VWD, von Willebrand disease; PK, pre-kallikrien; HMWK, high-molecular weight kininogen; dRVVT, dilute Russell viper venom test

the amount and clotting function of fibrinogen. An extremely prolonged TT usually indicates heparin effect. Reptilase, a snake venom protease, can clot fibrinogen in the presence of heparin and thus, can be used to identify heparin as the cause of a prolonged TT. Thrombin time will be prolonged in the presence of heparin whereas reptilase time will be normal. Heparin contamination in a sample can be confirmed by correction of a prolonged TT after treatment with heparinase, hepzyme, or mixing with protamine, an agent that antagonizes heparin.

Thrombin time is a useful screening test for quantitative, as well as qualitative abnormalities of fibrinogen. Because the TT is a function of the available fibrinogen, the test can be used to estimate fibrinogen levels. In addition, it allows for detection of inhibitors against thrombin or fibrin.

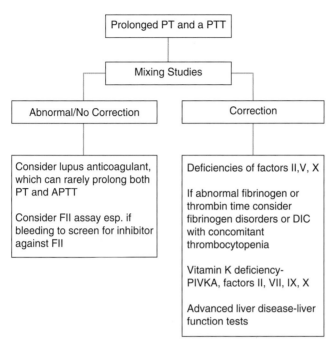

Figure 16-4 ▪ Pathway for investigation of prolonged aPPT and PT.
aPTT, activated partial thromboplastin time; PT, prothrombin time; DIC, disseminated intravascular coagulation; PIVKA; proteins induced by vitamin K absence

Fibrinogen

Fibrinogen plays a pivotal role in the hemostatic balance and has numerous functional interactions in both primary and secondary hemostasis. In primary hemostasis, it acts as a key ligand for platelet aggregation. It is the substrate during secondary hemostasis that, when cleaved by thrombin through excision of fibrinopeptides A and B, assembles by polymerization and cross-linking to form the fibrin clot. A number of methods are available for the measurement of fibrinogen concentration. Most automated coagulation analyzers now provide a measure of fibrinogen concentration, calculated from the degree of change of light scatter or optical density during measurement of the PT (PT-derived fibrinogen). Although this is simple and cheap, it is inaccurate in some patients, such as those with disseminated intravascular coagulation (DIC), liver or renal disease, dysfibrinogenemia, following thrombolytic therapy, and in those with markedly raised or reduced fibrinogen concentrations. The recommended method for measuring the level of functional fibrinogen or fibrinogen activity was originally described by von Clauss.[36] The Clauss fibrinogen assay is a quantitative, clot-based, functional assay. It measures the ability of fibrinogen to form fibrin after being exposed to a high concentration of purified thrombin, which makes fibrinogen the rate-limiting step in the clotting reaction. Plasma samples are pre-diluted which minimizes assay interference from substances like heparin and FDPs. The diluted plasma is incubated at 37°C prior to the addition of the pre-warmed (37°C) thrombin reagent. From the exact moment of the addition of thrombin, the time to clot is measured. The resulting clotting times in seconds is compared with a standard dilution curve to determine the concentration of clottable fibrinogen. This assay is sensitive to abnormalities in fibrinogen function or the presence of inhibitors of fibrin formation, such as FDPs.

Euglobulin Clot Lysis Test

The euglobulin clot lysis time (ECLT) is a screening test for excessive fibrinolysis. Citrated plasma is treated to precipitate the euglobulin fraction, which contains fibrinogen and activators of plasminogen, as well as a portion of fibrinolytic inhibitors, such as PAI-1. Clot lysis time is measured after the euglobulin fraction is re-dissolved and the fibrinogen is clotted. Hyperfibrinolysis produces shortening of the ECLT. There are specific assays for inhibitors of the fibrinolytic system, including PAI-1 and α2-antiplasmin. Deficiencies of these proteins can be either congenital or acquired and can be the cause of rare bleeding conditions.

Tests of Platelet Function

Platelet Count and Morphology

Platelets are discoid anucleated cells originating from fragmentation of megakaryocyte cytoplasm. Each megakaryocyte produces several thousand of platelets, leading to a rather stable intra-individual platelet count of 150,000–400,000 µ/L during the whole life. Platelets normally circulate for 10 days, constantly surveying the integrity of the vessel wall. Senescent platelets are eliminated by macrophages. Performing an accurate platelet count and a correct morphology analysis requires that an appropriate sample from the patient, mixed with the adequate amount of a suitable anticoagulant be delivered to the laboratory without undue delay.

Platelets are 1.5–3 µm sized small elements of round or oval shape and have a mean volume of 7–11 fL. There is a wide heterogeneity in platelet size. Platelet cytoplasm contains small azurophilic granules either scattered throughout the cytoplasm or centrally concentrated.

Platelets are prone to artifactual in vitro activation and to desensitization. Most functional tests have to be performed relatively quickly (less than 2 hours from sampling). Review of the platelets on a well-prepared and stained blood smear should give a visual estimate that matches the measured value. Excess of ethylenediaminetetraacetic acid (EDTA) has deleterious effects on platelet morphology in stained blood films. It causes them to swell and then disintegrate, producing platelet fragments, which may be counted as platelets leading to artificially high platelet count. The analysis of platelet morphology should systematically be done when examining any blood smear. Platelet size should be compared to the size of the red cells. The number of platelet granulations, their staining, and their distribution in the platelet cytoplasm should be carefully studied. Platelet clumps are generally detected in the tail of the film. The smear should also be searched for satellites of platelets. Platelets can appear gray or as exhausted, because they have released the content of alpha granules. Several mechanisms can induce this release, including coagulation activation during blood collection, vigorous blood/anticoagulant mixing, or true DIC.

Characteristics of platelet morphology in pediatrics

Platelet anisocytosis is more pronounced in neonates than in adults due to the substantial presence of platelets with large size at birth. Platelet size varies inversely with prematurity. In neonates, small megakaryocytes with only one nucleus or bare megakaryocyte nuclei may be present.[37]

Bleeding Time

The skin bleeding time (BT) has been clinically used for almost a century and has been modified several times in attempts to improve reliability. The BT is an approximate measure of the interaction of normal platelets with the blood vessel wall. Briefly, a constant blood pressure of 40 mm Hg is applied to the upper arm, and a disposable, sterile, automated template device is applied to inflict standardized cuts into the forearm. Excess blood is then removed with filter paper at regular intervals, and the time for the cessation of bleeding recorded. Normal bleeding times are less than 10 minutes. Harker and Slichter originally demonstrated that the BT is an approximate measure of the relationship between platelet number and function.[38] With normally functioning platelets, the BT begins to prolong at a platelet count of less than 100,000/μL. The most widely used method is the modified Ivy BT performed with a template.

The clear advantages of the bleeding time are that it is a simple test of natural hemostasis including the important contribution of the vessel wall. The disadvantages are that bleeding time results can be both poorly reproducible and insensitive to milder forms of platelet dysfunction. The consensus is that the test does not necessarily correlate well with the bleeding risk and that an accurate clinical history is more valuable.

Platelet Functional Analyzer (PFA-100)

Current platelet function tests are often viewed as inaccurate and unreliable (BT) or labor intensive and time consuming (platelet aggregation studies). Widespread experience with the PFA-100 instrument is increasing, but how the test should be used within normal laboratory practice remains to be fully defined. The PFA-100 uses test cartridges containing collagen/adenosine diphosphate (CADP)-coated membranes or collagen/epinephrine (CEPI)-coated membranes with a small aperture (150 μm). Citrated whole blood is aspirated under high shear (5000 to 6000/seconds) from the sample reservoir through a capillary tube onto the membrane, and blood flow is monitored through the aperture. The instrument monitors the drop in flow rate as platelets form a hemostatic plug that seals the aperture and stops blood flow. This parameter is recorded as the closure time (CT) with either cartridge. The maximal value obtainable is 300 seconds.

To ensure optimal PFA-100 performance and data interpretation, mandatory daily instrument checks; ensuring the quality of blood sampling; ensuring consistency in anticoagulation, 3.8% (0.129 mol/L) or 3.2% (0.105 mol/L) sodium citrate; checking for cartridge batch variation and testing within 4 hours of sampling is required. Transport through pneumatic vacuum transport system ("tube system") is not recommended.[39] Ideally, a full blood count should also be performed to help interpret the results, as the test is sensitive to platelet count and hematocrit. A platelet count of less than $80\text{-}100 \times 10^9$/L and a hematocrit of less than 30% lead to a prolonged CT.[39] A control group within each laboratory setting should be established. Each laboratory should also ideally establish their own reference ranges on both cartridges using normal volunteers from their institution. Typical normal ranges vary when obtained with either 3.2% or 3.8% trisodium citrate and needs to be noted when reporting out the results.

The intra-individual coefficient of variation (CV) for PFA-100 has been reported as approximately 10%, which, although acceptable for a platelet function test, may cause problems with values obtained close to the upper normal range cut-off values. The advantages of the test are that it is simple, rapid, and does not require specialist training (apart from training in the manipulation of blood samples). Within a typical population of patients tested, the overall negative predictive value of the test can be high (more than 90%), although the test is clearly not 100% sensitive to all platelet defects and can miss mild defects. The test is particularly useful in pediatric settings where the availability of blood is often a limiting factor. Given the high shear conditions to which platelets are exposed to during the test, it is not surprising that the test is highly von Willebrand factor (VWF) dependent and is useful not only for detecting von Willebrand disease (VWD), but also for monitoring therapy, particularly with 1-desamino-8-D-arginine vasopressin (DDAVP). A number of studies suggest that the PFA-100 is a potential in vitro replacement of the bleeding time. The disadvantages are that, like the in vivo bleeding time false negative results are sometimes obtained; for example, in patients with storage pool disease, primary secretion defects and in mild type 1 VWD. Diagnosis of these disorders could therefore be missed if relying on the PFA-100 as a screening test alone. In patients with apparently normal platelet function, the instrument has also been shown to occasionally give false-positive results, which then require further detailed testing. A recent ISTH Scientific and Standardization Committee (SSC) document by Hayward and colleagues provides a useful up-to-date consensus review of the utility of the test.[40]

Platelet Aggregation

Platelet aggregation is the most useful in vitro test of platelet function currently available, and it is still the gold standard to detect platelet disorders and to initiate a more precise characterization.

Platelets are known to aggregate under a variety of conditions and in the presence of a number of different agonists. Platelet aggregation can be performed in whole blood by impedance technique or in platelet-rich plasma (PRP) by the turbidometric technique. Anticoagulated whole blood may also be used in some commercial multichannel impedance-based aggregometers, such as the Chronolog or Multiplate aggregometers. These have the significant advantage that the blood does not require further processing for analysis. Additionally, whole blood platelet aggregation can be combined with the release of adenosine triphosphate (ATP) by using a lumi-aggregometer.

Different dosages of a panel of agonists added to an aliquot of the patient's sample trigger platelet activation, shape change, and primary and secondary aggregation events by changes in optical density (PRP) or impedance (whole blood), and this is recorded on the aggregation trace.[41] By using a panel of agonists at differing concentrations, it is possible to detect a number of classic platelet defects.

Modern instruments usually offer multichannel capability and computer analysis and storage of data, although samples and reagents still have to be prepared manually. A typical panel of agonists (stored in frozen aliquots) are adenosine diphosphate (ADP) (0.1–20 µmol/L), epinephrine (1.0–10 µmol/L), collagen (1–5 µg/mL) which usually mediates a steep aggregation curve but after a characteristic lag phase of more than 1 minute, arachidonic acid (1.0–2.0 mmol/L) and ristocetin (0.5–1.5 mg/mL) and lastly, thrombin (0.1–0.5 IU/mL). Ristocetin is not strictly an agonist but stimulates platelet agglutination through binding of plasma VWF to glycoprotein (Gp) Ib and therefore will also give abnormal results in VWD; usually used at a single low and high dose.

Platelet function testing presents many challenges in ensuring that accurate and meaningful results are obtained. First, unlike other tests, there are no widely available internal or external quality control measures available. To minimize the potential artifact occurrence, it is important to control pre-analytical variables, including drug therapy, improper sample collection, sample handling, transit, age of the sample, and test procedures.[42] Readers are encouraged to read ISTH's most recent SSC communication regarding platelet aggregation testing and methodology.[43]

Platelet Flow Cytometry

Whole blood flow cytometry offers a very attractive and reliable test for the diagnosis of various platelet receptor, granular, and other defects. Resting platelets constitutively express many surface glycoproteins that are easily identifiable by flow cytometry. Platelets undergo changes in antigenic expression on the cell surface with activation.[44,45] One of the major benefits of flow-cytometry is that it has the ability to quantitatively measure both the activation state of circulating platelets and the function of different pathways of platelet activation by stimulation with specific agonists and measuring changes in antigenic characteristics. Immunophenotyping of platelets by flow cytometry may be performed on platelets in whole blood, on washed platelets, or in PRP.

▍LABORATORY EVALUATION OF THROMBOPHILIA

Thrombophilia is the term used to describe the tendency to develop thrombosis, which can be acquired or inherited. This term should not be considered a disease, but a risk factor for (venous or arterial) thrombosis. It is important to recognize that the presence of thrombophilia in an individual is not absolutely predictive of thrombosis but that its presence determines a patient's risk for initial and subsequent (or recurrent) venous thromboembolism (VTE), which influences (primary and secondary) VTE prevention strategies.

Currently, there is no single laboratory global assay that will 'screen' for the presence of thrombophilia. Specific coagulation testing consists of a battery of complex (clot and DNA-based) thrombophilia assays to detect presence of an inherited or acquired thrombophilia. As discussed later, multiple pre-analytical conditions affect results of these assays (eg, anticoagulants, acute thrombosis, liver disease, etc.), so interpretation of results needs to be within the context of the circumstances before an individual is labeled with a diagnosis. This is especially true for abnormal clot-based assays. In general, specialized coagulation thrombophilia assays can be broadly divided into assays that detect a clot-based endpoint (eg, lupus anticoagulant, PS activity), chromogenic assays (eg, PC and anti-thrombin activities), or variants of enzyme linked immunosorbent assays (ELISAs; eg, anti-phospholipid antibodies). An ideal approach to testing consists of performing activity assays with reflexive antigenic assays if indicated (eg, a low anti-thrombin activity is typically followed up by performing an anti-thrombin antigen, primarily to classify the type of deficiency).

Factors Affecting Results of Coagulation Testing

Effect of Type of Anticoagulant in Specimen Collection Tube

Standard specimen collection tubes contain citrate for optimal results. Specimens may inadvertently be collected in EDTA, which will result in falsely reduced protein levels and a reduced APC-R ratio.

Effect of Specimen Processing

Specimens should be double centrifuged as soon as possible after collection in order to minimize the amount of residual platelets. The presence of residual platelets can result in a false-negative test for lupus anticoagulant.

Effect of Acute Thrombosis

During the acute thrombotic episode, levels of anti-thrombin, PC, and PS may be transiently reduced;[46] thus, if testing is not repeated, remote from the time of the thrombotic event and in the absence of anticoagulant therapy, the patient may be misdiagnosed as having a congenital deficiency.

Effect of Anticoagulants

Heparin therapy can falsely reduce anti-thrombin levels. Although most lupus anticoagulant reagents (eg, dilute Russell viper venom time (dRVVT) and STACLOT) contain heparin neutralizers that can neutralize up to 1 U/mL of heparin, presence of excess heparin may result in a false-positive test result, which impacts the duration of secondary prophylaxis. Thus, positive results of lupus anticoagulant testing performed while on heparin should be reconfirmed when the patient is off heparin. Protein C and S levels are lowered by vitamin K antagonist therapy (eg, warfarin) since they are vitamin K-dependent proteins. In addition, vitamin K antagonist (VKA) therapy may result in a false-positive lupus anticoagulant with certain assays (eg dRVVT). Because the majority of anticoagulant activity assays rely on generation of thrombin to achieve an endpoint of clot detection, presence of direct thrombin inhibitors (eg, argatroban, lepirudin, bivalirudin) interfere

Table 16-2 THROMBOPHILIA TESTING*	
Thrombophilia	Laboratory Tests
Factor V Leiden mutation	PCR or screening with APC-R assay
Prothrombin G20210A mutation	PCR
Protein C deficiency	Chromogenic or clotting assay
Protein S deficiency	Clotting assay or immunologic assay of total and free protein S antigen
Anti-thrombin deficiency	Chromogenic or clotting assay
Antiphospholipid antibodies	Phospholipid-based clotting assays (PTT-LA, dRVVT,) with confirmatory assay using exogenous excess phospholipids ELISA assay for IgM and IgG anticardiolipin and β2-glycoprotein antibodies
Elevated factor VIII	One-stage clotting assay, chromogenic assay

*PCR, polymerase chain reaction; APC-R, activated protein C resistance; PTT, partial thromboplastin time; dRVVT, dilute Russel viper venom time; ELISA, enzyme linked immunosorbent assay.

with this endpoint and delay clot formation. This can lead to a false-positive lupus anticoagulant or falsely reduced PC and S levels. Results of chromogenic assays are likely more reliable. The most common assays employed for testing are listed in Table 16-2.

Effect of Liver Disease

The majority of anticoagulant and pro-coagulant proteins are produced in the liver. In advanced liver disease, levels of both the anticoagulant and pro-coagulant proteins are reduced.

Factors Affecting Molecular (DNA-Based) Testing

The main patient-related factors affecting currently available DNA-based testing include liver and hematopoietic stem cell transplantation, the type of anticoagulant in the collection tube, and the white blood cell count.

Effect of liver transplantation: Anticoagulant proteins are produced in the liver. A patient with thrombophilia (eg, APC-R) who receives a liver transplant from an unaffected donor may be "cured" of APC-R, yet will still carry the FVL mutation in their peripheral blood genomic DNA, resulting in discordant results. In contrast, patients previously unaffected with APC-R, who receive a liver from an individual with APC-R, will test negative for the FVL mutation, yet have APC-R on protein-based testing.

Effect of hematopoietic stem cell transplantation (HSCT): A carrier of FVL mutation who receives HSCT from an unaffected donor will still have APC-R, but peripheral blood genomic DNA testing will be negative for FVL mutation.

Lupus Anticoagulant Testing

Lupus anticoagulation testing is an important component of laboratory testing for neonatal and pediatric VTE and antiphospholipid antibody syndrome (APS). Refer to Table 16-3 for the classification criteria of APS.

Table 16-3 **REVISED SAPPORO CLASSIFICATION CRITERIA FOR ANTIPHOSPHOLIPID ANTIBODY SYNDROME (APS)***	
APS is present if at least one of the following clinical criteria and one of the laboratory criteria are present:	
Clinical Criteria	Laboratory Criteria
1. Vascular Thrombosis • One or more clinical episodes of arterial, venous, or small vessel thrombosis in any tissue or organ, without significant evidence of inflammation in the vessel wall	1. Lupus anticoagulant present in plasma, on two or more occasions, at least 12 weeks apart, detected according to ISTH guidelines (see text) 2. Anticardiolipin antibody of IgG and/or IgM isotype in serum or plasma, present in medium or high titer (ie, >40 GPL or MPL, or > the 99th percentile), on two or more occasions, at least 12 weeks apart, measured by standard ELISA
2. Pregnancy morbidity • One or more unexplained deaths of a morphologically normal fetus beyond the 10th week of gestation with normal fetal physiology • One or more pre-mature births of a morphologically normal neonate before the 34th week because of eclampsia or placental insufficiency or • Three or more unexplained consecutive spontaneous abortions before the 10th week of gestation, with maternal anatomic, hormonal and paternal and maternal chromosomal causes excluded	3. Anti-β2-glycoprotein I antibody of IgG and/or IgM isotype in serum or plasma, (in titer > 99th percentile), present on two or more occasions, at least 12 weeks apart, measured by standard ELISA.

*ISTH, International Society of Thrombosis and Haemostasis; ELISA, enzyme linked immunosorbent assay
MPL refers to IgM Phospholipid Units. One MPL unit is 1 microgram of IgM antibody.
GPL refers to IgG Phospholipid Units. One GPL unit is 1 microgram of IgG antibody.

Antiphospholipid syndrome requires the combination of at least one clinical and one laboratory criterion.[47]

Antiphospholipid antibodies (aPLs) are a heterogeneous group of autoantibodies directed against glycoproteins bound to anionic phospholipids. Antiphospholipid antibodies were initially described in the setting of syphilis as a result of their ability to produce false-positive serologic assays for syphilis. The high prevalence of aPLs in patients with systemic lupus erythematosus (SLE) and the association of aPLs with a false-positive Venereal Disease Research Laboratory (VDRL) remain the explanation for the inclusion of a false-positive VDRL in diagnostic criteria for SLE.[48]

The lupus anticoagulant was first described in the 1950s as a cause of a bleeding diathesis in patients with SLE who presented with prolonged clotting times.[49] As a result of their clinical presentation the term "lupus anticoagulant" was coined. This name has subsequently proven to be a misnomer given the observation that many patients with these abnormalities do not have lupus and the principal clinical manifestation is a pro-coagulant rather than anticoagulant effect. In fact, the bleeding diathesis in the originally described patients was likely due to a rare effect where the lupus anticoagulant had specificity for prothrombin producing an acquired bleeding disorder.

In clinical laboratory practice, aPL evaluation (the laboratory component of APS) usually consists of a combination of the following: anticardiolipin antibody assay, anti-beta 2 glycoprotein I assay (ELISA based testing), and at least two lupus anticoagulant assays with an appropriate confirmatory test (clot based testing). The "anticoagulant" term reflects the prolongation of phospholipid-dependent clotting assays, which is due to the lupus anticoagulant's specificity for phospholipids. Lupus anticoagulants produce their laboratory effect by prolonging clotting times in assays within which phospholipid content is limited. Although many assays are available, all are based on this fundamental principle. The presence of a lupus anticoagulant can be confirmed by demonstrating normalization of clotting times with the addition of exogenous phospholipid.

Screening Tests

As no single assay detects a lupus anticoagulant, laboratories should heed consensus recommendations to run a minimum of two screening tests that use different test principles as recommended by ISTH.[50] Dilute Russell viper venom time and any aPTT test performed with silica as an activator and low phospholipid content is the second test of choice because of its sensitivity for lupus anticoagulant.[51,52] Kaolin and Ellagic acid as activators are not recommended due to their insensitivity for lupus anticoagulant, respectively. Kaolin Clotting Time (KCT) has a poorer reproducibility compared with the other tests available[53] and is therefore, also not recommended.

Lupus Sensitive aPTT

All lupus anticoagulant sensitive reagents contain a low concentration of phospholipid—often referred to as being "phospholipid limited." In aPTT-based assays, activation of the contact factors of coagulation occurs on negatively charged surfaces, such as silica. Platelet-poor plasma is incubated with the reagent for a pre-determined time. Calcium is added and the clotting time in seconds is determined. The lupus anticoagulant antibody binds to the phospholipid contained in the reagent causing a prolongation in the clot times. As a sole diagnostic test, a prolonged result does not confirm the presence of a lupus anticoagulant since other conditions may also cause prolonged clotting times.[54]

Dilute Russell Viper Venom Time

Dilute Russell viper venom time (dRVVT) is widely used in clinical laboratories and is believed to be specific for detecting lupus anticoagulant.[55] An International External Quality Assessment Program for laboratories working in the field of thrombosis showed that dRVVT is the most robust test in detecting lupus anticoagulant.[53] The dRVVT activates FX to FXa directly in the presence of a low concentration of phospholipid. The dRVVT reagent is added to the plasma and the clotting time in seconds is determined. Most commercial dRVVT reagents neutralize unfractionated heparin (up to 1 unit/mL) and low molecular weight heparin within the therapeutic range.[54] Commercial manufacturers often have a confirmation reagent with a higher concentration of phospholipid available to run in parallel with the dRVVT. The calculated ratio of the dRVVT test/dRVVT confirm that the patient sample is compared to a specified cutoff ratio to determine the presence of a lupus anticoagulant. If the ratio is greater than the established cutoff then the lupus anticoagulant is confirmed. Caution is needed in the interpretation of these assays because of the potential for oral anticoagulants to produce a "falsely positive" test. In principle, these tests do not require performance of the mixing test and the results may be interpreted according to the specific cut-off values by calculating either the percentage correction (screen-confirm/screen ×100) or the lupus anticoagulant ratio (screen/confirm).[56] Both the percentage correction and the lupus anticoagulant ratio may benefit from normalization of results against a pooled normal plasma (PNP) run in parallel with the test plasmas (screen/confirm) of patient divided by (screen/confirm) of PNP. Use of normalization ratios is the best way to compensate for inter-assay and intra-assay variation.

Platelet Neutralization Procedure

The platelet neutralization procedure is often used to confirm the presence of a lupus anticoagulant. The correction or neutralization of the of the patient's lupus-sensitive aPTT after the addition of a platelet membrane preparation is determined, and confirms the presence of a lupus anticoagulant. Both platelet membrane preparations and commercial kits are available commercially.[54]

Standardization

Because of the heterogeneity of lupus anticoagulants, there is no one diagnostic assay for detecting the lupus anticoagulant since some tests are more sensitive than others to lupus anticoagulants. Given epitope variation, expert panels, such as the ISTH have developed recommendations for standardized patient testing of lupus anticoagulants[57] to maximize diagnostic sensitivity.

Interpretation of Results

Interpreting qualitative results is challenging because of the variation of test nomenclature, heterogeneity of lupus anticoagulant, and the variety of available assays. Lupus anticoagulants are generally reported as positive or negative. False-positive results may be obtained in some patients receiving therapeutic dose anticoagulation, particularly those on warfarin. Prolongation of the screening assay with a failure to correct the confirmatory assay may be due to other non-specific inhibitors of coagulation, specific inhibitors of coagulation, and/or deficiencies of individual coagulation factors. Generally speaking, clinically important lupus anticoagulants will be persistently positive in the laboratory tests. Clinical importance is generally assigned to an antibody that is present on two occasions separated by a minimum of 12 weeks or within 5 years of detection of lupus anticoagulant and a clinical event suggestive of APS. This is especially important to remember in pediatrics as many viral and bacterial infections in childhood may induce production of aPLs, which tend to be transient and generally not associated with clinical manifestation of APS. Considerable reported evidence suggests some infectious agents are often "triggers" for APS.[58]

Quality Control

A positive and negative lupus anticoagulant control should be included with each run of patient samples. Controls should be retested with a reagent change or major instrument adjustment. Strong positive, weak positive, and negative lupus anticoagulant controls are available through commercial manufacturers and are preferred to the traditional plasma samples of local lupus anticoagulant-positive patients. It is recommended that each laboratory determine a reference interval specific for their reagent and instrument combination using accepted laboratory principles.[59] Reference intervals should be verified with a change in reagent lot number, instrument, collection system, or at least once per year. Better precision can be achieved when laboratories determine their own cutoff levels for positive results. An appropriate way to establish the cut-off level for lupus anticoagulant test, such as dRVVT or aPTT using a lupus-sensitive reagent is to determine the geometric mean ±2 standard deviation (SD) of 40 healthy individuals.

Antiphospholipid Antibody Profiles

A lupus anticoagulant result should always be considered in the context of a full laboratory aPL profile comprising anticardiolipin (aCL) and anti-β 2glyco-protein I (aβ2GPI) antibodies by ELISAs. The presence of medium-high titers aCL and aβ2GPI of the same isotype (most often IgG) is in agreement with a positive LA and identifies patients at high risk for thrombosis.[60] Less informa-tion is available for the correlations with fetal losses. Isolated lupus anticoagu-lant positivity is significantly more frequent in subjects without clinical events or may be false positive especially if identified as mild in potency or if it is diagnosed for the first time.[61]

Non-Criteria aPLs

The modified Sopporo classification (Table 16-3) considers IgA aCL, IgA aβ2GPI, and anti-phosphatidylserine antibodies, antiphosphatidylethanol-amine antibodies against prothrombin alone and antibodies to phosphatidyl-serine-prothrombin complex as non-criteria aPLs. While the presence of these antibodies is undoubtedly frequent, they are not specific to the diagnosis of APS. It is, however, reasonable to label a patient meeting all other clinic criteria of APS with persistently positive non-criteria aPLs as "features associated with APS" or "non-criteria features of APS."[47]

Sources of Error

The rates of false-positive and false-negative detections remain relatively high. The former are of particular concern because they qualify the patients for long and unnecessary oral anticoagulant treatment.

False-negative lupus anticoagulant testing may be caused by:

- Pre-analytic factors leading to either delay in processing or platelet activation—both of these effects can cause platelet-derived phospho-lipid to neutralize the lupus anticoagulant. Of note, weak lupus antico-agulants may be lost during the freezing and thawing performed.
- Ineffective centrifugation leading to excess platelet-derived phospholipid in the test system.

False-positive lupus anticoagulant testing may be caused by:

- Prolongation of the clotting time in clot-based lupus-sensitive assays, such as aPTT and dRVVT due to factor deficiencies or specific factor inhibitors.
- Prolongation of the clotting time by oral anticoagulant therapy, such as VKAs. The interpretation of results is difficult because of the prolonged basal clotting time. To avoid misinterpretation, it is recommended to perform laboratory procedures 1-2 weeks after discontinuation of treatment or when the international normalized ratio (INR) is less than 1.5. Bridging VKA discontinuation with low molecular weight heparin (LMWH) is recommended with the last dose of LMWH administered more than 12 hours before the blood is drawn for lupus anticoagulant testing. Alternatively, if the INR is between 1.5 and < 3.0, a 1:1 dilution of patient plasma and pooled normal plasma can be considered. The interpretation of results may still be difficult and the lupus anticoagulant titer will be diluted at least 2-fold.
- Lupus anticoagulant detection during acute thromboembolic events. Caution should be exercised in interpretation of the results of tests performed close to a thromboembolic event as patients may be treated with full doses of unfractionated heparin and/or VKAs. Furthermore, acute-phase reactants as FVIII may be increased during acute events.

ASSAYS RELATED TO ANTICOAGULANT ACTIVITY

Anti-factor Xa Assay

The anti-factor Xa (anti-Xa) assay is a functional assay that facilitates the measurement of AT-catalyzed inhibition of factor Xa by unfractionated heparin (UFH) and direct inhibition of FXa by LMWH. While automated methods for the determination of the abilities of UFH and LMWH to inhibit FXa have been available since the 1970s, their cost prohibited their widespread clinical use until relatively recently. The anti-Xa assay is used to guide the determination of therapeutic aPTT ranges in the clinical management of UFH therapy. As a result, the anti-Xa assay is commonly viewed as a heparin assay, despite the fact that it actually provides a measure of UFH *effect* as opposed to a measure of UFH *concentration*. UFH molecules are chemically or enzymatically altered to produce smaller fractions of lower molecular weight. The resultant LMWHs have greater specificity, producing increased anti-Xa activity relative to anti-IIa activity.[62] Therefore, aPTT measurement of LMWH activity is insensitive; activity must be measured using a direct anti-Xa assay.

The basic principle of the anti-Xa assay utilizes UFH's or LMWH's AT-catalyzed inhibition of Xa.[63] Prior to performing an anti-Xa assay, each laboratory must create a standard curve for UFH and/or LMWH using a pool of normal plasma spiked with varying amounts of UFH and/or LMWH. To this plasma pool, known quantities of Xa are added, and after a period of incubation, the amount of residual Xa is measured. The reagent contains an excess of activated FX (± exogenous AT), which is inhibited by the heparin:anti-thrombin complex. The amount of heparin in the test plasma is inversely proportional to the amount of factor Xa. Residual Xa is available to cleave a chromogenic substrate, resulting in a color change that can be detected optically.

The clinical utility of the anti-Xa assay in monitoring UFH was largely realized due to the observation that a proportion of patients exposed to therapeutic doses of UFH failed to achieve expected prolongation of the aPTT. Levine et al. report the outcomes of a study comparing the anti-Xa assay to the aPTT in a cohort of patients requiring large doses of UFH.[64] They demonstrated that ongoing escalations of UFH doses could be avoided by the use of anti-Xa assays, when aPTT results may indicate subtherapeutic levels of anticoagulation. Outcome measures such as incidence of major bleeding and recurrent thrombosis did not differ between patients managed by the aPTT and those managed by the anti-Xa assay, although the study was likely underpowered.

The anti-Xa level can be used as a primary measure of UFH effect, as well as a tool to validate aPTT measurement of UFH therapy. Therapeutic UFH therapy reflects an anti-Xa assay of between 0.35 and 0.7 U/mL or protamine titration (0.2-0.4 U/mL). Dosage of UFH therapy should be titrated to achieve this target anti-Xa assay range. Ignjatovic et al. report in vitro and ex vivo data suggesting that UFH monitoring using the aPTT titrated to an anti-Xa assay of 0.35-0.7 U/mL is associated with significant age-related variation.[65,66] This effect was especially apparent in younger children, suggesting that therapeutic aPTT ranges of 78-200 seconds were associated with an anti-Xa assay of 0.35-0.7 U/mL from in vitro samples in children aged 1-5 years, and were often un-recordable in ex vivo samples. Chan et al. and Kuhle et al. both reported poor correlation between the aPTT and anti-Xa assay in ex vivo pediatric samples.[67,68] Across a population of infants and children ranging from neonates to 18-year-old adolescents, agreement between the aPTT and anti-Xa assay was 0.09 and 0.22, respectively. Chan reported that the level of agreement was further reduced when only infants less than 2 years of age were analyzed.[67] The mechanism for the discrepancies between anti-Xa and aPTT are yet to be determined, but may reflect the variable anti-IIa to anti- Xa effect of UFH reported by Newall et al.[69]

Recommendations for the management of LMWH therapy in adults state that routine laboratory monitoring is generally unnecessary. The predictability of weight-adjusted dosing of LMWH in infants and children appears to be reduced compared to adults, making laboratory monitoring of therapy in infants and children necessary. Current guidelines for the management of LMWH therapy in infants and children recommend an anti-Xa level be measured 4-6 h following subcutaneous injection of the LMWH. Ongoing dosing of LMWH should be titrated to achieve an anti-Xa level of 0.5-1.0 U/mL.[70]

Relevance to Pediatrics

In vivo studies of UFH therapy in pediatric patients conducted by Ignjatovic et al.[65] demonstrated a lack of correlation between two anti-Xa assays: one assay did not have exogenous anti-thrombin, but did have added dextran sulfate while the other assay contained exogenous anti-thrombin.[71] The added dextran sulfate causes any heparin in the test plasma that is bound to proteins to be released. Some of this protein-bound heparin may not have been free to catalyze AT without the influence of dextran sulfate. As a result, this assay may overestimate the heparin activity in test plasma. Exogenous AT is added to ensure that the heparin present in test plasma has sufficient AT to catalyze. However, for a patient deficient in AT (ie, most pediatric patients) this exogenous AT may contribute to the non-physiological measurement of anti-Xa activity. Further investigation is required before recommendations can be made regarding which methodology is most appropriate for pediatric use. In vivo analysis of UFH therapy in pediatric patient plasma samples also suggests that the ratio between UFH inhibition of thrombin (IIa) and Xa varies with age. Infants and younger children have significantly greater anti-Xa activity than older children and adults for a given dose of UFH. This finding raises significant implications regarding the choice of an optimal method for monitoring UFH therapy in the pediatric population.

GLOBAL COAGULATION ASSAYS

Plasma based clotting assays, such as aPTT and PT, are commonly employed to detect aberrations in the coagulation cascade. While these are considered the "gold standard," they only assess the initiation of clot formation, when only 3-5% of thrombin has been generated. Thrombin generation is dependent on several key players in the coagulation cascade, including, but not limited to cellular elements, platelets, fibrin polymerization, and the components in the fibrinolytic cascade. Therefore, sufficient clot formation is a continuous process and is better studied by global coagulation assay.

The evaluation of coagulation has come a long way from assays such as the PT and aPTT, and global assays are now regaining an interest as they lend the ability to assess the rate and total thrombin generated, individual hemostatic potential, whole blood clot formation and/or fibrin polymerization, and clot structure and stability. The tests that fit these characteristics may be grouped into three categories based on what is measured. Thrombin generation assay (TGA) is an example of a global assay that measures thrombin generation. Clot formation is measured by assessing physical properties of the developing clot using assays, such as thromboelastography (TEG) and APTT wave form analysis. The CloFAL or clot formation and lysis assays measure both clot formation and thrombin generation, as the name suggests. The TGA and TEG will be discussed further as both have seen the most technological advances. The ISTH endorses both assays. A standardized protocol has been developed for TGA using a calibrated automated thrombogram (CAT).[72] Similarly, the official communication from the SSC of the ISTH standardizing the methodology for TEG/Thromboelastometry in hemophilia was recently published.[73]

Thromboelastography

Thromboelastography, first described in 1948, has undergone several modifications and is now currently available via two manufacturers, TEG (Haemonetics, Braintree, Massachusetts, USA) and ROTEM (Pentapharm GmbH, Munich, Germany). TEG analyzes whole blood under low shear conditions. While other conventional tests provide information up until the first fibrin strands in the developing clot, TEG begins to evaluate clot formation at this point, and collects data as clotting continues, through to eventual clot lysis.

The basic principle of TEG involves incubation of whole blood or platelet rich plasma in a heated sample cup containing a suspended pin. The pin and the cup or the cup alone oscillates, and as the blood clots, the motion of the cup is transmitted to the pin, which is recorded via a computer. There are minor mechanical differences between the two instruments, and the activators used differ with respect to potency. In the TEG, a sensor (pin) is connected with a torsion wire and clot formation generates a physical connection between the cup and sensor that is recorded via a mechanical-electrical transducer.

The TEG curve (Figure 16-5) is represented by the following five parameters: (i) R time, the time from the start of the test until clot formation. (ii) K-time (K), the period from the start of clot formation until the curve reaches an amplitude of 20 mm; indicating clot kinetics. (iii) α-angle, the angle between the baseline and the tangent to the TEG curve, reflecting the rate of clot formation. (iv) Maximal amplitude (MA) is a direct measure of the strength of the clot. (v) Ly 30 is the difference between MA and the amplitude after 30 minutes and reflects the degree of fibrinolysis at 30 minutes.

The initial clinical utility of TEG was to decrease the transfusion requirements in patients with complicated surgical procedures, but its application has now expanded to include coagulation disorders. Thromboelastography has defined the phenotypic variation seen in adult and pediatric patients with

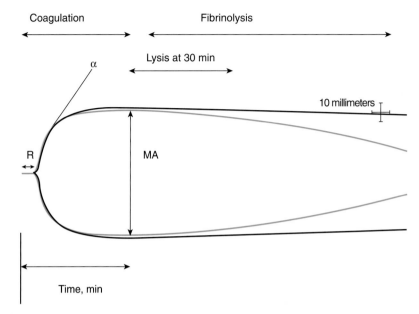

Figure 16-5 ▪ Normal TEG tracing showing parameters in TEG analysis.
R, reaction time; α- angle, speed of clot formation; MA, maximum amplitude, Clot lysis
at 30 minutes

severe hemophilia and in those with rare bleeding disorders.[74,75] The information gleaned from TEG can be used to individualize treatment. Management of bleeding in hemophilia patients with inhibitors remains a great challenge. The use of TEG to individualize therapy in patients with inhibitors leads to cost-effective care without compromising efficacy.[76] Other areas where TEG has been instrumental include coagulopathy of trauma, solid organ transplantation, and monitoring of new oral anticoagulants.

Thrombin Generation Assay

Thrombin is the final product and the key enzyme of the coagulation system. Thrombin measurement reflects the overall coagulation capacity of each individual. Other assays like D-dimer (cross-linked fibrin has formed), F1+2 (prothrombin has been split) and thrombin–anti-thrombin complex (TAT; active thrombin was present) are markers of ongoing coagulation activation while TGA represents an individual's potential to generate thrombin, should coagulation triggering conditions arise. These technical developments of the TGA make it potentially applicable to clinical laboratories.

The TGA, originally developed by Hemker et al.[77] is measured in platelet-rich or platelet-poor plasma, using a fluorescent substrate to establish a TG

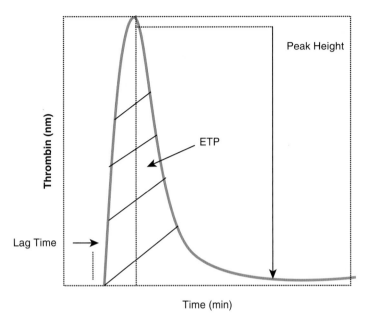

Figure 16-6 ▪ Normal TG tracing showing a standard TGA curve.
Lag time, time to initial thrombin burst; ETP, endogenous thrombin potential: Total
amount of thrombin formed; Peak height, peak thrombin formed.

curve (Figure 16-6), using CAT (Diagnostica Stago, Inc. Parsippany, NJ, USA). It
measures the rate and extent of thrombin and is based on the premise that the
thrombin thus generated promotes formation of a stable hemostatic plug. From
the TG curve, various parameters describing thrombin activity can be deduced,
including lag time (time until thrombin burst occurs; min), peak value of thrombin (nM), and the area under the curve (or endogenous thrombin potential
(ETP), which represents the total amount of thrombin generated; nM/min).

Correlations between the TG parameters and clinically observed bleeding
in patients with hemophilia and other inherited bleeding disorders have been
published.[72] This correlation between clinical bleeding risk and thrombin generating capacity led to the evaluation of this technology as a surrogate marker
for by-passing therapy in hemophilia patients with anti-FVIII/FIX alloantibodies.[78] It has also been shown that TGA is sensitive to hypercoagulability.[79,80]

Activated Clotting Time

Though not considered a "classic" global coagulation assay, the activated clotting
time (ACT) is a test of whole blood coagulation, incorporating the importance
of platelets and phospholipids, and gives a single parameter for interpretation.
ACTs are indicative of inhibition of contact and common pathway activation

rather than inhibition of the extrinsic coagulation pathway.[81] Unfractionated heparin is the anticoagulant of choice in most cardiac and surgical centers because it has a short half-life and is easily reversed. During longer procedures the short half-life of heparin, blood component replacement/dilution, and the patient's individual interaction can alter the effective time course of heparin. The point-of-care ACT test has been the preferred test in catheterization labs and cardiac operating rooms because it has a number of advantages over laboratory tests,[82] including:

- Shorter time between sampling and results.
- Smaller blood sample size.
- Availability to have test performed by non-lab personnel at bedside.
- Decreased risk of sample degradation with time.

The ACT tube has an activator substance that will activate factor XII through contact activation. The main activator substances used are celite, kaolin, or glass beads. The principle of the test is to completely activate the intrinsic coagulation cascade and measure the time it takes for generation of a fibrin clot. The machine heats the sample to 37°C. Depending on the type of machine being used, movement is created whether through either rotation of the sample tube, a plunger or through pressure. As a clot forms it imparts resistance onto a plunger or onto a free rolling bar in the sample tube or impedes flow of the blood.[83] The end result is the time taken for the sample to form a clot. Because it is non-specific, variables like hypothermia, hemodilution, platelet count, fibrinogen activity, and various coagulopathies can alter the result.[84]

The ACT is a commonly used point-of-care coagulation test during extracorporeal life support. Monitoring and stabilizing the coagulation profile of cardiac patients, particularly those on extracorporeal life support, is one of the major challenges in successfully supporting these patients over a period of days to weeks.

FUTURE DIRECTIONS

The currently available laboratory-based techniques to measure the hemostatic system vary from biological clot-based assays to chromogenic assays and immunological measurements of proteins. All are in vitro tests that do not really measure the hemostatic system in its functional reality. There remains an urgent need for further research to develop better and novel methods of assessing the hemostatic system in pediatrics. With recently advanced neonatal care and increased survival of very young, low-birth-weight, and sometimes extremely sick premature infants, the issue of validated reference values for all hemostatic proteins and assays in premature neonates deserves urgent attention. New devices and techniques for hemostasis assessment should be approached with structured, age-related research in order to define specific age-related reference values. Global coagulation assays appear promising but their widespread use is limited by lack of standardization. Clinical trials of novel long-acting factor concentrate, which seem to be the future of bleeding disorder therapies, are ongoing. These trials would be most informative with the use of global assays, in addition to the assessment of bleeding phenotype, enabling individualized therapy for such patients.

TRAINING MODULE

1. You are consulting on a new patient who was recently diagnosed with DVT of the right femoral vein. He is a 15-year-old WM who weighs 90 kg and who developed leg pain and swelling after a football injury to his knee that required bracing. After DVT was diagnosed, he was placed on heparin infusion and transitioned to warfarin. Current INR is 2.4. Thrombophilia testing was performed prior to discharge from the hospital.

Factor V Leiden	Homozygous normal
Prothrombin gene mutation	Homozygous normal
Factor VIII	200%
Protein S activity	40%
Protein C activity	30%
Anti-thrombin	85%
Lupus anticoagulant	Negative

Based on these results, the most likely contributed to his thrombosis is:

a. Inherited Protein C deficiency
b. Inherited Protein S deficiency
c. Immobility
d. Obesity
e. Elevated FVIII

2. A 5-month-old Caucasian female had open heart surgery 7 days ago. She is on an unfractionated heparin infusion at prophylactic dosing. Her total WBC was 13,000/mm^3 with 50% segmented neutrophils, 3% bands, 10% monocytes, and 37% lymphs. Hemoglobin was 10.5 g/dL and platelet count 45,000/mm^3. Her PT is 13 seconds, PTT 45 seconds, fibrinogen 350 mg/dL, and D-Dimers are mildly elevated. Her ALT is 35 U/L, AST 37 U/L, and creatinine 1.0 mg/dL. She has a catheter in her right femoral vein, which is not flushing adequately, and a Doppler sonogram shows partial occlusion of the right femoral vein.

The next best step in this patient's management is to:

a. Test for heparin-induced thrombocytopenia without altering current anticoagulation.
b. Remove the femoral catheter.
c. Discontinue unfractionated heparin and begin warfarin.
d. Test for heparin-induced thrombocytopenia and begin an alternative anticoagulant agent.
e. Discontinue unfractionated heparin and begin enoxaparin.

3. A teenage girl is on chronic warfarin therapy. The INR has been stable for the last 6 months, but is now 1.4. She denies missing any doses except for the day before her routine lab test, and a pill count suggests that no other doses have been missed. Which is the most likely reason for the drop in INR?

a. She has started to drink alcohol on the weekends.
b. She was prescribed an antibiotic for a sinus infection the week before.
c. She has a gene polymorphism making her resistant to warfarin.
d. She started a diet this month consisting of mostly fruits and vegetables.
e. She missed the dose the day before the test.

4. Which aspect of the endothelium has anticoagulant properties?

a. Release of thrombomodulin
b. Release of VWF and cleavage by ADAMTS-12
c. Vasoconstriction
d. Release of Tissue Factor

5. A 4-year-old white female is brought to you ER at a large tertiary medical center for nose bleeds, easy bruising and altered mental status. She has been staying with her grandparents while her parents are out of town. She has never had any bleeding issues in the past and even underwent tonsillectomy 6 months ago without incident. Family history is negative for bleeding disorders, but grandfather is on warfarin for atrial fibrillation. Labs have been drawn and stat head CT is being performed. You suspect warfarin toxicity due to accidental ingestion of grandfather's medications. CT confirms intracranial hemorrhage. CBC shows hemoglobin of 8.9 g/dL and platelets of 250,000. PT is markedly prolonged and corresponds to INR of 10.5. PTT is also prolonged at 60 seconds.

What is the best management for this child?

a. Give oral Vitamin K at a dose of 5 mg
b. Give FFP at a dose of 10 cc/kg
c. Give rFVIIa at a dose of 90 mcg/kg
d. Give a Prothrombin Complex Concentrate (PCC) at a dose of 50 units/kg
e. Pump the child's stomach

6. Which inherited thrombophilia is most likely to lead to a venous thromboembolic event prior to age 40?

a. Heterozygous Factor V Leiden gene mutation
b. Double heterozygous MTHFR polymorphism

   c. Heterozygous Prothrombin Gene mutation

   d. Heterozygous Protein S activity

   e. Heterozygous Anti-thrombin activity

7. A 12-year-old white male was diagnosed with DVT of the right lower extremity after knee surgery. He has been on anticoagulation for last 3 months and you are asked to provide recommendation for duration of therapy. Which of the following scenarios would require prolonged or indefinite anticoagulation therapy.

   a. Lupus anticoagulant was positive at diagnosis and remains positive

   b. At diagnosis the FVIII activity level was 300% and it is now 150%

   c. He tested positive for heterozygous Factor V Leiden mutation

   d. His protein C activity is 60%

   e. His mother had a DVT in the post-partum period

REFERENCES

1. Davie EW, Ratnoff OD. Waterfall sequence for intrinsic blood clotting. *Science*. 1964;145(3638):1310-1312.
2. Macfarlane RG. An enzyme cascade in the blood clotting mechanism, and its function as a biochemical amplifier. *Nature*. 1964;202:498-499.
3. Lord ST. Fibrinogen and fibrin: scaffold proteins in hemostasis. *Curr Opin Hematol*. 2007;14(3):236-241.
4. Wolberg AS. Thrombin generation and fibrin clot structure. *Blood Rev*. 2007;21(3):131-142.
5. Oliver JA, Monroe DM, Roberts HR, Hoffman M. Thrombin activates factor XI on activated platelets in the absence of factor XII. *Arterioscler Thromb Vasc Biol*. 1999;19(1):170-177.
6. Lerant I, Kovacs T, Papp B, Mandl J, Lambin P, Machovich R. Interaction of thrombin with endothelial cells in the presence of fibrinogen and alpha 2-macroglobulin. *Haematologia*. 1990;23(3):161-169.
7. Sie P, Ofosu F, Fernandez F, Buchanan MR, Petitou M, Boneu B. Respective role of antithrombin III and heparin cofactor II in the in vitro anticoagulant effect of heparin and of various sulphated polysaccharides. *Br J Haematol*. 1986;64(4):707-714.
8. Mascellani G, Liverani L, Bianchini P, et al. Structure and contribution to the heparin cofactor II-mediated inhibition of thrombin of naturally oversulphated sequences of dermatan sulphate. *Biochem J*. 15 1993;296 (Pt 3):639-648.
9. Prager NA, Abendschein DR, McKenzie CR, Eisenberg PR. Role of thrombin compared with factor Xa in the procoagulant activity of whole blood clots. *Circulation*. 1995;92(4):962-967.
10. Weitz JI, Hudoba M, Massel D, Maraganore J, Hirsh J. Clot-bound thrombin is protected from inhibition by heparin-antithrombin III but is susceptible to inactivation by antithrombin III-independent inhibitors. *J Clin Invest*. 1990;86(2):385-391.
11. Eisenberg PR, Siegel JE, Abendschein DR, Miletich JP. Importance of factor Xa in determining the procoagulant activity of whole-blood clots. *J Clin Invest*. 1993;91(5):1877-1883.

12. Bendayan P, Boccalon H, Dupouy D, Boneu B. Dermatan sulfate is a more potent inhibitor of clot-bound thrombin than unfractionated and low molecular weight heparins. *Thromb Haemost.* May 1994;71(5):576-580.

13. Dahlback B. The protein C anticoagulant system: inherited defects as basis for venous thrombosis. *Thromb Res.* 1995;77(1):1-43.

14. Broze GJ, Jr. Tissue factor pathway inhibitor. *Thromb Haemost.* 1995;74(1):90-93.

15. Lindahl AK. Tissue factor pathway inhibitor: from unknown coagulation inhibitor to major antithrombotic principle. *Cardiovasc Res.* 1997;33(2):286-291.

16. Sandset PM, Bendz B. Tissue factor pathway inhibitor: clinical deficiency states. *Thromb Haemost.* 1997;78(1):467-470.

17. Lindahl AK, Jacobsen PB, Sandset PM, Abildgaard U. Tissue factor pathway inhibitor with high anticoagulant activity is increased in post-heparin plasma and in plasma from cancer patients. *Blood Coagul Fibrinolysis.* 1991;2(6):713-721.

18. Collen D, Lijnen HR. Basic and clinical aspects of fibrinolysis and thrombolysis. *Blood.* 15 1991;78(12):3114-3124.

19. Francis CW, Marder VJ. Physiologic regulation and pathologic disorders of fibrinolysis. *Hum Pathol.* 1987;18(3):263-274.

20. Bajzar L. Thrombin activatable fibrinolysis inhibitor and an antifibrinolytic pathway. *Arterioscler Thromb Vasc Biol.* 2000;20(12):2511-2518.

21. Andrew M, Paes B, Milner R, et al. Development of the human coagulation system in the full-term infant. *Blood.* 1987;70(1):165-172.

22. Andrew M, Paes B, Johnston M. Development of the hemostatic system in the neonate and young infant. *Am J Pediatr Hematol Oncol.* 1990;12(1):95-104.

23. Andrew M, Vegh P, Johnston M, Bowker J, Ofosu F, Mitchell L. Maturation of the hemostatic system during childhood. *Blood.* 15 1992;80(8):1998-2005.

24. Monagle P, Barnes C, Ignjatovic V, et al. Developmental haemostasis. Impact for clinical haemostasis laboratories. *Thromb Haemost.* 2006;95(2):362-372.

25. Massicotte MP, Sofronas M, deVeber G. Difficulties in performing clinical trials of antithrombotic therapy in neonates and children. *Thromb Res.* 2006;118(1):153-163.

26. Reverdiau-Moalic P, Delahousse B, Body G, Bardos P, Leroy J, Gruel Y. Evolution of blood coagulation activators and inhibitors in the healthy human fetus. *Blood.* 1996;88(3):900-906.

27. Schwarz HP, Muntean W, Watzke H, Richter B, Griffin JH. Low total protein S antigen but high protein S activity due to decreased C4b-binding protein in neonates. *Blood.* 1988;71(3):562-565.

28. Corrigan JJ, Jr., Sleeth JJ, Jeter M, Lox CD. Newborn's fibrinolytic mechanism: components and plasmin generation. *Am J Hematol.* 1989;32(4):273-278.

29. Ignjatovic V, Ilhan A, Monagle P. Evidence for age-related differences in human fibrinogen. *Blood Coagul Fibrinolysis.* 2011;22(2):110-117.

30. Rajasekhar D, Barnard MR, Bednarek FJ, Michelson AD. Platelet hyporeactivity in very low birth weight neonates. *Thromb Haemost.* 1997;77(5):1002-1007.

31. Mazurier C, Daffos F, Forestier F. Electrophoretic and functional characteristics of the von Willebrand factor in human fetal plasma. *Br J Haematol.* 1992;81(2):263-270.

32. Lisman T, Platto M, Meijers JC, Haagsma EB, Colledan M, Porte RJ. The hemostatic status of pediatric recipients of adult liver grafts suggests that plasma levels of hemostatic proteins are not regulated by the liver. *Blood.* 10 2011;117(6):2070-2072.

33. Monagle P, Ignjatovic V, Savoia H. Hemostasis in neonates and children: pitfalls and dilemmas. *Blood Rev.* 2010;24(2):63-68.

34. Koepke JA. Performance guidelines for the partial thromboplastin time test. *Ric Clin Lab.* 1989;19(4):359-362.

35. Adcock DM, Marlar RA. Activated partial thromboplastin time reagent sensitivity to the presence of the lupus anticoagulant. *Arch Pathol Lab Med.* 1992;116(8):837-840.

36. Clauss A. [Rapid physiological coagulation method in determination of fibrinogen]. *Acta Haematol.* 1957;17(4):237-246.

37. Levine RF, Olson TA, Shoff PK, Miller MK, Weisman LE. Mature micromegakaryocytes: an unusual developmental pattern in term infants. *Br J Haematol.* Aug 1996;94(2): 391-399.

38. Harker LA, Slichter SJ. The bleeding time as a screening test for evaluation of platelet function. *N Engl J Med.* 27 1972;287(4):155-159.

39. Harrison P. The role of PFA-100 testing in the investigation and management of haemostatic defects in children and adults. *Br J Haematol.* 2005;130(1):3-10.

40. Hayward CP, Harrison P, Cattaneo M, et al. Platelet function analyzer (PFA)-100 closure time in the evaluation of platelet disorders and platelet function. *J Thromb Haemost.* 2006;4(2):312-319.

41. Kottke-Marchant K, Corcoran G. The laboratory diagnosis of platelet disorders. *Arch Pathol Lab Med.* 2002;126(2):133-146.

42. Hayward CP, Eikelboom J. Platelet function testing: quality assurance. *Semin Thromb Hemost.* 2007;33(3):273-282.

43. Cattaneo M, Cerletti C, Harrison P, et al. Recommendations for the standardization of light transmission aggregometry: a consensus of the working party from the platelet physiology subcommittee of SSC/ISTH. *J Thromb Haemost.* 10 2013.

44. Michelson AD, Benoit SE, Kroll MH, et al. The activation-induced decrease in the platelet surface expression of the glycoprotein Ib-IX complex is reversible. *Blood.* 15 1994;83(12):3562-3573.

45. Michelson AD, Furman MI. Laboratory markers of platelet activation and their clinical significance. *Curr Opin Hematol.* 1999;6(5):342-348.

46. Kovacs MJ, Kovacs J, Anderson J, Rodger MA, Mackinnon K, Wells PS. Protein C and protein S levels can be accurately determined within 24 hours of diagnosis of acute venous thromboembolism. *Clin Lab Haematol.* 2006;28(1):9-13.

47. Miyakis S, Lockshin MD, Atsumi T, et al. International consensus statement on an update of the classification criteria for definite antiphospholipid syndrome (APS). *J Thromb Haemost.* 2006;4(2):295-306.

48. Abo SM, DeBari VA. Laboratory evaluation of the antiphospholipid syndrome. *Ann Clin Lab Sci.* 2007;37(1):3-14.

49. Triplett DA. Antiphospholipid antibodies. *Arch Pathol Lab Med.* 2002;126(11):1424-1429.

50. Pengo V, Tripodi A, Reber G, et al. Update of the guidelines for lupus anticoagulant detection. Subcommittee on Lupus Anticoagulant/Antiphospholipid Antibody of the Scientific and Standardisation Committee of the International Society on Thrombosis and Haemostasis. *J Thromb Haemost.* 2009;7(10):1737-1740.

51. Tripodi A, Biasiolo A, Chantarangkul V, Pengo V. Lupus anticoagulant (LA) testing: performance of clinical laboratories assessed by a national survey using lyophilized affinity-purified immunoglobulin with LA activity. *Clini Chem.* 2003;49(10):1608-1614.

52. Jennings I, Kitchen S, Woods TA, Preston FE, Greaves M. Potentially clinically important inaccuracies in testing for the lupus anticoagulant: an analysis of results from three surveys of the UK National External Quality Assessment Scheme (NEQAS) for Blood Coagulation. *Thromb Haemost.* 1997;77(5):934-937.

53. Urbanus RT, Derksen RH, de Groot PG. Current insight into diagnostics and pathophysiology of the antiphospolipid syndrome. *Blood Rev.* 2008;22(2):93-105.

54. Teruya J, West AG, Suell MN. Lupus anticoagulant assays: questions answered and to be answered. *Arch Pathol Lab Med.* 2007;131(6):885-889.

55. Galli M, Finazzi G, Bevers EM, Barbui T. Kaolin clotting time and dilute Russell's viper venom time distinguish between prothrombin-dependent and beta 2-glycoprotein I-dependent antiphospholipid antibodies. *Blood.* 15 1995;86(2):617-623.

56. Jacobsen EM, Barna-Cler L, Taylor JM, Triplett DA, Wisloff F. The Lupus Ratio test–an interlaboratory study on the detection of Lupus anticoagulants by an APTT-based, integrated, and semi-quantitative test. Fifth International Survey of Lupus Anticoagulants–ISLA 5. *Thromb Haemost.* 2000;83(5):704-708.

57. Tripodi A. Laboratory testing for lupus anticoagulants: a review of issues affecting results. *Clin Chem.* 2007;53(9):1629-1635.

58. Shoenfeld Y, Blank M, Cervera R, Font J, Raschi E, Meroni PL. Infectious origin of the antiphospholipid syndrome. *Ann Rheum Dis.* Jan 2006;65(1):2-6.

59. Pierangeli SS, Harris EN. Clinical laboratory testing for the antiphospholipid syndrome. *Clin Chim Acta.* 1 2005;357(1):17-33.

60. Levine SR, Salowich-Palm L, Sawaya KL, et al. IgG anticardiolipin antibody titer > 40 GPL and the risk of subsequent thrombo-occlusive events and death. A prospective cohort study. *Stroke.* 1997;28(9):1660-1665.

61. Genvresse I, Luftner D, Spath-Schwalbe E, Buttgereit F. Prevalence and clinical significance of anticardiolipin and anti-beta2-glycoprotein-I antibodies in patients with non-Hodgkin's lymphoma. *Eur J Haematol.* 2002;68(2):84-90.

62. Hirsh J, Raschke R. Heparin and low-molecular-weight heparin: the Seventh ACCP Conference on Antithrombotic and Thrombolytic Therapy. *Chest.* 2004;126(3 Suppl):188S-203S.

63. Olson JD, Arkin CF, Brandt JT, et al. College of American Pathologists Conference XXXI on laboratory monitoring of anticoagulant therapy: laboratory monitoring of unfractionated heparin therapy. *Arch Pathol Lab Med.* 1998;122(9):782-798.

64. Levine MN, Hirsh J, Gent M, et al. A randomized trial comparing activated thromboplastin time with heparin assay in patients with acute venous thromboembolism requiring large daily doses of heparin. *Arch Int Med.* 1994;154(1):49-56.

65. Ignjatovic V, Summerhayes R, Than J, Gan A, Monagle P. Therapeutic range for unfractionated heparin therapy: age-related differences in response in children. *J Thromb Haemost.* 2006;4(10):2280-2282.

66. Ignjatovic V, Furmedge J, Newall F, et al. Age-related differences in heparin response. *Thromb Res.* 2006;118(6):741-745.

67. Chan AK, Black L, Ing C, Brandao LR, Williams S. Utility of aPTT in monitoring unfractionated heparin in children. *Thromb Res.* 2008;122(1):135-136.

68. Kuhle S, Eulmesekian P, Kavanagh B, et al. Lack of correlation between heparin dose and standard clinical monitoring tests in treatment with unfractionated heparin in critically ill children. *Haematologica.* 2007;92(4):554-557.

69. Newall F, Ignjatovic V, Johnston L, et al. Age is a determinant factor for measures of concentration and effect in children requiring unfractionated heparin. *Thromb Haemost.* 2010;103(5):1085-1090.

70. Monagle P, Chan AK, Goldenberg NA, et al. Antithrombotic therapy in neonates and children: Antithrombotic Therapy and Prevention of Thrombosis, 9th ed: American College of Chest Physicians Evidence-Based Clinical Practice Guidelines. *Chest.* 2012;141(2 Suppl):e737S-e801S.

71. Ignjatovic V, Summerhayes R, Gan A, et al. Monitoring Unfractionated Heparin (UFH) therapy: which Anti-Factor Xa assay is appropriate? *Thromb Res.* 2007;120(3): 347-351.

72. Dargaud Y, Beguin S, Lienhart A, et al. Evaluation of thrombin generating capacity in plasma from patients with haemophilia A and B. *Thromb Haemost.* 2005;93(3): 475-480.

73. Chitlur M, Rivard GE, Lillicrap D, et al. Recommendations for performing thromboelastography/thromboelastometry in hemophilia: communication from the SSC of the ISTH. *J Thromb Haemost.* 2014;12(1):103-106.

74. Sorensen B, Ingerslev J. Whole blood clot formation phenotypes in hemophilia A and rare coagulation disorders. Patterns of response to recombinant factor VIIa. *J Thromb Haemost.* 2004;2(1):102-110.

75. Chitlur M, Warrier I, Rajpurkar M, et al. Thromboelastography in children with coagulation factor deficiencies. *Br J Haematol.* 2008;142(2):250-256.

76. Young G, Blain R, Nakagawa P, Nugent DJ. Individualization of bypassing agent treatment for haemophilic patients with inhibitors utilizing thromboelastography. *Haemophilia.* 2006;12(6):598-604.

77. Hemker HC, Giesen P, Al Dieri R, et al. Calibrated automated thrombin generation measurement in clotting plasma. *Pathophysiol Haemost Thromb.* 2003;33(1):4-15.

78. Dargaud Y, Lienhart A, Negrier C. Prospective assessment of thrombin generation test for dose monitoring of bypassing therapy in hemophilia patients with inhibitors undergoing elective surgery. *Blood.* 16 2010;116(25):5734-5737.

79. Dargaud Y, Trzeciak MC, Bordet JC, Ninet J, Negrier C. Use of calibrated automated thrombinography +/− thrombomodulin to recognise the prothrombotic phenotype. *Thromb Haemost.* Nov 2006;96(5):562-567.

80. Besser M, Baglin C, Luddington R, van Hylckama Vlieg A, Baglin T. High rate of unprovoked recurrent venous thrombosis is associated with high thrombin-generating potential in a prospective cohort study. *J Thromb Haemost.* 2008;6(10):1720-1725.

81. Despotis GJ, Summerfield AL, Joist JH, et al. Comparison of activated coagulation time and whole blood heparin measurements with laboratory plasma anti-Xa heparin concentration in patients having cardiac operations. *J Thorac Cardiovasc Surg.* 1994;108(6):1076-1082.

82. Spinler SA, Wittkowsky AK, Nutescu EA, Smythe MA. Anticoagulation monitoring part 2: Unfractionated heparin and low-molecular-weight heparin. *Ann Pharmacother.* 2005;39(7-8):1275-1285.

83. Hattersley PG. Activated coagulation time of whole blood. *JAMA.* 1966;196(5):436-440.

84. Ammar T, Scudder LE, Coller BS. In vitro effects of the platelet glycoprotein IIb/IIIa receptor antagonist c7E3 Fab on the activated clotting time. *Circulation.* 1997; 95(3):614-617.

PEDIATRIC TRANSFUSION MEDICINE

17

Daniel K. Noland

LEARNING OBJECTIVES

1. Explain the special transfusion needs related to pediatric size (ie, aliquots) and immaturity of the immune system (ie, irradiation).
2. Characterize disorders unique to (ie, NAIT-neonatal alloimmune thrombocytopenia) and common in (ie, sickle cell disease) pediatric populations including current methods of transfusion support.
3. Elucidate common transfusion reactions encountered in pediatric treatment environments.

INTRODUCTION

This chapter is designed to address the common questions and requests a pathology resident or other laboratory trainee might encounter while rotating through a pediatric blood bank. To comprehensively address each issue would be the work of a book, not a chapter. The aim here, therefore, is to provide an immediately acceptable answer. The hope is that you will be intrigued enough by pediatric transfusion medicine to delve further and use the references in finding more complete answers.

BLOOD PRODUCT REQUESTS

Aliquots

Possibly the most frequent request in pediatric transfusion medicine is for a partial unit of a blood product (aliquot or divide) for a smaller patient. While standard doses in adults tend to be in whole units, pediatric dosing is usually done in milliliters per kilogram (mL/kg). Typical packed red blood dosing, for instance, is 10-15 mL/kg of patient weight, which should translate into a 2-3 g/dL increase in hemoglobin.[1] Platelets are expected to increase in count by 50-100 thousand with a dose of 5-10 mL/kg. A plasma dose of 10-15 mL/kg should increase circulating clotting factors by 15-20%. Finally, if fibrinogen is selectively needed, 1-2 unit per 10 kg of cryoprecipitated Anti-Hemophilic Factor (AHF) is expected to raise the level 60-100 mg/dL.

Any service providing red cells to patients smaller than 20 kg (300 mL typical additive solution leukoreduced unit[2] at dose of 15 mL/kg) must have a way to provide sterilely produced aliquots or divides. Products prepared in such a manner have a 28 day out-date or their original expiration date, whichever comes first. Some blood centers initially process blood products into "pedipacks." For example, a set of two to three 75 mL each bags of plasma, all from one donor, would expire after 1 year of frozen storage.[2] Aliquots and divides prepared using an open system expire 24 hours after being made (see section Whole Blood later).

Irradiation

The purpose of X-ray or gamma irradiation is to prevent transfusion associated graph versus host disease (TA-GVHD). Standard dose (25 Gray) irradiation prevents TA-GVHD by cross-linking the DNA of donor T-cells so they cannot replicate.[3] Settings for which irradiated cellular products are indicated include congenital immunodeficiency disorders and intra-uterine transfusions. Oncology patients with hematologic malignancies, undergoing chemotherapy, or receiving bone marrow transplants should also receive irradiated cellular blood products.[4] The other clearly indicated group is recipients who are generally immuno-competent but being transfused products from blood relatives or HLA matched individuals. Neonates have, by definition, an incomplete immune system. Whether this puts them at increased risk for TA-GVHD remains a matter of controversy. There are no documented cases of TA-GVHD in neonates without additional risk factors (ie, extreme prematurity, unrecognized DiGeorge syndrome).[5] Currently, most pediatric hospitals make an individual determination as to whether to irradiate all cellular blood products for their neonates. Irradiating blood products does not prevent allo-immunization to red cell or HLA antigens.

Washed Blood Products

Washed red blood cells are indicated in two main circumstances: recurrent allergic reactions and hyperkalemia. Since standard saline washing removes 98% of plasma from a red cell unit, IgA deficient patients or those known to have recurrent allergic reactions should receive these products. Potassium concentration increases with length of red cell storage. Small patients undergoing cardiovascular surgery, appear to be at increased risk for hyperkalemic arrest. Also, patients who are sick enough to require transfusion often have electrolyte disturbances including hyperkalemia. Washing in an open system gives the red blood cells (rbcs) a 24-hour expiration.[4] Because potassium can re-accumulate rapidly after washing, some authors recommend transfusion within the first 12 hours of that window.[2] Another group looked at blood one day after expiration, and measured the potassium that accumulated after washing.[6] Without irradiation they concluded that a unit should not accumulate more than 5 mEq/L for at least 6 hours. After irradiation, the safe window was only 3 hours.

Platelet Transfusion

There is little controversy that bleeding patients with thrombocytopenia can benefit from platelet transfusion. Much of the literature debate focuses on the prophylactic use of platelet transfusions in patients with a failure of production. After chemotherapy or hematopoietic stem cell transplant, failure of the bone marrow to produce normal numbers of platelets is predictable. The first set of multiple studies to address when or if these patients should receive platelets were conducted in the 1960s.[7,8] From this early work, a prophylactic transfusion threshold of 20,000/μL was widely adopted and mortality from hemorrhage in cases of hematologic malignancy dropped to less than 1%.[9] More recent studies indicate that a prophylactic platelet trigger at 10,000/μL is equivalent in reducing bleeding risk,[10-13] and the American Society of Clinical Oncology and the British Committee for Standards in Hematology have adopted this threshold.[14] In practice, many centers increase this threshold for conditions associated with increased bleeding risks: intracranial mass lesions, uncontrolled hypertension, recent gastrointestinal hemorrhage, or the immediately post-operative state. Sub-group analysis of recent platelet dose study, indicated that pediatric patients were more likely than adults to have grade 2 or 3 bleeding after stem cell transplant.[15] The authors did not necessarily recommend increasing the prophylactic threshold beyond 10,000/μL, however, because the bleeding occurred over a large range of platelet counts.

Prophylactic transfusion thresholds tend to be higher in two situations: neonates and prior to invasive procedures. Expert opinion supports a 30,000/μL platelet transfusion trigger in neonates who are stable and not bleeding. Stable yet bleeding pre-mature infants are transfused below 50,000/μL. Finally, experts recommend 100,000/μL as the cut-off for sick, premature infants with active bleeding. Infants prior to an invasive procedure are also transfused according to the 50,000 and 100,000/μL cut-offs.[1] In all patients, 50,000 μL is often used as the platelet transfusion threshold prior to surgery, central line placement, bronchoscopy, endoscopy, or solid organ biopsy despite some retrospective data, it is not superior to 20,000 µL in preventing procedural bleeding.[16]

Platelets are available for 5 days, whether manufactured from whole blood (random) or collected by apheresis (single donor). Many pediatric centers use apheresis platelets, to minimize the number of donors to which a recipient is exposed. One reason to limit exposures is to decrease the rate of allo-immunization and "platelet refractoriness" in which platelet transfusions fail multiple times to raise the platelet count. A single aliquot of 10 mL/kg of platelets should raise a pediatric patient's platelet count to 50,000-100,000/µL.[1] If a platelet count rises in a sample drawn within an hour of transfusion and later falls, then a consumptive process (splenic sequestration, on-going bleeding, thrombosis, etc.) is occurring.[2] If the platelet count is not increased in 1 hour, one must consider immunologic destruction more likely. Commercially available ELISAs are excellent screening tools to determine whether the patient's immune system is targeting HLA epitopes or platelet specific antigens. Many of the oncology patients that become platelet refractory have already been HLA-typed for current or future stem-cell transplant. These results can be forwarded to your blood provider, who can look for platelets that are HLA matched on a 1A (best) to 4B (worst) scale. If the patient is reacting to a platelet specific antigen, transfused platelets should be negative for that antigen (if typing reagents are available) and/or cross-matched.

Fresh Blood

There are a number of detrimental effects that occur, the longer blood is stored: the cells become less pliable and more prone to aggregating, loss of 2,3-diphosphoglycerate and ATP lead to decreased oxygen delivery, and potassium as well as other molecules leak into the supernatant.[17,18] These cumulative effects are known as the storage lesion and have long been theorized to affect clinical outcome. Multiple retrospective studies have associated "older" blood with poor clinical outcomes.[18-21] There are three fundamental issues with the retrospective studies: 1) as observational studies they cannot prove causation; 2) higher acuity patients receive more transfusions and are therefore more likely to receive older units; and 3) defining what constitutes exposure to "old" blood.[22] Even the use of multivariate analysis does not invalidate the first two points. The problem with defining exposure is that most patients received more than one transfusion. In addition, questions have not been answered as to what constitutes old. Four days? Seven? Fourteen? What constitutes enough old blood? Any? More old than fresh? In 2012, the ARIPI trial[23] compared (in double-blind, randomized controlled trial) transfusing blood stored for 7 days or less versus standard care of premature, very low-birth weight infants in Canada (mean age 15 days, median 13). The authors found no increased risk for any of the primary clinical outcomes (necrotizing enterocolitis, intraventricular hemorrhage, retinopathy of prematurity, bronchopulmonary dysplasia, and death). Similar studies are ongoing in adults (ABLE) and pediatric ICUs (ABC-PICU).[22] Until prospective and randomized data are available, each pediatric transfusion medicine service must collaborate with clinical departments in determining what day of storage cut-off should be set for which specialized populations (eg, cardiac surgery patients, chronically exchanged patients with sickle cell disease, etc.)

TRANSFUSION REACTIONS

The most important step in mitigating transfusion reactions, once they begin, is for the bedside team to recognize they are occurring. The transfusion should be halted and supportive care begun. A clerical check to confirm the correct patient is getting the correct blood product should be followed by urine and blood samples being sent to the blood bank (along with any remaining portion of the implicated unit). Laboratory personnel should check for hemolysis, hemoglobinuria, and run a Direct Antiglobulin Test(DAT) on the post-transfusion sample. Positive testing necessitates testing the pre-transfusion (ie, type and screen) sample to see whether the positive DAT was present and whether the strength of the reaction has changed.

Transfusion Related Acute Lung Injury

Transfusion Related Acute Lung Injury (TRALI) is the most common fatal transfusion reaction, constituting 37% of transfusion related deaths reported to the FDA from 2008-2012.[24] Reported estimates of the frequency of TRALI range from 1:400 to 1:50,000 units transfused.[25] This extremely wide estimated range reflects the variability in clinical recognition of TRALI, with resultant underreporting in many cases. TRALI may be more common in critically ill patients. This concept is illustrated by at least one prospective cohort study that found an 8% incidence of acute lung injury within 6 hours of transfusion in ICU patients.[26] Both one-hit (anti-HLA or anti-neutrophil antibodies) and two-hit mechanisms (antibodies in conjunction with endothelial/leukocyte priming) have been proposed as the etiology of TRALI. Indeed, as TRALI is a clinical syndrome, more than one mechanism can potentially result in a final common pathway of pulmonary endothelial damage and capillary leak. The one-hit hypothesis is predicated on the effects of a biologic response modifier, either anti-HLA antibodies (which are found in 15-26% of units from multiparous donors) or anti-neutrophil antibodies or neutrophil-activating lipid mediators (ie, white cell priming lipids) present within transfused units. Any of these potential biologic modifiers can then further activate or attack circulating and pulmonary leukocytes or pulmonary endothelium directly and ultimately stimulate complement activation and pulmonary injury.[27] In the two-hit hypothesis, the previous mechanisms are preceded by an additional hit which involves priming of the pulmonary endothelium via a precipitating event in the recipient that activates the endothelium and leads to neutrophil sequestration. This precipitating event or "first hit" is a system primer that reduces the threshold with respect to the effects of the biologic response modifier and usually is a clinical condition, which involves systemic activation of inflammatory and/or hemostatic systems (eg, sepsis, Disseminated Intravascular Coagulation (DIC), hypoperfusion etc.). Whether precipitated by a one or two hit mechanism, the net result is rapid development of a pulmonary capillary congestion and increased permeability. Clinically this manifests as rapid (eg, within minutes to several hours after transfusion) development of dyspnea, tachypnea, hypoxemia, and increased oxygen requirements secondary to pulmonary injury/edema that necessitates administration of higher FIO_2 via supplemental oxygen administration and intubation with mechanical ventilatory support in 70-80% of patients.

With ventilatory and hemodynamic supportive management, most patients recover within 48-96 hours, however, mortality rates of 5-25% have been reported.[25] Although TRALI can occur with any blood components, it is more common in patients receiving plasma-containing components. One study estimated the fatality rate from TRALI as 4.9 deaths per million plasma units transfused, 3.1 per apheresis platelet units, and 0.4 per red cell unit.[28] The SHOT trial in Great Britain demonstrated that the majority of TRALI cases were related to transfusion of blood components derived from leukocyte antibody positive female donors.[29] After adoption of a policy in the United Kingdom to minimize the transfusion of FFP and platelets from female donors, both suspect cases (36 to 11) and TRALI related deaths (7 to 0) decreased between 2003 and 2012.[24] AABB guidelines for 2014 included a similar restriction for the United States, "Plasma shall be from males, females who have not been pregnant, or females who have been tested since their most recent pregnancy."[30]

Acute Hemolytic Transfusion Reactions

Acute Hemolytic Transfusion Reactions (AHTR) have traditionally resulted from ABO incompatible red cell infusions. Between 2008 and 2012, however, 31 non-ABO hemolytic transfusion reactions were reported to the FDA compared to only 22 ABO hemolytic transfusion reactions.[24] If the recipient's antibody fixes compliment, then intravascular hemolysis occurs.[4] The membrane attack complex (C5b-9) is formed and causes red cell lysis. The resulting plasma free hemoglobin can be as high as 200 mg/dL or more (normal pediatric range: 0-100 mg/dL). In AHTRs, therefore, it is important to look for a pink or red discoloration to the plasma in transfusion reaction samples sent to the blood bank. Once haptoglobin is saturated, free hemoglobin molecules move through the glomerulous causing hemoglobinuria. Thus, a recipient urine sample should be obtained as soon as possible during a transfusion reaction work-up. Meanwhile, compliment 3a, 5a, and other inflammatory mediators can precipitate the profound hypotension and shock that are clinical hallmarks of AHTRs. Other reactions commonly seen in this medical emergency include: fever, chills, anxiety, DIC, dyspnea, chest pain, and flank pain. Life threatening reactions are less common if the antibody only fixes C3 or does not fix compliment at all, because such antibodies result in extra-vascular hemolysis. However, any hemolytic transfusion reaction can constitute a medical emergency. Therefore, AHTR should always be considered in the differential especially since they can present initially with minimal symptoms (eg, mild hypotension, fever).

Delayed Hemolytic Transfusion Reactions

Days (anamnestic) to weeks (de novo alloimmunity) after a transfusion, the recipient immune system can form antibodies against the transfused red blood cells. Such reactions usually result in IgG mediated extravascular clearance of donated red cells. While this decreases the effective half-life of the transfusion, in most cases Delayed Hemolytic Transfusion Reactions (DHTRs) result in few clinical symptoms. Often they will be detected on follow-up antibody screen (tested every three days to look for new clinically significant antibodies), DAT, or by the unexpectedly quick drop in hemoglobin. Other laboratory findings are associated with the hemolysis (increased LDH, unconjugated hyperbilirubinemia, and decreased haptoglobin) and the body's response to it (increased reticulocyte count). If the antibody targets Kell or Duffy blood group antigens, then hemolysis is more likely to be intravascular. Even if intravascular, DHTRs are less likely to be life-threatening than AHTRs because less compliment and other pro-inflammatory cytokines are generated.

Allergic Transfusion Reactions

Allergic reactions occur with 1-3% of transfusions.[31] Because they are so common and usually self-limited, it has been suggested that one can continue a transfusion if all symptoms resolve quickly with anti-histamine treatment (usually diphenhydramine).[4] Mild transfusion reactions present with symptoms, such as: pruritis, urticaria, and flushing. On the other end of the spectrum, severe anaphylactic allergic reactions occur rarely, but can be life-threatening. Symptoms associated with severe allergic reactions include: fevers, chills, dyspnea, wheezing, and/or laryngeal edema. True analphylactic reactions occur from antibodies to: IgA, haptoglobin, or compliment factor four (C4). Treatment with fluid resuscitation, epinephrine, steroids, vasopressors, or intubation may be required. Patients who have had severe allergic reactions should receive washed RBCs for future transfusions. Pre-transfusion treatment with diphenhydramine was not shown to prevent allergic reactions in at least one randomized trial.[32] Despite this, diphenhydramine pre-treatment is still in wide clinical use.

Infectious Complications

The infusion of bacterially contaminated blood is an uncommon cause of febrile transfusion reactions (approximately 1:2,000 units contaminated with bacteria).[32,33] The risk of sepsis is much greater (ie, 40 fold) from platelets (stored at 20-24°C) than from RBCs (stored at 4°C). This complication accounts for 11% of transfusion-related fatalities reported to the FDA 2008-2012.[34] To enhance blood safety, rapid bacterial screening of all platelet products was introduced in the United States in 2004. A review of the American Red Cross experience using culture-based screening for bacterial contamination of apheresis platelet products has demonstrated a rate of sepsis in 1:75,000 units and a fatality rate of 1:500,000 units.[34] It had been previously estimated that infusion of bacterial contaminated components results in 20 deaths per million units transfused.[33] The Gram negative septic shock associated with RBC transfusion is related to the effects of endotoxin produced by pathogenic bacteria that grow at 4°C (eg, *Yersinia enterocolitica*) which have been isolated at a frequency of 1:50,000 red cell units.[35]

The risk of transmission of lipid enveloped viruses, such as HIV (1:1.5 million), HTLV I/II (1:2.5 million), Hepatitis B (1:765,000) and Hepatitis C (1: 1.1 million) has greatly decreased over time,[36,37] with utilization of more sensitive immunoassays and the use of nucleic acid amplification testing (NAT).[34] Hepatitis D is problematic only when there is ongoing or prior HBV infection whereas transmission of either the enterically-transmitted Hepatitis A or E via transfusion is rare. Compared to transmission rates for these viruses, other blood-borne infectious diseases, such as: syphilis, Epstein-Barr virus, leishmaniasis, Lyme disease, brucellosis, B-19 parvovirus (increased prevalence in hemophiliacs), tick-borne encephalitis virus, Colorado Tick fever virus, and human herpes viruses as well as parasitic diseases (eg, malaria, babesiosis, toxoplasmosis and Chagas' disease) and possibly vCJD are rarely (ie, as compared to transmission rates for the lipid enveloped viruses) transmitted via transfusion in the United States. However, these pathogens can result in significant transfusion risks in some areas of the world and with ever increasing international travel and immigration, these pathogens can potentially increase transfusion risks in the United States. An example is West Nile virus (WNV) which was first identified in the United States in 1999, and was transmitted via either transplant or transfusion transmission. Introduction of WNV NAT testing potentially prevented 1500 cases of transfusion-transmitted WNV in 2003.[38]

Febrile Non-Hemolytic Transfusion Reactions

There are many reasons for a fever during transfusion: AHTR, bacterial contamination of the unit, the patient's underlying condition, etc. Febrile Non-Hemolytic Transfusion Reaction (FNHTR), therefore, is a diagnosis of exclusion.[4] Other causes of fever ruled out, the fever must still meet criteria: over 38°C by oral thermometer and an increase of at least 1°C from pre-transfusion measurements.[31] Interestingly, a FNHTR can also be diagnosed on the basis of chills and/or rigors alone. Most FNHTR can be treated with anti-pyretics and are without long-term sequelae. However, rigors can be problematic when patients cardiac and/or respiratory systems are already inadequate. The estimated incidence of FNHTRs is higher in platelets (0.06 to 2.2%) than red cells(0.04 to 0.44%).[4] Pre-storage leukocyte filtration is also thought to reduce the incidence.[8]

Hyperhemolysis Syndrome in Sickle Cell Disease

Patients with sickle cell disease (SCD) are at risk for many complications of transfusion. One syndrome which is mostly seen in SCD (but also reported in thalassemia, myelofibrosis, lymphoma,etc) is hyperhemolysis syndrome.[39] Patients present with fever, pain, and other symptoms that can closely resemble a sickle cell pain crisis.[40] The anemia can be severe and even life threatening as a brisk hemolysis of both transfused cells and bystander red cells occurs. The laboratory findings include: anemia with a hemoglobin often below pre-transfusion levels, reticulocytopenia, and multiple markers of hemolysis. However, the DAT is often negative.[39,40] Since the DAT reflects intravascular hemolysis, this finding supports one proposed mechanism for hyperhemolysis: red cell destruction via peripheral macrophages.[40] No evidence based treatment guidelines for this disorder have been established, but current interventions include: IVIG, steroids, and avoiding additional transfusions.

▌VARIOUS TREATMENT PROTOCOLS

Leukocyte reduction

There are three main advantages to leukocyte reduced blood products: 1) fewer febrile transfusion reactions (FNHTRs), 2) less Human Leukocyte Antigen (HLA) alloimmunization, and 3) leukocyte reduced products are CMV "reduced risk."[4] Pre-storage (at the time of collection or shortly thereafter) leukocyte reduction is generally considered superior to bedside filtration because fewer cytokines accumulate and adequate leukoreduction (to less than 5 times 10^6 white cells per unit) is more likely to occur. Many pediatric hospitals and some adult institutions provide only leukoreduced blood products. When not universally available, such products are best reserved for those at high risk for FNHTRs, HLA alloimmunzation or CMV infection. When leukoreduction was first introduced, there was controversy over whether it was as effective as blood from CMV seronegative donors at preventing CMV infection. Studies showing leukoreduction's effectiveness in at risk populations (such as very low birth weight neonates[41] and stem cell transplant recipients[42]) continue to accumulate. However, research is still ongoing and not all physicians taking care of CMV at risk populations consider leukocyte reduction alone sufficient.

Whole Blood

Whole blood is often used to fill extra-corporeal circuits in both the Intensive Care Unit (Extra-Corporeal Membrane Oxygenation and Continual Veno-Venous Hemofiltration) and Operating Room (bypass). At least two studies have indicated fresh (less than 48 hours old) whole blood may reduce coagulation abnormalities after bypass.[43,44] The logistical difficulty of maintaining a fresh whole blood inventory, however, regularly means that some hospitals are not able or willing to provide this product. Patients are then transfused with whole blood reconstituted from compatible red cells and plasma products.

Preservative Solutions

The addition of additive solutions (AS1 and AS3) allows an expiration date of 42 days. However, these solutions also introduce mannitol and adenine, two substances that cause nephrotoxicity at high concentrations in laboratory animals.[2] Additionally, mannitol can act as a diuretic and cause changes in intracerebral pressure. Especially in neonatal patients at high risk for intracerebral hemorrhage, this theoretical risk is excessive for some physicians. For the subset of hospitals still using it, obtaining units persevered in more traditional solutions (ie, CPD, CPDA-1, or C2PD) can be difficult in the 21st century when most units are stored in additive solution. For standard volume transfusions, there is a randomized single-blind clinical trial in very low birth weight infants showing transfusions from additive solution units that are just as safe as those containing CPDA-1.[45]

Granulocytes

Granulocyte infusion can be a useful adjunct to therapy in a neutropenic patient with a documented infection which has not responded to 24 to 48 hours of standard antimicrobial therapy, when the neutropenia is considered to be reversible.[2] In 2005, a meta-analysis was performed regarding using granulocytes to treat infections in neutropenic patients.[46] The authors concluded that the odds ratio favored transfusing granulocytes to prevent mortality (RR = 0.64). Survival was improved more (mortality RR = 0.37) in those studies where dose was at least $1 \times 10^{10}/m^2$. The data was so heterogeneous, however, that the study was called inconclusive. All studies were conducted at least 25 years ago, mortality data was collected at widely varying time points, the number of granulocytes transfused differed, and even the definitions of what constituted neutropenia were discordant. Only 4 of 8 studies in the 2005 analysis included children and the majority of the patients were adults with AML. By contrast, a 2011 study by the same database looked at only granulocyte transfusion in neutropenic neonates.[47] Unfortunately but not surprisingly, there were fewer studies (4 vs. 8) and patients (44 vs. 310) available to perform an analysis in neonates. The authors were unable to recommend for or against transfusion of granuloctyes in neutropenic newborns.

Based on the adult studies, the AABB requires that 75% of products for non-neonates contain 1×10^{10} granulocytes.[3] Because this is difficult to obtain in un-stimulated donors, granulocyte donors are often stimulated with steroids or Granulocyte-Colony-Stimulating-Factor (G-CSF). Granulocyte products should also be ABO-compatible and cross-matched, unless the apheresis technique used yields less than two milliliters of red blood cells in an entire product. These products are stored at room temperature. Granulocytes should be transfused as soon as possible, because they expire after 24 hours.[2,3]

Apheresis

The 2013 American Society for Apheresis Guidelines recognize four categories of indication for therapeutic apheresis.[48] Category I includes "disorders for which apheresis is accepted as first line therapy either as primary standalone treatment or in conjunction with other modes of treatment." Similarly, category II indications are those "for which apheresis is accepted as second-line therapy either as primary standalone treatment or in conjunction with other modes of treatment." By contrast, category III indications are those where the "optimum role of apheresis therapy is not established" and "treatment should be individualized." Finally, category IV includes disease states "in which published evidence demonstrates or suggests apheresis is ineffective or even harmful" and recommends IRB approval before beginning treatment.

Published therapeutic apheresis complication rates are higher in children than adults. The adverse event rate in pediatrics is reported as 5.6 to 55%.[49,50] The rate of side effects in adult apheresis is reported as 4.3 to 28%. Also, the common indications for apheresis vary in children and adults (see Table 17-1). Three of the five top indications for plasma exchange are the same in children

Table 17-1	**FIVE MOST COMMON INDICATIONS FOR TPE IN US CHILDREN (2003-10) VERSUS CANADIAN ADULTS (2010)**	
	Pediatric[1]	Adult[2]
1	Myasthenia Gravis (29%)	TTP/HUS(25%)
2	Thrombotic Thrombocyopenic Purpura (27%)	Myasthenia Gravis (21%)
3	Guillain-Barre Syndrome (19%)	Chronic Inflammatory Demyelinating Polyneuropathy(6%)
4	ANCA Positive Vasculitis (10%)	ANCA Positive Vasculitis (5%)
5	Rasmussen's Encephalitis (5%)	Waldenstrom's (5%)

[1] Pediatric data from Weiss et al. *J Clin Apher.* 27:287-294 (2012), extracted from database covering 70% of US freestanding children's hospitals.

[2] Adult data from Canadian Apheresis Group as reported by Clark, W.F. *J Clin Apher.* 27:112-116 (2012).

Note: Pediatric data is per hospital admission diagnosis in patients receiving apheresis (total 506) and adult data is per TPE procedure (total 9246).

and adults, however, so it is logical that the guidelines developed mainly via studies in adults apply to pediatrics. There is little choice until a larger body of pediatric transfusion medicine literature is published.

There are many physiologic differences between children and adults that affect therapeutic apheresis. The most obvious is size. Smaller children make obtaining adequate vascular access more difficult. Whether peripheral access or dual-lumen dialysis compatible catheter, they are all harder to place in smaller veins. Also, central lines are more difficult to keep open in children. To maintain patency, these catheters are packed with heparin. However, there is fear regarding the heparin causing systemic anticoagulation if accidently flushed into small patients, especially tiny infants.

Another issue of size is priming the circuit. Although modern apheresis machines operate by continuous flow, an aliquot of patient whole blood must replace the initial saline prime. While this approximately 200 mL (depending on instrument choice and blood warmer use) of extra-corporeal volume is usually tolerated by adults, it constitutes a much larger portion of what is contained in a 25 kg child's veins. So pediatric transfusion medicine physicians prime with: pRBC(66%), whole blood(42%), or albumin(17%).[51]

Manual Exchanges

Different apheresis services have different comfort levels with using automated apheresis instruments in small infants (less than 10-15 kg). An alternative with a long tradition (especially in Neonatal Intensive Care Units) is to use a two way stopcock, whole blood (either fresh or reconstituted), and a syringe to remove and replace aliquots of blood. A two blood volume exchange is generally used to treat disorders of the plasma compartment (such as hyperbilirubinemia) compared to a one volume exchange to treat anemia or coagulopathies.[52]

Massive Transfusion

An adult trauma patient who arrives to the emergency department with abnormal coagulation testing (PT or PTT) has a worse prognosis, independent of his or her injury severity score (ISS).[53] The question is whether the coagulopathy of trauma can be corrected to help the patient survive. In 2007, medical personnel in the armed services published retrospective data showing the closer the wounded came to receiving one unit of plasma for every unit of pRBCs, the more likely they were to survive.[54] It is unknown whether this was survivor bias. Did those who were less severely wounded survive to get the plasma? In 2008, a group at Vanderbilt published a case control series comparing outcomes before and after a trauma protocol of 10 pRBCs, 4 units of plasma, and 2 single-donor platelets was implemented.[55] Even though ISS were comparable (worse but not statistically significant in protocol group), there was less blood product utilization in the first 24 hours and better 30 day mortality with the protocol in place. There have been many published massive transfusion cohorts since then.[56-58] Multiple authors argue that civilian centers should adopt the military 1 pRBC:1 plasma:1 platelet protocol.[56,58] In 2010 the AABB convened a 17 member expert panel to perform a "systemic review and meta-analysis."[59] The panel came to two conclusions: 1) they "suggest that plasma be transfused to trauma patients requiring massive" transfusion, and 2) that "we cannot recommend for or against the transfusion of plasma at plasma:RBC ratio of 1:3 or more."

There is even less evidence in pediatric massive transfusion. If one compares three published protocols, there is no agreement regarding: 1) what constitutes a massive transfusion/when to initiate the protocol or 2) what ratio of blood products to utilize in pediatrics.[60-62] In the absence of more data, it seems logical to implement a massive transfusion protocol for pediatric trauma patients. The chapter author is aware of at least one survey and a separate multi-center study currently attempting to clarify the most beneficial way to apply a massive transfusion protocol to pediatric trauma.

Transfusion-Associated Hyperkalemic Cardiac Arrest

One complication of massive transfusion in children, especially infants and neonates, is Transfusion-Associated Hyperkalemic Cardiac Arrest (TAHCA). One literature review found nine cases of TAHCA.[63] Risk factors possibly associated with the arrests included: older age of red blood cells, rate (more than overall volume) of infusions, use of smaller gauge central lines, and the presence of co-morbities, such as anemia. The review also presented some recommended interventions to prevent TAHCA, such as: use of larger bore (22 gauge or lower) peripheral IV catheters, avoiding rapid infusers, checking and treating metabolic abnormalities more often, transfusing as soon as possible after irradiation, and considering washing RBCs, as indicated.

OTHER CONSIDERATIONS IN PEDIATRIC TRANSFUSION MEDICINE

Hemolytic Disease of the Newborn

Asymptomatic hemorrhage in one pregnancy can lead to maternal production of IgG to paternal red cell antigens in subsequent pregnancies. Naturally occurring ABO antibodies are the exception and are already present as a result of environmental antigens (no paternal exposure required). The resulting antibody-mediated red cell destruction in subsequent pregnancies leads to anemia. The anemia has many deleterious effects on the fetus, especially when severe. To compensate, there is increased erythropoiesis in the liver leading to decreased albumin production.[64] The cardiovascular failure from the anemia and the loss of oncotic pressure from hypoalbuminemia result in a deadly generalized edema with pericardial and pleural effusions known as hydrops fetalis.

Prior to the advent of Rhesus immune globin Rh D alloimmunization occurred in approximately 1% of pregnancies. In 2003, that number had decreased to 6.8 cases per 1,000 live births.[64] While Rh remains the most common cause, severe HDN can also be caused by antibodies to Kell, Duffy, Kidd, and MNS blood group antigens.[65] Fortunately, current therapy including modern intrauterine transfusion techniques developed in the 1980's has led to perinatal survival rates approaching 95% in experienced hands.[66] Red cell units for intrauterine transfusion should be: irradiated, CMV reduced risk, ABO compatible with both mother and fetus, and most often are included as one of the specialized populations for which units less than 5-7 days old are indicated.

Neonatal Alloimmune Thrombocytopenia

There are at least a dozen causes of neonatal thrombocytopenia. The most clinically important is neonatal alloimmune thrombocytopenia (NAIT).[67] When immune causes of thrombocytopenia are suspected, maternal platelet count should be reviewed. Maternal thrombocytopenia indicates Neonatal

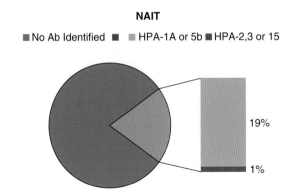

NAIT

■ No Ab Identified ■   ■ HPA-1A or 5b ■ HPA-2,3 or 15

19%

1%

Figure 17-1 ■ Causative antibodies in NAIT. Data from Chakravorty.[67]

Autoimmune Thrombocytopenia, due to mom's systemic lupus erythematosus, idiopathic thrombocytopenic purpura, etc. Normal maternal platelet count indicates NAIT. Mom lacks a human platelet antigen (HPA) that the neonate expresses. Maternal antibodies cross the placenta and recognize the child's platelets as foreign. The gold standard diagnostic test is the monoclonal antibody-specific immobilization of platelet antigens. Some experts also recommend genotyping the infant for the most common HPA targets (HPA-1a,2,3,5b, and 15), but these only account for 20% of causative antibodies (see Figure 17-1). Research testing on the remaining 80% sometimes identifies antibodies to minor antigens, such as 6w or 9w, but the causative antibody remains unknown in the majority of cases.[68] The main goal of therapy is to maintain platelet count of 50,000/μL or greater for the first week of life and avoid the most devastating complication: intracranial hemorrhage (ICH).[67] This is accomplished with platelets negative for the causative HPA (if known) and IVIG administration. IVIG is thought to inhibit peripheral destruction of platelets, but it can take up to 36 hours to raise the platelet count.[67] Testing, especially if sent out to a reference laboratory, may also take some time to get back. If available, pediatric transfusion medicine practitioners should consider HPA-1a and 5b negative platelets empirically. British Committee for Standards in Hematology guidelines recommends not delaying treatment if antigen negative platelets are not available.[67] Maternal platelets should, by definition, be free of the causative HPA, but can be logistically difficult to obtain and wash or plasma reduce in a clinically relevant time-frame. Unlike with HDN, NAIT can be severe in the first pregnancy.

Neonatal Alloimmune Neutropenia

The maternal immune system can react to human neutrophil antigens (HNAs) similarly to how it reacts to HPAs and red cell antigens.[69] The resulting Neonatal Alloimmune Neutropenia (NAIN) can be asymptomatic, though omphalitis and mild skin infections are common.[70] Despite absolute neutrophil counts that are often less than 500×10^6 per liter, severe infectious complications, such as pneumonia and meningitis are rare.[71] Antibiotics alone are usually sufficient treatment for NAIN related infections. However, IVIG and G-CSF have been used successfully in severe cases.[69,70] Mean duration of neutropenia is 11 weeks.[69]

SUMMARY

For many years, a large number of pediatric transfusion medicine treatments were extrapolated from adults, based on expert opinion, or from small and retrospective studies. The recent RECESS trial looked at the effect of red blood storage age on MODS (primary) and mortality (secondary) in patients undergoing cardiac surgery.[72] The authors found no statistical difference in either outcome with changes in length of red cell storage. While the median patient age was 72-73 years, inclusion criteria was 12 years or older and at least one 14-year-old was included. Currently, encouraging work is being done in length of red cell storage and massive transfusion that is pediatric specific.[22] I hope in engaging this chapter, the reader is intrigued enough follow the field of pediatric transfusion medicine as it continues to grow and mature.

TRAINING MODULE

1. According to 2012 FDA data, what is the most common fatal transfusion reaction:
   a. Acute Hemolytic Transfusion Reaction (AHTR)
   b. Transfusion Related Acute Lung Injury (TRALI)
   c. Allergic Transfusion Reaction (ATR)
   d. Septic Transfusion Reaction (STR)

2. Which of the following recipients do NOT require irradiated blood products:
   a. Patients with hematologic malignancies currently on chemotherapy
   b. A fetus receiving intra-uterine transfusion
   c. A patient receiving products from a genetically related family member
   d. Patients with sickle cell disease receiving a large volume transfusion

3. The American Society of Clinical Oncology and the British Committee for Standards in Hematology recommend what platelet count as a prophylactic transfusion trigger in non-bleeding patients:
   a. 5,000 per mm^3
   b. 10,000 per mm^3
   c. 20,000 per mm^3
   d. 30,000 per mm^3

REFERENCES

1. Josephson CD. Neonatal and pediatric transfusion practice. In: Robrack JD, Grossman BJ, Harris T, Hillyer CD, eds. *Technical Manual.* 17th ed. Bethesda, MD: AABB;2011:645-670.

2. Roseff SD ed. *Pediatric Transfusion: A Physician's Handbook.* 3rd ed. Bethesda, MD:AABB;2006.

3. Kakaiya R, Aronson CA, Julleis J. Whole blood collection and component processing at blood collection centers. In: Robrack JD, Grossman BJ, Harris T, Hillyer CD, eds. *Technical Manual.* 17th ed. Bethesda, MD:AABB;2011:187-226

4. King KE ed. *Blood Transfusion: A Physician's Handbook,* 10th ed. Bethesda, MD:AABB;2011.

5. Strauss RG: Data-driven blood banking practices for neonatal RBC transfusions. *Transfusion.* 2000;40:1528-1540.

6. Weiskopf RB, Schnapp S, Rouine-Rapp K, et al. Extracellular potassium concentrations in red blood cell suspensions after irradiation and washing. *Transfusion.* 2005;45:1295-1301.

7. Gaydos. The quantitative relation between platelet count and hemorrhage in patients with acute leukemia. *N Engl J Med.* 1962;266:905-909.

8. Parker RI. Transfusion in critically Ill children: indications, risks and challenges. *Crit Care Med.* 2014;42:675-690

9. Slichter SJ. Controversies in platelet transfusion therapy. *Ann Rev Med.* 1980; 31: 509-540.

10. Rubella. The threshold for prophylactic platelet transfusions in adults with acute myeloid leukemia. *New Engl J Med.* 1997;337: 1870-1875.

11. Zumberg. A prospective randomized trial of prophylactic platelet transfusion and bleeding incidence in haemopoietic stem cell transplant recipients: 10,000/uL vs 20,000/uL trigger. *Biol Blood Marrow Transplant.* 2002;8:569-576.

12. Wandt. Safety and cost-effectiveness of a 10x109/L trigger for prophylactic platelet transfusions compared with the traditional 20x109/L trigger: a prospective comparative trial in 105 patients with acute myeloid leukemia. *Blood.* 1998;91:3601-3606.

13. Heddle NM, Cook RJ, Tinmouth A, et al. SToP Study Investigators of the BEST collaborative: a randomized controlled trial comparing standard and low-dose strategies for transfusion of platelets (SToP) to patients with thrombocytopenia. *Blood.* 2009;113:1564-1573.

14. British Committee for Standards in Haematology (BCSH): guidelines for the use of platelet transfusions. *Br J Haematol.* 2003; 122: 10-23.

15. Josephson CD, Granger S, Assman SF, et al. Bleeding risks are higher in children versus adults given prophylactic platelet transfusions for treatment-induced hypoproliferative thrombocytopenia. *Blood.* 2012;120(4):748-760

16. Zeidler K, Arn K, Senn O, et al. Optimal preprocedural platelet transfusion threshold for central venous catheter insertions in patients with thrombocytopenia. *Transfusion.* 2011;51:2269-2276.

17. Vandromme MJ, McGwin Jr G, and Weinburg JA. Blood Transfusion in the Critically Ill: does storage age matter? *Scand J Trauma Resusc Emerg Med.* 2009;17: 35-41.

18. Purdy FR, Tweeddale MG, Merrick PM: Association of mortality with age of blood transfused in septic ICU patients. *Can J Anaesth*. 1997;44:1256-1261.

19. Vamvakas EC, Carven JH: Length of storage of transfused red cells and postoperative morbidity in patients undergoing coronary artery bypass graft surgery. *Transfusion*. 2000;40:101-109.

20. Murrell Z, Haukoos JS, Putnam B, et al. The effect of older blood on mortality, need for ICU care and length of ICU stay after major trauma. *Am Surg*. 2005;71:781-785.

21. Weinburg JA, McGwin, Marques MB, et al. Transfusions in the less severely injured: does age of transfused blood affect outcomes? *J Trauma*. 2008;65:794-8.

22. Lacroix J, Hebert P, Fergusson D, et al. The age of blood evaluation (ABLE) randomized controlled trial: study design. *Transfus Med Rev*. 2011;25(3):197-205.

23. Fergusson, DA, Herbert P, Hogan DL, et al. Effect of fresh red blood cell transfusions on clinical outcomes in premature, very low-birth-weight infants. *JAMA*. 2012;308(14):1443-1451.

24. Bolton-Maggs PH, Cohen H. Serious hazards of transfusion (SHOT) haemovigilance and progress is improving transfusion safety. *Br J Haematol*. 2013; 163:303-314.

25. Kleinman S, Caulfield T, Chan P, et al. Toward an understanding of transfusion related acute lung injury: statement of a consensus panel. *Transfusion*. 2004;44(12):1774-1789.

26. Gajic O, Rana R, Winters JL, et al. Transfusion-related acute lung injury in the critically ill: prospective nested case-control study. *Am J Respir Crit Care Med*. 2007;176:886-891.

27. McCullough J. Complications of transfusion. In: McCullough J, ed. *Transfusion Medicine*. New York, NY: McGraw-Hill. 1999:337-359.

28. Silliman CC, Paterson AJ, Dickey WO, et al. The association of biologically active lipids with the development of transfusion-related acute lung injury: a retrospective study. *Transfusion*. 1997;37:719-726.

29. Stainsby D, Jones H, Asher D, et al. Serious hazards of transfusion: a decade of hemovigilance in the UK. *Transfus Med Rev*. 2006;20:273-82.

30. Levitt J, Beaton MA, Benson K, et al. *Standards for Blood Banks and Transfusion Services*, 29th ed. Bethesda, MD:AABB; 2014.

31. Mazzei CA, Popovsky MA, and Kopko PM. Non-infectious complications of blood transfusion. In: Robrack JD, Grossman BJ, Harris T, Hillyer CD, eds. *Technical Manual*. 17th ed. Bethesda, MD:AABB;2011:727-757.

32. Kennedy L, Case L, Hurd D, et al. A prospective, randomized, double-blind controlled trial of acetaminophen and diphenhydramine pretransfusion medication versus placebo for the prevention of transfusion reactions. *Transfusion*. 2008;48:2285-2291.

33. Goodnough LT, Brecher ME, Kanter MH, et al. Transfusion Medicine: Blood Transfusion. *N Engl J Med*. 1999;340:438-447.

34. Goodnough LT, Shander A, Brecher ME. Transfusion medicine: looking to the future. *Lancet*. 2003;361:161-169.

35. Sazama K. Reports of 355 transfusion-associated deaths: 1976 through 1985. *Transfusion*. 1990;30:583-590.

36. Zou S, Stramer SL, Dodd RY. Donor testing and risk: current prevalence, incidence and residual risk of transfusion-transmissible agents in US allogeneic donations. *Transfus Med Rev*. 2012;26:119-128.

37. Stramer SL, Notari EP, Krysztof DE, Dodd RY. Hepatitis B virus testing by minipool nucleic acid testing: does it improve blood safety? Transfusion. 2013;53(10p2):2449-2458.

38. Kleinman S, Glynn SA, Busch M, et al. The 2003 West Nile virus United States epidemic: the America's Blood Centers experience. *Transfusion.* 2005;45:469-479.

39. Santos B, Portugal R, Nogueira C, et al. Hyperhemolysis syndrome in patients with sickle cell anemia: report of three cases. Transfusion 2015;55:1394-1398.

40. Uhlmann EJ, Shenoy S, and Goodnough LT. Successful treatment of recurrent hyperhemolysis syndrome with immunosuppression and plasma-to-red blood cell exchange transfusion. Tranfusion. 2014;54:384-388.

41. Delany M, Mayock D, Knezevic A, et al. Postnatal cytomegalovirus infection: a pilot comparative effectiveness study of transfusion safety using leukoreduced-only transfusion strategy. *Transfusion.* 2016;56(8):1945-1950.

42. Kekre N, Tokessy M, Mallick R et al. Is cytomegalovirus testing of blood products still needed in the era of universal leukoreduction? Biol Blood Marrow Transplant. 2013;19:1719-1724.

43. Manno CS, Hedberg KW, Kim HC et al. Comparison of the hemostatic effects of fresh whole blood, stored whole blood, and components after open heart surgery in children. *Blood.* 1991;77(5):930-936.

44. Greenwald CE, McCrindle BW, Crawford-Lean L, et al. Reconstituted fresh whole blood improves clinical outcome compared with stored component blood therapy for neonates undergoing cardiopulmonary bypass for cardiac surgery: a randomized controlled trial. *J Thor Cardiovasc Surg.* 2008;136(6):1442-1449.

45. Strauss RG, Burmeister LF, Johnson K et al. AS-1 red cells for neonatal transfusions: A randomized trial assessing donor exposure and safety. *Transfusion.* 1996;36:873-878.

46. Pammi M and Brocklehurst P. Granulocyte transfusions for neonates with confirmed or suspected sepsis and neutropenia (review). *Cochrane Database Syst Rev.* 2011;(10):CD003956.

47. Stanworth S, Massey E, Hyde C, et al. Granulocyte transfusions for treating infections in patients with neutropenia or neutrophil dysfunction (Review). *Cochrane Database Syst Rev.* 2005;(3):CD005339.

48. Schwartz J, Winters JL, Padmanabhan A, et al. Guidelines on the use of therapeutic apheresis in clinical practice- evidence-based approach from the Writing Committee of the American Society for Apheresis: the sixth special issue. *J Clin Apher.* 2013;28: 145-284.

49. Michon B, Moghrabi A, Winikoff R et al. Complications of apheresis in children. *Transfusion.*2007;47:1837-1842.

50. De Silvestro G, Tison T, Vicarioto M, et al. The Italian registry of pediatric therapeutic apheresis: a report on activity during 2005. *J Clin Apher.* 2009;24:1-5.

51. Delaney M, Capocelli KE, Eder AF, et al. An international survey of pediatric apheresis practice. *J Clin Apher.* 2014;29:120-126.

52. Wong EC and Luban NL: Intrauterine, neonatal, and pediatric transfusion. In: Mintz, PD ed. *Transfusion Therapy: Clinical Principles and Practice.* 2nd ed. Bethesda, MD: AABB Press; 2005: 159-201.

53. Brohi K, Singh J, Heron M, et al. Acute Traumatic Coagulopathy. *J Trauma.* 2003; 54(6):1127-1130.

54. Borgman MA, Spinella PC, Perkins JG, et al. The ratio of blood products transfused affects mortality in patients receiving massive transfusions at a combat support hospital. *J Trauma.* 2007:63(4):805-813.

55. Cotton BA, Gunter OL, Isbell J, et al. Damage control hematology: the impact of a trauma exsanguination protocol on survival and blood product utilization. *J Trauma.* 2008;64(5):1177-1182.

56. Duchesne JC, Hunt JP, Wahl G, et al. Review of current blood transfusions strategies in a mature level i trauma center: were we wrong for the last 60 years? *J Trauma.* 2008;65(2):272-278.

57. Kashuk JL, Moore EE, Johnson J, et al. Postinjury life threatening coagulopathy: is 1:1 fresh frozen plasma: packed cells the answer? *J Trauma.*2008;65(2):261-271.

58. Holcomb JB, Wade CE, Michalek JE, et al. Increased plasma and platelet to red blood cell ratios improves outcome in 466 massively transfused civilian trauma patients. *Ann Surg.* 2008;248(3):447-458.

59. Roback JD, Caldwell S, Carson J, et al. Evidence-based practice guidelines for plasma transfusion. *Transfusion.* 2010;50(6):1227-1239.

60. Dehmer JJ, Adamson WT. Massive transfusion and blood product use in the pediatric trauma patient. *Semin Pediatr Surg.* 2010;19(4):286-291.

61. Hendrickson JE, Shaz BE, Pareira G, et al. Implementation of a pediatric trauma massive transfusion protocol: one institution's experience. *Transfusion.* 2012;52:1228-1236.

62. Dressler AM, Finck CM, Carroll CL et al. Use of a massive transfusion protocol with hemostatic resuscitation for severe intraoperative bleeding in a child. *J Ped Surg.* 2010;45:1530-1533.

63. Lee AC, Reduque LL, Luban NLC et al. Transfusion-associated hyperkalemic cardiac arrest in pediatric patients receiving massive transfusion. *Transfusion.* 2014;54:244-254.

64. Moise Jr KJ. Management of Rhesus Alloimmunization in pregnancy. *Obstet Gynecol.* 2008;112(1): 164-176.

65. Prenatal typing of Rh and Kell blood group antigens: The edge of a watershed. *Transfus Med Rev.* 2003;17(1):31-44.

66. Lindenburg IT, Smits-Wintjens VE, van Klink JM, et al. Long-term neurodevelopmental outcome after intrauterine transfusion for hemolytic disease of the fetus/newborn: the LOTUS study. *Am J Obstet Gynecol.* 2012;141:e1-e8.

67. Chakravorty S and Roberts I. How I manage neonatal thrombocytopenia. *Br J Haematol.* 2012;156(2):155-162.

68. Risson DC, Davies MW, Williams BA. Review of neonatal alloimmune thrombocytopenia. *J Pediatr Child Health.* 2012;48(9):816-822.

69. Mraz GA, Crighton GL, Christie DJ. Antibodies to human neutrophil antigen HNA-4b implicated in a case of neonatal alloimmune neutropenia. *Transfusion.* 2016;56: 1161-1165.

70. Bux J, Jung KD, Kauth T, et al. Serological and clinical aspects of granulocyte antibodies leading to alloimmune neonatal neutropenia. *Transfus Med.* 1992;2:143-149.

71. Reil A, Sachs UJ, Siahanidou T et al. HNA-1d: a new human neutrophil antigen located on Fcγ receptor IIIb associated with neonatal immune neutropenia. *Transfusion.* 2013;53:2145-153.

72. Steiner ME, Ness PM, Assman DJ et al. Effects of Red-Cell Storage Duration on Patients Undergoing Cardiac Surgery. *NEJM.* 2015;372(15):1419-1429.

ANSWERS AND EXPLANATIONS

Chapter 1—Daily Issues in the Practice of Pediatric Laboratory Medicine

1. Which of the following is true about small sample volumes?

Answer: b. They can affect sample integrity for add-on tests. Small sample volumes are prone to evaporation effects, making sample integrity poor for adding on tests later. The other three answers are all false. Small samples should not be collected in regular sized tubes **a.**, they do affect instrumentation that can be used **c.** and when mislabeled are often allowed to be corrected **d.**, which is not common outside of pediatric labs.

2. Heelstick samples:

Answer: a. Should be collected from the side of the heel. This is always true. The other answers are not. The heel should be warmed before collection **b.**, the capillary blood collected is fine for more chemistry analyses **c.**, and fingerstick devices should never be used to perform a heelstick **d.**

3. When collecting multiple samples involving multiple tubes in a single blood collection opportunity:

Answer: c. For a capillary collection in micro-collection tubes, collect non-anticoagulated tubes last. When doing capillary collection, heel or fingerstick, clotting starts immediately, so anticoagulated tubes are collected first and non-anticoagulated tubes are collected last when it won't matter if it's clotting. The other answers are not true.

4. Send out testing:

Answer: b. Should be managed to prevent over-utilization. Sendout testing in any lab should be managed to prevent over-utilization, but it's extremely important in a pediatric lab where sendout testing is likely to be extensive **a.** Sendout testing does not include testing performed in-house **c.**, and it comprises an increasingly large part of the lab budget with the growth of expensive molecular genetic testing **d.**

5. A CLIA validation of LDTs includes:

Answer: b. A. plus a reference interval study. A CLIA validation of an LDT requires all of these things except a clinical utility study **d.**

Chapter 2—Common Tests and Consideration Important in Pediatric Medicine

1. As part of a work up for abdominal pain in a 4-year-old female, a complete metabolic panel is ordered. Physical exam was unremarkable. All the results are normal, except for alkaline phosphatase, which was 1,238 U/L (normal range: 85-370 U/L). What should the physician do with these results?

Answer: c. Order alkaline phosphatase isoenzymes. If bone and liver isoenzymes are equally elevated, then retest the patient in 4 months. Transient hyperphosphatemia occurs in 2-5% of healthy children and shows as a non-specific elevation of alkaline phosphatase with both bone and liver forms elevated. Elevation will have returned to normal in a few months.

2. A 3-month-old male presents with suspected new-onset diabetes type 1. To confirm the diagnosis, an A1C is ordered for this patient. However, the lab rejects the sample. Why?

Answer: b. The value of HbF is too high in a 3-month-old to report an accurate A1C. Hemoglobin F is high at birth and normalizes by about 6 months of age. It is not detected by immunoassay A1C methods and so A1C values may be falsely low. It is also true that A1C cutoffs for diabetes diagnosis were established in adults, and A1C may not be a good diagnostic test in children, but it continues to be used as such.

3. Which of the following is a common problem specifically encountered in pediatric laboratory testing?

Answer: a. Need for age-specific reference intervals

4. A 3-day-old newborn is screened for kernicterus risk prior to discharge. His total serum bilirubin at the hospital places him in the intermediate risk zone, and he is discharged with orders to have total serum bilirubin measured 24 hours later as an outpatient. The result from the outpatient laboratory is 3.5 mg/dL higher than at the hospital, moving him to the high risk zone. What could explain this increase?

Answer: d. All of the above

5. Which of the following is true about lead exposure?

Answer: c. Historically, many children were exposed to lead from lead gasoline.

Chapter 3—Inborn Errors of Metabolism

1. Explain how data acquisition in tandem mass spectrometry using precursor ion scanning is performed.

Answer: All acylcarnitine species lose a neutral molecule of butyl-carnitine with a m/z of 85 when fragmented in the collision cell of a tandem mass spectrometer. The precursor ions are 85 m/z units larger than the product ions, thus the mass selection quadrupole mass spectrometers (MS1 and MS3) are set to detect any precursor and product ions that are 85 m/z units apart.

2. What is the precursor ion common to all carnitine esters?

Answer: m/z 85

3. What is an isobaric compound when referring to mass analysis?

Answer: Compounds that have the same mass/charge ratio are isobaric. They must be separated chromatographically, as they cannot be distinguished apart in a mass spectrometer.

4. List the two carnitine esters that primarily contribute to the C4 component.

Answer: Butyryl- and isobutyryl-carnitines contribute to the C4-carnitine component.

5. List the carnitine esters that might contribute to the C5 component.

Answer: Isovaleryl- and 2-methylbutyryl-carnitines may contribute to the C5 component.

6. List the enzymes implicated by elevations of C4, C5, C6, C8, C10, C14, and C18 carnitine esters.

Answer: The following enzymes are implicated: short-chain acyl CoA dehydrogenase, isobutyryl CoA dehydrogenase, isovaleryl CoA dehydrogenase, 2-methylbutyryl CoA dehydrogenase, medium-chain acyl CoA dehydrogenase, very long chain acyl CoA dehydrogenase.

7. What is the difference between a C14 ester and a C14:1 carnitine ester?

Answer: Both are 14 carbon fatty acyl-carnitines. C14 is completely saturated, and C14:1 in mono-unsaturated, with a single double bond between 2 carbons.

8. How likely is it that all of these enzymes are deficient?

Answer: It is unlikely that all these enzymes are deficient.

9. Is there a diagnosis that can unify these biochemical findings?

Answer: Yes, a diagnosis of multiple acyl CoA dehydrogenase deficiency, also known as glutaric acidemia, type 2, would unify all these biochemical findings. This disorder results from defects in the electron transport chain ETF/ETF-QO enzymes on which all these dehydrogenases rely to transfer electrons, and thus effects many dehydrogenases, especially in the fatty acid oxidation pathway.

10. What molecules would be found in urine organic acid analysis in a patient with this condition?

Answer: Urine organic acid would show elevated excretion or ethylmalonic acid, glutaric acid, and multiple acylglycines including isovalerylglycine, and often hexanoyl- and suberylglycines. 3-hydroxyisovaleric acid is often present as well.

Chapter 4—Diagnostic Approach to the Patient with a Suspected Inborn effort of Metabolism

1. List a common reason other than IEM that may lead to the following laboratory results on day of life 2.

Answer: a. A low glucose may also be caused by many things, including fasting, liver disease, infections, maternal diabetes, and birth stress.

b. A high ammonia in a newborn may be caused by immature liver function or by delayed processing of the sample for ammonia analysis.

c. An elevated lactate may be caused by sepsis, seizures, asphyxia, or by preanalytical errors in blood sample processing.

d. Sample degradation can be a cause of low CO_2.

Each of these results may be secondary to an IEM but there are more common reasons for these circumstances. Neonatal hypoglycemia is very common during the transition from placental to oral feeding. 40 mg/dL represents a common threshold where intervention (glucose bolus) is considered. Mild increases in plasma ammonia occur transiently in the neonatal period and may also be secondary to delayed sample transport. Transiently elevated lactate in the neonatal period may occur due to lung immaturity, prolonged tourniquet use during sample collection, or delayed specimen transport. Finally, the most common cause for apparent hypocapnia in a newborn is diffusion of CO_2 from very low volume specimens with very high surface/volume ratios.

2. Which of the following metabolic disorders is associated with a characteristic odor?

Answer: a, b, and **d.** Isovaleric acidemia, trimethylaminuria, and MSUD are associated with the odor of sweaty feet, rotten fish, and maple syrup, respectively. Methylmalonic acidemia is not associated with a characteristic odor.

3. Which of the following metabolic disorders are associated with hyperammonemia?

Answer: a, b, and **c.** These are associated with hyperammonemia. Citrullinemia and OTC deficiency are urea cycle disorders. Toxins that accumulate in propionic acidemia are thought to inhibit early reactions of the urea cycle and cause what can be considerable hyperammonemia in affected patients.

4. Which of the following metabolic disorders are associated with dysmorphic features?

Answer: e. None of these disorders are typically associated with dysmorphic features. In general, inborn errors of metabolism are not characterized by outward physical dysmorphology.

5. Amino acid profiles are most commonly performed by which of the following technique

Answer: d. Amino acid profiles are most commonly performed using LC-photometric/fluorescent detection. The use of mass spectrometry is increasing.

6. Acylcarnitine profiles are most commonly performed using which of the following techniques?

Answer: b. Acylcarnitine profiles are most commonly performed using MS/MS of butyl derivatives using precursor ion scanning butyl derivatives of various acylcarnitine species are detected using their common fragment ion of m/z 85. This approach does not allow distinction of isomeric esters, such as butyryl and isobutyrylcarnitine.

7. Organic acid profiles are most commonly performed using which of the following techniques?

Answer: c. Organic acid profiles are most commonly performed using GC/MS. Compounds are volatilized through formation of trimethylsilyl derivatives. Mass spectra of these derivatives are highly reproducible across MS platforms.

8. Which of the following techniques may be employed to detect MSUD?

Answer: b. MSUD is most diagnosed using plasma amino acid profile. However, increased excretion of branched-chain amino acids and branched-chain keto acids in urine may also yield a diagnosis.

9. Which of the following techniques may be employed to detect MCAD deficiency?

Answer: a. MCAD deficiency is most commonly and definitively detected using acylcarnitine profile. In addition to acylcarnitine profiling, a urine organic acid profile may also contain elevated amounts of medium-chain dicarboxylic acids as well as medium chain glycine conjugates that indicate MCAD deficiency.

10. Which of the following techniques may be employed to detect methylmalonic acidemia?

Answer: e. Methylmalonic acidemia is definitively diagnosed using a urine organic acid profile. The most distinct feature is increased excretion of methylmalonic acid. An acylcarnitine profile also effectively detects methylmalonic acidemia via increased propionyl (C3) carnitine. A urine organic acid profile is still necessary to distinguish propionic from methylmalonic acidemia.

Chapter 5—Newborn Screening

1. The best marker for newborn screening for Tyrosinemia type I is:

Answer: d. Succinylacetone. Succinylacetone is only produced when the enzyme block is at fumarylacetoacetate hydrolase, resulting in tyrosinemia type 1. The only other possible answer (E. tyrosine) is incorrect because many things can cause an elevated tyrosine in the newborn period.

2. Second-tier tests are helpful to:

Answer: a. Decrease the number of false positives. When a positive newborn screening result is obtained on the initial test, retesting with a second test, the second-tier test, can rule out some of those positives and thus decrease the false positive rate.

3. The newborn screen results of a 5-days old baby boy, born full term after an uncomplicated pregnancy, are abnormal for an elevated C5-carnitine. What are the possible causes of elevated C5-carnitine? (Select all that apply)

Answer: a, c, and **d.** These are all possibilities with an elevated C5-carnitine.

4. Which metabolic disorder identified by newborn screening may have a clinical presentation that can be seen in non-accidental trauma?

Answer: c. Glutaric acidemia, type 1. This disorder may present with subdural hematomas and retinal hemorrhages, leading to a suspicion of child abuse.

5. Newborn screening for SCID (Severe Combined Immunodeficiencies) is performed by measuring T-cell receptor excision circles (TREC); they are:

Answer: c. Circular DNA byproducts. TREC (T-cell receptor excision circles) are small circular pieces of DNA that have been lost from the T cell genes as T cells undergo t cell receptor gene rearrangement during maturation in the thymus. In SCID, the absence of mature T cells also predicates and absence of TREC.

Chapter 6—Cystic Fibrosis and Seat Testing

1. Cystic fibrosis is an autosomal recessive disease, and has a frequency in the Caucasian population of:

Answer: d. CF has a frequency of 1 in 2,500 live births in the Caucasian population. CF is one of the most common life-shortening genetic defects in the Caucasian population.

2. A 1-month-old girl with a sweat chloride result of 35 mmol/L is interpreted as:

Answer: b. Intermediate, possible CF. There is a different interpretive reference interval for children under 6 months of age, which reflects the fact that sweat chloride is lower in the newborn period and gradually rises through childhood. Under 6 months the intermediate range is: 30-59 mmol/L and after 6 months of age it is 40-59 mmol/L.

3. The CFTR mutation F508del results in abnormal protein folding and trafficking. This primary function places this mutation into what Class?

Answer: b. Class II. See Table 6-1, page 137 for description of mutation classifications.

4. Non-classic CF patients

Answer: c. Non-classic CF patients have clinical disease limited to one organ system.

Chapter 7—Pediatric Reference Intervals

1. Which statement describes an appropriate approach to determining reference intervals when changing to a new vendor's chemistry analyzer?

Answer: b. The laboratory will be able to perform transference studies by using a small number of samples in each age/gender sub-group, confirming the validity of this approach using statistical analyses.

Statement **a**: unfortunately, currently no vendor is providing such a service.

Statement **c**: reference intervals need to be establish from all age groups.

Statement **d**: reference intervals for all tests need to be validated on the new instrument before transference can be accomplished.

2. Which of the following statements regarding establishing reference intervals is true?

Answer: d. The laboratory will be able to use the current reference intervals since all tests are currently performed in the laboratory and chemistry analytes have less variance across vendors than immunoassay methods.

Statement **a**: decision limits are available in national guidelines

Statement **b**: Using left-over samples is acceptable if they are samples from areas where the patients are generally healthy

Statement **c**: parametric approach can only be used in parameters following Gaussian distribution

3. Which statement regarding reference intervals is true?

Answer: a. The laboratory can exchange specimens with another laboratory for the purpose of establishing reference intervals if the samples have been anonymized

Statement **b**: All specimen types used in the laboratory should be used when establishing reference intervals

Statement **c**: Reference intervals established in another country can be used when statistical analysis for transference is performed

Statement **d**: All reference intervals should be verified before being used

Chapter 8—Maternal-Fetal Testing

1. Which of the following statements is true about hemolytic disease of the newborn (HDN)?

Answer: c. HDN can be diagnosed by measuring bilirubin in amniotic fluid. The other choices are incorrect, **a.** HDN is caused by maternal IgG antibodies, **b.** HDN is usually seen in the second pregnancy of an Rh- mother with an Rh+ fetus, **d.** the larger the fetomaternal hemorrhage, the more risk of sensitization to the fetal antigens and **e.** delta OD 450 is an old method no longer in use due to its lack of sensitivity.

2. Currently, the American College of Obstetrics and Gynecology recommends that all pregnant women be screened for gestational diabetes using which of the following?

Answer: a. A two-step method with a 50 g OGTT screen and 100 g OGTT diagnostic test. The other choices are incorrect, **b.** not recommended by anyone to use as a screen, **c.** IADPSG proposed method, **d.** HgA1C not recommended for screening for gestational diabetes, **e.** ADA and ACOG do not agree on this.

3. Which is true about maternal serum screening for Down syndrome?

Answer: c. Sensitivity is highest when 1st and 2nd trimester biochemical tests are incorporated with ultrasound measurements.

4. Which of the following changes to thyroid function occur during pregnancy?

Answer: e. TSH decreases in the 1st trimester

5. Abnormal fetal heart patterns, intrapartum fever, severe fetal growth restriction and C-section for fetal compromise are indications for measuring which of the following:

Answer: b. Cord blood gases

Chapter 9—Pediatric Toxicology and Therapeutic Drug Monitoring

1. The antidote for acetaminophen toxicity is:

Answer: b. *N*-acetyl-cysteine. Deferoxamine is used to treat acute iron poisoning, naloxone is an antidote for opioid overdose and leucovorin is used to rescue if methotrexate concentrations are in the toxic range.

2. The current (2014), CDC, reference level for action for lead is:

Answer: a. 5 μg/dL. The CDC dropped the action level to this level recently as differences in cognitive ability were found in children even at these low levels.

3. The most commonly used specimen for drug screening is:

Answer: c. Urine. Blood is the second most common and the other sample types are much less common.

4. Approximately, how many half-lives are needed for a drug to reach steady-state concentration?

Answer: a. Five half-lives. See Figure 9-3, page 224.

5. Benzoylecgonine is measured to detect the use of:

Answer: d. Cocaine. Benzoylecgonine is a metabolite of cocaine, and given cocaine's very short half-life, the metabolite is used to detect cocaine presence.

Chapter 10—Lipids and Lipoproteins

1. Chylomicrons are formed in which of the lipid metabolism pathways?

Answer: a. Exogenous pathway. In the exogenous pathway, dietary lipids are absorbed in the small intestine. Fatty acids are reassembled into TG and combine with ApoB-48, cholesterol, phospholipids and cholesterol esters to form chylomicrons.

2. A well appearing 3-year-old male presents for investigation of small, elevated 'bumps' on the knees and elbows with lipid profile notable for TC = 752 mg/dL, TG = 97 mg/dL, and LDL-C = 660 g/dL. Both parents report taking lipid-lowering drugs because their LDL-C >250 mg/dL. Which dyslipidemia is most consistent with this scenario?

Answer: c. Homozygous familial hypercholesterolemia (FH). In this case the child presents at a very early age with visible fat deposits (xanthomas), markedly elevated TC and LDL-C with normal TG and parental history of significant elevation in LDL-C. This case is representative for a child with homozygous familial hypercholesterolemia.

3. A 10-year-old female undergoes lipid screening at the time of a routine well child visit and school physical. She is within normal limits for height and weight for age. History and physical exam are unremarkable. Her non-fasting lipid profile shows: TC = 163 mg/dL; HDL-C = 62 mg/dL; TG = 95 mg/dL. Calculate her non-HDL-C.

Answer: d. 101 mg/dL. Non-HDL-C is the recommended first line test for universal lipid screening in children, as it does not require fasting and elevated non-HDL-C is a predictor of increased CVD risk. Non-HDL-C = TC – HDL-C.

Chapter 11—Point of Care Testing in the Pediatric Setting

1. Which of the following technologies is NOT encountered in POCT devices?

Answer: e. Sequencing/polymerase chain reaction. These are sophisticated molecular genetic techniques that are not amenable to usage in simple point of care devices.

2. Which of the following is not an advantage of POCT?

Answer: c. Cost effectiveness. In general POC devices are significantly more expensive that main lab analyses.

3. Which of the following statement about capillary blood collection is false?

Answer: b. "Arterializing" capillary blood is done by warming the skin not cooling it. Warming the skin increases blood flow and increases the arterial blood that's present.

4. Which of the following POCT does not require confirmatory testing?

Answer: e. Activated clotting time. All the others are basically screening tests that should be confirmed, especially if results are not consistent with the clinical picture. The activated clotting time is only available as a POC test.

5. True or False. "Off-label" use of a CLIA-waived POCT device only requires CLIA certification and adherence to manufacturer guidelines

Answer: b. False. Off-label use of any in vitro diagnostic requires a full CLIA validation of the assay.

Chapter 12—Pediatric Laboratory Testing for Specific Endocrine Conditions

1. Using Figure 12-1 (adrenal steroidogenic pathway), androstenedione is not likely to be elevated in which of the following disorders?

Answer: a. 17-hydroxylase deficiency. Looking at Figure 12-1, a block at 17-hydroxylase should cause elevations of pregnenolone and progesterone and nothing else. Deficiencies of 21-hydroxylase or 11-beta hydroxylase would cause blocks that would back up and cause an elevated androstenedione.

2. An elevated 17-OHP result on a newborn screen:

Answer: b. Suggests the need for follow-up testing. 17-OH-progesterone is used on newborn screen testing to screen for CAH, but many things can elevate 17-OH-progesterone in the newborn period, including prematurity and other steroid interferences. Thus elevated 17-OH-progesterone on a newborn screen requires additional follow-up testing.

3. Which of the following does not cause variability in IGF-1 measurements?

Answer: b. Pulsatile release of IGF-1. IGF-1 is not released in a pulsatile fashion. In addition, the rest of the answers do affect the variability in IGF-1 measurements.

Chapter 13—Molecular Diagnostic Testing

1. The key components of PCR include:

Answer: d. Key components of PCR include DNA polymerase, dNTPs, template DNA, oligonucleotide primer, divalent cations (e.g., Mg^{2+}) and pH buffering (e.g., 10 mM Tris). ddNTPs are used in Sanger sequencing.

2. Next-generation sequencing (NGS) is clinically useful in 2015 because:

Answer: b. A single NGS assay can be cheaper than sequencing multiple genes by Sanger.

3. Which of the following tests can potentially be used to determine a patient's identity through the identification of short tandem repeats (STRs)?

Answer: a. Whole exome sequencing can identify STRs. However, it is important to remember that the STR profile that is sequenced can only be linked back to a patient's identity with access to an STR database. Even then, the patient's STR profile must have been previously characterized and stored.

b. Is incorrect because STRs used for identity testing are within introns, sequencing of exons will not reveal these STRs.

c. Is incorrect because quantitative analysis of EBV by PCR amplifies portions of the EBV genome. The patient's genome is not amplified or sequenced.

d. Is incorrect because FISH for MYCN will demonstrate the number of copies of the MYCN gene in a cell. It does not identify STRs.

e. Is incorrect because hybridization assays for CFTR mutations target specific mutations in the exons of the gene. No STR data is contained in these regions.

Chapter 14—Pediatric Microbiology

1. An 8-year-old child is suspected of having group A *Streptococcus* pharyngitis but rapid antigen testing for this organism is negative. Which of the following statements is correct?

Answer: b. It is uncertain whether the child has group A Streptococcus and confirmatory culture should be performed before concluding that the child does not have disease.

2. A neonate is suspected of having early onset sepsis and blood cultures reveal a Gram-negative rod that grows on chocolate, sheep blood, and MacConkey agar. The organism grows on MacConkey as a lactose fermenter, is indole-positive, and oxidase-negative. What is the identity of this organism?

Answer: c. *Escherichia coli.*

3. A child is suspected of having *Kingella kingae* septic arthritis, however, synovial fluid cultures are negative. Which of the following culture techniques can help to improve the yield of *K kingae* from synovial fluid cultures.

Answer: d. Inject some specimen in blood culture bottles and incubate in a standard blood culture system.

Chapter 15—Pediatric Hematology and Hemoglobinopathies

1. A 2-year-old male presents to the hematology clinic for evaluation of persistent microcytic anemia. The peripheral blood smear shows microcytic, hypochromic anemia with frequent target cells and elliptocytes. There is prominent anisopoikilocytosis and no discernable polychromasia. The CBC shows normal WBC and platelets, decreased RBC, MCH, MCHC, and increased RDW. Newborn screen was reportedly normal.

Based on the above scenario, which of the following tests will be most useful in diagnosing the cause for the microcytic anemia?

Answer: b. The scenario described above is most consistent with iron deficiency anemia and serum ferritin would be the most useful diagnostic test. The differential diagnosis for IDA includes anemia of inflammation, sideroblastic anemia and thalassemia trait. Serum ferritin is expected to be low only in IDA and will be normal or increased in the other three conditions. Evaluation for hemoglobinopahy or thalassemia would be helpful in differentiating IDA from β-thalassemia trait, however, the above hematologic indices are not typical of thalassemia as the RBC is decreased and the RDW is increased. The newborn screen is usual abnormal in a patient with α-thalassemia. Haptoglobin is useful in the diagnosis of anemia due to hemolysis, however, the lack of polychromasia would be unusual for a hemolytic anemia. Serum iron is not as useful in differentiating IDA from the other conditions as serum iron is reduced in both IDA and anemia of inflammation. Serum iron is increased in sideroblastic iron and normal in thalassemia trait.

2. Which of the following β-globin disorders would be expected to result in the sickling disorder of least severity if inherited in combination with the Hb S mutation?

Answer: d. Hb E in combination Hb S will produce a mild Sickle Cell Disease (SCD). Hb E is associated with an alternate splicing site in the mRNA that results in decreased expression of the gene. This will lead to relatively increased levels of Hb S in the cell and results in a mild sickling phenotype. β°-thalassemia inherited with Hb S will result in a severe SCD due to the fact that there is no normal β-globin chain production and virtually all the intracellular hemoglobin is Hb S. Hb D-Punjab interacts directly with Hb S to increase the polymerization of the Hb S chains and will result in a severe SCD comparable to homozygous Hb S. Hb C in compound heterozygosity with Hb S results in a moderately severe SCD that is milder than homozygous Hb S doe to the fact that Hb C polymerizes less readily than Hb S.

3. Which of the following conditions is associated with hemolysis, hyperbilirubinemia, and decreased haptoglobin?

Answer: c. Hereditary spherocytosis results in relative rigidity of spherocytes with entrapment and increased destruction of the red cells by the reticuloendothelial system (extravascular hemolysis). Immune thrombocytopenic purpura is associated with autoantibodies to platelet antigens and can be associated with increased risk of bleeding, but not hemolysis. Deletional HPFH and homozygous δβ-thalassemia can both result in 100% Hb F. While homozygous δβ-thalassemia is associated with hemolytic anemia, HPFH is not. Anemia of inflammation is associated with ineffective erythropoiesis due to pathologic iron homeostasis and is not associated with hemolysis.

Chapter 16—Pediatric Coagulation

1. You are consulting on a new patient who was recently diagnosed with DVT of the right femoral vein. He is a 15-year-old WM who weighs 90 kg and who developed leg pain and swelling after a football injury to his knee that required bracing. After DVT was diagnosed, he was placed on heparin infusion and transitioned to warfarin. Current INR is 2.4. Thrombophilia testing was performed prior to discharge from the hospital.

Factor V Leiden	Homozygous normal
Prothrombin gene mutation	Homozygous normal
Factor VIII	200%
Protein S activity	40%
Protein C activity	30%
Antithrombin	85%
Lupus anticoagulant	Negative

Based on these results, the most likely contributor to his thrombosis is:

Answer: c. Although he does have low protein C and S activity levels, he was on warfarin at the time of testing. These are both Vitamin K dependent proteins and will be low when on warfarin. This will need to be rechecked when off of warfarin for at least a month. The effect of warfarin on protein S especially can last for up to 4 weeks. Although he does have elevated FVIII activity, it is not >250% and it was obtained in the acute setting. This is more likely an acute phase reactant and a result of the DVT. It will also have to be rechecked prior to stopping anti-coagulation. If FVIII remains elevated after 3-6 months, he has increased risk of Post-thrombotic syndrome and recurrent DVT. Although obesity is a risk factor, the most important contributor is an orthopedic injury requiring immobilization of the leg.

2. A 5-month-old Caucasian female had open heart surgery 7 days ago. She is on an unfractionated heparin infusion at prophylactic dosing. Her total WBC was 13,000/mm^3 with 50% segmented neutrophils, 3% bands, 10% monocytes, and 37% lymphs. Hemoglobin was 10.5 g/dL and platelet count 45,000/mm^3. Her PT is 13 seconds, PTT 45 seconds, fibrinogen 350 mg/dL, and D-Dimers are mildly elevated. Her ALT is 35 U/L, AST 37 U/L and creatinine 1.0 mg/dL. She has a catheter in her right femoral vein, which is not flushing adequately, and a Doppler sonogram shows partial occlusion of the right femoral vein.

The next best step in this patient's management is to:

Answer: d. Although heparin-induced thrombocytopenia (HIT) is extremely rare in children it is most common in infants after open heart surgery who have been previously exposed to unfractionated heparin. Because this child has evidence of thrombosis as well, unfractionated heparin must be discontinued while assessing for HIT, but another form of anticoagulation must be initiated to prevent further thrombotic complications. Enoxaparin is a low molecular weight heparin and has cross reactivity with unfractionated heparin. Warfarin cannot be initiated without a bridge with another anticoagulant. Removing the femoral catheter is not emergent and may not be necessary as the thrombus is nonocclusive.

3. A teenage girl is on chronic warfarin therapy. The INR has been stable for the last 6 months, but is now 1.4. She denies missing any doses except for the day before her routine lab test, and a pill count suggests that no other doses have been missed. Which is the most likely reason for the drop in INR?

Answer: d. Because she had never had a problem achieving therapeutic INR in the past, a genetic polymorphism for warfarin resistance is unlikely. This should be considered in children in whom it is very difficult to anticoagulate initially with anything other than very high doses of warfarin. Alcohol use and the use of most antibiotics usually increase the INR. Missing one dose of warfarin does not typically decrease an INR between 2 and 3 down to 1.4. Discontinuing warfarin will usually drop the INR to <1.5 in 3-5 days. Therefore, the most likely reason for this new warfarin resistance is the increase in vitamin K containing foods in her diet.

4. Which aspect of the endothelium has anticoagulant properties?

Answer: a. All but A are procoagulant properties of the endothelium. When endothelial cell-associated thrombomodulin is activated, it can, in turn, activate protein C, the active form of which, in association with protein S inactivates FVIIIa and

FVa, quenching thrombin production. Vasoconstriction and release of VWF are steps involved in primary hemostasis. Secondary hemostasis in initiated by release of tissue factor upon vessel injury.

5. A 4-year-old white female is brought to you ER at a large tertiary medical center for nose bleeds, easy bruising and altered mental status. She has been staying with her grandparents while her parents are out of town. She has never had any bleeding issues in the past and even underwent tonsillectomy 6 months ago without incident. Family history is negative for bleeding disorders, but grandfather is on warfarin for atrial fibrillation. Labs have been drawn and stat head CT is being performed. You suspect warfarin toxicity due to accidental ingestion of grandfather's medications. CT confirms intracranial hemorrhage. CBC shows hemoglobin of 8.9 g/dL and platelets of 250,000. PT is markedly prolonged and corresponds to INR of 10.5. PTT is also prolonged at 60 seconds.

   What is the best management for this child?

Answer: d. For a symptomatic patient with INR >10, bleeding needs to be controlled and warfarin reversed. Oral vitamin K will reduce INR by half in about 24 hours. IV formulations are faster (12 hours), but not fast enough for this child with life threatening bleeding. Vitamin K should be given but in IV form and in addition to an agent that will replace factors. FFP and PCCs are both good choices to give to an actively bleeding patient with warfarin overdose as they replace all Vitamin K dependent factors inhibited by warfarin. However, 10 cc/kg of FFP will likely not be enough. She will need 15-30 cc/k g which is a large volume for this child. PCCs are effective in small volumes; unfortunately, they are not readily available at all small centers. rFVIIa has been shown to be effective but is associated with thrombotic risk and is only replacing the FVII being inhibited by the warfarin. In order for the INR to be markedly elevated the warfarin will have had to have been in the child's system for over 24 hours. Pumping her stomach will have little utility at reversing her coagulopathy.

6. Which inherited thrombophilia is most likely to lead to a venous thromboembolic event prior to age 40?

Answer: e.

Inherited thrombophilia	Frequency in Population	Risk of thrombosis
Factor V Leiden	Heterozygous state: 3-8% of Caucasians 1.2% African American Rare in Asian	Heterozygous state 3-5 X increase over a lifetime Minimal increased risk of recurrent events Homozygous 18 X increased risk Combined with prothrombin gene 30-50 X increased risk

Prothrombin Gene mutation	Heterozygous state: 2% of US Caucasians; 0.5% African Americans	Heterozygous state 3 X increased risk over lifetime Possible increased risk of recurrent events in children, but not adults Homozygous increased but unclear Combined with Factor V Leiden 30-50 X increased risk
Antithrombin deficiency	Heterozygous 1 in 500 to 5000	50% risk of even prior to age 40 Increased risk of recurrent events (10-17% per year) Homozygous state not compatible with life
Protein S deficiency	Heterozygous state 1 in 800 to 3000	Heterozygous 31 X increased risk prior to age 55 Increased risk of recurrent events (44% in 5 years) Homozygous early purpura fulminans VTE,
Protein C deficiency	Heterozygous state 1 in 500 to 600 Homozygous state 1 in 1,000,000	Heterozygous 24 X increased risk prior to age 55 Increased risk of recurrent events (37% in 5 years) Homozygous—purpura fulminans as neonate
MTHFR polymorphisms: C677T (thermolabile) and A1298C	Heterozygous state 35% of population Homozygous state 12-20% of population	Debatable significance unless leads to elevated plasma homocysteine
PAI-1 polymorphism	Heterozygous state 12% of population	Debatable significance unless PAI-1 activity also elevated

7. A 12-year-old white male was diagnosed with DVT of the right lower extremity after knee surgery. He has been on anticoagulation for last 3 months and you are asked to provide recommendation for duration of therapy. Which of the following scenarios would require prolonged or indefinite anticoagulation therapy.

Answer: a. Family history of a provoked DVT is not an indication for chronic anticoagulation therapy. Indications would be persistently elevated FVIII activity, strong thrombophilia (protein C, S, or AT deficiency), and antiphospholipid antibody syndrome. Although the protein C activity is technically low for an adult, it is normal for a pre-teen. Normal adult levels are not achieved until adolescence. If there is a concern for inherited Protein C deficiency, antigen testing as well as activity testing should be repeated in a couple of years. Heterozygous Factor V Leiden is a mild thrombophilia and will not require indefinite anticoagulation, as risk of recurrence is not higher for these patients. However, they will need DVT prophylaxis in high risk situations. Antiphospholipid antibody syndrome is defined as the persistence of APLAs or lupus anticoagulant for 12 weeks in the context of a thrombotic event. This is associated with high risk of recurrent events.

Chapter 17—Pediatric Transfusion Medicine

1. According to 2012 FDA data, what is the most common fatal transfusion reaction:

Answer: b. Transfusion Related Acute Lung Injury (TRALI)

2. Which of the following recipients do NOT require irradiated blood products:

Answer: d. Patients with sickle cell disease receiving a large volume transfusion

3. The American Society of Clinical Oncology and the British Committee for Standards in Hematology recommend what platelet count as a prophylactic transfusion trigger in non-bleeding patients:

Answer: b. 10,000 per mm^3

Index

Note: Page numbers followed by *f* denote figures; page numbers followed by *t* denote tables.